Tumors
of the
Lymph Nodes and Spleen

Atlas
of
Tumor Pathology

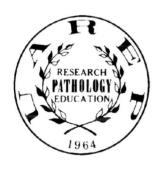

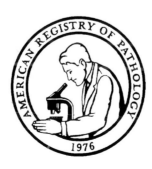

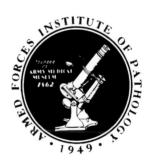

ATLAS OF TUMOR PATHOLOGY

Third Series
Fascicle 14

TUMORS OF THE LYMPH NODES AND SPLEEN

by

ROGER A. WARNKE, M.D.
Professor of Pathology
Co-Director, Immunodiagnosis Laboratory
Stanford University Medical Center
Stanford, California 94305

LAWRENCE M. WEISS, M.D.
Director, Surgical Pathology
Division of Pathology
City of Hope National Medical Center
Duarte, California 91010

JOHN K. C. CHAN, M.B.B.S., M.R.C.Path
Consultant Pathologist
Department of Pathology
Queen Elizabeth Hospital
Kowloon, Hong Kong

MICHAEL L. CLEARY, M.D.
Associate Professor of Pathology
Director, Molecular Diagnostics Laboratory
Stanford University Medical Center
Stanford, California 94305

RONALD F. DORFMAN, M.B.B.Ch., F.R.C.Path
Professor of Pathology
Stanford University Medical Center
Stanford, California 94305

Published by the
ARMED FORCES INSTITUTE OF PATHOLOGY
Washington, D.C.

Under the Auspices of
UNIVERSITIES ASSOCIATED FOR RESEARCH AND EDUCATION IN PATHOLOGY, INC.
Bethesda, Maryland
1995

Accepted for Publication
1994

Available from the American Registry of Pathology
Armed Forces Institute of Pathology
Washington, D.C. 20306-6000
ISSN 0160-6344
ISBN 1-881041-18-2

ATLAS OF TUMOR PATHOLOGY

EDITOR
JUAN ROSAI, M.D.
Department of Pathology
Memorial Sloan-Kettering Cancer Center
New York, New York 10021-6007

ASSOCIATE EDITOR
LESLIE H. SOBIN, M.D.
Armed Forces Institute of Pathology
Washington, D.C. 20306-6000

EDITORS' NOTE

The Atlas of Tumor Pathology has a long and distinguished history. It was first conceived at a Cancer Research Meeting held in St. Louis in September 1947 as an attempt to standardize the nomenclature of neoplastic diseases. The first series was sponsored by the National Academy of Sciences-National Research Council. The organization of this Sisyphean effort was entrusted to the Subcommittee on Oncology of the Committee on Pathology, and Dr. Arthur Purdy Stout was the first editor-in-chief. Many of the illustrations were provided by the Medical Illustration Service of the Armed Forces Institute of Pathology, the type was set by the Government Printing Office, and the final printing was done at the Armed Forces Institute of Pathology (hence the colloquial appellation "AFIP Fascicles"). The American Registry of Pathology purchased the Fascicles from the Government Printing Office and sold them virtually at cost. Over a period of 20 years, approximately 15,000 copies each of nearly 40 Fascicles were produced. The worldwide impact that these publications have had over the years has largely surpassed the original goal. They quickly became among the most influential publications on tumor pathology ever written, primarily because of their overall high quality but also because their low cost made them easily accessible to pathologists and other students of oncology the world over.

Upon completion of the first series, the National Academy of Sciences-National Research Council handed further pursuit of the project over to the newly created Universities Associated for Research and Education in Pathology (UAREP). A second series was started, generously supported by grants from the AFIP, the National Cancer Institute, and the American Cancer Society. Dr. Harlan I. Firminger became the editor-in-chief and was succeeded by Dr. William H. Hartmann. The second series Fascicles were produced as bound volumes instead of loose leaflets. They featured a more comprehensive coverage of the subjects, to the extent that the Fascicles could no longer be regarded as "atlases" but rather as monographs describing and illustrating in detail the tumors and tumor-like conditions of the various organs and systems.

Once the second series was completed, with a success that matched that of the first, UAREP and AFIP decided to embark on a third series. A new editor-in-chief and an associate editor were selected, and a distinguished editorial board was appointed. The mandate for the third series remains the same as for the previous ones, i.e., to oversee the production of an eminently practical publication with surgical pathologists as its primary audience, but also aimed at other workers in oncology. The main purposes of this series are to promote a consistent, unified, and biologically sound nomenclature; to guide the surgical pathologist in the diagnosis of the various tumors and tumor-like lesions; and to provide relevant histogenetic, pathogenetic, and clinicopathologic information on these entities. Just as the second series included data obtained from ultrastructural (and, in the more recent Fascicles, immunohistochemical) examination, the third series will, in addition, incorporate pertinent information obtained with the newer molecular biology techniques. As in the past, a continuous attempt will be made to correlate, whenever possible, the nomenclature used in the Fascicles with that proposed by the World Health Organization's International Histological Classification of Tumors. The format of the third series has been changed in order to incorporate additional items and to ensure a consistency of style throughout. Close cooperation between the various authors and their respective liaisons from the editorial board will be emphasized to minimize unnecessary repetition and discrepancies in the text and illustrations.

To its everlasting credit, the participation and commitment of the AFIP to this venture is even more substantial and encompassing than in previous series. It now extends to virtually all scientific, technical, and financial aspects of the production.

The task confronting the organizations and individuals involved in the third series is even more daunting than in the preceding efforts because of the ever-increasing complexity of the matter at hand. It is hoped that this combined effort—of which, needless to say, that represented by the authors is first and foremost—will result in a series worthy of its two illustrious predecessors and will be a suitable introduction to the tumor pathology of the twenty-first century.

Juan Rosai, M.D.
Leslie H. Sobin, M.D.

ACKNOWLEDGMENTS

We are indebted to the innumerable pathologists who have shared their interesting cases with us through the years. They have enriched our diagnostic experience and provided us with most of the case examples illustrated in this Fascicle. We would especially like to thank the pathologists who provided unusual examples of previously published cases, which are individually acknowledged in the respective figure legends.

We are grateful to the various heads of our respective departments and to our colleagues for their longstanding support and encouragement, particularly during the preparation of this Fascicle. We also thank colleagues who have provided editorial assistance during the preparation of individual sections. Many individuals including technologists, residents, fellows, and colleagues have made invaluable contributions to our hematopathology programs.

We would especially like to acknowledge the pioneering work of the previous authors of Fascicles on Tumors of the Hematopoietic System, initially Dr. Henry Rappaport and more recently Drs. Robert Lukes and Robert Collins, in addition to the exceptional contributions to hematopathology made by Professor Karl Lennert. We have derived much inspiration from their teachings, publications, and concepts of lymphomagenesis. We were saddened by the recent death of Dr. Lukes.

We thank Ms. Eileen Maisen for secretarial assistance, Mr. Phil Verzola and Ms. Rebecca Horne for photographic assistance, and Ms. Eva Pfendt for the double-label immunohistochemistry.

We are grateful to the reviewers of this Fascicle who provided an in-depth analysis and made numerous helpful suggestions. We also wish to express our appreciation to the editorial staff, Ms. Dian Thomas, Mr. Andrew Male, and Ms. Audrey Kahn, for their remarkable patience and assistance in the preparation of this Fascicle.

Roger A. Warnke, M.D.
Lawrence M. Weiss, M.D.
John K. C. Chan, M.B.B.S., M.R.C.Path
Michael L. Cleary, M.D.
Ronald F. Dorfman, M.B.B.Ch., F.R.C.Path

Permission to use copyrighted illustrations has been granted by:

American Medical Association:
    Arch Pathol 1969;87:63–70. For figure 18-18.

Blackwell Science:
    Histopathology 1981;5:697–709. For figure 18-27.

Churchill Livingstone:
    Burkitt's Lymphoma 1970:11. For figure 10-2.

JB Lippincott:
    Ann Surg 1928;87:467–71. For figure 10-1.
    Cancer 1961;14:258–269. For figure 10-3.
    Cancer 1972;30:1174–88. For figures 18-19 and 18-26.
    Cancer 1982;49:1994–8. For figure 18-21.
    Cancer 1991;68:1988–93. For figure 9-1.

Karger:
    Frontiers of Radiation Therapy and Oncology, vol 28, 1994:3. For figure 2-1.

Taylor & Francis:
    Ultrastruct Pathol 1981;2:101–19. For figure 18-40.

Times-Mirror International:
    Immunology 1993:3.4. For figure 2-15.

WB Saunders:
    Semin Diagn Pathol 1990;7:19–73. For figures 18-19 and 18-25.

Williams & Wilkins:
    Am J Pathol 1985;119:351–6. For figure 6-37.

TUMORS OF THE LYMPH NODES AND SPLEEN

Contents

TUMORS OF THE LYMPH NODES AND SPLEEN

1

INTRODUCTION

In the third series of the Atlas of Tumor Pathology, tumors of the hematopoietic system are separated into those of the bone marrow and those of the lymphoid system. Every effort has been made to use consistent terminology in both Fascicles. Furthermore, different aspects of the same general topic are covered separately in the two volumes. For example, plasma cell tumors that manifest in the bone marrow (multiple myeloma) are largely covered in the bone marrow Fascicle whereas plasma cell tumors that present in extramedullary sites are discussed here (plasma cell neoplasms and amyloidosis). Leukemias are covered in both Fascicles but are here restricted to extramedullary leukemias and mastocytosis as well as leukemias in the differential diagnosis of lymphomas. The section on normal anatomy and function focuses on the lymph nodes and spleen, reserving bone marrow anatomy for that Fascicle.

Although the authors use the morphologic terminology of the Working Formulation (much of it adapted from the Lukes and Collins classification) and the Kiel classification, we also incorporate newer concepts. For example, most lymphomas previously designated as intermediate lymphocytic, diffuse small cleaved cell (Working Formulation) and centrocytic (Kiel classification) are here designated mantle cell lymphomas in the section on small lymphocytic lymphomas. The cytologic and clinical separation of immunoblastic lymphomas from nonimmunoblastic large cell lymphomas is difficult; thus, these lymphomas are discussed together in one section. Because of their morphologic and clinical diversity, a separate section is devoted to post-thymic T-cell lymphomas. Similarly, a separate section is devoted to nodular lymphocyte predominance Hodgkin's disease (nodular paragranuloma) in recognition of recent information indicating that this subtype is distinctly different from the classic forms of Hodgkin's disease, namely, nodular sclerosis and mixed cellularity. In addition, because of their special features, a separate section is devoted to lymphomas that arise in the immunocompromised.

Since the publication of the first and second series' Fascicles, there have been considerable advances in our understanding of the immune system's response to antigenic stimulation and tumor production. There continues to be dynamic change in our understanding of the cellular and molecular events that take place in lymphoid hyperplasia and neoplasia, and the phenotypic and genotypic parameters in the diagnostic evaluation of a lymphoid lesion continue to evolve. A separate section summarizes many of these cellular and molecular features.

The occurrence of two distinct morphologic types of lymphoma in the same patient has been referred to as composite or discordant lymphoma. In light of recent information, many of these combinations are discussed in a separate section as examples of tumor progression (transformation) or differentiation.

While current treatment modalities make considerable use of these morphologic categories of lymphoma, it is possible that newer modes of therapy that capitalize on the dynamic interplay between tumor cells and responding host cells will render some, if not all, of these categorizations obsolete over time.

NORMAL ANATOMY AND FUNCTION
OF LYMPH NODES AND SPLEEN

The lymphoid tissues of the body can be divided into primary, secondary, and tertiary lymphoid organs. The primary lymphoid organs of bone marrow and thymus are the sites capable of producing functionally mature but naive lymphocytes from nonfunctioning precursors. The secondary lymphoid organs, including the lymph nodes, spleen, and Peyer's patches, are the predominant sites of secondary lymphoid differentiation: the proliferation and differentiation of antigen-specific B and T lymphocytes in response to exogenous antigen. Tertiary "lymphoid tissues" include all other tissues of the body (such as skin, respiratory tract, and reproductive tract) that normally contain few lymphoid elements but in the setting of inflammation can be induced by antigen to recruit unique populations of primarily memory lymphocytes (13). In these sites previously stimulated memory and effector precursor cells can be restimulated, leading to further clonal expansion; terminal effector responses of B and T lymphocytes also occur (13).

LYMPH NODES

Gross Anatomy

Lymph nodes are generally ovoid, encapsulated aggregates of precisely structured lymphoreticular tissue. They range in size from a few millimeters to greater than 1 cm in largest dimension and occur at intervals along lymphatic vessels. They are most frequent along major vessels at the base of the extremities, and in the retroperitoneum, mesentery, mediastinum, and neck; they also occur in other locations such as subcutaneous tissue, hilum of organs such as lung, and within salivary glands. Although the grayish tan cut surface of lymph nodes often does not reveal clues to pathology, in some instances accentuated architectural features are seen: prominent nodules in reactive follicular hyperplasia or follicular lymphoma, pigmented paracortical regions in dermatopathic lymphadenopathy, or foci of necrosis in necrotizing lymphadenitis. In addition, lymph nodes removed from particular sites often have certain gross features: fatty replacement in axillary nodes, fibrosis in inguinal nodes, and pigment in mediastinal nodes.

Microscopic Anatomy

See figure 2-1 for a schematic diagram of the microscopic anatomy.

Primary B-Cell Follicles. Deeply hematoxyphilic compact nodules of small lymphocytes within a network of follicular dendritic cell processes reside in the outer regions (cortex) of lymph nodes and are termed primary (resting) follicles (figs. 2-2, 2-3) (17). They are present as early as the second trimester of human fetal life. The virgin (naive) and memory B cells that comprise these nodules (fig. 2-4) express a high concentration of surface immunoglobulin composed of either kappa or lambda light chains in combination with mμ and delta heavy chains; only a few small B cells have gamma or alpha heavy chains (15). The normal ratio of kappa to lambda B cells in humans is approximately 2 to 1 (fig. 2-5) (7). When fetal B cells arrive in follicles, most express surface molecules that are not commonly found on B cells after the first year of life, such as CD5 and CD10 (22). The immunoglobulin on B cells that express CD5 in adult life often has an affinity for auto-antigens and these cells may be elevated in various disease states such as rheumatoid arthritis. Many low-grade diffuse B-cell lymphoproliferative disorders, particularly chronic lymphocytic leukemia, express the CD5 antigen.

Secondary B-Cell Follicles. Secondary B-cell follicles result from the stimulation of B cells by antigens, especially T-cell–dependent antigens (9). They are composed of a central, pale-staining germinal center and a deeply hematoxyphilic corona of small lymphocytes comprising the mantle zone (figs. 2-2, 2-4, 2-6) (17). The germinal center can be further subdivided into a pale zone and a dark zone. The dark zone lies nearest the paracortical T zone and is rich in proliferating large lymphoid cells/centroblasts (fig. 2-7) which are also associated with tingible body macrophages. The pale zone, together with the focally

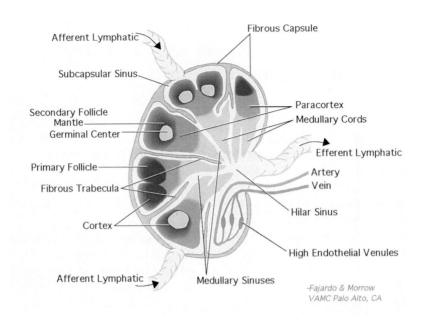

Figure 2-1
STRUCTURE OF A HUMAN LYMPH NODE
(Plate 1 [Fig. 1] from Fajardo LF. Lymph nodes and cancer. A review. In: Meyer JL, ed. Lymphatic systems and cancer. Mechanisms and clinical management. Basel:Karger, 1994:3. [Meyer J, ed. Frontiers of radiation therapy and oncology. Vol. 28.])

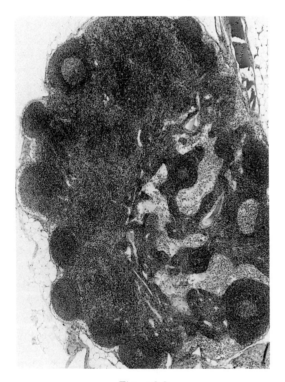

Figure 2-2
NORMAL LYMPH NODE

Note the primary and secondary follicles in the cortex adjacent to the paracortical T zone. The subcapsular sinus connects to the medullary sinuses via trabecular sinuses (right).

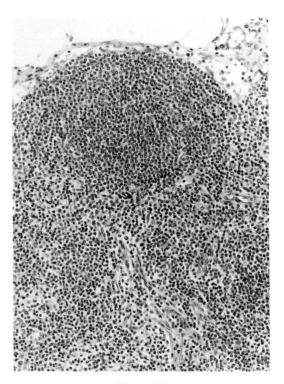

Figure 2-3
PRIMARY FOLLICLE

The nodule of small lymphocytes at top merges with the paracortical T zone at bottom.

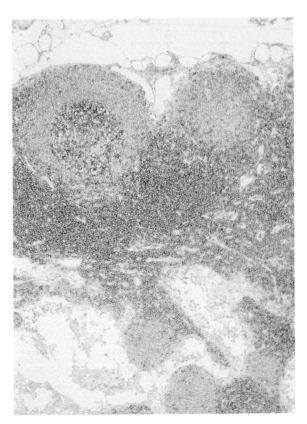

Figure 2-4
LYMPH NODE

B cells predominate in the primary and secondary folli-cles as well as in the medullary cords (labeled blue with L26/CD20) whereas T cells predominate in the paracortex (labeled red with Leu-22/CD43).

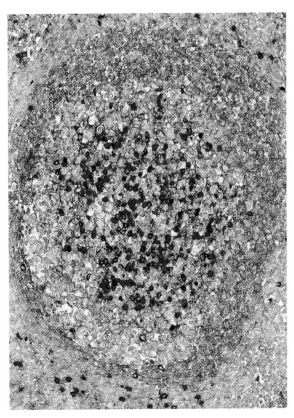

Figure 2-5
SECONDARY FOLLICLE

The germinal center of this follicle demonstrates an unusu-ally large number of cells containing abundant cytoplasmic immunoglobulin. The ratio of kappa-expressing to lambda-ex-pressing cells appears normal at approximately 2-3 to 1 (kappa cells labeled red and lambda cells labeled blue). The admixture of kappa and lambda cells in the mantle cannot easily be discerned in this paraffin section.

thickened mantle zone, is often polarized toward the site of antigen entry, such as the subcapsular sinus of lymph nodes or the epithelium of mu-cosa-associated lymphoid tissues (tonsils [fig. 2-6] or Peyer's patches). The pale zone is rich in small cleaved cells/centrocytes, follicular den-dritic cells (dendritic reticulum cells) (fig. 2-8), and CD4-positive (helper/inducer) T cells. Mas-sive cell death by apoptosis occurs in the pale zone of the germinal center (see below for discus-sion of affinity maturation and *bcl*-2 expression) and is accompanied by tingible body macro-phages. Cells undergoing apoptotic cell death lack expression of the *bcl*-2 protein; this dis-tinguishes germinal center cells from mantle zone B cells, which do express this antigen (fig. 2-9). Cells in the germinal center also express CD10.

B cells of the germinal center generally express low to undetectable levels of surface immuno-globulin but the complex network of cell pro-cesses of follicular dendritic cells contains readily detectable levels of immunoglobulin in the form of immune complexes (16) which stain for kappa, lambda, gamma, alpha, and mµ chains (fig. 2-10). The cell processes of the dendritic cells also react with antibodies against complement receptors CR1 (CD35) and CR2 (CD21) (fig. 2-8). Immuno-globulin may be detected in the cytoplasm of some germinal center cells, particularly plasmacytoid cells (basophilic centrocytes); in experimental an-imals, the number of these cells increases with the intensity of antigenic stimulation (fig. 2-5). These cells may stain for mµ, gamma, alpha or, occasionally, delta heavy chains and also stain for J (joining) chain (5).

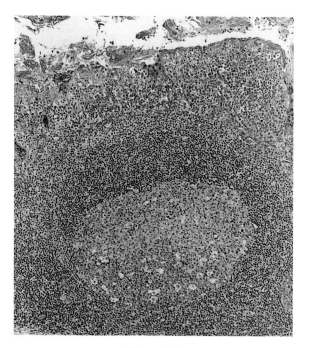

Figure 2-6
SECONDARY FOLLICLE

Note the polarization of the mantle as well as the pale zone of the germinal center toward the site of antigen entry from the epithelial surface of the tonsil at top.

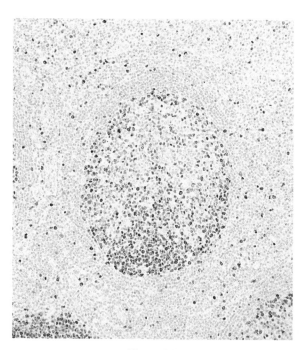

Figure 2-7
SECONDARY FOLLICLE

Proliferating cells labeled with the paraffin-reactive antibody MIB-1 (against the Ki-67 antigen) are concentrated in the dark zone of the germinal center at bottom, away from the site of antigen entry from the tonsillar surface at top.

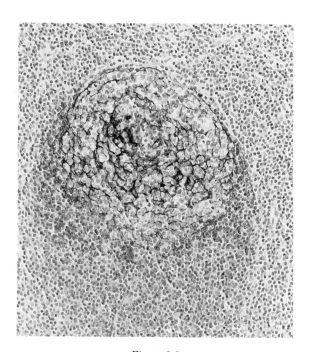

Figure 2-8
SECONDARY FOLLICLE

Staining for the CR1 complement receptor (CD35) highlights the follicular dendritic cell processes of the germinal center. The proliferative pole at the bottom shows fewer stained cell processes.

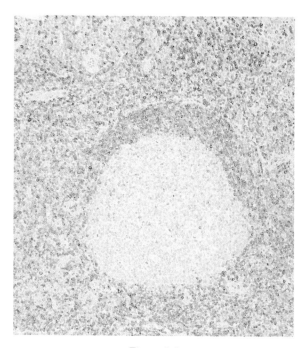

Figure 2-9
SECONDARY FOLLICLE

The *bcl*-2 protein, which blocks programmed cell death (apoptosis), is strongly expressed on the mantle B lymphocytes and adjacent T lymphocytes but expressed on few cells in the germinal center.

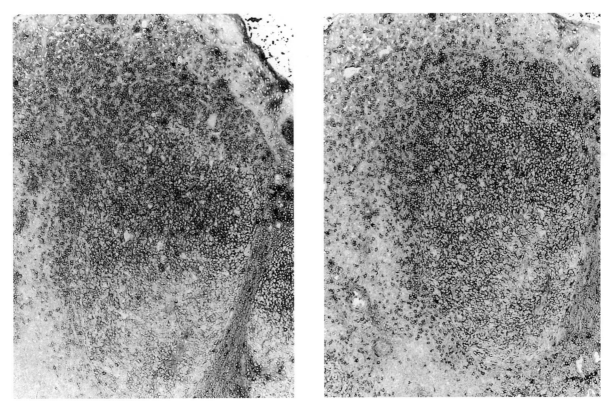

Figure 2-10
SECONDARY FOLLICLE
Staining for kappa (left) and lambda (right) light chains shows membrane-labeled small lymphocytes in the mantle. Most of the staining in the germinal center is localized to the follicular dendritic cell processes and is in the form of immune complexes. Scattered, intensely labeled plasma cells are also present near the surface of the tonsil.

Mantle zone B cells are similar morphologically and phenotypically to primary follicle B cells. In contrast to germinal center B cells, these cells express immunoglobulin, lack J chain, and show a low proliferative rate. In addition, they express CD21, CD32, CD35, and *bcl*-2 protein and do not express CD10 and CD38.

Medullary Cords. In addition to the follicles, B cells, and especially plasma cells, predominate in the medullary cords, which lie central to the cortex and paracortex and extend to the hilum (fig. 2-4).

Paracortex. The lymphoid tissue between the B-cell follicles and the medulla is rich in T cells and is termed the paracortex (figs. 2-2, 2-4). In unstimulated lymph nodes, these T cells have the appearance of small lymphocytes and are cytologically indistinguishable from small B lymphocytes of primary follicles or the mantle zone of secondary follicles (fig. 2-11). There is a wide variation in distribution of the two major

subsets of T cells: CD4-positive (helper/inducer) and CD8-positive (cytotoxic/suppressor) cells (fig. 2-12). The CD4 to CD8 ratio may vary from 2 to 1 to greater than 10 to 1 and may also be reversed, as in the initial phase of certain viral infections (14). The ratio is profoundly altered in the late phase of human immunodeficiency virus (HIV) infection. Many of the paracortical T cells express CD45RO, which is associated with a memory function, an apparently short lifespan, and a capacity to elaborate a wide variety of cytokines (fig. 2-13). Most of the remaining paracortical T cells express CD45RA, which is associated with a virgin/naive status, an apparently long lifespan, and a capacity to mainly elaborate IL-2 (fig. 2-13) (1,4).

When the number of large T-lymphoid cells is increased with antigenic stimulation, a mottled appearance to the paracortex is often seen on low-power examination. With intense antigenic

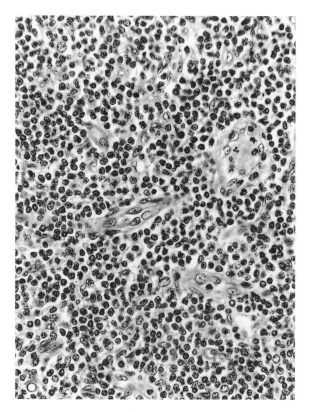

Figure 2-11
PARACORTEX (T ZONE)
Note the small lymphocytes surrounding the high endothelial venules (HEV), a morphologic marker for the T zone.

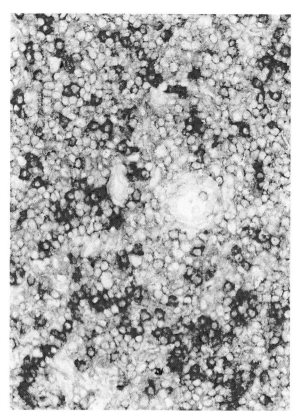

Figure 2-12
PARACORTICAL T ZONE
Surrounding the high endothelial venule at center is an admixture of CD4 (labeled blue) and CD8 (labeled red) expressing T cells.

stimulation, as occurs with infection by the Epstein-Barr virus, the paracortex may contain virus-infected B immunoblasts as well as large numbers of reactive T immunoblasts (21).

A cellular marker of the paracortex is the interdigitating dendritic cell (interdigitating reticulum cell), which presents processed antigen in combination with class II histocompatibility antigens. These cells have pale, often irregularly shaped vesicular nuclei and rather abundant, pale-staining cytoplasm that interdigitates with T lymphocytes through long, delicate processes (fig. 2-14). These interdigitating dendritic cells have many phenotypic similarities to the antigen-presenting cells of skin, the Langerhans cells. They are bone marrow derived and express many markers of myelomonocytic differentiation; they also show strong nuclear staining for S-100 protein (fig. 2-14). An additional marker for the T-cell–rich paracortex of lymph nodes is the high endothelial venule, a postcapillary vessel lined by cuboidal en-

dothelium (fig. 2-11). These specialized vessels are the site of entry of B and T lymphocytes into lymphoid tissues from the blood through a complex array of molecular interactions (13).

Sinuses. Afferent lymphatics enter the subcapsular sinus, which connects with medullary sinuses via radial sinuses (see fig. 2-2). These radial sinuses run parallel to trabeculae, hence the alternative term of trabecular sinuses. The sinuses are traversed by reticular cells and reticulin fibers. Within the sinuses are many macrophages, which are the first cells of the lymph node to encounter foreign antigens.

Vasculature and Cellular Trafficking. Most arterial vessels enter the lymph node at the hilum; however, a few enter the convex surface of the capsule. Arterioles reach the cortex where they break up into capillaries which empty into venules. The venules enter veins traversing from the cortex to the medulla to exit at the hilum.

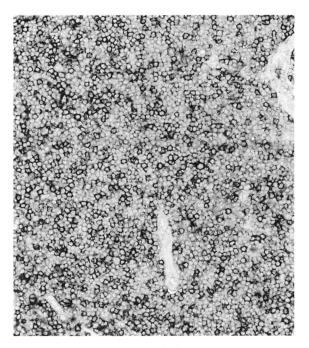

Figure 2-13
PARACORTICAL T ZONE
The T cells in the paracortical region of this mesenteric lymph node comprise an admixture of virgin (labeled blue with 4KB5/CD45RA) and memory (labeled red with OPD4/CD45RO) cells.

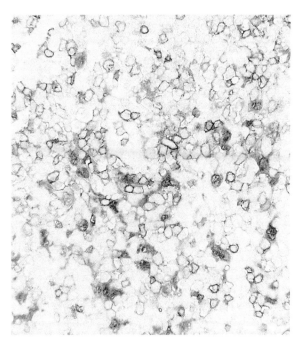

Figure 2-14
INTERDIGITATING DENDRITIC CELLS
The T cells (labeled blue with Leu-22/CD43) are often adjacent to the dendritic antigen-presenting cells (nuclei labeled brown by their expression of S-100 protein).

Mesenteric lymph nodes differ from the peripheral lymph nodes: several arteries penetrate the capsule rather than a single artery entering at an invaginated hilum. The sinuses are more often ectatic and filled with lymph (2).

Naive B and T cells emigrating from the bone marrow and thymus localize preferentially to the secondary lymphoid organs such as the lymph nodes, spleen, and Peyer's patches. Their migratory properties appear to be determined in ontogeny as a function of their differentiation. There is likely continuous traffic between the different secondary lymphoid organs until lymphocytes respond to antigen or die. When antigen accumulates in a secondary lymphoid organ, antigen-specific lymphocytes accumulate and through a complex series of events, memory and effector lymphocytes are generated. These memory and effector lymphocytes may display different migratory properties, such as predilection for skin or intestines, particularly when these tissues are involved in the immune response. Such tissue-selective homing enhances the efficiency

of the immune system by targeting tissues most similar to those in which the antigen initially entered the body; it may also reduce autoimmune cross reactions with tissue components in unrelated tissues (13).

Changes Following Antigenic Stimulation. The immune system produces a wide variety of lymphocytes bearing clonally determined antigen receptors. In response to stimulation with a specific antigen, the immune system provides a microenvironment that brings together antigen and those rare lymphocytes that can react with it (13). It also promotes and regulates clonal expansion and differentiation of the appropriate responding lymphocytes. Finally, it disperses the effector and memory lymphocytes to appropriate sites in the body to fight acute invasion and prevent reinvasion. These principal functions of the immune response are compartmentalized within lymph nodes and other secondary lymphoid tissues, and the various lymphoid organs are connected through a system of targeted lymphocyte trafficking and recirculation.

Antigen-presenting cells play an important role in bringing together antigen and reactive lymphocytes in the different microenvironments of the lymph nodes and spleen. Various cell types are capable of presenting foreign antigens including macrophages, interdigitating dendritic cells, and follicular dendritic cells; however, the route of immunization and the nature of the antigen determine which cells respond and the nature of the immunologic reaction. Within minutes, antigen can be identified in the subcapsular sinus of the draining lymph nodes; by 4 hours, there is a peak accumulation localized to macrophages in the sinuses (11,12). There is an initial accumulation of polymorphonuclear leukocytes within 4 to 14 hours. At approximately 24 hours, antigen begins to localize on the web of follicular dendritic cell processes in primary follicles. During the first 24 to 48 hours following antigenic stimulation, antigen-specific lymphocyte clones are retained in those lymphoid organs that drain the site of entry of antigen and are concomitantly depleted from the recirculating and peripheral pools.

The first site of antigen-specific B-cell proliferation is the T zone of the lymph node (9). This occurs on the second day following immunization and is largely over in 4 days. Thus, the initial proliferation of B cells takes place in regions rich in interdigitating dendritic cells that are active in T-cell–dependent B-cell activation by presenting antigen to T cells in conjunction with class II histocompatibility antigens. The B cells also express class II antigens and may present antigen directly to T cells. This extrafollicular B-cell response is important in recruiting naive cells into T-cell–dependent antibody responses and in generating short-lived plasma cells. It is also important in initiating T-cell activation and inducing specific T-cell migration to follicles.

However, the follicles are the major site of B-cell activation and proliferation in response to most antigens (8). Antigen-specific "blasts" are first identified in primary follicles at 36 hours following immunization. By 72 hours, the blasts form a small confluent center which displaces the small lymphocytes into a mantle. Over the next 24 hours these blasts express various B antigens, but not surface immunoglobulin, and collect in a region of the follicle nearest the T zone that forms the dark zone of germinal centers. These proliferating B cells have cell cycle times of 6 to 7 hours. It has been suggested that the somatic hypermutation mechanism, which acts on immunoglobulin V region genes and is responsible for the selection of B-cell clones with an increased affinity for antigen (affinity maturation), is selectively activated in the dark zone (10). Nondividing small cleaved cells/centrocytes accumulate in the pale zone of the germinal center, an area rich in follicular dendritic cells, and come to greatly outnumber the residual proliferating B-cell blasts. There is a high death rate among these small cleaved cells/centrocytes and their intensely basophilic nuclear debris is taken up by macrophages of the germinal center (tingible body macrophages). As indicated previously, most B cells in the germinal center that are destined to undergo programmed cell death do not express the *bcl*-2 protein.

The germinal center reaction peaks in about 1 week and gradually subsides over the following 2 weeks. In the final stage of the follicular response, a small cluster of blasts may persist for weeks, presumably in response to small amounts of persistent antigen on follicular dendritic cells. While these cellular events are taking place in the follicular and paracortical regions of the lymph node, a variable accumulation of plasma cells occurs in the medullary cords, starting on the third to fifth day.

SPLEEN

Gross Anatomy

Though the normal weight of the spleen is often reported to be approximately 150 g, the weight varies considerably in relationship to age, sex, body height, weight, and body surface area. The mean weight at age 29 is 125 g for males and 103 g for females (with a standard deviation from the mean of approximately 25 percent) (6). The weight of the spleen decreases after the seventh decade (6). Another presumptive age-related finding is the hyalinization of splenic arterioles, although this finding may be observed in spleens removed from young individuals (18). The spleen is encapsulated by a thin rim of white connective tissue, indented medially at the hilus, where it is penetrated by vessels and nerves which follow the extensive branching network of fibrous trabeculae. Single or multiple accessory spleens occur in about 10 percent of

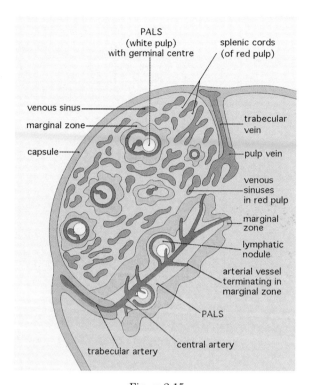

Figure 2-15
STRUCTURE OF HUMAN SPLEEN
(Fig. 3.8 from Roitt IM, Brostoff J, Male DK. Immunology. 3rd ed. St. Louis: Mosby, 1993:3.4.)

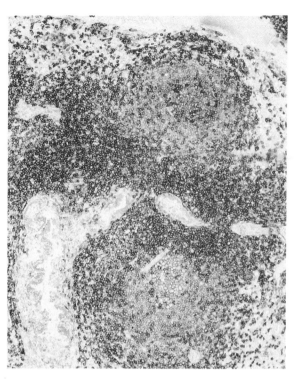

Figure 2-16
SPLENIC WHITE PULP
The T cells predominate in the periarteriolar lymphoid sheath (labeled red with Leu-22/CD43). The follicles, which tend to occur at arterial branch points, are labeled blue (L26/CD20).

individuals. In addition, following traumatic rupture, small nodules of splenic tissue may grow on the peritoneal surface as implants (splenosis).

In contrast to the cut surface of lymph nodes which offers few clues to the pathologic diagnosis, the cut surface of the spleen typically shows an expanded or increased number of white pulp nodules (Malpighian corpuscles) when involved by lymphoma and a homogenous red cut surface when heavily infiltrated by leukemia (see chapter 20).

Microscopic Anatomy

See figure 2-15 for a schematic diagram of the microscopic anatomy (3,18,19).

White Pulp. The white pulp comprises the lymphoid compartment of the spleen and consists of both follicular B-cell–rich areas as well as T-cell–rich periarteriolar lymphoid sheaths.

Periarteriolar T-Cell–Rich Lymphoid Sheaths. The splenic counterpart to the paracortical region of lymph nodes is the lymphoid sheath, which surrounds splenic arteries as they exit the

fibrous trabeculae (fig. 2-16). The reticular meshwork tends to be arranged circumferentially around the central artery. T cells of similar composition and phenotype to those in the paracortical regions of lymph nodes predominate in these areas, which also contain interdigitating cells and macrophages. The lymphoid sheaths become attenuated when the arterial vessels become small arterioles.

Primary and Secondary B-Cell Follicles. Primary and secondary follicles are often located at arterial branch points at the periphery of the T zone and have the identical histologic and phenotypic features of primary and secondary follicles of lymph nodes (fig. 2-16). Because the spleen is part of the vascular rather than lymphatic system and lacks afferent lymphatics, it is relatively protected from exogenous antigen. This is probably why the normal adult spleen has a greater number of primary rather than secondary follicles. The marginal zone, which surrounds the primary follicle and the mantle zone

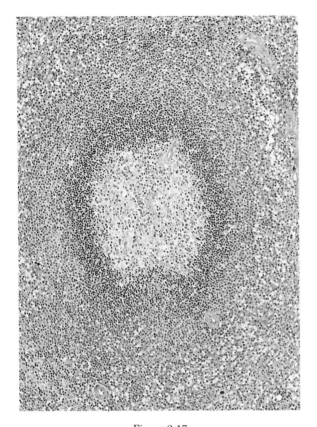

Figure 2-17
SPLENIC SECONDARY FOLLICLE
The central germinal center is surrounded by a thin mantle of small lymphocytes internal to a prominent marginal zone.

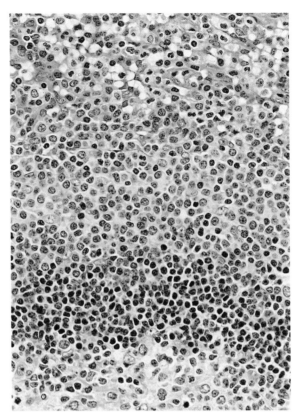

Figure 2-18
SPLENIC MARGINAL ZONE
The marginal zone lymphocytes are set apart by pale-staining cytoplasm. The nuclei are slightly larger and more irregular than those of the small lymphocytes in the mantle adjacent to germinal center cells (bottom).

of secondary follicles, consists of a corona of medium-sized lymphoid cells with prominent pale cytoplasm (fig. 2-17). The nuclear chromatin of the intermediate-sized marginal zone cells is somewhat less condensed than that of small lymphocytes (fig. 2-18). Marginal zone lymphocytes are admixed with a variable number of plasma cells, T cells, and macrophages. Marginal zone B lymphocytes express surface immunoglobulin with mμ heavy chain and little, if any, delta heavy chain. These cells typically have avid receptors for the Fc portion of IgG, and stain for complement receptors I and II (CD35 and CD21) and alkaline phosphatase. In contrast to mantle zone B-lymphocytes, marginal zone B cells generally lack expression of the CD45 isoform recognized by Ki-B3 as well as CD23 (19). Some intermediate-sized lymphoid cells can also be identified in Peyer's patches and infiltrating the epithelium overlying their follicles. Marginal

zone type B cells can occasionally be seen in lymph nodes, particularly in the mesentery, where collections of these cells may be polarized toward the subcapsular sinus.

Red Pulp. The splenic pulp is red owing to the large volume of erythrocytes. It is composed of four vascular structures: slender and nonanastomosing arterial vessels; a reticular meshwork consisting of thin plates of cellular tissue lying between the sinusoids comprising splenic cords; large, thin-walled venous vessels called sinusoids; and pulp veins which drain the sinusoids.

Cords. The reticular meshwork consists of a branching system of cords lying between the sinuses (20). After the central artery distributes branches to the white pulp and marginal zone, the attenuated main stem runs on into the cords of the red pulp, branching into straight nonanastomosing slender vessels or penicilli, which

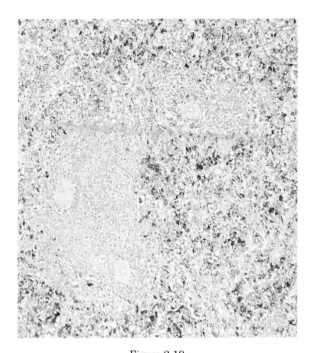

Figure 2-19
SPLENIC MACROPHAGES
Macrophages are preferentially located in the marginal zone and red pulp cords of the spleen (labeled brown with KP-1/CD68).

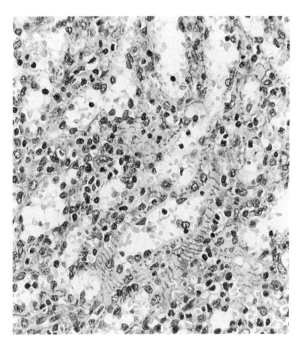

Figure 2-20
SPLENIC RED PULP
PAS stain highlights the distinctive ring fibers and bridging fibers.

open directly into the reticular meshwork of the cords. Shortly before they terminate, they may run through a sheath of macrophages. Erythrocytes, granulocytes, and other blood cells may be present in the sheath. Well-developed sheaths, which may contain many splenic macrophages, possess extraordinary phagocytic capacity, are likely major sites of clearance of blood-borne particles, and may even control splenic blood flow. These macrophage sheaths are not highly developed in the human spleen and the splenic clearance functions in man are also handled by marginal zone and red pulp macrophages (fig. 2-19). The red pulp cords also contain lymphoid cells with predominant populations of CD8-reactive T cells and natural killer cells.

Sinuses. The sinuses are lined by tapered endothelial cells separated by slit-like spaces and surrounded by distinctive ring fibers and bridging fibers (fig. 2-20). These endothelial cells contain tight junctional complexes and lie on a fenestrated basement membrane. They stain for endothelial markers (fig. 2-21) as well as CD8.

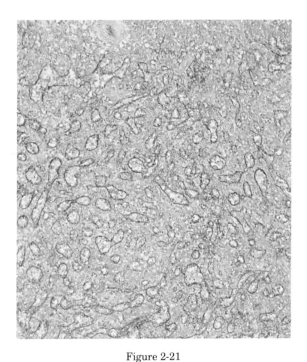

Figure 2-21
SPLENIC RED PULP
Factor VIII–related antigen is present on the endothelial cells that line the sinusoids.

Vasculature and Cellular Trafficking. The specialized vasculature of the spleen makes it ideally suited for a variety of functions including differentiation of reticulocytes, platelets, and monocytes and modification or removal of abnormal erythrocytes. It can sequester monocytes, facilitating their transformation into macrophages and is a reservoir for erythrocytes, granulocytes, and platelets. Not only is the spleen an enormous reservoir of phagocytic function but a major site of antibody production, particularly in response to blood-borne antigens.

Changes Following Antigenic Stimulation, Particularly of Marginal Zone B Cells. Since the B cells of the marginal zone are bathed in a blood-sinusoidal system, they are ideally situated to respond to blood-borne antigens before these antigens reach the macrophages in the red pulp (10). Experimental evidence in rodents indicates that nonrecirculating marginal zone B cells, in contrast to recirculating B cells, are vital in immunologic responses to pure polysaccharide antigens such as *Streptococcus pneumoniae, Neisseria meningitidis,* and *Haemophilus influenzae* type B (6,10). When activated by antigen, marginal zone B cells migrate to adjacent T-cell–rich areas and probably to follicles before entering the cell cycle. In addition, the macrophages of rodent marginal zones can take up and retain carbohydrate macromolecules, a property not shared by dendritic cells or red pulp macrophages. Thus, the overwhelming sepsis that may complicate splenectomy, particularly in children, may relate to deficiency of specialized macrophages and B cells in the marginal zones.

REFERENCES

1. Beverley PC. Functional analysis of human T cell subsets defined by CD45 isoform expression. Semin Immunol 1992;4:35–41.
2. Davies JD. Gut-associated lymph nodes. In: Whitehead R, ed. Gastrointestinal and esophageal pathology. Edinburgh: Churchill Livingstone, 1989:611–6.
3. Grogan TM, Rangel CS, Richter LC, Wirt DP, Villar HV. Further delineation of the immunoarchitecture of the human spleen. Lymphology 1984;17:61–8.
4. Janossy G, Bofill M, Rowe D, Muir J, Beverley PC. The tissue distribution of T lymphocytes expressing different CD45 polypeptides. Immunology 1989;66:517–25.
5. Korsrud FR, Brandtzaeg P. Immunohistochemical evaluation of J-chain expression by intra- and extrafollicular immunoglobulin-producing human tonsillar cells. Scand J Immunol 1981;13:271–80.
6. Lampert IA. The spleen. In: McGee JO, Isaacson PG, Wright NA, eds. Oxford textbook of pathology, Vol 2b. Pathology of systems. New York: Oxford University Press, 1992:1794.
7. Levy R, Warnke R, Dorfman RF, Haimovich J. The monoclonality of human B-cell lymphomas. J Exp Med 1977;145:1014–28.
8. Liu YJ, Johnson GD, Gordon J, MacLennan IC. Germinal centres in T-cell-dependent antibody responses. Immunol Today 1992;13:17–21.
9. _____, Zhang J, Lane PJ, Chan EY, MacLennan IC. Sites of specific B cell activation in primary and secondary responses to T cell-dependent and T cell-independent antigens. Eur J Immunol 1991;21:2951–62.
10. MacLennan IC, Liu YJ, Oldfield S, Zhang J, Lane PJ. The evolution of B-cell clones. Curr Top Microbiol Immunol 1990;159:37–63.
11. Nossal GJ, Abbot A, Mitchell J. Antigens in immunity. XIV. Electron microscopic radioautographic studies of antigen capture in the lymph node medulla. J Exp Med 1968;127:263–76.
12. _____, Abbot A, Mitchell J, Lummus Z. Antigens in immunity. XV. Ultrastructural features of antigen capture in primary and secondary lymphoid follicles. J Exp Med 1968;127:277–90.
13. Picker LJ, Butcher EC. Physiological and molecular mechanisms of lymphocyte homing. Annu Rev Immunol 1992;10:561–91.
14. _____, Weiss LM, Medeiros LJ, Wood GS, Warnke RA. Immunophenotypic criteria for the diagnosis of non-Hodgkin's lymphoma. Am J Pathol 1987;128:181–201.
15. Stein H, Bonk A, Tolksdorf G, Lennert K, Rodt H, Gerdes J. Immunohistologic analysis of the organization of normal lymphoid tissue and non-Hodgkin's lymphomas. J Histochem Cytochem 1980;28:746–60.
16. Szakal AK, Kosco MH, Tew JG. Microanatomy of lymphoid tissue during humoral immune responses: structure function relationships. Annu Rev Immunol 1989;7:91–109.
17. Van der Valk P, Meijer CJ. The histology of reactive lymph nodes. Am J Surg Pathol 1987;11:866–82.
18. Van Krieken JH, de Velde J. Normal histology of the human spleen. Am J Surg Pathol 1988;12:777–85.
19. _____, von Schilling C, Kluin PM, Lennert K. Splenic marginal zone lymphocytes and related cells in the lymph node: a morphologic and immunohistochemical study. Hum Pathol 1989;20:320–5.
20. Weiss L. The spleen. In: Weiss L, ed. Histology: cell and tissue biology. New York: Elsevier Biomedical, 1983:544–68.
21. _____, Movahed LA. In situ demonstration of Epstein-Barr viral genomes in viral-associated B cell lymphoproliferations. Am J Pathol 1989;134:651–9.
22. Westerga J, Timens W. Immunohistological analysis of human fetal lymph nodes. Scand J Immunol 1989;29:103–12.

3

EVALUATION OF LYMPHOID LESIONS

Advances in the staging and treatment of malignant lymphomas have necessitated a high degree of accuracy in the diagnosis and classification of these neoplasms. Fortunately, a greater degree of diagnostic precision has resulted from recent advances in the immunology and molecular biology of malignant lymphomas as well as new diagnostic reagents and methods. Although most lymphoid lesions can be accurately diagnosed by conventional methods, many present problems in differential diagnosis and may require one or more special studies. The proper handling of specimens for adjunctive diagnostic studies, the pitfalls in the fixation and processing of lymphoid lesions which may compromise the accuracy of diagnosis, and a morphologic approach to the differential diagnosis of these lesions are discussed here. We provide a catalogue of antibodies and a panel approach to their use in differential diagnosis, a catalogue of molecular probes for the identification of clonal populations in lymphoid lesions, and a list of recurrent chromosomal abnormalities in the most studied lymphoma subtypes. Finally, we comment on the role of electron microscopy and fine needle aspiration in the differential diagnosis of lymphoid lesions.

HANDLING THE FRESH SPECIMEN

Clinical Correlation

Knowledge of the patient's history and clinical diagnosis or differential diagnosis is critical in the optimal handling of each fresh specimen (9). The surgeon should be encouraged to excise the largest and most abnormal-appearing lymph node. If an infectious disease is suspected, a portion from one pole can be taken in the sterile environment of the operating room and submitted for appropriate microbiologic studies. Otherwise, the specimen should be submitted to the pathologist intact in saline or culture medium in a Petri dish or other specimen container to avoid desiccation of the cortex of the lymph node. Most lymph node biopsies yield enough tissue for routine histology so that fresh cells or frozen tissue

can be reserved for phenotypic and genotypic studies. Touch imprint preparations obtained from the cut surface of the biopsy can be air-dried for Giemsa staining or immediately wet-fixed in alcohol for staining with hematoxylin and eosin. A sterile portion may be saved for possible cytogenetic studies. When the amount of tissue is limited, the most important consideration is submitting ample tissue for proper fixation and paraffin embedding. However, it is almost always possible to save a small portion of tissue for frozen section phenotypic or genotypic study. The allocation of limited amounts of tissue should be dictated by appropriate clinical information.

Technical Considerations in the Choice of Ancillary Studies

Table 3-1 summarizes the types of specimens that may be used for ancillary special studies. Although comparable phenotyping results often can be obtained by either cell suspension or slide-based methods, generally we prefer to phenotype leukemias and other disorders already in suspension with cell suspension methods and to phenotype lymphomas and other disorders in tissues with tissue section methods (6). Tissue section immunostains are less amenable to quantitation of number of stained cells or antigen density than cells stained in suspension and evaluated by flow cytometry or stained cell monolayers assessed by image analysis (5–7). However, tissue section methods permit simple collection and storage of samples with little initial processing and preserve the topography of the positive and negative cell populations. The stored samples can be reused several times for additional studies, including genotyping. Phenotypic studies on fixed paraffin-embedded tissue sections offer excellent correlation with architectural as well as cellular details. Although fewer antigens are preserved in fixed and embedded tissues than in fresh frozen tissues, new markers reactive with fixation-resistant epitopes continue to be produced. In addition, novel methods, such as microwaving for unmasking antigenic reactivity after fixation, are often helpful in improving the antigen detection

Table 3-1
TYPES OF SPECIMENS SUITABLE FOR ANCILLARY DIAGNOSTIC STUDIES

Studies	Sterile Cells	Non-sterile Cells	Touch Imprints	Cytospin Preparations	Frozen Tissue	Paraffin-Embedded Fixed Tissue
Microbial culture	+	+/–				
Chromosomal analysis	+	+/–				
Phenotyping by flow cytometry	+	+				
Slide-based phenotyping						
Surface immunoglobulin			+/–	+	+	+/–
Cytoplasmic immunoglobulin			+	+	+/–	+
Other surface antigens			+	+	+	+,+/–
Cytoplasmic/nuclear antigens			+	+	+	+,+/–
Antigen receptor rearrangements						
Southern blotting	+	+			+	+/–
Polymerase chain reaction	+	+			+	+/–

+ = suitable for special study.
+/– = less than ideal for special study because of interstitial immunoglobulin or altered/destroyed protein, RNA, or DNA or less than optimal probes.

threshold and increasing the spectrum of antibodies that work on routine paraffin sections (8).

Just as immunologic phenotyping reagents and methods continue to evolve, newer molecular methods for identifying clonal populations of T- and B-lineage cells using the polymerase chain reaction (PCR) may eventually supplant the more standard Southern blot method (1–4).

As with all laboratory tests, ancillary studies should be carefully controlled and interpreted with caution by experienced pathologists. The results of special studies must be closely correlated with histopathology. To provide the best patient care at the least cost, it is critical that the pathologist regularly replace older, less efficient methods with newer, more efficient and, ideally, cost-effective methods.

Role of Frozen Section Diagnosis

Because the diagnosis of lymphoid neoplasms may be difficult even in optimally fixed and processed tissues, we discourage clinicians from requesting a frozen section diagnosis in suspected hematolymphoid lesions. In exceptional cases, when rapid diagnosis is essential for patient care, touch imprints or scrape preparations, in conjunction with frozen sections, are useful. Frozen sections may reveal architectural features but touch imprints are essential in assessing cytologic features. It is often difficult or impossible to distinguish follicular hyperplasia from follicular lymphoma or accurately identify a poorly differentiated large cell neoplasm in frozen sections. In contrast, a diagnosis of lymphoblastic lymphoma or Burkitt's lymphoma may be obvious in cytologic preparations. Although imprint preparations often facilitate the identification of Reed-Sternberg cells, we believe that a diagnosis of Hodgkin's disease based on frozen section should only be rendered when the clinical situation mandates an immediate diagnosis.

More frequently and more appropriately, in our opinion, surgical pathologists are requested to perform frozen sections to assess adequacy of a specimen for diagnosis and the optimal allocation of tissue for routine and special studies when the amount is limited. In addition, if a lymph node removed from a patient strongly suspected of harboring lymphoma shows changes in the frozen sections consistent with a reactive process, the surgeon may elect to search further for a more abnormal-appearing node. The frozen section remnant can be left frozen and retained for possible phenotypic or genotypic studies if the cut surface is covered with additional freezing medium and refrozen (see below).

Specimen Transport

To avoid irreversible drying artifacts, lymph nodes, and particularly small samples such as needle biopsies, should not be transported on dry towels or surgical sponges but rather on wet gauze or in a container in saline or culture medium (9). Storage of a lymph node at 4°C for 24 hours or occasionally longer is often satisfactory for morphologic assessment and a surprising number of cellular antigens are also preserved (6). Although cooling a specimen to 4°C delays autolysis, the slicing of lymph nodes at 2 to 3 mm intervals enhances cellular preservation for optimal fixation. An ammonium sulfate–based transport medium such as Michel's may be used for lymphoid organs but some antigens are not preserved by this method and the morphologic preservation is often suboptimal.

Optimal Freezing for Immunologic Studies

Representative tissue should be frozen whenever lymphoma is a reasonable possibility because most of the ancillary studies in hematopathology can be performed on frozen tissue (6,7). Snap freezing in liquid nitrogen or in an isopentane and dry ice mixture is ideal, but satisfactory results may also be obtained if a less than 2-mm slice is frozen on a rapid-freeze chuck accessory in a cryotome. Tissue can be frozen in embedding medium in electron microscopy embedding capsules or on a cryostat chuck. The use of plastic capsules permits easy storage and avoids desiccation of specimens. Tissue frozen in O.C.T. on a chuck or on a solid block must be wrapped in foil or plastic for storage to avoid desiccation. Frozen tissue is ideally stored at -70°C, but storage at -20°C is suitable for many antigens. Since many microtomes and refrigerator freezing compartments feature automatic defrost cycles, it is critical to transfer frozen tissue to a noncycling freezer for safekeeping. An alternative is to freeze and store short-term in an automatic cryobath.

FIXATION AND PROCESSING

Fixation

Despite recent advances in immunology and molecular biology, most diagnostic hematopathology rests primarily on the histologic assessment of sections prepared from paraffin-embedded fixed tissues. The most critical factors in the preparation of optimal histologic sections include adequate fixation and technical precision (11,13). Adequate fixation is the most critical since tissue blocks can be reinfiltrated, recleared, and redehydrated but inadequate fixation can seldom be reversed. Lymph nodes should be sliced completely at 2- to 3-mm intervals. Many laboratories employ two fixatives for the routine fixation of lymph nodes: a metal-based fixative and neutral-buffered formaldehyde. The particular metal fixative varies according to the preference of the surgical pathologist but is commonly B5, neutral Zenker's solution, or zinc sulphate. Although B5 yields excellent nuclear detail, close attention must be paid to the time of fixation, mercuric chloride crystals must be removed from sections, the cost is relatively high, and mercury is an environmental hazard. In addition, nonspecific staining may be encountered with immunologic stains on tissues overfixed in B5 or Zenker's fixative. Zinc sulfate is an attractive second fixative as it often yields good nuclear detail, is low in cost, and requires no special precautions for disposal. Alcohol-based fixatives have been promoted for enhanced preservation of some antigens as well as enhanced preservation of DNA for certain molecular studies. However, morphology may be suboptimal after alcohol fixation, particularly in small biopsy specimens. A more detailed discussion of different fixatives is provided by Banks and Larsson (10,17). Plastic embedding may be used to enhance cytologic detail; technical modifications have been made to preserve immunoreactivity for many antigens (12,14). Methods employing cold acetone fixation followed by methyl benzoate and xylene treatment prior to paraffin embedding (AMeX and ModAMeX) have also been used to preserve morphology and enhance antigenicity (15,18).

Artifacts of Fixation and Processing

Several articles have indicated that fixation and processing artifacts are often accentuated in lymphoid lesions (10,11,13). Many of these artifacts are listed in Table 3-2. When lymph node sections are suboptimal for no apparent reason, a carefully recut hematoxylin and eosin stained section from the same paraffin block on the following day may sometimes show remarkable improvement. Perhaps the single most important factor for optimal

Table 3-2

COMMON ERRORS IN FIXATION AND PROCESSING OF LYMPHOID TISSUE*

Step	Problem	Consequence
Transport	Drying of specimen	Dark, amorphous edge in stained section; if long delay to fixation, central autolysis
Blocking	>3 mm thick or encapsulated	Soft, unfixed core may fragment; cells in center show ballooning and pale staining
Fixation	Overfixation in mercuric chloride–based fixative	Brittle tissue may shatter; nuclear staining may be diminished
Dehydration	Aqueous contamination or inadequate time	Sections may crumble, tear, or explode; may show numerous small cracks ("dry earth effect"); faint staining with blurred nuclear chromatin
Clearing	Excessive time, alcohol contamination	Brittle tissue may shatter; compressed, wrinkled sections will not ribbon
Infiltration	Paraffin too hot	Hard, shrunken tissue may shatter; homogenous muddy staining with poor nuclear and cytoplasmic detail
Embedding	Delay in embedding after removal from paraffin bath	Air spaces around tissue in block make for difficult paraffin sectioning
Sectioning	Improper knife angle, defective knife edge, section too thick	"Venetian-blind" or "shutter" effect; lines across sections; diminished cytologic detail
Floating section	Uneven on bath	Folds or tears
Drying	Too hot	"Bubbled" nuclei; antigen loss
Staining	Inadequate eosin rinse	Overall red hue with obscured detail

*From references 10,11,13.

histology is the thickness of the section, which should be one cell layer thick irrespective of the microtome setting. As mentioned, Romanovsky, Papanicolaou, or hematoxylin and eosin stained touch imprint preparations may be invaluable for cytologic assessment. These imprints can also be used for enzyme histochemical and immunological studies. If air-dried imprints are stored at -20°C, many antigens are retained for up to a week or longer (one notable exception being terminal deoxynucleotidyl transferase [TdT]). Air-dried imprints that are carefully stored in air-tight containers at -70°C retain some antigens for months to years.

Routine and Histochemical Stains

We find that hematoxylin and eosin staining is adequate for assessing most lymphoid lesions. Special stains that may be helpful in diagnosis include Giemsa, periodic acid–Schiff (PAS), reticulin, and methyl-green pyronin. The Giemsa stain highlights nuclear features; demonstrates cytoplasmic granules, particularly in

mast cells and myeloid cells; and is very useful in identifying plasmacytoid features in cells. PAS demonstrates mucin and glycogen, for example, when carcinoma, seminoma, or Ewing's sarcoma is included in a differential diagnosis. Cytoplasmic and "nuclear" immunoglobulin inclusions also stain with PAS, particularly those rich in carbohydrates such as IgM and IgA (see fig. 7-9). In addition, PAS highlights basement membranes of blood vessels. The reticulin stain may be useful in delineating architecture; for example, in accentuating follicles and residual sinuses. The methyl-green pyronin stain demonstrates cytoplasmic RNA, thus highlighting plasmacytoid cells.

In our experience, enzyme histochemistry has a limited role in routine lymph node evaluation, apart from the invaluable naphthol ASD chloroacetate esterase (Leder) stain which identifies cells of myeloid and mast cell lineage in paraffin-embedded material (see figure 19-14). This enzyme is destroyed by acid decalcification of bone lesions but can be retained by decalcification in

Table 3-3

DIFFERENTIAL DIAGNOSIS BASED UPON RECOGNITION OF PREDOMINANT PATTERN IN LYMPH NODE AT LOW MAGNIFICATION

Follicular/ Nodular	Interfollicular/ Paracortical	Diffuse	Sinus	Mixed/Other
NON-NEOPLASTIC				
Reactive follicular hyperplasia Explosive follicular hyperplasia (HIV) Progressive transformation of germinal centers Castleman's disease Rheumatoid lymphadenopathy Luetic lymphadenitis Kimura's disease	Immunoblastic proliferations Viral lymphadenitis (EBV, CMV, herpes) Post-vaccination lymphadenitis Drug sensitivity, e.g., Dilantin	Immunoblastic proliferations Viral lymphadenitis (EBV, CMV, herpes) Post-vaccination lymphadenitis Drug sensitivity e.g., Dilantin	Sinus hyperplasia Rosai-Dorfman disease Lymphangiogram effect Whipple's disease Vascular transformation of sinuses Hemophagocytic syndrome	Mixed hyperplasia Dermatopathic lymphadenopathy Toxoplasmosis Cat scratch disease Systemic lupus erythematosus Kawasaki's disease Kikuchi's lymphadenitis Granulomatous lymphadenitis Inflammatory pseudotumor
UNCERTAIN IF NEOPLASTIC				
Nodular lymphocyte predominance HD		Angioimmunoblastic lymphadenopathy	Langerhans' cell histiocytosis	Systemic Castleman's disease
NEOPLASTIC				
Nodular sclerosing HD Follicular lymphoma Mantle cell lymphoma Monocytoid B-cell lymphoma CLL/SLL with proliferation centers	Interfollicular HD T-zone lymphoma Mixed cellularity HD Small cell B/T lymphoma/leukemia Large cell B/T lymphoma Lymphoblastic lymphoma/leukemia Burkitt's lymphoma Plasmacytoma Nonlymphoid leukemia Mastocytosis Histiocytic neoplasms Nonhematolymphoid neoplasms	Mixed cellularity HD Small cell B/T lymphoma/leukemia Large cell B/T lymphoma Lymphoblastic lymphoma/leukemia Burkitt's lymphoma Plasmacytoma Anaplastic large cell lymphoma Nonlymphoid leukemia Mastocytosis Histiocytic neoplasms Nonhematolymphoid neoplasms	Anaplastic large cell lymphoma Sinusoidal large cell lymphoma Mastocytosis Nonlymphoid leukemia Histiocytic neoplasms Nonhematolymphoid neoplasms	Mucosa-associated lymphoid tissue lymphoma Monocytoid B-cell lymphoma

ethylenediaminetetraacetic acid (EDTA). Although mercuric chloride–containing fixatives are said to destroy this enzyme, it may be detected if the iodine or sodium thiosulfate steps to remove crystals are eliminated. In addition, myeloperoxidase, Sudan black B, and nonspecific esterase stains on air-dried imprints help evaluate myeloid or monocytic differentiation. Such stains may be especially helpful in the diagnosis of T-cell lymphoma since many of the paraffin T-cell–associated markers also react with myelomonocytic cells.

PATTERN RECOGNITION IN THE MORPHOLOGIC DIFFERENTIAL DIAGNOSIS

As in other areas of pathology, an accurate morphologic diagnosis of a lymphoid lesion requires integration of both architectural and cellular features (16). Evaluation at low magnification commonly provides a recognizable pattern and cellular staining characteristics suggestive of a particular lymphoma; this can be confirmed by medium- and high-power examination. The predominant patterns of many benign and malignant lesions of lymph nodes as well as those of uncertain nature are described in Table 3-3. The size of lymphoid cells is categorized by comparing the neoplastic cell nuclei with those of histiocytes or endothelial cells: small, medium, and large cells refer to cells with nuclei smaller, approximately the same size, or larger than those of reactive histiocytes or endothelial cells. More detailed diagnostic features and differential diagnoses are discussed in the following chapters.

IMMUNOHISTOCHEMICAL STUDIES

Markers Used on
Fixed Paraffin-Embedded Tissues

Table 3-4 lists many of the leukocyte markers detected in routinely fixed and paraffin-embedded tissue sections. The antibodies are grouped by their predominant pattern of normal cell reactivity. Their reactivity with hematolymphoid neoplasms is also summarized. Newly produced markers reactive with fixation-resistant epitopes and antigenic determinants unmasked after usual formaldehyde fixation continue to modify the list of antibodies that can be used in this setting (28). Most of the leukocyte markers listed in Table 3-4 are not repeated in Table 3-5 although they can be used on fresh cells in suspension, cells fixed on slides, or in frozen sections. With few exceptions, monoclonal antibodies that stain well in paraffin sections stain as well or better in acetone-fixed frozen sections. Antigenic determinants embedded in the cell membrane or within the cytoplasm or nucleus are more easily detected in cell monolayers or tissue sections than in cells in suspension, which require a permeable cell membrane. Polyclonal antisera often contain a significant number of unwanted reactivities that limit their application to fresh cells in suspension or in tissue sections but polyclonal anti-immunoglobulin antibodies are preferable to monoclonal ones because of their wider reactivity. Nevertheless, antibodies generated by immunization with highly purified antigens may work well in both fresh and fixed tissues (70,80).

It is beyond the scope of this chapter to discuss in any detail the methods for immunohistochemical staining (44,51). In general, a variety of indirect three-stage methods can be used suc-

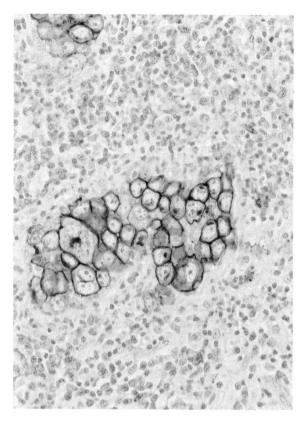

Figure 3-1
MEMBRANE AND PARANUCLEAR/GOLGI
STAINING PATTERN
Many leukocyte markers stain the cell membrane. In this example of a pleomorphic large cell lymphoma involving sinuses, the lymphoma cells also show paranuclear/Golgi staining for CD20 with antibody L26. (Immunoperoxidase with hematoxylin counterstain)

cessfully to label a wide range of leukocyte markers. On occasion, a more specific method, for example, using specific conjugates to detect the mμ chain of certain mouse monoclonal antibodies like Leu-M1 and Leu-7, may be useful (67).

Although most paraffin section reactive leukocyte markers stain the cell membrane (fig. 3-1), a perinuclear or Golgi pattern of staining may be observed with some (figs. 3-1, 3-2), or in certain cell types such as macrophages. A Golgi pattern is commonly seen with CD15 (fig. 3-2) and CD30, with or without associated cell membrane staining. Cytoplasmic staining for immunoglobulins (Ig) results from the production of specific Ig by plasma cells; in Hodgkin cells and histiocytes it is generally due to the uptake of interstitial Ig (fig. 3-3). Cytoplasmic staining

Table 3-4

PRINCIPAL ANTIBODIES EMPLOYED IN
IMMUNOHISTOCHEMICAL STAINING OF PARAFFIN TISSUE SECTIONS

CD Antigen and/ or Antibody	Predominant Normal Cell Reactivity	Reactivity in Neoplasms	Comment/Caution
LEUKOCYTES			
CD45RB (PD7) Leukocyte common antigen*	B cells and most T cells, macrophages, myeloid cells	Most lymphomas and leukemias	Plasma cell neoplasms and Reed-Sternberg cells usually unreactive, some lymphoblastic and anaplastic large cell lymphomas unreactive (42,56,63,64,145)
B LYMPHOCYTES			
Immuno-globulin (polyclonal)	B cells and plasma cells	B cell and plasma cell neoplasms	Diffuse cytoplasmic staining for both light chains seen in macrophages, Reed-Sternberg cells, and degenerated cells (attributed to passive uptake); cytoplasmic Ig often detectable in paraffin sections; surface Ig often requires frozen tissue (70)
CD79 (mb-1/B29) (Ig associated)	B cells (B29 absent in plasma cells)	Most B lymphomas, B leukemias from pre-B-cell stage	Associated with antigen receptor (Ig) on B cells in a similar manner as CD3 on T cells; antibodies cross react with all mammalian species tested (78,82)
CD20 (L26)	B cells, sometimes macrophages	Most B-cell lymphomas, L&H cells in NLPHD, some Reed-Sternberg cells in ~ 20 % of classic Hodgkin's disease, rare T-cell lymphomas	Does not work well in acid decalcified tissues particularly if Bouin fixed (unless microwaved), plasma cell neoplasms usually unreactive, some thymomas may stain (27,34,76,101)
CD45RA (4KB5, MB1)	B cells and subpopulation of T cells	Most B-cell lymphomas, few T-cell lymphomas, L&H cells in NLPHD, some myeloid leukemias	Plasma cell neoplasms usually unreactive (34,39,100,114)
CDw75 (LN1)	B cells (mainly germinal center cells)	Many B-cell lymphomas, some T-cell lymphomas, L&H cells in NLPHD; Reed-Sternberg cells in classic Hodgkin's disease (some cases)	Works better in mercuric chloride–containing fixatives (75,97)
CD74 (LN2 and MB3)	B cells, interdigitating dendritic cells, some macrophages, Langerhans cells	Many B-cell lymphomas, some T-cell lymphomas, Reed-Sternberg cells, many myeloid leukemias, Langerhans' cell histiocytosis	Works better in mercuric chloride–containing fixatives (75,97)
MB2	B cells, some macrophages	Most B-cell lymphomas, some T-cell lymphomas, some myeloid leukemias	Plasma cell neoplasms unreactive, many nonhematolymphoid neoplasms reactive (114)
T LYMPHOCYTES			
CD3 (polyclonal)	T cells	Many T-cell lymphomas	May require prolonged proteolytic digestion or wet heat pretreatment, may see nonspecific cytoplasmic staining in macrophages and plasma cells (77,80)
βF1 (TCR beta chain)	T cells	Many T-cell lymphomas	Requires proteolytic digestion, more sensitive in frozen sections (125)

Table 3-4 (continued)

PRINCIPAL ANTIBODIES EMPLOYED IN IMMUNOHISTOCHEMICAL STAINING OF PARAFFIN TISSUE SECTIONS

CD Antigen and/ or Antibody	Predominant Normal Cell Reactivity	Reactivity in Neoplasms	Comment/Caution
		T LYMPHOCYTES (continued)	
CD43 (Leu-22, MT1, DFT1)	T cells, plasma cells, some macrophages, granulocytes, erythroid cells, Langerhans cells	Most T-cell lymphomas, ~1/3 B-cell lymphomas, myeloid leukemias, many plasma cell neoplasms, Langerhans' cell histiocytosis	Can be exploited especially for diagnosis of small cell B-lymphoma/ leukemia (21,95,98,99,114,127,137)
CD45RO (UCHL1, A6, OPD4)	Major T-cell subset, some macrophages, granulocytes	Many T-cell lymphomas, few B-cell lymphomas, myeloid leukemias, some plasma cell cell neoplasms	May see nonspecific cytoplasmic staining (23,99,102,115,156)
CD57 (Leu-7, HNK1)	Subset of germinal center T-cells, some natural killer cells	Few lymphoblastic lymphomas, some natural killer cell neoplasms	CD56 in frozen sections better marker for natural killer cells, IgM isotype may benefit from isotype-specific detection, subset of reactive T-cells ring L&H cells in NLPHD (57,96,112,131)
		HODGKIN'S DISEASE ASSOCIATED	
CD15 (LeuM1)	Granulocytes, some macrophages	Reed-Sternberg cells in most cases of classic Hodgkin's disease, large cells in some B- and T-cell lymphomas, some myeloid leukemias	Many carcinomas reactive, CMV-infected cells reactive, IgM isotype may benefit from isotype-specific detection, L&H cells usually unreactive in paraffin sections (20,55,130,135)
CD30 (BerH2)	Some activated B and T cells, some plasma cells	Reed-Sternberg cells in most cases of classic Hodgkin's disease, most cases of anaplastic large cell lymphoma, some B- and T-cell lymphomas, many plasma cell neoplasms; L&H cells usually unreactive in paraffin sections	Less sensitive in mercuric chloride–containing fixatives, embryonal carcinomas and few other non-hematolymphoid neoplasms reactive, cytoplasmic staining may be non-specific, staining of plasma cells may be abolished by prior wet heat treatment (such as microwave) (103,128,134)
		ACCESSORY CELLS	
CD68 (KP1)	Macrophages, myeloid cells	True histiocytic neoplasms, many myeloid leukemias; dot-like staining in some small cell B-lymphomas and leukemias, especially hairy cell leukemia, mastocytosis	Reactive in granular cell tumors, some melanomas, malignant fibrous histiocytomas, and renal cell carcinomas PGM1 (CD68) does not stain myeloid cells (33,117,118,146)
Lysozyme (polyclonal)	Macrophages, myeloid cells	True histiocytic lymphomas, myeloid leukemias	Reactive with many non-hematolymphoid neoplasms (62)
S-100 protein (polyclonal/ monoclonal)	Langerhans cells, interdigitating (IDRC) and sometimes follicular dendritic cells	Langerhans' cell histiocytosis, IDRC tumors, rare T-cell lymphomas, true histiocytic lymphomas, myeloid leukemias, Rosai-Dorfman disease	Reactive with many non-hematolymphoid neoplasms (138,142)
Mac-387	Macrophages, myeloid cells	True histiocytic lymphomas, myeloid leukemias	Reactive with some squamous cell carcinomas (24,25,43)

Table 3-4 (continued)

**PRINCIPAL ANTIBODIES EMPLOYED IN
IMMUNOHISTOCHEMICAL STAINING OF PARAFFIN TISSUE SECTIONS**

CD Antigen and/ or Antibody	Predominant Normal Cell Reactivity	Reactivity in Neoplasms	Comment/Caution
		MISCELLANEOUS	
bcl-2	Nongerminal center B cells most T cells, plasma cells	Overexpressed in most follicular lymphomas and some diffuse large B-cell lymphomas, also expressed in many other lymphomas and leukemias	Works best in B5 and Bouin fixed tissues (unless microwaved); most useful in differentiating benign from malignant follicular lesions, i.e, non-neoplastic germinal center B-cells unreactive (45,60,66)
EBV-latent membrane protein (LMP-1)	EBV-infected cells	Reed-Sternberg cells in some cases of classic Hodgkin's disease, i.e., those containing EBV DNA; most immunodeficiency-associated lymphomas	(37,104)
Myeloperoxidase (polyclonal)	Myeloid cells	Myeloid leukemias	Most sensitive and specific marker for myeloid neoplasms (111)
Epithelial membrane antigen	Plasma cells	In Hodgkin's disease, mainly NLPHD type; plasma cell neoplasms; many anaplastic large cell lymphomas and some other B and T large cell lymphomas	Many epithelial tumors reactive (32,36,110)

NLPHD = nodular lymphocyte predominance Hodgkin's disease.
*All of the above markers produce cell membrane and/or Golgi staining except: 1) CD74 (LN2): nuclear membrane staining; 2) S-100 protein: nuclear +/– cytoplasmic staining; 3) MB2, CD68 (KP1), Mac-387, Ig, lysozyme, *bcl*-2, and myeloperoxidase: diffuse cytoplasmic staining.

may be nonspecific for some markers, such as leukocyte common antigen and S-100 protein. A nuclear pattern of staining is characteristic for S-100 protein and the proliferation marker Ki-67 (figs. 3-4, 3-5). Thus, pathologists must be familiar with both the pattern of cell staining (figs. 3-1–3-6) and the pattern of reactivity with different cell types for the various leukocyte markers.

Many of the paraffin section–reactive markers summarized in Table 3-4 have a less specific staining profile than similar markers that are not paraffin section reactive (i.e., lineage associated rather than lineage restricted). For this reason it is especially important to apply several markers in a panel when approaching problems in differential diagnosis (Table 3-6). A panel approach increases the sensitivity and specificity of the study and helps detect patterns of nonspecific staining.

Markers Used on Fresh Cells or Frozen Tissues

Over 1000 different monoclonal antibodies to leukocyte antigens have been produced and many have been assigned to more than 100 cluster designations based on the recognition of a particular well-defined leukocyte antigen by more than one antibody (58). Table 3-5 groups the principal markers employed in the staining of fresh cells in suspension or fixed on slides as cell monolayers or in frozen tissue. Although this table emphasizes normal and neoplastic cell reactivity, additional information regarding the antigen and its function can be found in recent publications (59). If a particular differential diagnosis requires fresh cells or tissue, we generally prefer frozen section studies over cell suspension studies since

23

Table 3-5

**PRINCIPAL ANTIBODIES EMPLOYED IN STAINING
FRESH CELLS IN SUSPENSION OR IN CYTOSPINS AND FROZEN SECTIONS**

CD Antigen or Antibody	Predominant Normal Cell Reactivity	Reactivity in Neoplasms	Comment/Caution
LEUKOCYTES			
CD45 (2D1, L3B12, T29/33)	Hemato-lymphoid cells	Nearly all lymphomas and leukemias	Some plasma cell neoplasms unreactive, few precursor cell neoplasms unreactive, some anaplastic large cell lymphomas unreactive (22,154)
CD11A/18 (LFA-1α and β)	Hemato-lymphoid cells	Many lymphomas and leukemias	Many intermediate and high-grade B lineage lymphomas lack expression of the alpha and/or beta chain of LFA-1 (85,90)
B LYMPHOCYTES			
Immuno-globulins (Ig)	B cells (Ig staining of normal germ-inal center cells weak to absent)	Most B-cell lymphomas and leukemias, plasma cell neoplasms	Precursor B lymphomas and leukemias do not express Ig except for cytoplasmic mμ chains in pre-B tumors; some follicular and diffuse large cell lymphomas of B-lineage lack expression; monoclonal anti-Ig reagents less sensitive than polyclonal reagents; detection of cytoplasmic Ig often better in fixed and processed tissues; neoplasms show Ig light chain expression restricted to either kappa chains or lambda chains (50,70,133,141)
CD79 (mb-1/B29) (Ig associated)	B cells (B29 absent in plasma cells)	Most B lymphomas, B leukemias from pre-B-cell stage	Associated with antigen receptor (Ig) on B cells in a similar manner as CD3 on T cells, antibodies cross react with all mammalian species tested (78,82)
CD19 (B4, Leu-12)	B cells	Most B lymphomas, and leukemias, few myeloid leukemias	Earliest expressed B-cell differentiation antigen, most plasma cell neoplasms unreactive (87,91)
CD20 (B1, Leu-16, L26)	B cells	Most B lymphomas, B leukemias, Reed-Sternberg cells in some cases of classic Hodgkin's disease	Most plasma cell neoplasms unreactive, cytoplasmic reactivity may be seen in macrophages (92)
CD22 (Leu-14)	B cells	Most B lymphomas, most B leukemias	Expressed early in B-cell differentiation in the cytoplasm and arrives at the cell membrane at about the same time as Ig; may be undetectable on the surface in some chronic lymphocytic leukemias; most plasma cell neoplasms unreactive (81,129)
CD24 (BA1)	B cells	Most B lymphomas, most B leukemias	Most plasma cell neoplasms unreactive, granulocytes reactive, nonhematolymphoid neoplasms may be reactive (19)
CD37	B cells	Most B lymphomas, many B leukemias, some T lymphomas	Most plasma cell neoplasms unreactive, reactivity with subset of T-cell lymphomas may be useful in diagnosis (72)
B-LYMPHOCYTE SUBSETS			
CD10 (J5) (CALLA)	Precursor B cells, germinal center B cells	Many precursor B leukemias, some precursor T leukemias, many follicular lymphomas, subset of the other	May be useful in separating follicular from other low-grade B lymphomas; expressed by subset of myeloma; reactive with some non-hematolymatolymphoid neoplasms, e.g. Ewing's sarcoma and malignant fibrous histiocytoma (123,124)

Table 3-5 (continued)

PRINCIPAL ANTIBODIES EMPLOYED IN STAINING
FRESH CELLS IN SUSPENSION OR IN CYTOSPINS AND FROZEN SECTIONS

CD Antigen or Antibody	Predominant Normal Cell Reactivity	Reactivity in Neoplasms	Comment/Caution
B-LYMPHOCYTE SUBSETS (continued)			
CD21 (B2)	Mantle and marginal zone B cells, follicular dendritic cells	Most lymphomas of mantle and marginal zone B cells, follicular dendritic cell tumors	C3d (CR2) complement receptor, receptor for EBV (93,140)
CD23	Mantle zone B cells, subset of follicular dendritic cells	CLL/small lymphocytic lymphoma often reactive, mantle cell lymphomas often unreactive	Low affinity Fc receptor for IgE, upregulated by EBV infection (139)
CD32	Mantle zone B cells, many macrophages, plasma cells	Most lymphomas of mantle zone B cells, subset of follicular and other B lymphomas, myeloid leukemias, plasma cell neoplasms	Low affinity Fc receptor for IgG, reactivity with many follicular lymphomas may be useful in diagnosis (89,116,157)
CD35 (TO5)	Mantle and marginal zone B cells follicular dendritic cells, some macrophages	Most lymphomas of mantle and marginal zone B cells, follicular dendritic cell tumors	C3b (CR1) complement receptor (47)
CD38 (OKT10, Leu-17)	Lymphoid progenitor cells, NK cells, plasma cells	Some B and T lymphomas especially of progenitor cells, plasma cell neoplasms	One of few markers commonly expressed by plasma cell neoplasms (120,136)
T LYMPHOCYTES			
CD2 (OKT11, Leu-5)	T cells, NK cells	Most T lymphomas and leukemias, few myeloid leukemias	Sheep erythrocyte receptor (143)
CD3 (OKT3, Leu-4)	T cells	Most T lymphomas and leukemias	Associated with antigen receptor in a multimolecular complex, T-lymphoblastic lymphomas and leukemias more often show cytoplasmic rather than surface expression (61,73,119)
CD5 (OKT1, Leu-1)	T cells, weak expression by small B-cell subset	Most T lymphomas and leukemias, many diffuse small B-cell neoplasms	CD5 reactive B cells may be elevated in autoimmune disorders, expression of CD5 by many diffuse small B-cell neoplasms useful in diagnosis (26,41,121,144)
CD7 (3A1, Leu-9)	Most T cells, NK cells	Many T lymphomas and leukemias, some myeloid leukemias	Earliest expressed antigen in T-cell ontogeny and one of best T markers for lymphoblastic neoplasms; most commonly deleted antigen in post-thymic T-cell malignancy, particularly mycosis fungoides (53,71)
T-cell receptor beta chain (WT1, βF1)	T cells	Most T lymphomas and leukemias	Some T lymphomas, especially thymic ones, lack expression; few of the cases that lack expression show the alternative γδ receptor (94,107)
T-LYMPHOCYTE SUBSETS			
CD1A (NA134, OKT6, Leu-3)	Cortical thymocytes, Langerhans cells	Many thymic T lymphomas and leukemias, Langerhans' cell histiocytosis	Reliable marker for many precursor T-cell neoplasms; thymomas are rich in CD1A-positive thymocytes (83,120)

Table 3-5 (continued)

PRINCIPAL ANTIBODIES EMPLOYED IN STAINING
FRESH CELLS IN SUSPENSION OR IN CYTOSPINS AND FROZEN SECTIONS

CD Antigen or Antibody	Predominant Normal Cell Reactivity	Reactivity in Neoplasms	Comment/Caution
T-LYMPHOCYTE SUBSETS (continued)			
CD4 (OKT4, Leu-3)	Most helper/inducer T cells, class II MHC restricted T cells, many macrophages, many dendritic cells including follicular dendritic and Langerhans cells	Many post-thymic T lymphomas, often lacking or expressed together with CD8 on T-precursor neoplasms, many accessory cell neoplasms, some myeloid leukemias	HIV receptor, generally predominates in reactive and neoplastic disorders; may be one of myelomonocytic markers expressed in some plasma cell neoplasms (61,68,120,122,155)
CD8 (OKT8, Leu-2)	Most cytotoxic/suppresor T cells, class I MHC restricted, subset of NK cells, splenic sinus lining cells	Minority of post-thymic T lymphomas, often lacking or expressed together with CD4 on T-precursor neoplasms	Generally minority of T-subset neoplasms, but may predominate in early phase of some viral infections and in late phase of HIV infection (68,120)
T-cell receptor delta chain	Few T cells	Few T lymphomas and leukemias (predominantly thymic ones)	Reactive and neoplastic γ/δ T cells generally lack expression of both CD4 and CD8 (106)
MYELOMONOCYTIC CELLS			
CD11c (Leu-M5)	Myelomonocytic cells	Hairy cell leukemia, monocytoid B-cell lymphoma, few small B-cell lymphomas/leukemias, few T-cell lymphomas, some myeloid leukemias especially M4 and M5, Langerhans' cell histiocytosis	Sensitive but not totally specific marker for hairy cell leukemia or monocytoid B-cell lymphoma (74,129)
CD13 (My7)	Myelomonocytic cells, many macrophages, interdigitating dendritic cells	Most myeloid leukemias from M1-M5, few B-lymphoblastic leukemias, rare T-lymphoblastic leukemias	Some nonhematolymphoid cells (49)
CD14 (Mo2, Leu-M3)	Monocytes and macrophages, dendritic cells including follicular, interdigitating and Langerhans cells	Many M4 or M5 leukemias	My4 antibody but not others such as Leu-M3 reacts with some B-cell lymphomas and rare T-cell lymphomas (38,49)
CD33 (My9)	Early myeloid cells and all monocytes	Most myeloid leukemias	B and T lymphomas unreactive (48)
NATURAL KILLER CELLS			
CD16 (Leu-11)	NK cells, granulocytes	Many NK proliferative disorders	IgG Fc receptor III (96,105,131)
CD56 (Leu-19, NKH1)	NK cells, few T cells	Many NK proliferative disorders, many nasal non-B-lymphomas, plasma cell neoplasms	Reactivity with neoplastic but few reactive plasma cells may be useful for diagnosis; reacts with neural and neuroendocrine cells and their neoplasms (54,65,96,153)

Table 3-5 (continued)

PRINCIPAL ANTIBODIES EMPLOYED IN STAINING
FRESH CELLS IN SUSPENSION OR IN CYTOSPINS AND FROZEN SECTIONS

CD Antigen or Antibody	Predominant Normal Cell Reactivity	Reactivity in Neoplasms	Comment/Caution
		MISCELLANEOUS	
CD25 (TAC)	Activated T cells, B cells, and monocytes	Adult T-cell lymphoma/leukemia, hairy cell leukemia, most anaplastic large cell lymphomas, Reed-Sternberg cells in many cases of Hodgkin's disease, some other B and T lymphomas	Low affinity interleukin-2 receptor (69,132,150)
CD34 (HPCA1)	Progenitor cells, endothelial cells	Some myeloid leukemias, some lymphoblastic leukemias	Useful in identifying some difficult to classify hematolymphoid neoplasms; useful for diagnosis of vascular tumors (30)
Ki-67	Cells not in G0 phase of cell cycle (proliferating cells)	Cells not in G0 phase of cell cycle	General correlation with grade of lymphoma, most consistent correlation in lymphomas is between high proliferation fraction and adverse survival in low-grade B lymphoma, may be useful in diffentiating proliferating tumor cells from nonproliferating host cells (46,109,151)
TdT	Precursor cells in marrow, cortical thymocytes	Most lymphoblastic lymphomas and leukemias of a T or B lineage, some myeloid leukemias	Useful as marker of precursor cell lymphoma/leukemia (126)

architectural features are still evident and focal lesions may be appreciated. In addition, various cells differ in their susceptibility to destruction during the preparation of cell suspensions: lymphoid infiltrates in sclerotic stroma or fibrous extranodal sites have the potential for enrichment of certain populations and depletion of others, increasing the possibility of spurious interpretations. However, potential problems in cell suspension studies in which neoplastic cells are admixed with significant numbers of nonneoplastic cells can often be circumvented by gating on cell size or by dual labeling (152). For frozen section immunohistochemistry, a panel approach should be used (Table 3-6).

Differential Diagnosis with Panels of Markers

Just as patient history and the clinical differential diagnosis are important for the optimal handling of a fresh specimen, they are also critical, along with histologic findings, in formulating an approach to a diagnostic problem that includes lymphoma. Panels of antibodies, applied to either paraffin or frozen tissue sections, are used to assess the differential diagnosis of lymphomas (Table 3-6) (29,79,88,108,147). Our general approach is to construct panels in which at least one marker for each diagnostic possibility is expected to be positive if it is present and at least one marker is expected to be negative. Confidence in the reactivity of an appropriate marker is reinforced by lack of reactivity with one or more additional markers. Tissue section immunohistochemical studies are ideally suited for this approach since additional antibody stains are relatively easy to perform if an initial panel of markers does not help resolve a diagnostic problem. A panel approach is especially important in paraffin section studies since many of the paraffin-reactive leukocyte markers are either less sensitive or less specific than many of the markers available for studies on fresh cells or tissue. For example, the T-cell markers CD43 and CD45RO

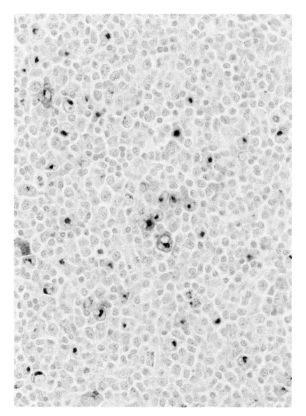

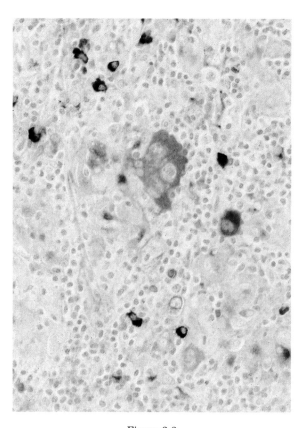

Figure 3-2
PARANUCLEAR/GOLGI STAINING PATTERN
Antibodies to CD15 (in this example Leu-M1 is used to stain a case of Hodgkin's disease) often label the paranuclear/Golgi region. Weak cytoplasmic staining is also seen in some of the Hodgkin cells as well as fine granular cytoplasmic staining in some histiocytes. (Immunoperoxidase with hematoxylin counterstain)

Figure 3-3
CYTOPLASMIC STAINING PATTERN
In this example of Hodgkin's disease, the neoplastic cells show cytoplasmic staining of variable intensity for lambda light chains. Plasma cells in the background infiltrate show intense cytoplasmic staining while histiocytes show weak staining. A similar pattern of staining is seen for kappa light chains. (Immunoperoxidase with hematoxylin counterstain)

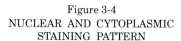

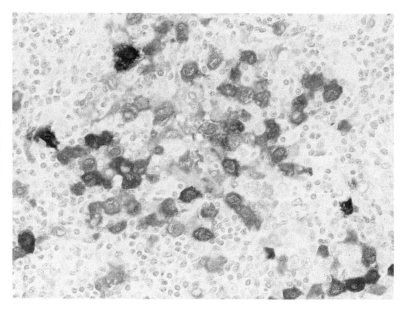

Figure 3-4
NUCLEAR AND CYTOPLASMIC
STAINING PATTERN
Nuclear staining, with or without cytoplasmic staining, is characteristic for S-100 protein. The neoplastic cells in this example of Langerhans' cell histiocytosis show intense labeling. (Immunoperoxidase with hematoxylin counterstain)

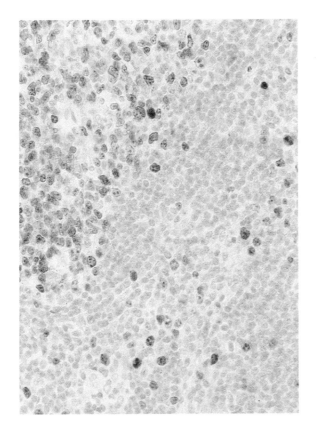

Figure 3-5
NUCLEAR STAINING PATTERN

The nuclei of proliferating cells are stained in the germinal center and paracortex of tonsil with antibody MIB-1 which is reactive with a fixation-resistant epitope of the Ki-67 molecule. This marker requires microwave pretreatment of paraffin sections. Also note the more intense labeling of nucleoli and chromocenters. (Immunoperoxidase with hematoxylin counterstain)

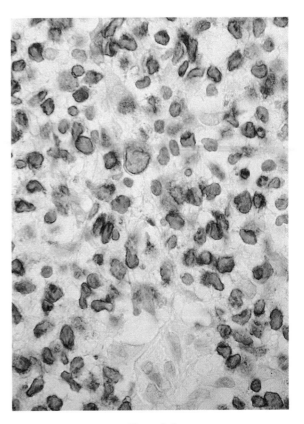

Figure 3-6
NUCLEAR MEMBRANE AND
CYTOPLASMIC STAINING PATTERN

The nuclear membrane and cytoplasm of some of these follicular lymphoma cells show intense labeling with an antibody to the *bcl*-2 protein which is overexpressed as a consequence of the t(14;18) translocation. (Immunoperoxidase with hematoxylin counterstain)

also stain histiocytes and granulocytes and their neoplasms. CD3 and beta-F1 are much more specific for T cells.

One of the most common diagnostic problems in paraffin section studies is differentiating non-Hodgkin's lymphoma, carcinoma, and melanoma (88). If the initial panel, including antibodies against leukocyte common antigen, low molecular weight keratin, and S-100 protein, is unreactive, then additional leukocyte, epithelial, or melanocytic markers may be applied. In the few unresolved cases, fresh tissue may be used for frozen section phenotypic or molecular studies. Alternatively, electron microscopy may be performed. In general, we do not perform molecular or ultrastructural studies at the outset since they typically examine smaller samples and are

more time-consuming and expensive than phenotypic studies.

We also use paraffin section staining in the differential diagnosis of non-Hodgkin's lymphoma and Hodgkin's disease since it facilitates the identification of the staining pattern of the atypical cells, particularly if they are infrequent, as compared to cell suspension studies (flow cytometry) (40,86). If the results with an initial panel of markers do not help resolve the diagnostic dilemma, additional lineage markers may be applied to paraffin sections or fresh tissue (29). Occasionally, T-cell lymphoma may have to be distinguished from Hodgkin's disease by molecular studies showing a major rearranged band (149). As with all diagnostic procedures, the number of special studies performed should be

Table 3-6

**EXAMPLES OF AN APPROACH TO THE DIFFERENTIAL DIAGNOSIS OF
LYMPHOMAS WITH PANELS OF ANTIBODIES APPLIED TO TISSUE SECTIONS***

Differential Diagnosis	Example of a Marker Panel	Comment
PARAFFIN		
Non-Hodgkin's lymphoma (NHL) vs carcinoma vs melanoma	CD45RB, keratin, S-100	If neoplasm is unreactive, additional panel of markers such as CD20, CD43, HMB-45, EMA, and CD30 may be useful; additional studies on fresh tissue may be required
NHL vs Hodgkin's disease (HD)	CD15, CD30, CD45RB, CD45RA, CD43	Atypical cells of classic HD will typically react with first two and not other markers; most NHL will stain for CD45RB and one or more lineage markers; some cases will require additional paraffin or occasionally frozen section markers
Nodular lymphocytic predominance (NLP) vs classic HD	CD15, CD30, CD45RB, CD45RA, EMA, CD57	Atypical cells of classic HD will typically react with first two and not other markers, while NLPHD will show opposite pattern; subset of T cells reactive with CD57 ring the atypical cells in NLP but not classic HD
Plasmacytoid neoplasms vs hyperplasia	Kappa chains, lambda chains	Because of potential technical and interpretive problems, additional phenotypic or sometimes genotypic studies on fresh tissue may be required
Follicular lymphoma vs follicular hyperplasia	Kappa chains, lambda chains, *bcl*-2	Monotypic staining pattern and/or *bcl*-2 staining in follicle centers supports lymphoma; additional phenotypic or sometimes genotypic studies on fresh tissue may be required
Small cell lymphoma vs hyperplasia	CD20, CD43, CD45RO, kappa, lambda	Many small cell (B) lymphomas show anomalous expression of CD43; some also show a monotypic Ig pattern
Plasma cell neoplasm vs lymphoma with plasmacytoid features	CD20, CD45RB, HLA-DR, kappa, lambda	Plasma cell neoplasms lack expression of first three markers
FROZEN		
B-cell (Ig+) lymphoma vs hyperplasia	kappa, lambda, mμ; CD19, CD20 or other pan-B; CD5, CD43	In most lymphomas the monotypic but interstitial Ig or Ig in macrophages (κ,λ,γ,α) may cause interpretive problems; inclusion of mμ and delta stains often helpful; "anomalous" expression of CD5 or CD43 in B-cell population also supports a diagnosis of lymphoma
Ig-negative B-lineage lymphoma vs hyperplasia	kappa, lambda, mμ; CD19, CD20 or other pan-B; CD5, CD32, CD43, Ki-67, *bcl*-2	Lack of Ig on FDC or *bcl*-2 and/or CD32 expression in follicular lesions supports lymphoma; Ig-negative B-lineage population outside follicles also supports a diagnosis of lymphoma
T-cell lymphoma vs hyperplasia	CD2, 3, 4, 5, 7, 8, 37; βF-1	Altered CD4/CD8 ratio not generally helpful in diagnosis; lack of expression or co-expression of both subset antigens may be observed in 10-20 percent of post-thymic T lymphomas; lack of expression of one or more pan-T antigens is observed in up to 80 percent of post-thymic T lymphomas; 10–20 percent of post-thymic T lymphomas may show anomalous expression of pan-B marker CD37
T-lymphoblastic vs post-thymic T-cell lymphoma	CD1, 2, 3, 4, 5, 7, 8; βF-1; TdT	Most T lymphoblastic lymphomas express multiple pan-T markers and show expression of CD1 and/or CD4+CD8+/CD4-CD8- phenotypes; nearly all lymphoblastic lymphomas show nuclear staining for TdT

*The panels listed above are not the exact panels that we use in our practice but are based on our own experience as well as that published in the literature. In addition, only some of the most common differential diagnostic problems are presented.

tailored to the importance of the clinical distinction. For example, an aggressive diagnostic approach with time-consuming and expensive ancillary studies might be inappropriate when the patient is elderly, or has other serious medical problems, a poor performance status, or limited treatment options.

The identification of a markedly predominant kappa-expressing or lambda-expressing B-lineage population (90 percent or greater predominance of one light chain over the other) provides strong support for malignancy (70). Plasmacytoid or plasma cell neoplasms often stain more reliably in fixed paraffin-embedded sections (fig. 16-5) than in acetone-fixed frozen sections. In contrast, many other B-lineage neoplasms, particularly if they express surface but only little cytoplasmic immunoglobulin, may not react for light chains after fixation and processing (an exception is illustrated in figs. 7-16, 7-17). In some cases, light chain monotypia of a plasmacytoid subpopulation indicates the neoplastic nature of a largely unstained predominant B-lineage population. Fortunately, additional markers to suggest malignancy can be applied to paraffin sections, such as *bcl*-2 for follicular B-cell proliferations (fig. 3-6) (45,66) and CD43 for diffuse B-cell proliferations. CD43 is anomalously expressed in most small B-cell lymphomas (see figs. 7-18–7-20) and leukemias, Burkitt's lymphomas, and many intermediate and other high-grade B-cell lymphomas (98,127). Anomalous CD43 expression is rarely, if ever, seen in reactive B-cell populations. Plasma cell neoplasms may only react with anti-light chain antibodies and frequently lack reactivity for leukocyte common antigen (LCA) and B-lineage markers.

While the alteration or loss of immunoglobulin may complicate the identification of a monotypic B-cell population in paraffin sections, the same is true of too much immunoglobulin in the form of interstitial immunoglobulin or immunoglobulin within macrophages in frozen sections (108). Fortunately, mμ and delta are the most frequently expressed heavy chains in lymphomas and are less prevalent in serum than other heavy and light chains (51,133). In addition, there are a number of phenotypic criteria for the diagnosis of B-lineage lymphomas other than light chain restriction (see Table 3-6) (108).

With the exception of a limited number of antibodies to particular T-cell receptor beta-chain V regions, which can be used to identify clonal populations of T cells in fresh tissues (31,113), no equivalent to B-cell light chain monotypia exists for T cells. Nevertheless, lack of expression or markedly diminished expression of one or more pan-T antigens may be observed in frozen sections in 80 percent of post-thymic T-cell lymphomas (52,108). In addition, a subset of cases of post-thymic T-cell lymphoma may lack expression of both T-subset antigens (CD4 and CD8), show anomalous coexpression of both subset antigens, or show anomalous expression of a pan-B marker such as CD37 (108). Most T-lymphoblastic lymphomas that may be confused with other undifferentiated neoplasms of childhood or occasionally with post-thymic T-cell lymphomas have a distinctive immunophenotype (148). TdT is an excellent marker for lymphoblastic disease if a myelomonocytic process is not in the differential. Molecular studies using probes to antigen receptor genes are especially useful for differentiating T-cell lymphoma from hyperplasia (35,84).

ANTIGEN RECEPTOR GENES AND ANALYSIS OF THEIR REARRANGEMENTS

Theoretical Background

The use of antigen receptor gene rearrangements as diagnostic markers is based on the fact that these genes undergo a series of programmed deletions during the course of normal lymphoid cell development (fig. 3-7). These rearrangements cause the shuffling of various gene segments whose combinations account for the antigen specificity of their fully assembled protein products: the immunoglobulin or T-cell receptor molecules. With few exceptions, the configuration of fully assembled receptor genes is fixed and stable in a given lymphocyte and its progeny. Non-neoplastic lymphoid tissues consist of mixed populations of lymphocytes, each with its own characteristic pattern of rearranged receptor genes, and not sufficiently abundant to be detected using currently employed molecular techniques. Detectable gene rearrangements appear only when an individual lymphocyte clonally expands to more than a few percent of the total population, a process invariably associated with neoplastic growth (see below for discussion of clonality versus malignancy).

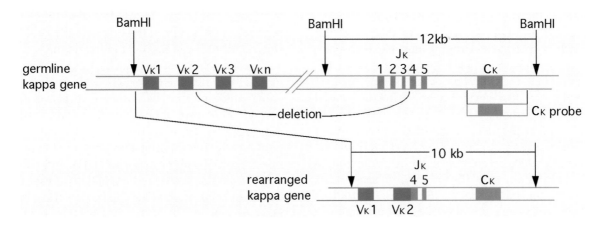

Figure 3-7

SCHEMATIC REPRESENTATION OF IMMUNOGLOBULIN GENE REARRANGEMENT

The germline configuration of the kappa light chain gene (upper line) consists of numerous variable gene segments (V-kappa, 1-n), five joining gene segments (J-kappa, 1-5), and a single constant region gene segment (C-kappa). To assemble a functional light chain gene (lower line), select V and J segments are juxtaposed with each other by deletion of the intervening DNA. The deletion reconfigures restriction enzyme cutting sites upstream of J-kappa, changing the size of the BamH1 fragment detected with a C-kappa hybridization probe (12 kb germline versus 10 kb rearranged in figure).

Technical Aspects

Most analyses of clonality are currently performed using the Southern blot procedure, the technical aspects of which have been described elsewhere (162,165). This technique involves enzymatic treatment and hybridization analysis of DNA isolated from lesional tissues. Generally, 1 to 3 weeks are required to perform the procedure. Two separate enzyme digestions for analyses of the immunoglobulin heavy chain (BamH1 and EcoR1) and beta-T-cell receptor (BamH1 and BglII) genes are always performed to minimize problems with spurious bands. Single enzyme digestions are adequate for immunoglobulin light chain gene analysis. In most laboratories, a lymphoid clone needs to constitute at least 5 percent of the total cell population to result in a detectable rearrangement.

As a general rule, molecular tests require fresh or frozen tissues that have not been subjected to fixation. Most fixatives alter cellular DNA rendering it unsuitable for subsequent enzymatic procedures. Exceptions to this rule are polymerase chain reaction (PCR)–based tests which require small fragments of DNA that may remain following fixation. However, it is best to check with the individual laboratory when contemplating PCR since many are not prepared to analyze fixed specimens. Snap-frozen tissues, with or without O.C.T. compound, are suitable for molecular studies that

are not affected by freeze artifacts. Fresh tissues may be refrigerated for up to 24 hours prior to analysis. For Southern blot analyses, a minimum of 32 mm³ of tissue or at least 10 million cells are required. PCR procedures require substantially less tissue.

DNA probes used in various gene rearrangement analyses for the identification of clonal lymphoid populations are listed in Table 3-7 and have been described in detail elsewhere (158). Only rearrangements detected with the immunoglobulin light chain probes are lineage specific since these are rarely if ever observed in non-B cells. Rearrangements of immunoglobulin heavy chain and T-cell receptor beta-chain genes are useful clonal markers in spite of their lineage infidelity. Other receptor gene probes are not useful diagnostically since the V gene repertoires are too limited and rearrangements are frequently detected in non-neoplastic tissues.

PCR analysis of gene rearrangements is based on the use of primers homologous to highly conserved sequences in the immunoglobulin and T-cell receptor genes that flank the sites where various gene segments are joined to each other (fig. 3-8). PCR may be associated with a higher false negative rate since not all gene segments have conserved sequences recognized by these generic amplification primers. This rate may be

Table 3-7

MOLECULAR PROBES USED IN THE IDENTIFICATION OF CLONAL POPULATIONS OF B AND T LYMPHOCYTES AND POPULATIONS HARBORING CHROMOSOMAL TRANSLOCATIONS

Gene Probes	Southern Blotting	PCR	Comments
Ig GENE PROBES			
Ig heavy chain	+	+	All B lineage and occasional T lineage
Ig kappa	+		High specificity for B lineage
Ig lambda	+		High specificity for B lineage
TCR GENE PROBES			
Beta	+	+	All T lineage and occasional B lineage
Gamma	+	+	Not diagnostically useful due to restricted V gene repertoires
Delta	+		
TRANSLOCATION PROBES			
t(14;18)	+	+	Two 18q21 cluster regions containing most but not all breakpoints
t(11;14)	+		Widely scattered 11q13 breakpoints with moderate clustering
t(3;v)(q27;v)	+		Clustered within or near BCL-6/LAZ-3 gene
t(2;5)(p23;q35)	+	+	NPM-ALK fusion gene and transcript

v = variable sites.

reduced by using mixtures of more than one set of primers. PCR has the advantage of requiring less time to perform but does not offer a significant increase in sensitivity since the signal-to-noise ratio is limited by the background of nonclonally rearranged genes, which are also amplified by the generic primers.

Applications

Gene rearrangement analysis is most frequently used to provide objective evidence for the clonality of a lymphoid proliferation. Monoclonality is diagnostic of neoplasia although not necessarily synonymous with malignancy, as a variety of indolent disorders, particularly those involving extranodal sites such as skin, can contain monoclonal lymphoid cells (165). In spite of this caveat, gene rearrangement analysis often provides critical support for a diagnosis of malignancy, particularly in T-cell lymphomas, since no reliable phenotypic marker of T-cell clonality is yet available. As detailed elsewhere, gene rearrangement is best employed as a diagnostic modality only if an unequivocal diagnosis cannot be

attained with more conventional techniques (159). This approach is cost-effective and provides maximal sensitivity and specificity. The usual profiles of antigen receptor gene configurations in various lymphoproliferative lesions are shown in Table 3-8.

Gene rearrangements can be used as lineage markers, taking into consideration limitations in the specificity of certain probes (Table 3-7). They may also serve as markers for longitudinal assessment of residual disease status, although Southern blot techniques are not sensitive enough to warrant this approach in most cases. PCR has the promise of a highly sensitive method for longitudinal assessment of patients with malignant lymphoma although it has not yet been widely applied or tested.

Interpretation

In spite of the objective nature of most molecular tests, i.e., the presence or absence of a band, their interpretation may not be straightforward. Commonly encountered gene rearrangement patterns and their probable interpretations are

A. Antigen receptor gene rearrangement   B. Translocation breakpoint cluster

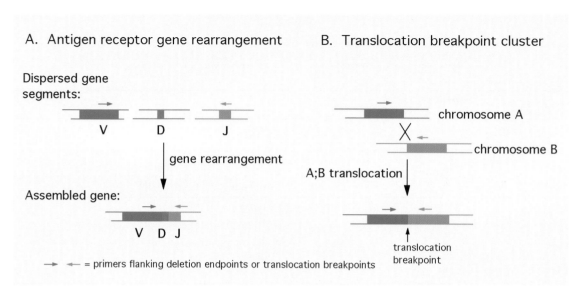

Figure 3-8
DIAGNOSTIC APPLICATIONS OF POLYMERASE CHAIN REACTION

The experimental rationale for PCR detection of rearranged antigen receptor genes (left) is based on the use of generic primers homologous to conserved DNA sequences present in variable (V) and joining (J) gene segments. These primers result in the amplification of sequences spanning the V-D-J junction, which varies in size and sequence composition among fully assembled receptor genes in different lymphocytes. Detection of translocation breakpoint junctions (right) employs a pair of primers homologous to DNA sequences that flank the breakpoint cluster sites on different chromosomes. Amplification products are only produced in cells carrying the appropriate translocation that juxtaposes the two sequences recognized by the primers. Similar strategies may be employed for detection of chromosomal deletions, e.g., those that activate the TAL/SCL gene in lymphoblastic lymphoma (see chapter 11).

summarized in Table 3-9. The most important consideration is to avoid the erroneous conclusion that a clone is present when in fact it is not since this would lead to an inappropriate diagnosis of malignancy. A number of technical artifacts and sources of false positive results have been described by others (160,161,163,164) and will not be detailed here. Frequent causes of false positive results include incomplete digestion of DNA resulting in so-called partial digestion products and individual variation in positions of germline bands, i.e., polymorphisms. False negative results occur if sampling is inadequate or if the clone is present below the threshold of detection for the technique as performed by the individual laboratory. In general, DNA rearrangement analyses should be performed by a laboratory that is skilled in these techniques and the findings should be interpreted by an experienced molecular pathologist. Molecular results should always be interpreted in the context of other pathologic and clinical information. We are very reluctant to reach a diagnosis of malignancy on the basis of molecular findings alone.

COMMON CHROMOSOMAL ABNORMALITIES

A number of consistent chromosomal translocations occur with certain types of malignant lymphomas (Table 3-10). Each translocation is associated with one, or a few, select morphologic subtypes of lymphoma but generally is not entirely specific for those subtypes, as discussed in detail in the following chapters. Since cytogenetic aberrations are, in general, confined to neoplastic cells, they constitute useful markers for lymphoma cells. Most chromosomal translocations in lymphomas result from errors in the rearrangement of antigen receptor genes in progenitor B or T lymphocytes. Molecular studies show that these types of translocations result in deregulated expression of cellular oncogenes following their juxtaposition with antigen receptor genes (fig. 3-9) (167–169). Probes for some of these oncogenes (most notably *bcl*-2, *myc*, and *bcl*-1) or their flanking chromosomal DNA may be used for molecular cytogenetic studies. For example, rearrangement of the *bcl*-2 gene is the molecular hallmark of the

Table 3-8

USUAL ANTIGEN RECEPTOR GENE STATUS IN VARIOUS LYMPHOPROLIFERATIVE LESIONS

Abnormality	IgH	Igκ	Igλ	TCRβ	TCRγ	TCRδ
Normal lymphoid tissue	G	G	G	G	Rp	Rp
Reactive lymphoid tissue	G	G	G	G	Rp	Rp
Lymphoid hyperplasia in a setting of immunodeficiency	G/R	Rp	G	G	Rp	Rp
B-cell lymphoma	R	R	G/R	G/R	G/Rp	G/Rp
T-cell lymphoma	G/R	G	G	R	R	R
Hodgkin's disease, classic type	G/R	G	G	G	Rp	Rp
Hodgkin's disease, nodular lymphocyte predominance	G	G	G	G	Rp	Rp

G = germline band; R = rearranged band; Rp = polyclonal rearranged bands.
Some T-cell lymphomas may lack detectable TCR gene rearrangements. AILD-like T-cell lymphomas show a fairly high frequency of simultaneous IgH gene rearrangements (30 to 40 percent).

Table 3-9

COMMONLY ENCOUNTERED GENE REARRANGEMENT PATTERNS AND THEIR INTERPRETATION

Antigen Receptor Gene Status					
IgH	Igκ	Igλ	TCRβ	TCRγ	Most Probable Interpretation
R	R	G	G	G	B-cell neoplasm
R	R	R	G	G	B-cell neoplasm
G	G	G	R	R	T-cell neoplasm
R	G	G	R	R	T-cell neoplasm
G	G	G	G	G	No molecular support for lymphoma

R = rearranged band; G = germline band.

t(14;18) chromosomal translocation and its detection using Southern blot techniques is technically less cumbersome in many cases than conventional cytogenetic analysis of lymph nodes involved by follicular lymphoma (173).

Translocation breakpoints that are clustered in their genomic distribution may be detected using PCR techniques (fig. 3-8), an approach with great advantages in sensitivity and specificity, particularly for longitudinal assessment of residual disease status (170,172). Application of PCR to detect translocation breakpoint DNA junctions has led to the surprising observation that at least one translocation, the t(14;18), can be detected at extremely low levels in reactive lymphoid tissues from normal individuals, most of whom will presumably not develop lymphoma (166,171). In view of this finding, PCR is not a specific screening test for lymphoma and perhaps may even be limited in its use for longitudinal assessment of minimal residual disease status in patients with t(14;18)-carrying lymphomas. It is currently not clear whether t(14;18) is exceptional with regard to its prevalence in the general population. However, these findings underscore the cautious approach that should be pursued in the application and interpretation of current and yet to be developed molecular diagnostic tests.

Table 3-10

RECURRENT CHROMOSOMAL ABNORMALITIES IN LYMPHOMAS

Chromosomal Abnormality	Most Frequent Types of Lymphoma	Antigen Receptor Gene	Oncogene
t(8;14)(q24;q32)	Small noncleaved cell lymphoma	IgH	c-*myc*
t(2;8)(2p12;q24)	(Burkitt's and non-Burkitt's), some	Igκ	c-*myc*
t(8;22)(q24;q11)	diffuse large cell lymphomas (B-cell type)	Igλ	c-*myc*
t(14;18)(q32;q21)	Follicular lymphoma, subset of large B-cell lymphomas	IgH	*bcl*-2
t(11;14)(q13;q32)	Mantle cell lymphoma	IgH	*bcl*-1 (PRAD 1)
t(3;v)(q27;v)*	Large cell lymphoma	IgH, Igκ, Igλ, others	*bcl*-6 (LAZ 3)
t(14;v)(q11;v)	Lymphoblastic lymphoma, adult T-cell leukemia/lymphoma	TCRα/TCRδ	Several (see Table 11-1)
t(14;v)(q32;v)	Occasional small lymphocytic lymphoma, diffuse large cell lymphoma, others	IgH	*bcl*-3, unknown
t(7;v)(q35;v)	Lymphoblastic lymphoma (T-cell type)	TCRβ	Several (see Table 11-1)
t(2;5)(p23;q35)	Anaplastic large cell lymphoma, others	NA**	NPM-ALK fusion gene

*Variable.
**NA = not applicable.

ELECTRON MICROSCOPY

In the past, electron microscopy was very helpful in distinguishing undifferentiated carcinoma or malignant melanoma from large cell lymphoma, and lymphoblastic lymphoma from other small round cell malignancies of childhood. Electron microscopy has largely been supplanted by immunologic studies in most institutions because of lower cost and relative ease of performance. Nevertheless, an occasional diagnostic problem still may benefit from electron microscopy; thus, we recommend fixing 1-mm cubes of fresh biopsy tissue in glutaraldehyde. Ultrastructural studies may also be performed on fixed tissue obtained from paraffin blocks although such fixation is usually suboptimal, particularly if a metal fixative was used. A method for processing fresh frozen tissue for electron microscopy has also been described (174). The presence of junctions of any type between neoplastic cells (with exceptions) militates against a diagnosis of lymphoma. However, the identification of such junctional attachments may be helpful in supporting the rare diagnosis of a follicular dendritic cell neoplasm. Moreover, the identification of cytoplasmic organelles, such as melanosomes or neurosecretory granules, may help support other specific diagnoses.

ASPIRATION CYTOLOGY

Fine needle aspiration is increasingly used in surgical pathology, and there is frequent pressure on pathologists to provide both initial and follow-up diagnoses based on aspirate specimens from lymph nodes. It is beyond the scope of this brief section to address the role of fine needle aspiration in the diagnosis and classification of hematolymphoid neoplasms (175). We believe that aspiration cytology should be used for the initial diagnosis only in restricted circumstances: if the patient is a poor candidate for surgical biopsy and the high morbidity or mortality of the procedure offsets any uncertainty in the diagnosis or classification of lymphoma, or if the cytologic findings, particularly when combined with special studies, are essential for the rapid diagnosis of some lymphomas, such as lymphoblastic or small noncleaved cell, which may present as medical emergencies. However, since a definitive diagnosis of many lymphomas depends on both architectural as well as cytologic features, it is important to request sufficient tissue for ancillary studies that may be required for diagnosis and classification. Aspiration cytology may play a prominent role in the staging and follow-up of patients with well-documented malignant lymphoma and may include selected phenotypic or genotypic studies useful in the management of such patients.

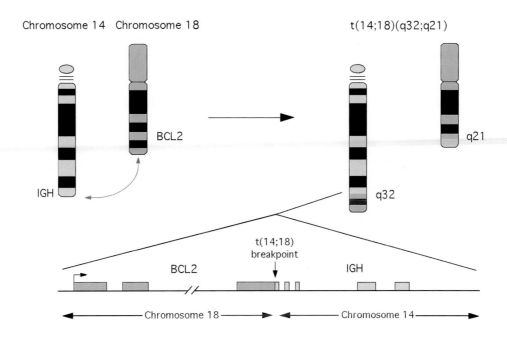

Chromosome 14   Chromosome 18

t(14;18)(q32;q21)

Figure 3-9
SCHEMATIC ILLUSTRATION OF CHROMOSOMAL TRANSLOCATION
The t(14;18) chromosomal translocation is a model for several translocations in lymphomas that result in juxtaposition of a cellular proto-oncogene with immunoglobulin or T-cell receptor genes. The *bcl*-2 gene on chromosome 18 is translocated to chromosome 14 directly adjacent to the immunoglobulin heavy chain gene.

REFERENCES

Handling the Fresh Specimen

1. Bahler DW, Berry G, Oksenberg J, Warnke RA, Levy R. Diversity of T-cell antigen receptor variable genes used by mycosis fungoides cells. Am J Pathol 1992;140:1–8.
2. _____, Campbell MJ, Hart S, Miller RA, Levy S, Levy R. Ig VH gene expression among human follicular lymphomas. Blood 1991;78:1561–8.
3. Campbell MJ, Zelenetz AD, Levy S, Levy R. Use of family specific leader region primers for PCR amplification of the human heavy chain variable region gene repertoire. Mol Immunol 1992;29:193–203.
4. Deane M, McCarthy KP, Wiedemann LM, Norton JD. An improved method for detection of B-lymphoid clonality by polymerase chain reaction. Leukemia 1991;5:726–30.
5. Mason DY, Biberfeld P. Technical aspects of lymphoma immunohistology. J Histochem Cytochem 1980;28:731–45.
6. Rouse RV, Warnke RA. Special application of tissue section immunologic staining in the characterization of monoclonal antibodies and in the study of normal and neoplastic tissues. In: Weir DM, Herzenberg LA, Blackwell CC, Herzenberg LA, eds. Handbook of experimental immunology. 4th ed. Edinburgh: Blackwell, 1986:116.1–116.10.
7. Sheibani K. Immunohistochemical analysis of lymphoid tissue. In: Knowles DM, ed. Neoplastic hematopathology. Baltimore: Williams & Wilkins, 1992:197–213.
8. Shi SR, Key ME, Kalra KL. Antigen retrieval in formalin-fixed, paraffin-embedded tissues: an enhancement method for immunohistochemical staining based on microwave oven heating of tissue sections. J Histochem Cytochem 1991;39:741–8.
9. Weiss LM, Dorfman RF, Warnke RA. Lymph node work-up. In: Fenoglio-Preiser C, ed. Advances in pathology, Vol. 1. Chicago: Year Book Medical Publishers, 1988:111–30.

Fixation and Processing and Pattern Recognition

10. Banks PM. Technical factors in the preparation and evaluation of lymph node biopsies. In: Knowles DM, ed. Neoplastic hematopathology. Baltimore: Williams & Wilkins, 1992:367–84.
11. Beard C, Nabers K, Bowling MC, Berard CW. Achieving technical excellence in lymph node specimens: an update. Lab Med 1985;16:468–75.
12. Beckstead JH. Optimal antigen localization in human tissues using aldehyde-fixed plastic-embedded sections. J Histochem Cytochem 1985;33:954–8.
13. Bowling MC. Lymph node specimens: achieving technical excellence. Lab Med 1979;10:467–76.
14. Casey TT, Olson SJ, Cousar JB, Collins RD. Plastic section immunohistochemistry in the diagnosis of hematopoietic and lymphoid neoplasms. Clin Lab Med 1990;10:199–213.

15. Delsol G, Chittal S, Brousset P, et al. Immunohisto-chemical demonstration of leucocyte differentiation antigens on paraffin sections using a modified AMeX (ModAMeX) method. Histopathology 1989;15:461–71.

16. Dorfman RF, Warnke R. Lymphadenopathy simulating the malignant lymphomas. Hum Pathol 1974;5:519–50.

17. Larsson LI. Tissue preparation methods for light microscopic immunohistochemistry. Appl Immunohisto-chem 1993;1:2–16.

18. Sato Y, Mukai K, Watanabe S, Goto M, Shimosato Y. The AMeX method. A simplified technique of tissue processing and paraffin embedding with improved preservation of antigens for immunostaining. Am J Pathol 1986;125:431–5.

Immunohistochemical Studies

19. Abramson CS, Kersey JH, LeBien TW. A monoclonal antibody (BA–1) reactive with cells of human B lymphocyte lineage. J Immunol 1981;126:83–8.

20. Arber D, Weiss L. CD15: a review. Appl Immuno-histochem 1993;1:17–30.

21. _____, Weiss L. CD43: a review. Appl Immuno-histochem 1993;1:88–96.

22. Battifora H, Trowbridge IS. A monoclonal antibody useful for the differential diagnosis between malignant lymphoma and nonhematopoietic neoplasms. Cancer 1983;51:816–21.

23. Berti E, Aversa GG, Soligo D, et al. A6—a new 45RO monoclonal antibody for immunostaining of paraffin-embedded tissues. Am J Clin Pathol 1991;95:188–93.

24. Brandtzaeg P. The new monoclonal antibody (Mac 387) that reacts with macrophages on paraffin sections detects the well-known leukocyte L1 antigen [Letter]. J Histochem Cytochem 1988;36:1203–6.

25. _____, Jones DB, Flavell DJ, Fagerhol MK. Mac 387 antibody and detection of formalin resistant myelomonocytic L1 antigen. J Clin Pathol 1988;41:963–70.

26. Burns BF, Warnke RA, Doggett RS, Rouse RV. Expression of a T-cell antigen (Leu-1) by B-cell lymphomas. Am J Pathol 1983;113:165–71.

27. Cartun RW, Coles FB, Pastuszak WT. Utilization of monoclonal antibody L26 in the identification and confirmation of B-cell lymphomas. A sensitive and specific marker applicable to formalin-and B5-fixed, paraffin-embedded tissues. Am J Pathol 1987;129:415–21.

28. Cattoretti G, Pileri S, Parravicini C, et al. Antigen unmasking on formalin-fixed, paraffin-embedded tissue sections. J Pathol 1993;171:83–98.

29. Chittal SM, Caveriviere P, Schwarting R, et al. Monoclonal antibodies in the diagnosis of Hodgkin's disease. The search for a rational panel. Am J Surg Pathol 1988;12:9–21.

30. Civin CI, Strauss LC, Brovall C, Fackler MJ, Schwartz JF, Shaper JH. Antigenic analysis of hematopoiesis III. A hematopoietic progenitor cell surface antigen defined by a monoclonal antibody raised against KG-Ia cells. J Immunol 1984;133:157–65.

31. Clark DM, Boylston AW, Hall PA, Carrel S. Antibodies to T cell antigen receptor beta chain families detect monoclonal T cell proliferation. Lancet 1986;2:835–7.

32. Cordell J, Richardson TC, Pulford KA, et al. Production of monoclonal antibodies against human epithelial membrane antigen for use in diagnostic immunocyto-chemistry. Br J Cancer 1985;52:347–54.

33. Davey FR, Cordell JL, Erber WN, Pulford KA, Gatter KC, Mason DY. Monoclonal antibody (Y1/82A) with specificity towards peripheral blood monocytes and tissue macrophages. J Clin Pathol 1988;41:753–8.

34. _____, Gatter KC, Ralfkiaer E, Pulford KA, Krissansen GW, Mason DY. Immunophenotyping of non-Hodgkin's lymphomas using a panel of antibodies on paraffin-embedded tissues. Am J Pathol 1987;129:54–63.

35. Davis RE, Warnke RA, Dorfman RF, Cleary ML. Utility of molecular genetic analysis for the diagnosis of neoplasia in morphologically and immunophenotypically equivocal hematolymphoid lesions. Cancer 1991;67:2890–9.

36. Delsol G, Al ST, Gatter KC, et al. Coexpression of epithelial membrane antigen (EMA), Ki-1, and interleukin-2 receptor by anaplastic large cell lymphomas. Diagnostic value in so-called malignant histiocytosis. Am J Pathol 1988;130:59–70.

37. _____, Brousset P, Chittal S, Rigal HF. Correlation of the expression of Epstein-Barr virus latent membrane protein and in situ hybridization with biotinylated BamHI-W probes in Hodgkin's disease. Am J Pathol 1992;140:247–53.

38. Dimitriu-Bono A, Burmester GR, Waters SJ, Winchester RJ. Human mononuclear phagocyte differentiation antigens. I. Patterns of antigenic expression on the surface of human monocytes and macrophages defined by monoclonal antibodies. J Immunol 1983;130:145–52.

39. Dobson CM, Myskow MW, Krajewski AS, Carpenter FH, Horne CH. Immunohistochemical staining of non-Hodgkin's lymphoma in paraffin sections using the MB1 and MT1 monoclonal antibodies. J Pathol 1987;153:203–12.

40. Dorfman RF, Gatter KC, Pulford KA, Mason DY. An evaluation of the utility of anti-granulocyte and anti-leukocyte monoclonal antibodies in the diagnosis of Hodgkin's disease. Am J Pathol 1986;123:508–19.

41. Engleman EG, Warnke R, Fox RI, Dilley J, Benike CJ, Levy R. Studies of a human T-lymphocyte antigen recognized by a monoclonal antibody. Proc Natl Acad Sci USA 1981;78:1791–5.

42. Falini B, Pileri S, Stein H, et al. Variable expression of leucocyte-common (CD45) antigen in CD30 (Ki1)-positive anaplastic large-cell lymphoma: implications for the differential diagnosis between lymphoid and non-lymphoid malignancies. Hum Pathol 1990;21:624–9.

43. Flavell DJ, Jones DB, Wright DH. Identification of tissue histiocytes on paraffin sections by a new monoclonal antibody. J Histochem Cytochem 1987;35:1217–26.

44. Gatter KC, Cordell JL, Falini B, et al. Monoclonal antibodies in diagnostic pathology: techniques and applications. J Biol Response Mod 1983;2:369–95.

45. Gaulard P, d'Agay MF, Peuchmaur M, et al. Expression of the bcl-2 gene product in follicular lymphoma. Am J Pathol 1992;140:1089–95.

46. Gerdes J. Ki-67 and other proliferation markers useful for immunohistological diagnostic and prognostic evaluations in human malignancies. Semin Cancer Biol 1990;1:199–206.

47. _____, Naiem M, Mason DY, Stein H. Human complement (C3b) receptors defined by a mouse monoclonal antibody. Immunology 1982;45:645–53.

48. Griffin JD, Linch D, Sabbath K, Larcom P, Schlossman SF. A monoclonal antibody reactive with normal and leukemic human myeloid progenitor cells. Leuk Res 1984;8:521–34.

49. _____, Ritz J, Nadler LM, Schlossman SF. Expression of myeloid differentiation antigens on normal and malignant myeloid cells. J Clin Invest 1981;68:932–41.

50. Grogan TM, Spier CM, Richter LC, Rangel CS. Immunologic approaches to the classification of non-Hodgkin's lymphomas. In: Bennett JM, Foon KA, eds. Immunologic approaches to the classification and management of lymphomas and leukemias. Boston: Kluwer Academic, 1988:31–148.

51. Hancock WH, Atkins RC. Immunohistological studies with monoclonal antibodies. In: Langone JJ, Van Vunakis H, eds. Methods in enzymology, Vol. 121. Orlando: Academic Press, 1986:828–48.

52. Hastrup N, Ralfkiaer E, Pallesen G. Aberrant phenotypes in peripheral T cell lymphomas. J Clin Pathol 1989;42:398–402.

53. Haynes B, Eisenbarth G, Fauci A. Human lymphocyte antigens: production of a monoclonal antibody that defines functional thymus-derived lymphocyte subsets. Proc Natl Acad Sci USA 1979;76:5829–33.

54. Hercend T, Griffin JD, Bensussan A, et al. Generation of monoclonal antibodies to a human natural killer clone. Characterization of two natural killer-associated antigens, NKH1A and NKH2, expressed on subsets of large granular lymphocytes. J Clin Invest 1985;75:932–43.

55. Hsu SM, Jaffe ES. Leu M1 and peanut agglutinin stain the neoplastic cells of Hodgkin's disease. Am J Clin Pathol 1984;82:29–32.

56. Jensen GS, Poppema S, Mant MJ, Pilarski LM. Transition in CD45 isoform expression during differentiation of normal and abnormal B cells. Int Immunol 1989;1:229–36.

57. Kamel OW, Gelb AB, Shibuya RB, Warnke RA. Leu7 (CD57) reactivity distinguishes nodular lymphocyte predominance Hodgkin's disease from nodular sclerosing Hodgkin's disease, T cell rich B cell lymphoma and follicular lymphoma. Am J Pathol 1993;142:541–6.

58. Knapp W, ed. Leukocyte typing IV: white cell differentiation antigens. Fourth International Workshop and Conference on Human Leukocyte Differentiation Antigens, Vienna, 21-25 February 1989. New York: Oxford University Press, 1989.

59. Knowles DM, Chadburn A, Inghirami G. Immunophenotypic markers useful in the diagnosis and classification of hematopoietic neoplasms. In: Knowles DM, ed. Neoplastic hematopathology. Baltimore: Williams & Wilkins, 1992:73–167.

60. Kondo E, Nakamura S, Onoue H, et al. Detection of bcl-2 protein and bcl-2 messenger RNA in normal and neoplastic lymphoid tissues by immunohistochemistry and in situ hybridization. Blood 1992;80:2044–51.

61. Kung PC, Goldstein G, Reinherz EL, Schlossman SF. Monoclonal antibodies defining distinctive human T-cell surface antigens. Science 1979;206:347–9.

62. Kurec AS, Cruz VE, Barrett D, Mason DY, Davey FR. Immunophenotyping of acute leukemias using paraffin-embedded tissue sections. Am J Clin Pathol 1990;93:502–9.

63. Kurtin PJ, Pinkus GS. Leukocyte common antigen—a diagnostic discriminant between hematopoietic and nonhematopoietic neoplasms in paraffin sections using

64. Lai R, Visser L, Poppema S. Tissue distribution of restricted leukocyte common antigens. A comprehensive study with protein- and carbohydrate-specific CD45R antibodies. Lab Invest 1991;64:844–54.

65. Lanier LL, Le AM, Civin CI, Loken MR, Phillips JH. The relationship of CD16 (Leu-11) and Leu-19 (NKH-1) antigen expression on human peripheral blood NK cells and cytotoxic T lymphocytes. J Immunol 1986;136:4480–6.

66. LeBrun DP, Kamel OW, Cleary ML, Dorfman RF, Warnke RA. Follicular lymphomas of the gastrointestinal tract. Pathologic features in 31 cases and bcl-2 oncogenic protein expression. Am J Pathol 1992;140:1327–35.

67. _____, Kamel OW, Dorfman RF, Warnke RA. Enhanced staining for Leu M1 (CD15) in Hodgkin's disease using a secondary antibody specific for immunoglobulin M. Am J Clin Pathol 1992;97:135–8.

68. Ledbetter JA, Evans RL, Lipinski M, Cunningham-Rundles C, Good RA, Herzenberg LA. Evolutionary conservation of surface molecules that distinguish T lymphocyte helper/inducer and cytotoxic/suppressor subpopulations in mouse and man. J Exp Med 1981;153:310–23.

69. Leonard WJ, Depper JM, Robb RJ, Waldmann TA, Greene WC. Characterization of the human receptor for T-cell growth factor. Proc Natl Acad Sci USA 1983;80:6957–61.

70. Levy R, Warnke R, Dorfman RF, Haimovich J. The monoclonality of human B-cell lymphomas. J Exp Med 1977;145:1014–28.

71. Link M, Warnke R, Finlay J, Amylon M, Dilley J, Levy R. A single monoclonal antibody identifies T-cell lineage of childhood lymphoid malignancies. Blood 1983;62:722–8.

72. Link MP, Bindl J, Meeker TC, et al. A unique antigen on mature B cells defined by a monoclonal antibody. J Immunol 1986;137:3013–8.

73. _____, Stewart SJ, Warnke RA, Levy R. Discordance between surface and cytoplasmic expression of the Leu-4 (T3) antigen in thymocytes and in blast cells from childhood T lymphoblastic malignancies. J Clin Invest 1985;76:248–53.

74. MacDonald SM, Pulford K, Falini B, Micklem K, Mason DY. A monoclonal antibody recognizing the p150/95 leucocyte differentiation antigen. Immunology 1986;59:427–31.

75. Marder RJ, Variakojis D, Silver J, Epstein AL. Immunohistochemical analysis of human lymphomas with monoclonal antibodies to B cell and Ia antigens reactive in paraffin sections. Lab Invest 1985;52:497–504.

76. Mason DY, Comans-Bitter WM, Cordell JL, Verhoeven MA, van Dongen JJ. Antibody L26 recognizes an intracellular epitope on the B-cell-associated CD20 antigen. Am J Pathol 1990;136:1215–22.

77. _____, Cordell J, Brown M, et al. Detection of T cells in paraffin wax embedded tissue using antibodies against a peptide sequence from the CD3 antigen. J Clin Pathol 1989;42:1194–200.

78. _____, Cordell JL, Tse AG, et al. The IgM-associated protein mb-1 as a marker of normal and neoplastic B cells. J Immunol 1991;147:2474-82.

79. _____, Gatter KC. The role of immunocytochemistry in diagnostic pathology. J Clin Pathol 1987;40:1042–54.

80. _____, Krissansen GW, Davey FR, Crumpton MJ, Gatter KC. Antisera against epitopes resistant to denaturation on T3 (CD3) antigen can detect reactive and neoplastic T cells in paraffin embedded tissue biopsy specimens. J Clin Pathol 1988;41:121–7.

81. _____, Stein H, Gerdes J, et al. Value of monoclonal anti-CD22 (p135) antibodies for the detection of normal and neoplastic B lymphoid cells. Blood 1987;69:836–40.

82. _____, van Noesel CJ, Cordell JL, et al. The B29 and mb-1 polypeptides are differentially expressed during human B cell differentiation. Eur J Immunol 1992;22:2753–6.

83. McMichael AJ, Pilch JR, Galfre G, Mason DY, Fabre JW, Milstein C. A human thymocyte antigen defined by a hybrid myeloma monoclonal antibody. Eur J Immunol 1979;9:205–10.

84. Medeiros LJ, Bagg A, Cossman J. Application of molecular genetics to the diagnosis of hematopoietic neoplasms. In: Knowles DM, ed. Neoplastic hematopathology. Baltimore: Williams & Wilkins, 1992.

85. _____, Weiss LM, Picker LJ, et al. Expression of LFA-1 in non-Hodgkin's lymphoma. Cancer 1989;63:255–9.

86. _____, Weiss LM, Warnke RA, Dorfman RF. Utility of combining antigranulocyte with antileukocyte antibodies in differentiating Hodgkin's disease from non-Hodgkin's lymphoma. Cancer 1988;62:2475–81.

87. Meeker TC, Miller RA, Link MP, Bindl J, Warnke R, Levy R. A unique human B lymphocyte antigen defined by a monoclonal antibody. Hybridoma 1984;3:305–20.

88. Michie SA, Spagnolo DV, Dunn KA, Warnke RA, Rouse RV. A panel approach to the evaluation of the sensitivity and specificity of antibodies for the diagnosis of routinely processed histologically undifferentiated human neoplasms. Am J Clin Pathol 1987;88:457–62.

89. Micklem KJ, Stross WP, Willis AC, Cordell JL, Jones M, Mason DY. Different isoforms of human FcRII distinguished by CDw32 antibodies. J Immunol 1990;144:2295–303.

90. Miedema F, Tromp JF, van't Veer MB, Poppema S, Melief CJ. Lymphocyte function-associated antigen 1 (LFA-1) is a marker of mature (immunocompetent) lymphoid cells. A survey of lymphoproliferative diseases in man. Leuk Res 1985;9:1099–104.

91. Nadler LM, Anderson KC, Marti G, et al. B4, a human B lymphocyte-associated antigen expressed of normal, mitogen-activated, and malignant B lymphocytes. J Immunol 1983;131:244–50.

92. _____, Ritz J, Hardy R, Pesando JM, Schlossman SF, Stashenko P. A unique cell surface antigen identifying lymphoid malignancies of B-cell origin. J Clin Invest 1981;67:134–40.

93. _____, Stashenko P, Hardy R, van Agthoven A, Terhorst C, Schlossman SF. Characterization of a human B cell-specific antigen (B2) distinct from B1. J Immunol 1981;126:1941–7.

94. Ng CS, Chan JK, Hui PK, Chan WC, Lo ST. Application of a T cell receptor antibody beta F1 for immunophenotypic analysis of malignant lymphomas. Am J Pathol 1988;132:365–71.

95. _____, Chan JK, Hui PK, Lo ST. Monoclonal antibodies reactive with normal and neoplastic T cells in paraffin sections. Hum Pathol 1988;19:295–303.

96. _____, Chan JK, Lo ST. Expression of natural killer cell markers in non-Hodgkin's lymphomas. Hum Pathol 1987;18:1257–62.

97. _____, Chan JK, Lo ST, Lo DS. Critical assessment of four monoclonal antibodies reactive with B-cells in formalin-fixed paraffin-embedded tissues. Histopathology 1987;11:1243–58.

98. Ngan BY, Picker LJ, Medeiros LJ, Warnke RA. Immunophenotypic diagnosis of non-Hodgkin's lymphoma in paraffin sections. Co-expression of L60 (Leu-22) and L26 antigens correlates with malignant histologic findings. Am J Clin Pathol 1989;91:579–83.

99. Norton AJ, Isaacson PG. An immunocytochemical study of T-cell lymphomas using monoclonal and polyclonal antibodies effective in routinely fixed wax embedded tissues. Histopathology 1986;10:1243–60.

100. _____, Isaacson PG. Detailed phenotypic analysis of B-cell lymphoma using a panel of antibodies reactive in routinely fixed wax-embedded tissue. Am J Pathol 1987;128:225–40.

101. _____, Isaacson PG. Monoclonal antibody L26: an antibody that is reactive with normal and neoplastic B lymphocytes in routinely fixed and paraffin wax embedded tissues. J Clin Pathol 1987;40:1405–12.

102. _____, Ramsay AD, Smith SH, Beverley PC, Isaacson PG. Monoclonal antibody (UCHL1) that recognises normal and neoplastic T cells in routinely fixed tissues. J Clin Pathol 1986;39:399–405.

103. Pallesen G, Hamilton-Dutoit SJ. Ki-1 (CD30) antigen is regularly expressed by tumor cells of embryonal carcinoma. Am J Pathol 1988;133:446–50.

104. _____, Hamilton DS, Rowe M, Young LS. Expression of Epstein-Barr virus latent gene products in tumour cells of Hodgkin's disease. Lancet 1991;337:320–2.

105. Perussia B, Trinchieri G, Jackson A, et al. The Fc receptor of IgG on human natural killer cells: phenotypic, functional, and comparative studies with monoclonal antibodies. J Immunol 1984;133:180–9.

106. Picker LJ, Brenner MB, Michie S, Warnke RA. Expression of T cell receptor delta chains in benign and malignant T lineage lymphoproliferations. Am J Pathol 1988;132:401–5.

107. _____, Brenner MB, Weiss LM, Smith SD, Warnke RA. Discordant expression of CD3 and T-cell receptor beta-chain antigens in T-lineage lymphomas. Am J Pathol 1987;129:434–40.

108. _____, Weiss LM, Medeiros LJ, Wood GS, Warnke RA. Immunophenotypic criteria for the diagnosis of non-Hodgkin's lymphoma. Am J Pathol 1987;128:181–201.

109. Pileri S, Gerdes J, Rivano M, et al. Immunohistochemical determination of growth fractions in human permanent cell lines and lymphoid tumours: a critical comparison of the monoclonal antibodies OKT9 and Ki-67. Br J Haematol 1987;65:271–6.

110. Pinkus GS, Kurtin PJ. Epithelial membrane antigen—a diagnostic discriminant in surgical pathology: immunohistochemical profile in epithelial, mesenchymal, and hematopoietic neoplasms using paraffin sections and monoclonal antibodies. Hum Pathol 1985;16:929–40.

111. _____, Pinkus JL. Myeloperoxidase: a specific marker for myeloid cells in paraffin sections. Mod Pathol 1991;4:733–41.

112. Poppema S. The nature of the lymphocytes surrounding Reed-Sternberg cells in nodular lymphocyte predominance and in other types of Hodgkin's disease. Am J Pathol 1989;135:351–7.

113. _____, Hepperle B. Restricted V gene usage in T-cell lymphomas as detected by anti-T-cell receptor variable region reagents. Am J Pathol 1991;138:1479–84.

114. _____, Hollema H, Visser L, Vos H. Monoclonal antibodies (MT1, MT2, MB1, MB2, MB3) reactive with leukocyte subsets in paraffin-embedded tissue sections. Am J Pathol 1987;127:418–29.

115. _____, Lai R, Visser L. Monoclonal antibody OPD4 is reactive with CD45RO, but differs from UCHL1 by the absence of monocyte reactivity. Am J Pathol 1991;139:725–9.

116. Pulford K, Ralfkiaer E, MacDonald SM, et al. A new monoclonal antibody (KB61) recognizing a novel antigen which is selectively expressed on a subpopulation of human B lymphocytes. Immunology 1986;57:71–6.

117. Pulford KA, Rigney EM, Micklem KJ, et al. KP1: a new monoclonal antibody that detects a monocyte/macrophage associated antigen in routinely processed tissue sections. J Clin Pathol 1989;42:414–21.

118. _____, Sipos A, Cordell JL, Stross WP, Mason DY. Distribution of the CD68 macrophage/myeloid associated antigen. Int Immunol 1990;2:973–80.

119. Reinherz EL, Hussey RE, Schlossman SF. A monoclonal antibody blocking human T cell function. Eur J Immunol 1980;10:758–62.

120. _____, Kung PC, Goldstein G, Levey RH, Schlossman SF. Discrete stages of human intrathymic differentiation: analysis of normal thymocytes and leukemic lymphoblasts of T-cell lineage. Proc Natl Acad Sci USA 1980;77:1588–92.

121. _____, Kung PC, Goldstein G, Schlossman SF. A monoclonal antibody with selective reactivity with functionally mature human thymocytes and all peripheral human T cells. J Immunol 1979;123:1312–7.

122. _____, Moretta L, Roper M, et al. Human T lymphocyte subpopulations defined by Fc receptors and monoclonal antibodies: a comparison. J Exp Med 1980;151:969–974.

123. Ritz J, Nadler LM, Ghan AK, Notis-McConarty J, Pesando J, Schlossman SF. Expression of common acute lymphoblastic leukemia antigen (cALLa) by lymphomas of B-cell and T-cell lineage. Blood 1981;58:648–652.

124. _____, Pesando JM, Notis-McConarty J, Lazarus H, Schlossman SF. A monoclonal antibody to human acute lymphoblastic leukaemia antigen. Nature 1980;283:583–5.

125. Said JW, Shintaku IP, Parekh K, Pinkus GS. Specific phenotyping of T-cell proliferations in formalin-fixed paraffin-embedded tissues. Use of antibodies to the T-cell receptor beta F1. Am J Clin Pathol 1990;93:382–6.

126. _____, Shintaku IP, Pinkus GS. Immunohistochemical staining for terminal deoxynucleotidyl transferase (TDT). An enhanced method in routinely processed formalin-fixed tissue sections. Am J Clin Pathol 1988;89:649–52.

127. _____, Stoll PN, Shintaku P, Bindl JM, Butmarc JR, Pinkus GS. Leu–22: a preferential marker for T–lymphocytes in paraffin sections. Staining profile in T– and B-cell lymphomas, Hodgkin's disease, other lymphoproliferative disorders, myeloproliferative diseases, and various neoplastic processes. Am J Clin Pathol 1989;91:542–9.

128. Schwarting R, Gerdes J, Durkop H, Falini B, Pileri S, Stein H. BER-H2: a new anti-Ki-1 (CD30) monoclonal antibody directed at a formol-resistant epitope. Blood 1989;74:1678–89.

129. _____, Stein H, Wang CY. The monoclonal antibodies alpha S-HCL 1 (alpha Leu-14) and alpha S-HCL 3 (alpha Leu-M5) allow the diagnosis of hairy cell leukemia. Blood 1985;65:974–83.

130. Sheibani K, Battifora H, Burke JS, Rappaport H. Leu-M1 antigen in human neoplasms. An immunohistologic study of 400 cases. Am J Surg Pathol 1986;10:227–36.

131. _____, Winberg CD, Burke JS, et al. Lymphoblastic lymphoma expressing natural killer cell-associated antigens: a clinicopathologic study of six cases. Leuk Res 1987;11:371–7.

132. _____, Winberg CD, van de Velde S, Blayney DW, Rappaport H. Distribution of lymphocytes with interleukin-2 receptors (TAC antigens) in reactive lymphoproliferative processes, Hodgkin's disease, and non-Hodgkin's lymphomas. An immunohistologic study of 300 cases. Am J Pathol 1987;127:27–37.

133. Stein H, Mason DY. Immunological analysis of tissue sections in the diagnosis of lymphoma. In: Hoffbrand AV, ed. Recent advances in haematology. Edinburgh: Churchill Livingstone, 1985:127–69.

134. _____, Mason DY, Gerdes J, et al. The expression of the Hodgkin's disease associated antigen Ki-1 in reactive and neoplastic lymphoid tissue: evidence that Reed-Sternberg cells and histiocytic malignancies are derived from activated lymphoid cells. Blood 1985;66:848–58.

135. _____, Uchanska-Ziegler B, Gerdes J, Ziegler A, Wernet P. Hodgkin's and Sternberg-Reed cells contain antigens specific to late cells of granulopoiesis. Int J Cancer 1982;29:283–90.

136. Strickler JG, Audeh MW, Copenhaver CM, Warnke RA. Immunophenotypic differences between plasmacytoma/multiple myeloma and immunoblastic lymphoma. Cancer 1988;61:1782–6.

137. Stross WP, Warnke RA, Flavell DJ, et al. Molecule detected in formalin fixed tissue by antibodies MT1, DF-T1, and L60 (Leu-22) corresponds to CD43 antigen. J Clin Pathol 1989;42:953–61.

138. Takahashi K, Isobe T, Ohtsuki Y, Sonobe H, Takeda I, Akagi T. Immunohistochemical localization and distribution of S-100 proteins in the human lymphoreticular system. Am J Pathol 1984;116:497–503.

139. Thorley-Lawson DA, Nadler LM, Bhan AK, Schooley RT. BLAST-2 [EBVCS], an early cell surface marker of human B cell activation, is superinduced by Epstein Barr virus. J Immunol 1985;134:3007-12.

140. Timens W, Boes A, Vos H, Poppema S. Tissue distribution of the C3d/EBV-receptor: CD21 monoclonal antibodies reactive with a variety of epithelial cells, medullary thymocytes, and peripheral T-cells. Histochemistry 1991;95:605–11.

141. Tubbs RR, Fishleder A, Weiss RA, Savage RA, Sebek BA, Weick JK. Immunohistologic cellular phenotypes of lymphoproliferative disorders. Comprehensive evaluation of 564 cases including 257 non-Hodgkin's lymphomas classified by the International Working Formulation. Am J Pathol 1983;113:207–21.

142. Vanstapel MJ, Gatter KC, de Wolf-Peeters C, Mason DY, Desmet VD. New sites of human S-100 immunoreactivity detected with monoclonal antibodies. Am J Clin Pathol 1986;85:160–8.

143. Verbi W, Greaves M, Schneider C, et al. Monoclonal antibodies OKT 11 and OKT 11A have pan-T reactivity and block sheep erythrocyte receptors. Eur J Immunol 1982;12:81–6.

144. Wang CY, Good RA, Ammirati P, Dymbort G, Evans RL. Identification of a p69,71 complex expressed on human T cells sharing determinants with B-type chronic lymphatic leukemic cells. J Exp Med 1980;151:1539–44.

145. Warnke RA, Gatter KC, Falini B, et al. Diagnosis of human lymphoma with monoclonal antileukocyte antibodies. N Engl J Med 1983;309:1275–81.

146. _____, Pulford KA, Pallesen G, et al. Diagnosis of myelomonocytic and macrophage neoplasms in routinely processed tissue biopsies with monoclonal antibody KP1. Am J Pathol 1989;135:1089–95.

147. _____, Weiss LM. A practical approach to the immunodiagnosis of lymphomas emphasizing differential diagnosis. In: Franks LM, ed. Cancer surveys, Vol. 4. Oxford: Oxford University Press, 1985:349–58.

148. Weiss LM, Bindl JM, Picozzi VJ, Link MP, Warnke RA. Lymphoblastic lymphoma: an immunophenotype study of 26 cases with comparison to T cell acute lymphoblastic leukemia. Blood 1986;67:474–8.

149. _____, Chang KL. Molecular biologic studies of Hodgkin's disease. Semin Diagn Pathol 1992;9:272–8.

150. _____, Michie SA, Medeiros LJ, Strickler JG, Garcia CF, Warnke RA. Expression of Tac antigen by non-Hodgkin's lymphomas. Am J Clin Pathol 1987;88:483–5.

151. _____, Strickler JG, Medeiros LJ, Gerdes J, Stein H, Warnke RA. Proliferative rates of non-Hodgkin's lymphomas as assessed by Ki-67 antibody. Hum Pathol 1987;18:1155–9.

152. Willman CL. Flow cytometric analysis of hematologic specimens. In: Knowles DM, ed. Neoplastic hematology. Baltimore: Williams & Wilkins, 1992:169–95.

153. Wong KF, Chan JK, Ng CS, Lee KC, Tsang WY, Cheung MM. CD56 (NKH1)-positive hematolymphoid malignancies: an aggressive neoplasm featuring frequent cutaneous/mucosal involvement, cytoplasmic azurophilic granules, and angiocentricity. Hum Pathol 1992;23:798–804.

154. Wood GS, Link M, Warnke RA, Dilley J, Levy R. Pan-leukocyte monoclonal antibody L3812. Characterization and application to research and diagnostic problems. Am J Clin Pathol 1984;81:176–83.

155. _____, Warner NL, Warnke RA. Anti-Leu-3/T4 antibodies react with cells of monocyte/macrophage and Langerhans lineage. J Immunol 1983;131:212–6.

156. Yoshino T, Mukuzono H, Aoki H, et al. A novel monoclonal antibody (OPD4) recognizing a helper/inducer T cell subset. Its application to paraffin-embedded tissues. Am J Pathol 1989;134:1339–46.

157. Zipf TF, Lauzon GJ, Longenecker BM. A monoclonal antibody detecting a 39,000 M.W. molecule that is present on B lymphocytes and chronic lymphocytic leukemia cells but is rare on acute lymphocytic leukemia blasts. J Immunol 1983;131:3064–72.

Analysis of Antigen Receptor Gene Rearrangements

158. Cleary M, Chao J, Warnke R, Sklar J. Immunoglobulin gene rearrangement as a diagnostic criterion of B-cell lymphoma. Proc Natl Acad Sci USA 1984;81:593–7.

159. Davis RE, Warnke RA, Dorfman RF, Cleary ML. Utility of molecular genetic analysis for the diagnosis of neoplasia in morphologically and immunophenotypically equivocal hematolymphoid lesions. Cancer 1991;67:2890–9.

160. Henni T, Gaulard P, Divine M, et al. Comparison of genetic probe with immunophenotype analysis in lymphoproliferative disorders: a study of 87 cases. Blood 1988;72:1937–43.

161. Kamat D, Laszewski M, Kemp J, et al. The diagnostic utility of immunophenotyping and immunogenotyping in the pathologic evaluation of lymphoid proliferations. Mod Pathol 1990;3:105–12.

162. Medeiros LJ, Bagg A, Cossman J. Application of molecular genetics to the diagnosis of hematopoietic neoplasms. In: Knowles DM, ed. Neoplastic hematopathology. Baltimore: Williams & Wilkins, 1992.

163. O'Connor N, Gatter K, Wainscoat J, et al. Practical value of genotypic analysis for diagnosing lymphoproliferative disorders. J Clin Pathol 1987;40:147–50.

164. Papadopoulos K, Bagg A, Bezwoda W, Mendelow B. The routine diagnostic utility of immunoglobulin and T-cell receptor gene rearrangements in lymphoproliferative disorders. Am J Clin Pathol 1989;91:633–8.

165. Sklar J. Antigen receptor genes: structure, function, and techniques for analysis of their rearrangements. In: Knowles DM, ed. Neoplastic hematopathology. Baltimore: Williams & Wilkins, 1992.

Analysis of Chromosomal Abnormalities

166. Aster J, Kobayashi Y, Shiota M, Mori S, Sklar J. Detection of the t(14;18) at similar frequencies in hyperplastic lymphoid tissues from American and Japanese patients. Am J Pathol 1992;141:291–9.

167. Cleary M. Oncogenic conversion of transcription factors by chromosomal translocations. Cell 1991;66:619–22.

168. Gaidano G, Dalla-Favera R. Protooncogenes and tumor suppressor genes. In: Knowles DM, ed. Neoplastic hematopathology. Baltimore: Williams & Wilkins, 1992.

169. LeBeau M. The role of cytogenetics in the diagnosis and classification of hematopoietic neoplasms. In: Knowles DM, ed. Neoplastic hematopathology. Baltimore: Williams and Wilkins, 1992.

170. Lee M, Chang K, Cabanillas F, Freireich E, Trujillo J, Stass S. Detection of minimal residual cells carrying the t(14;18) by DNA sequence amplification. Science 1987;237:175–8.

171. Limpens J, de Jong D, van Krieken J, et al. Bcl-2/JH rearrangements in benign lymphoid tissues with follicular hyperplasia. Oncogene 1991;6:2271–6.

172. Ngan BY, Nourse J, Cleary M. Detection of chromosomal translocation t(14;18) within the minor cluster region of bcl-2 by polymerase chain reaction and direct genomic sequencing of the enzymatically amplified DNA in follicular lymphomas. Blood 1989;73:1759–62.

173. Weiss L, Warnke R, Sklar J, Cleary M. Molecular analysis of the t(14;18) chromosomal translocation in malignant lymphomas. N Engl J Med 1987;317:1185–9.

Electron Microscopy and Aspiration Cytology

174. Minda JM, Lubensky IA, Pietra GG. Prolonged storage of tissues at low temperatures does not preclude their use for ultrastructural studies. Arch Pathol Lab Med 1992;116:56–9.

175. Pitts WC, Weiss LM. The role of fine needle aspiration biopsy in diagnosis and management of hematopoietic neoplasms. In: Knowles DM, ed. Neoplastic hematopathology. Baltimore: Williams & Wilkins, 1992:385–405.

4

NOMENCLATURE AND CLASSIFICATION OF LYMPHOID TUMORS

In 1832, Thomas Hodgkin described the gross pathologic findings in seven cases of lymphadenopathy (10). Additional cases were reported 33 years later by Samuel Wilkes (29), who named this lymphoid tumor Hodgkin's disease. The classic diagnostic cell and distinctive inflammatory background were described at the turn of the century by Sternberg in Vienna and Reed in Baltimore, Maryland (19,21). In 1926, six of Hodgkin's original cases were examined histologically, and three were confirmed to represent what is now widely known as Hodgkin's disease (6). But it was not until the mid-1940s that Jackson and Parker (11) proposed a classification system for Hodgkin's disease; this was replaced 20 years later by the classification of Lukes and Butler, modified at the Rye Conference and still in use today (13–15).

The recognition and subdivision of other lymphoid tumors has been and remains more problematic. In 1846, Virchow (25–27) provided one of the earliest accurate descriptions of leukemia and soon thereafter used the terms lymphoma and lymphosarcoma. Billroth (3) first proposed the term malignant lymphoma in 1871. From the late 1800s to about 1930, the major subdivisions of lymphoma were lymphosarcoma and Hodgkin's disease, and the term malignant lymphoma continues to be used to designate Hodgkin's and non-Hodgkin's lymphomas. Additional categories of lymphoid tumors presumed to derive from follicles or from reticular cells were described in the early part of this century (1,2,4,8,20,23). The lack of success in attempts to standardize nomenclature and classification led Willis (30) to comment in 1948, "nowhere in pathology has a chaos of names so clouded clear concept as in the subject of lymphoid tumors." An early classification of lymphomas by Gall and Mallory (7) in 1942 was supplanted by that of Rappaport (18) in 1966. This classification scheme was proved clinically relevant by a number of subsequent clinicopathologic studies (see chapter 5). Discussion of additional classification schemes for lymphomas other than Hodgkin's disease is also provided in chapter 5.

Attempts to improve the classification of lymphoid tumors through newer morphologic, immunologic, and molecular information and an immunologic framework for these tumors follow.

CLASSIFICATION BASED ON HISTOLOGIC FEATURES

Histology remains the most important criterion for current lymphoma classification. The clinically relevant classification system published by Rappaport in 1966 (18) divided lymphomas into those composed of small cells, those composed of large cells, and mixed tumors. Each type could be further subdivided based on a nodular (follicular) versus diffuse architectural pattern. Generally, lymphomas with a follicular pattern or those diffuse lymphomas composed of small cells are clinically less aggressive, more responsive to less aggressive forms of therapy, but also not as easily cured as those composed of large cells. The currently used terminology corresponds well to that used in hematology: chronic lymphocytic leukemia and acute lymphoblastic leukemia represent the morphologically identical leukemic counterparts of small lymphocytic lymphoma and lymphoblastic lymphoma, respectively.

A recurrent problem with classification by morphology alone has been the lack of adequate reproducibility (12,24). Stout (22) found an incidence of reticulum cell sarcoma of 57 percent, which he contrasted with an incidence of 4 percent and 94 percent in two similar large series reported at about the same time. After follicular lymphomas were accurately described, they were reproducibly identified in a high percentage of cases irrespective of the degree of expertise of the pathologist (12). Subcategories of follicular or diffuse lymphomas are poorly reproducible, even among experienced observers (5,9,16,17,28) or when the same case is assessed by the same experienced observer on two separate occasions (28).

Thus, lymphoma classification schemes that have a large number of categories are likely to have poor inter- and intraobserver reproducibility. Nevertheless, as the architectural and cytologic features of different morphologic subtypes of lymphoma have become better delineated and are supplemented by immunologic, molecular, or cytogenetic findings, the accuracy of classification may improve. In addition, availability of high quality histologic sections and careful attention to lymphoma cell size using an internal standard, such as the nucleus of a macrophage or endothelial cell, may improve reproducibility. Touch preparations are also helpful for evaluating cytologic details. Furthermore, some of the most clinically relevant distinctions are the most reproducible, such as follicular versus diffuse pattern and small cell versus large cell type. As will be emphasized in the following chapters, clinical features should always be correlated with histologic findings. For example, if a particular lymphoma diagnosis is being considered but that lymphoma rarely presents in the patient's age group or with the particular constellation of clinical findings, the histologic features should be reassessed and if confirmed, additional studies to support or refute the favored diagnosis may be indicated.

CLASSIFICATION BASED ON IMMUNOLOGIC FEATURES

It was hoped that the myriad of monoclonal antibodies reactive with lymphocytes would lead to an immunologic classification that would be more scientifically accurate and overcome the reproducibility problems inherent in the various morphologic classification schemes. Unfortunately, as Mason (35) has emphasized, such hopes are based on a fallacy which becomes apparent when one tries to imagine how this "hand over of power" from morphologists to immunohistologists might occur. In setting up studies to prove the validity of an immunophenotypic profile, investigators would be comparing immunophenotypic data (not necessarily highly reproducible among different laboratories and different methodologies) defined by the same subjective morphologic criteria that the studies are attempting to overcome.

A potentially more useful approach might be to compare the immunophenotypic profiles with the clinical features of a disease. A marker or combination of markers might correlate with distinctive clinical features. However, if such an immunoclinical correlation were found, it would only be of value if it were independent of other known clinical prognosticators (35). Studies attempting to identify clinically significant immunologic parameters, independent of morphologic and clinical parameters, have not been successful; there has been little if any agreement on any proposed prognostic indicators. For example, it has been difficult to substantiate the widely held assumption that aggressive lymphomas of T lineage have a worse clinical outcome than aggressive lymphomas of B lineage (33). Better knowledge of the functions and functional interactions of lymphocyte markers will facilitate the performance and validity of such studies: increased knowledge of the adhesive interactions between cell surface molecules on lymphoma cells and components of various endothelial cells and extracellular matrix should shed light on the migratory capabilities of these cells.

The investigation of markers that identify a more dynamic property of lymphomas, such as growth fraction, may be useful in classification. It is generally agreed that the growth fraction is lower in low-grade lymphomas than in intermediate- and high-grade lymphomas (42). In addition, several studies have identified a more proliferative subgroup among low-grade lymphomas which behaves more aggressively (31,34,36). However, whether growth fraction can be used to clinically subdivide particular intermediate- and high-grade lymphoma subgroups remains controversial. Nevertheless, this area of investigation holds real promise, particularly as functionally relevant markers are studied.

Some markers are already useful in classification. CD5 is nearly always expressed in cases of chronic lymphocytic leukemia, small lymphocytic lymphoma, and mantle cell lymphoma (intermediate lymphocytic/centrocytic/mantle zone lymphoma) but rarely expressed by follicular lymphomas or other lymphoma types (32,37,40, 41). Similarly, CD43 is frequently expressed in diffuse lymphomas and chronic lymphoid leukemias composed of small lymphoid cells and seldom expressed by follicular lymphomas (38,39). The following chapters provide additional examples of single markers or combinations of markers that can be used as adjuncts in lymphoma classification.

CLASSIFICATION BASED ON MOLECULAR FEATURES

Identification of genetic markers associated with the molecular events of antigen receptor gene rearrangements and chromosomal translocations has raised expectations that lymphoma classification might be based on criteria that are more reproducible, biologically meaningful, and clinically relevant. Although these expectations have been partially fulfilled, limitations to the application of molecular markers are now apparent. For example, gene rearrangements have been shown to lack specificity as lineage markers in lymphomas. A subset of otherwise indistinguishable B-cell lymphomas contain rearrangements of T-cell receptor genes and a subset of T-cell lymphomas may show rearrangements of immunoglobulin heavy chain genes (rearrangement of immunoglobulin light chain genes is rarely found in T-cell neoplasms) (44,46). Despite these limitations, molecular studies have been instrumental in identifying the lymphoid derivation of anaplastic large cell lymphomas which typically express few phenotypic markers (48,51), although a significant number of these unusual lymphomas may lack B- or T-cell gene rearrangements (48). In other settings, the lack of gene rearrangements has been helpful. For example, in an unusual group of lymphomas of the nasal cavity which often present with the clinical picture of lethal midline granuloma and express T-cell and natural killer cell markers, the absence of T-cell receptor rearrangements supports the possibility that they may represent malignancies of natural killer cells (52,54).

Despite their shortcomings as lineage markers, gene rearrangements have proven to be reliable clonal markers and in some settings may constitute the most sensitive and specific criteria to support a diagnosis of lymphoma, particularly of T lineage. However, detection of minor clonal lymphoid populations in otherwise complex tissues has revealed some interesting diagnostic pitfalls. It has become apparent that clonal populations of lymphoid cells may be observed in disorders that have a benign clinical course. This is particularly true of several indolent skin disorders (such as lymphomatoid papulosis) that occasionally evolve to malignant lymphoma (see chapter 12). Therefore, monoclonality within a lymphoid proliferation is not always predictive of malignant behavior, underscoring the fact that molecular studies must be interpreted in the context of other pathologic and clinical studies.

Chromosomal translocations are useful markers of malignancy but are not entirely specific for currently defined histologic categories of malignant lymphoma: the t(14;18) translocation is observed in both follicular and diffuse lymphomas that vary widely in their mixtures of small or large cells, thereby limiting its use in subclassification (53). Nevertheless, molecular characterization of this chromosomal translocation led to the identification of the *bcl-2* gene product and antibodies against this protein are useful diagnostic reagents for distinguishing follicular lymphoma and follicular hyperplasia (45, 47,49,50). Since *bcl-2* is involved in preventing cell death induced by a variety of cytotoxic agents, including chemotherapeutic drugs and radiotherapy, deregulated expression may prove to be an important diagnostic criterion regardless of morphologic subtype, although it is currently unclear whether it correlates with clinically important parameters. Cytogenetic studies suggest that genomic alterations in addition to t(14;18) actually determine the clinical behavior of follicular lymphomas (55). Further molecular characterization of these secondary changes may provide additional markers that could play a role in more meaningful classification. Similarly, although a t(8;14) abnormality is not entirely specific for small noncleaved cell lymphomas, the association with this subtype is very high (43). Thus, if this translocation or one of its variants is identified in a lymphoma other than small noncleaved cell, the morphologic features should be reexamined and correlated with appropriate clinical parameters.

Cytogenetic and molecular studies have provided vivid evidence of the multistep nature of lymphomagenesis. It is likely that a wide variety of genetic alterations in oncogenes and tumor suppressor genes determines the biologic and clinical features of any given malignant lymphoma, and that current morphologic categories are useful but not precise. Lymphomas will increasingly be defined by the genetic lesions underlying their pathogenesis; whether this will result in classification schemes more predictive of biologic behavior and response to therapy is unclear.

CLASSIFICATION IN THE CONTEXT OF LYMPHOID ONTOGENY

Precursor Cell Lymphomas and Leukemias

Lymphoid neoplasms of precursor cells are composed of medium-sized cells with nuclear features of immaturity (lymphoblasts) which generally arise in, and primarily involve, the primary lymphoid organs, bone marrow and thymus. The bone marrow is the major site of myelopoiesis and early B lymphocyte development throughout adult life, which may explain why the majority (approximately 85 percent) of acute lymphoblastic leukemias derive from B lineage (56). In contrast, the bone marrow elaborates pre-T cells, which migrate to the thymus where, under the influence of the thymic microenvironment there is rearrangement of the antigen receptor genes and subsequent expression of specific cell surface antigen receptor molecules. Cells expressing receptors reactive with self-antigens, which might lead to autoimmune disease, undergo apoptotic cell death in the thymic cortex while a few that survive undergo further differentiation and migrate to secondary lymphoid organs such as lymph nodes and spleen.

In contrast to the lymphoblastic leukemias, which mainly derive from B lineage, approximately 85 percent of lymphoblastic lymphomas derive from the T lineage and, not unexpectedly, frequently arise in or involve the thymus (61). The precursor B- and T-lineage lymphomas and leukemias are thought to be more prevalent in childhood because of the increased relative volume of the bone marrow and thymus or because more precursor cells are produced (59). Involvement of the bone marrow and, consequently, the peripheral blood, sometimes leads to uncertainty whether a lymphoid tumor is a leukemia or lymphoma. While such a distinction may have practical therapeutic and prognostic significance, separating lymphoid tumors composed of precursor B or T cells may be artificial and arbitrary (see chapter 11). In addition, lymphoid tumors composed of mature B cells or T cells may circulate through the bone marrow and present as leukemia. The most important diagnostic and therapeutic considerations are cell type and tumor burden (59). Thus, the terms leukemia and lymphoma do not precisely define subsets of lymphoid neoplasms, but they will continue to be used despite their shortcomings in taxonomic nomenclature. As our knowledge of lymphocyte maturation and its relationship to migration patterns evolves, we may eventually understand why particular precursor cell neoplasms primarily involve the bone marrow or thymus or alternatively present in peripheral sites such as gastrointestinal tract or skin.

B- and T-lineage lymphoblastic neoplasms appear to arise from, or at least retain many of the phenotypic and genotypic characteristics of, normal T- and B-precursor cell types (corresponding to antigen independent stages of differentiation) (59). However, much of our knowledge of presumptive stages of lymphocyte differentiation, particularly for those of B lineage, comes from the study of lymphomas and leukemias that may imperfectly reflect stages of normal differentiation (57,59,60,61). As lymphoid tumors are studied more carefully, more phenotypic or genotypic deviations from normal are found, a not surprising finding in view of their neoplastic nature. A schematic diagram for the differentiation of B-cell precursors is given in figure 4-1. In general, tumors that have a phenotype and genotype similar to the least differentiated precursor B cell manifest as leukemia whereas uncommon tumors that present as lymphomas correspond to a slightly more mature stage of development and are more apt to express CD10 and, especially, cytoplasmic mμ chains (pre-B-cell phenotype) (58).

A schematic diagram for the differentiation of T-cell precursors is given in figure 4-2. In general, T-cell lymphoblastic neoplasms that manifest as leukemia have phenotypes that are similar to the least mature, or occasionally, most mature, thymic precursor whereas those that present as lymphoma most frequently express a cortical thymocyte phenotype (62).

LYMPHOMAS AND LEUKEMIAS REFLECTIVE OF ANTIGEN-DEPENDENT STAGES OF LYMPHOCYTE DIFFERENTIATION

Although lymphoid tumors of precursor cells imperfectly mirror stages of normal antigen-independent B- and T-cell differentiation, they appear to correspond to such stages of differentiation better than tumors thought to correspond to

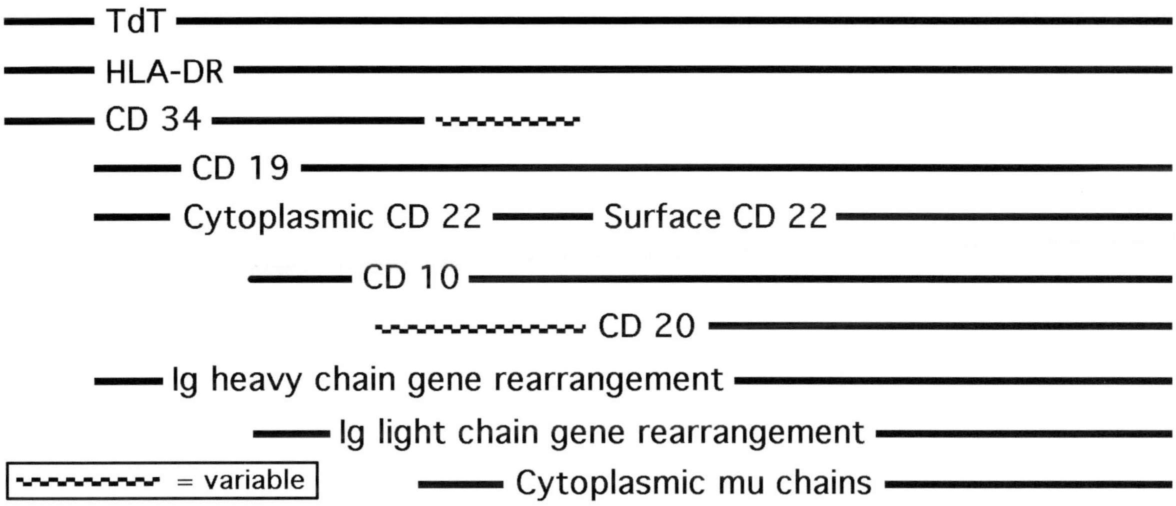

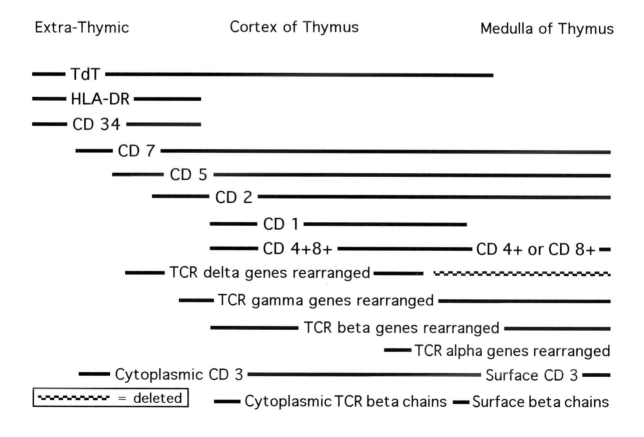

—— TdT ————————————————————————————
—— HLA-DR ————————————————————————————
—— CD 34 ————— ~~~~~~~~
   —— CD 19 ————————————————————————————
   —— Cytoplasmic CD 22 ——— Surface CD 22 ———————————
      —— CD 10 ————————————————————————
         ~~~~~~~~~ CD 20 ————————————————
   —— Ig heavy chain gene rearrangement ————————————
      —— Ig light chain gene rearrangement ————————
   [~~~~~~~~~ = variable]   —— Cytoplasmic mu chains ——————

Figure 4-1
B-CELL PRECURSORS

Extra-Thymic   Cortex of Thymus   Medulla of Thymus

—— TdT ————————————————————————————
—— HLA-DR ————
—— CD 34 ————
   —— CD 7 ————————————————————————————
      —— CD 5 ————————————————————————
      —— CD 2 ————————————————————————
         —— CD 1 ————————————
         —— CD 4+8+ ———————————— CD 4+ or CD 8+ —
   —— TCR delta genes rearranged ——— ~~~~~~~~~~~~~~~
      —— TCR gamma genes rearranged ————————————————
         —— TCR beta genes rearranged ——————————
            —— TCR alpha genes rearranged
—— Cytoplasmic CD 3 ———————————————————— Surface CD 3 ——
[~~~~~~~~~ = deleted]   —— Cytoplasmic TCR beta chains — Surface beta chains

Figure 4-2
T-CELL PRECURSORS

antigen-dependent maturational stages. Small noncleaved cell lymphomas are thought to arise from a cell in transition from a precursor B cell to a germinal center cell (73). These lymphomas share many features with lymphoblastic neoplasms: they are composed of medium-sized lymphoid cells, commonly occur in childhood, and may manifest as a leukemia (FAB L3 subtype of lymphoblastic leukemia). In contrast to lymphoblastic neoplasms, small noncleaved cell lymphomas do not express terminal deoxynucleotidyl transferase (TdT) and produce a surface immunoglobulin that typically includes mμ heavy chains, with or without delta chains; however, these lymphomas stain strongly for CD10 (common acute lymphoblastic leukemia antigen), which may also be expressed by normal and neoplastic germinal center cells (66). An additional link to germinal center cells is provided by the lack of expression of the homing-related molecules CD44 and Leu-8 by small noncleaved cells (66,75–77). A morphologic link to germinal centers was provided when Mann et al. (74) described selective involvement of germinal centers in about 20 percent of small noncleaved cell lymphomas. This involvement is often focal and may be easily overlooked, particularly if areas adjacent to a main tumor mass are not sampled.

The isotype of a tumor immunoglobulin has been used in attempts to link a particular B-cell tumor to a normal stage of B-cell development. Immature B cells can be divided into two major subsets based on expression of surface IgM or IgM plus IgD (80). Following binding of a specific antigen and through a series of activation and differentiation events, both antibody-secreting cells as well as memory cells are generated. Such memory B cells may express IgM, IgD, and IgG before losing their IgD and subsequently IgM (80). Since most lymphomas express IgM with or without IgD, they resemble immature or primary follicle B cells. Nevertheless, such lymphomas may represent highly proliferative small noncleaved cell lymphomas, follicular or diffuse lymphomas composed of predominantly small cells or large cells, or unusually indolent diffuse small cell lymphomas. Expression of IgG as a heavy chain provides a link to memory B cells and is most often seen in lymphomas of presumed follicular center cell origin composed predominantly of small cells, large cells, or admixtures.

These post-precursor cell lymphomas may have a highly complex architectural and cellular composition which mimics that of the normal immune system. The follicles of follicular lymphoma retain a complex network of follicular dendritic cells as well as a complement of intrafollicular T cells and are often surrounded by a mantle of normal polyclonal B cells together with interfollicular T cells (65,78,81). Whether antigen is present on their follicular dendritic cell processes is unknown, but there is little if any immunoglobulin deposited on these cell processes (81). Some of these lymphomas remain under host regulatory control, as evidenced by a significant incidence of spontaneous regression, a finding correlated with the number and type of host regulatory T cells (68,79). In regard to normal homing properties, follicular lymphomas that are predominantly composed of small cells nearly always circulate through, and involve, the bone marrow in contrast to those composed of large cells which less often infiltrate the bone marrow (70). As evidence of their capacity to differentiate into plasma cells, a subset of follicular lymphomas contains a population of monoclonal plasma cells producing the same immunoglobulin as the follicular component (71). Irrespective of how closely follicular lymphomas resemble normal secondary follicles, it is likely that newer forms of therapy will depend on one or more of their immunologic features. For example, effective treatment may include vaccination with a patient's particular tumor immunoglobulin (72).

Similarly, low-grade B-cell lymphomas of mucosa-associated lymphoid tissue are similar to the acquired lymphoid tissue from which they appear to derive. The bacterial organism *Helicobacter pylori* has been linked both to the hyperplastic lymphoid tissue that is acquired by the gastric mucosa as well as to low-grade B-cell lymphomas. Furthermore, the lymphoma cells from a given patient proliferate in culture in response to a particular strain of *H. pylori* and non-neoplastic T cells are required for this growth (69). Remarkably, eradication of *H. pylori* with antibiotic treatment has been shown to cause tumor regression in some patients (82).

Post-thymic T cells comprise numerous functional subgroups that give rise to an extremely heterogenous collection of T-cell lymphomas.

Most of these lymphomas lack expression of one or more normal T-cell differentiation antigens (77): the most conserved marker on precursor T-cell lymphomas, CD7, is least often expressed on post-thymic T-cell lymphomas. Two isoforms of the leukocyte common antigen, CD45RA and CD45RO, are associated with virgin and mem-ory T cells, respectively (63). Most post-thymic T-cell lymphomas express the phenotype of memory cells whereas the small number of T-cell lymphomas that express a virgin phenotype are frequently precursor T-cell neoplasms (64,67). On the other hand, most B-cell lymphomas do not exhibit a memory cell phenotype.

REFERENCES

History of, and Classification Based on Morphologic Features

1. Baehr G. The clinical and pathological picture of follicular lymphoblastoma. Trans Assoc Am Physicians 1932;47:330–8.
2. _____, Rosenthal N. Malignant lymph follicle hyperplasia of spleen and lymph nodes. Am J Pathol 1927;3:550–1.
3. Billroth T. Multiple lymphome. Erfolgreiche Behandlung mit Arsenik. Wein Med Wochenschr 1871;21:1066–7.
4. Brill NE, Baehr G, Rosenthal N. Generalized giant lymph follicle hyperplasia of the lymph nodes and spleen. A hitherto undescribed type. JAMA 1925;84:668–71.
5. Classification of non-Hodgkin's lymphomas. Reproducibility of major classification systems. NCI non-Hodgkin's Classification Project Writing Committee. Cancer 1985;55:91–5.
6. Fox H. Remarks on microscopical preparations made from some of the original tissue described by Thomas Hodgkin, 1832. Ann Med History 1926;8:370–4.
7. Gall EA, Mallory TB. Malignant lymphoma. A clinicopathologic survey of 618 cases. Am J Pathol 1942;18:381–429.
8. Ghon A, Roman B. Ueber das Lymphosarkom. Frankfurt Z Pathol 1916;19:1–138.
9. Hastrup N, Hamilton-Dutoit S, Ralfkiaer E, Pallesen G. Peripheral T-cell lymphomas: an evaluation of reproducibility of the updated Kiel classification. Histopathology 1991;18:99–105.
10. Hodgkin T. On some morbid appearances of the absorbent glands and spleen. Trans Med Chir Soc Lond 1832;17:68–114.
11. Jackson H Jr, Parker F Jr. Hodgkin's disease. II. Pathology. N Engl J Med 1944;231:35–44.
12. Jones SE, Butler JJ, Byrne GE Jr, Coltman CA Jr, Moon TE. Histopathologic review of lymphoma cases from the Southwest Oncology Group. Cancer 1977;39:1071–6.
13. Lukes RJ, Butler JJ. The pathology and nomenclature of Hodgkin's disease. Cancer Res 1966;26:1063–83.
14. _____, Butler JJ, Hicks EB. Natural history of Hodgkin's disease as related to its pathologic picture. Cancer 1966;19:317–44.
15. _____, Craver LF, Hall TC, Rappaport H, Rubin T. Report of the nomenclature committee. Cancer Res 1966;26:1311.
16. Metter GE, Nathwani BN, Burke JS, et al. Morphological subclassification of follicular lymphoma: variabil-ity of diagnoses among hematopathologists, a collaborative study between the Repository Center and Pathology Panel for Lymphoma Clinical Studies. J Clin Oncol 1985;3:25–38.
17. Nathwani BN, Metter GE, Miller TP, et al. What should be the morphologic criteria for the subdivision of follicular lymphomas? Blood 1986;68:837–45.
18. Rappaport H. Tumors of the hematopoietic system. In: Atlas of Tumor Pathology, 1st Series, Fascicle 8. Washington, DC: Armed Forces Institute of Pathology, 1966.
19. Reed DM. On the pathological changes in Hodgkin's disease, with especial reference to its relation to tuberculosis. Johns Hopkins Hosp Rep 1902;10:133–96.
20. Roulet F. Das Primare Retothelsarkom der Lymphknoten. Virchows Arch Pathol Anat 1930;277:15–47.
21. Sternberg C. Ueber eine eigenartige unter dem Bilde der Pseudoleukamie verlaufende Tuberculose des lymphatischen Apparates. Z fur Heilkunde, Berlin 1898;19:21–90.
22. Stout AP. The results of treatment of lymphosarcoma. N Y State J Med 1947;47:158–64.
23. Symmers D. Follicular lymphadenopathy with splenomegaly. A newly recognized disease of the lymphatic system. Arch Pathol 1927;3:816–20.
24. Symmers WS. Survey of the eventual diagnosis in 226 cases referred for a second histological opinion after an initial biopsy diagnosis of reticulum cell sarcoma. J Clin Pathol 1968;21:654–5.
25. Virchow R. Weisses Blut und Milztumoren. Med Zeitung, Berlin 1846;15:157–63.
26. _____. Die Cellularpathologie in igrer Begruendung auf physiologische und pathologische Gewebelehre. Berlin: Hirschwald, 1858.
27. _____. Die Krankgaftern Geschwuelste, Vol. 2. Berlin: Hirschwald, 1863:728–38.
28. Warnke RA, Strauchen JA, Burke JS, Hoppe RT, Campbell BA, Dorfman RF. Morphologic types of diffuse large-cell lymphoma. Cancer 1982;50:690–5.
29. Wilks S. Cases of enlargement of the lymphatic glands and spleen (or Hodgkin's disease), with remarks. Guy's Hosp Rep 1865;11:56–67.
30. Willis RA. The tumours of lymphoid tissue. In: Pathology of tumors. St. Louis: Mosby, 1948:760.

Classification Based on Immunologic Features

31. Bookman MA, Lardelli P, Jaffe ES, Duffey PL, Longo DL. Lymphocytic lymphoma of intermediate differentiation: morphologic, immunophenotypic, and prognostic factors. JNCI 1990;82:742–8.

32. Burns BF, Warnke RA, Doggett RS, Rouse RV. Expression of a T-cell antigen (Leu-1) by B-cell lymphomas. Am J Pathol 1983;113:165–71.

33. Kwak LW, Wilson M, Weiss LM, et al. Similar outcome of treatment of B-cell and T-cell diffuse large-cell lymphomas: the Stanford experience. J Clin Oncol 1991;9:1426–31.

34. Lardelli P, Bookman MA, Sundeen J, Longo DL, Jaffe ES. Lymphocytic lymphoma of intermediate differentiation. Morphologic and immunophenotypic spectrum and clinical correlations. Am J Surg Pathol 1990;14:752–63.

35. Mason DY. A new look at lymphoma immunohistology [Editorial]. Am J Pathol 1987;128:1–4.

36. Medeiros LJ, Picker LJ, Gelb AB, et al. Numbers of host helper T cells and proliferating cells predict survival in diffuse small-cell lymphomas. J Clin Oncol 1989; 7:1009–17.

37. _____, Strickler JG, Picker LJ, Gelb AB, Weiss LM, Warnke RA. Well-differentiated lymphocytic neoplasms. Immunologic findings correlated with clinical presentation and morphologic features. Am J Pathol 1987;129:523–35.

38. Ngan BY, Picker LJ, Medeiros LJ, Warnke RA. Immunophenotypic diagnosis of non-Hodgkin's lymphoma in paraffin sections. Co-expression of L60 (Leu-22) and L26 antigens correlates with malignant histologic findings. Am J Clin Pathol 1989;91:579–83.

39. Said JW, Stoll PN, Shintaku P, Bindl JM, Butmarc JR, Pinkus GS. Leu-22: a preferential marker for T-lymphocytes in paraffin sections. Staining profile in T- and B-cell lymphomas, Hodgkin's disease, other lymphoproliferative disorders, myeloproliferative diseases, and various neoplastic processes. Am J Clin Pathol 1989;91:542–9.

40. Strickler JG, Medeiros LJ, Copenhaver CM, Weiss LM, Warnke RA. Intermediate lymphocytic lymphoma: an immunophenotypic study with comparison to small lymphocytic lymphoma and diffuse small cleaved cell lymphoma. Hum Pathol 1988;19:550–4.

41. Sundeen JT, Longo DL, Jaffe ES. CD5 expression in B-cell small lymphocytic malignancies. Correlations with clinical presentation and sites of disease. Am J Surg Pathol 1992;16:130–7.

42. Weiss LM, Strickler JG, Medeiros LJ, Gerdes J, Stein H, Warnke RA. Proliferative rates of non-Hodgkin's lymphomas as assessed by Ki-67 antibody. Hum Pathol 1987;18:1155–9.

Classification Based on Molecular Features

43. Bloomfield CD, Arthur DC, Frizzera G, Levine EG, Peterson BA, Gajl-Peczalska KJ. Nonrandom chromosome abnormalities in lymphoma. Cancer Res 1983;43:2975–84.

44. Chen YT, Godwin TA, Mouradian JA. Immunohistochemistry and gene rearrangement studies in the diagnosis of malignant lymphomas: a comparison of 152 cases. Hum Pathol 1991;22:1249–57.

45. LeBrun DP, Kamel OW, Cleary ML, Dorfman RF, Warnke RA. Follicular lymphomas of the gastrointestinal tract. Pathologic features in 31 cases and bcl-2 oncogenic protein expression. Am J Pathol 1992;140:1327–35.

46. Medeiros LJ, Bagg A, Cossman J. Application of molecular genetics to the diagnosis of hematopoietic neoplasms. In: Knowles DM, ed. Neoplastic hematopathology. Baltimore: Williams & Wilkins, 1992.

47. Ngan BY, Chen-Levy Z, Weiss LM, Warnke RA, Cleary ML. Expression in non-Hodgkin's lymphoma of the bcl-2 protein associated with the t(14;18) chromosomal translocation. N Engl J Med 1988;318:1638–44.

48. O'Connor NT, Stein H, Gatter KC, et al. Genotypic analysis of large cell lymphomas which express the Ki-1 antigen. Histopathology 1987;11:733–40.

49. Pezzella F, Jones M, Ralfkiaer E, Ersboll J, Gatter KC, Mason DY. Evaluation of bcl-2 protein expression and 14;18 translocation as prognostic markers in follicular lymphoma. Br J Cancer 1992;65:87–9.

50. _____, Tse AG, Cordell JL, Pulford KA, Gatter KC, Mason DY. Expression of the bcl-2 oncogene protein is not specific for the 14;18 chromosomal translocation. Am J Pathol 1990;137:225–32.

51. Weiss LM, Picker LJ, Copenhaver CM, Warnke RA, Sklar J. Large-cell hematolymphoid neoplasms of uncertain lineage. Hum Pathol 1988;19:967–73.

52. _____, Picker LJ, Grogan TM, Warnke RA, Sklar J. Absence of clonal beta and gamma T-cell receptor gene rearrangements in a subset of peripheral T-cell lymphomas. Am J Pathol 1988;130:436–42.

53. _____, Warnke RA, Sklar J, Cleary ML. Molecular analysis of the t(14;18) chromosomal translocation in malignant lymphomas. N Engl J Med 1987;317:1185–9.

54. Wong KF, Chan JK, Ng CS, Lee KC, Tsang WY, Cheung MM. CD56 (NKH1)-positive hematolymphoid malignancies: an aggressive neoplasm featuring frequent cutaneous/mucosal involvement, cytoplasmic azurophilic granules, and angiocentricity. Hum Pathol 1992;23:798–804.

55. Yunis JJ, Frizzera G, Oken MM, McKenna J, Theologides A, Arnesen M. Multiple recurrent genomic defects in follicular lymphoma. A possible model for cancer. N Engl J Med 1987;316:79–84.

Precursor Cell Lymphomas and Leukemias

56. Chan LC, Pegram SM, Greaves MF. Contribution of immunophenotype to the classification and differential diagnosis of acute leukaemia. Lancet 1985;1:475–9.

57. Hurwitz CA, Loken MR, Graham ML, et al. Asynchronous antigen expression in B lineage acute lymphoblastic leukemia. Blood 1988;72:299–307.

58. Kamps WA, Poppema S. Pre-B-cell non-Hodgkin's lymphoma in childhood. Report of a case and review of the literature. Am J Clin Pathol 1988;90:103–7.

59. Magrath I. Lymphocyte ontogeny: a conceptual basis for understanding neoplasia of the immune system. In: Magrath IT, ed. The non-Hodgkin's lymphomas. Baltimore: Williams & Wilkins, 1990.

60. Mason DY. A new look at lymphoma immunohistology [Editorial]. Am J Pathol 1987;128:1–4.

61. Picker LJ, Weiss LM, Medeiros LJ, Wood GS, Warnke RA. Immunophenotypic criteria for the diagnosis of non-Hodgkin's lymphoma. Am J Pathol 1987;128:181–201.

62. Weiss LM, Bindl JM, Picozzi VJ, Link MP, Warnke RA. Lymphoblastic lymphoma: an immunophenotype study of 26 cases with comparison to T cell acute lymphoblastic leukemia. Blood 1986;67:474–8.

Lymphomas and Leukemias Reflective of Antigen-Dependent Stages of Lymphocytic Differentiation

63. Beverley PC. Functional analysis of human T cell subsets defined by CD45 isoform expression. Semin Immunol 1992;4:35–41.

64. Davey FR, Gatter KC, Ralfkiaer E, Pulford KA, Krissansen GW, Mason DY. Immunophenotyping of non-Hodgkin's lymphomas using a panel of antibodies on paraffin-embedded tissues. Am J Pathol 1987;129:54–63.

65. Dvoretsky P, Wood GS, Levy R, Warnke RA. T-lymphocyte subsets in follicular lymphomas compared with those in non-neoplastic lymph nodes and tonsils. Hum Pathol 1982;13:618–25.

66. Garcia CF, Weiss LM, Warnke RA. Small noncleaved cell lymphoma: an immunophenotypic study of 18 cases and comparison with large cell lymphoma. Hum Pathol 1986;17:454–61.

67. Hall PA, d'Ardenne AJ, Stansfeld AG. Paraffin section immunohistochemistry. I. Non-Hodgkin's lymphoma. Histopathology 1988;13:149–60.

68. Horning SJ, Rosenberg SA. The natural history of initially untreated low-grade non-Hodgkin's lymphomas. N Engl J Med 1984;311:1471–5.

69. Hussell T, Isaacson PG, Crabtree JE, Spencer J. The response of cells from low-grade B-cell gastric lymphomas of mucosa-associated lymphoid tissue to Helicobacter pylori. Lancet 1993;342:571–4.

70. Jones SE, Fuks Z, Bull M, et al. Non-Hodgkin's lymphomas. IV. Clinicopathologic correlation in 405 cases. Cancer 1973;31:806–23.

71. Keith TA, Cousar JB, Glick AD, Vogler LB, Collins RD. Plasmacytic differentiation in follicular center cell (FCC) lymphomas. Am J Clin Pathol 1985;84:283–90.

72. Kwak LW, Campbell MJ, Czerwinski DK, Hart S, Miller RA, Levy R. Induction of immune responses in patients with B-cell lymphoma against the surface-immunoglobulin idiotype expressed by their tumors. N Engl J Med 1992;327:1209–15.

73. Magrath I. Lymphocyte ontogeny: a conceptual basis for understanding neoplasia of the immune system. In: Magrath IT, ed. The non-Hodgkin's lymphomas. Baltimore: Williams & Wilkins, 1990.

74. Mann RB, Jaffe ES, Braylan RC, et al. Non-endemic Burkitt's lymphoma. A B-cell tumor related to germinal centers. N Engl J Med 1976;295:685–91.

75. Michie SA, Garcia CF, Strickler JG, Dailey MO, Rouse RV, Warnke RA. Expression of the Leu-8 antigen by B-cell lymphomas. Am J Clin Pathol 1987;88:486–90.

76. Picker LJ, Medeiros LJ, Weiss LM, Warnke RA, Butcher EC. Expression of lymphocyte homing receptor antigen in non-Hodgkin's lymphoma. Am J Pathol 1988;130:496–504.

77. , Weiss LM, Medeiros LJ, Wood GS, Warnke RA. Immunophenotypic criteria for the diagnosis of non-Hodgkin's lymphoma. Am J Pathol 1987;128:181–201.

78. Stein H, Gerdes J, Mason DY. The normal and malignant germinal centre. Clin Hematol 1982;11:531–59.

79. Strickler JG, Copenhaver CM, Rojas VA, Horning SJ, Warnke RA. Comparison of "host cell infiltrates" in patients with follicular lymphoma with and without spontaneous regression. Am J Clin Pathol 1988;90:257–61.

80. Tsiagbe VK, Linton PJ, Thorbecke GJ. The path of memory B-cell development. Immunol Rev 1992;126:113–41.

81. Warnke R, Levy R. The immunopathology of follicular lymphomas. A model of B-lymphocyte homing. New Engl J Med 1978;298:481–6.

82. Wotherspoon AC, Doglioni C, Diss TC, et al. Regression of primary low-grade B-cell gastric lymphoma of mucosa-associated lymphoid tissue type after eradication of Helicobacter pylori. Lancet 1993;342:575–7.

✧✧✧

5
MALIGNANT LYMPHOMAS OTHER THAN HODGKIN'S DISEASE (NON-HODGKIN'S LYMPHOMAS): AN OVERVIEW

Recognizing that the classification of non-Hodgkin's lymphomas (NHLs) has been the subject of controversy and heated debate during the past two decades, the authors have no intention of introducing new terminology, new concepts, or new classifications other than those already published with proven clinical utility. A brief review of current systems is nonetheless warranted.

Rappaport et al. (68) proposed a classification system in 1956 that was subsequently modified in 1966 (Table 5-1) (4,66). Jones et al. (42) demonstrated that the Rappaport classification was eminently applicable to clinicopathologic investigations. This was confirmed by subsequent studies at the National Cancer Institute (22,76) and other institutions (9,14). A single classification system allowed clinicians worldwide to compare the results of various therapeutic modalities. Rappaport's system was further revised to acknowledge the importance of clinicopathologic entities such as Burkitt's lymphoma and lymphoblastic lymphoma (59) and was adopted for use by the Lymphoma Pathology Panel for Clinical Trial Studies (23,50) which, for many years, served cancer chemotherapy groups throughout the United States and other countries. However, because of evolving concepts of the immune system and lymphoid physiology, the validity of Rappaport's terminology and the concepts inherent in his classification were questioned (26,54), with the result that five new classifications were proposed: the British National Lymphoma Investigation (3), Lukes and Collins (56), Dorfman (24–26), a European consortium representing the Kiel classification (31), and the World Health Organization (55). Meetings designed to resolve the differences of opinion and controversy resulting from these new classifications were held in Florence, Italy (1974) and Warrenton, Virginia (1975). These efforts failed mainly because inadequate clinical data were available to resolve the controversial issues.

A collaborative international study was sponsored by the National Cancer Institute in the late 1970s to evaluate these six classification systems. The clinical records and biopsy slides of 1175 cases of NHL, uniformly staged and treated at the Istituto Nazionale Tumori, Milan, Italy; Stanford University Medical Center, Stanford, California; Tufts New England Medical Center, Boston, Massachusetts; and the University of Minnesota, Minneapolis, Minnesota were reviewed. At the completion of this remarkable multi-institutional study, the major conclusion was that all six classifications were valuable and comparable in reproducibility and clinical correlation. An outgrowth of this study was a new terminology defining lymphomas, published in 1982 as "A Working Formulation of Non-Hodgkin's Lymphomas for Clinical Usage" (Table 5-2) (19,60). This formulation was not proffered as a new classification but as a means of translation from one classification system to another. Nonetheless, since its inception, most hematopathologists and clinicians in the United States have adopted the Working Formulation as their primary classification system. In 1988, a long-term follow-up of 1153 patients included in the initial 1982 National Cancer Institute–sponsored study concluded that the Working Formulation for NHL is a simple and useful system for selecting treatment and reporting results (81). Many pathologists and clinicians in Europe and elsewhere use the Kiel classification system, but in this Fascicle the terminology of the Working Formulation (Table 5-2) is used and includes analogous terms of the updated Kiel system (Table 5-3) (83).

Table 5-1

RAPPAPORT CLASSIFICATION OF MALIGNANT LYMPHOMAS

Nodular	Diffuse
Lymphocytic, well differentiated	
Lymphocytic, poorly differentiated	
Mixed cell (lymphocytic-histiocytic)	
Histiocytic	
Undifferentiated	

Table 5-2

A WORKING FORMULATION OF NON-HODGKIN'S LYMPHOMAS FOR CLINICAL USAGE: RECOMMENDATIONS OF AN EXPERT INTERNATIONAL PANEL

Low grade

Malignant lymphoma
  Small lymphocytic
    consistent with chronic lymphocytic
    leukemia; plasmacytoid

Malignant lymphoma, follicular
  Predominantly small cleaved
    diffuse areas; sclerosis

Malignant lymphoma, follicular
  Mixed, small cleaved and large cell
    diffuse areas; sclerosis

Intermediate grade

Malignant lymphoma, follicular
  Predominantly large cell
    diffuse areas; sclerosis

Malignant lymphoma, diffuse
  Small cleaved
    sclerosis

Malignant lymphoma, diffuse
  Mixed, small and large cell
    sclerosis; epithelioid cell component

Malignant lymphoma, diffuse
  Large cell
    cleaved; noncleaved; sclerosis

High grade

Malignant lymphoma
  Large cell, immunoblastic
    plasmacytoid; clear cell; polymorphous;
    epithelioid cell component

Malignant lymphoma
  Lymphoblastic
    convoluted; nonconvoluted

Malignant lymphoma
  Small noncleaved
    Burkitt's; follicular areas

Miscellaneous

Composite

Mycosis fungoides

Histiocytic

Extramedullary plasmacytoma

Unclassifiable

Other

The Working Formulation is a compromise system that falls short of accomplishing the ideals proposed by Rappaport in 1975 (67) that "a histological classification should be clinically useful, scientifically accurate, reproducible, easily taught and readily learned." Major shortcomings in the Working Formulation include the lack of separation of lymphomas based on cell lineage and the omission of several recently recognized clinicopathologic entities. Moreover, a recent report by Hastrup et al. (37) maintains that the reproducibility of the classification of Suchi et al. (84) and the updated Kiel classification for peripheral T-cell lymphomas are inadequate. The application of immunologic and molecular genetic techniques to biopsy material from patients with suspected lymphoma has proven invaluable in separating reactive disorders and in elucidating the lineage of the lymphoma cells. Presumably, lymphomas derived from different cell lineages have unique biologic characteristics. Nonetheless, as emphasized by the authors of the updated Kiel classification, "the basis of lymphoma classification must remain morphological, at least in the foreseeable future" (83). Therapeutic decisions are still primarily based on histologic subtype in addition to clinical and pathologic staging procedures and not on the B or T lineage of lymphomas. A recent proposal for a consensus classification does take into account cell lineage and recently described clinicopathologic entities (Table 5-4) (36). Nonetheless, it is not yet known if this classification will have clinical utility. Recently described entities such as the monocytoid B-cell lymphoma (62,79) and closely related lymphomas (41), intravascular (angiotropic) lymphomas (58,78), and anaplastic large cell lymphoma (45) have been included for discussion by us under appropriate categories in the ensuing chapters.

EPIDEMIOLOGY

The advent of newer diagnostic methodologies, particularly paraffin section immunohistochemistry, has clearly demonstrated that in the past malignant lymphomas were underdiagnosed. Studies performed at Oxford University and Stanford University (34,87) have indicated that a significant percentage of "anaplastic tumors" represent large cell lymphomas. Immunophenotyping studies

Table 5-3

UPDATED KIEL CLASSIFICATION OF NON-HODGKIN'S LYMPHOMAS

B Cell	T Cell
Low grade	**Low grade**
Lymphocytic:* chronic lymphocytic and pro-lymphocytic leukemia; hairy-cell leukemia	Lymphocytic: chronic lymphocytic and prolymphocytic leukemia
	Small, cerebriform cell: mycosis fungoides, Sézary's syndrome
Lymphoplasmacytic/cytoid (LP immunocytoma)	Lymphoepithelioid (Lennert's lymphoma)
Plasmacytic	Angioimmunoblastic (AILD, LgX)
Centroblastic/centrocytic*	T zone
- follicular +/-	
- diffuse	
Centrocytic*	Pleomorphic, small cell (HTLV-1+/-)
High grade	**High grade**
Centroblastic	Pleomorphic, medium and large cell (HTLV-1+/-)
Immunoblastic*	Immunoblastic (HTLV-1+/-)
Large cell anaplastic (Ki-1+)*	Large cell anaplastic (Ki-1+)
Burkitt's lymphoma	
Lymphoblastic*	Lymphoblastic
Rare types	**Rare types**

*Indicates some degree of correspondence, either in morphology or in functional expression, between categories in two columns.

have shown that some cases previously regarded as Hodgkin's disease are actually NHLs (46). In addition, some lesions previously regarded as "pseudolymphoma" or as preneoplastic have been shown to be NHL.

NHLs account for more than 3 percent of cancers and 3.1 percent of all cancer deaths in the United States, based on current cancer statistics (80). More than 37,000 cases were diagnosed in the United States in 1991, with 19,000 deaths (11,21). NHL is four times more common than Hodgkin's disease and accounts for ten times as many deaths (39). It is more common in men, with a ratio of 1.3 to 1 (60), and is more common in whites. The median age at diagnosis is approximately 55 years. However, high-grade lymphomas, especially Burkitt's and lymphoblastic lymphomas, have a higher incidence in young children and NHL is the third most common cause of cancer mortality in children under the age of 15, after leukemia and tumors of the central nervous system. Follicular lymphomas are rare in children and adolescents (30,63,90) as are diffuse low-grade lymphomas (small lymphocytic and mantle cell lymphomas).

The 1982 International Lymphoma Study (60) revealed geographic differences in the distribution of different types of lymphoma in the United States and Europe. In the United States, 49 percent of lymphomas were low grade, 38 percent intermediate grade, and only 12 percent high grade. In Milan, the corresponding categories were 18 percent, 53 percent, and 30 percent (39). Low-grade lymphomas are uncommon in Asians (35,61).

Most NHLs are B-cell lymphomas, representing all follicular lymphomas and between 80 and 90 percent of diffuse lymphomas. Asians, however, have a much higher incidence of T-lineage NHL than Western populations. True histiocytic tumors account for less than 1 percent of cases.

Recent epidemiologic studies have shown an increase in the incidence and mortality rates of NHL, even after considering improvements in diagnostic accuracy. Since the early 1970s, incidence rates have increased 3 to 4 percent per year, among whites and blacks, both within the United States and internationally, in both sexes, and over all age groups except the very young (21). Since the 1980s, a greater increase has occurred among young and middle-aged men, due in large part to a markedly increased incidence of NHL in patients with human immunodeficiency virus (HIV) infection.

There is also an increased incidence of NHL in patients with other immunodeficiency states, e.g.,

Table 5-4

LIST OF LYMPHOID NEOPLASMS RECOGNIZED BY THE INTERNATIONAL LYMPHOMA STUDY GROUP*

B-CELL NEOPLASMS

I. Precursor B-cell neoplasm: B-precursor lymphoblastic leukemia/lymphoma

II. Peripheral B-cell neoplasms
   1. B-cell chronic lymphocytic leukemia/prolymphocytic leukemia/small lymphocytic lymphoma
   2. Lymphoplasmacytoid lymphoma/immunocytoma
   3. Mantle cell lymphoma
   4. Follicle center lymphoma, follicular
      Provisional cytologic grades: small cell, mixed small and large cell, large cell
      Provisional subtype: diffuse, predominantly small cell type
   5. Marginal zone B-cell lymphoma
      Extranodal (MALT type +/- monocytoid B cells)
      Provisional category: nodal (+/- monocytoid B cells)
      Provisional category: splenic (+/- villous lymphocytes)
   6. Hairy cell leukemia
   7. Plasmacytoma/myeloma
   8. Diffuse large cell B-cell lymphoma
      Subtype: primary mediastinal (thymic) B-cell lymphoma
   9. Burkitt's lymphoma
   10. Provisional category: high-grade B-cell lymphoma, Burkitt's-like

T-CELL AND PUTATIVE NK-CELL** NEOPLASMS

I. Precursor T-cell neoplasm: T-precursor lymphoblastic lymphoma/leukemia

II. Peripheral T-cell and NK-cell neoplasms
   1. T-cell chronic lymphocytic leukemia/prolymphocytic leukemia
   2. Large granular lymphocytic leukemia (LGL)
   3. Mycosis fungoides/Sézary's syndrome
   4. Peripheral T-cell lymphoma provisional subtypes: medium-sized cell, mixed medium and large cell, large cell, lymphoepithelioid cell
   5. Angioimmunoblastic T-cell lymphoma (AILD)
   6. Angiocentric lymphoma
   7. Intestinal T-cell lymphoma (+/- enteropathy associated)
   8. Adult T-cell lymphoma/leukemia (ATL/L)
   9. Anaplastic large cell lymphoma (ALCL), CD30+, T- and null-cell types
   10. Provisional subtype: anaplastic large-cell lymphoma, Hodgkin's-like

UNCLASSIFIABLE
   1. B-cell lymphoma, unclassifiable (low grade/high grade)
   2. T-cell lymphoma, unclassifiable (low grade/high grade)
   3. Malignant lymphoma, unclassifiable

*From reference 35.
**NK = natural killer.

congenital immunodeficiency disorders such as ataxia telangiectasia and Wiskott-Aldrich syndrome, in addition to patients subjected to long-term immunosuppressive therapy for the prevention of transplant rejection or for the management of autoimmune disorders such as rheumatoid arthritis, systemic lupus erythematosus, and celiac disease. Also disturbing is the increasing incidence of NHL in patients treated for Hodgkin's disease with combined modality therapy. This incidence is 30 times the expected rate in the normal population and is still rising after 20 years (85).

The etiology and pathogenesis of NHL have been subjects of intense investigation and some speculation for many years. HTLV-1, the human T-cell leukemia/lymphoma virus, characterized as a c-RNA retrovirus,was first isolated in 1980 from a patient in the United States with a cutaneous T-cell lymphoma (64). This proved to be the first link between a retrovirus and human cancer. Adult T-cell leukemia/lymphoma is endemic in several areas of the world including southwestern Japan (86), the Caribbean (17), and the southeastern United States (7,8,13).

The successful establishment of cell lines in tissue cultures of African Burkitt's lymphoma by Epstein, Achong, and Barr (28) led to the discovery of the Epstein-Barr virus (EBV). Although EBV-DNA and EBV nuclear antigen can be detected in the lymphoma cells of 90 percent of children with African Burkitt's lymphoma, a causal relationship between the two has yet to be established. Moreover, EBV infection has been identified in a minority of non-African cases of Burkitt's lymphoma (52). EBV has also been identified in a variety of other NHLs, including almost all cases of post-transplantation lymphoma (65); approximately 50 percent of lymphomas arising in the setting of HIV infection (including 100 percent of the primary central nervous system lymphomas) (53); some cases of post-thymic T-cell lymphoma, particularly angiocentric forms arising in the upper respiratory tract (57,89); and occasional cases of head and neck B-lineage lymphomas (89). However, similar to the situation in Burkitt's lymphoma, a causal link has not yet been established. Nonetheless, these findings do suggest a role for EBV in the pathogenesis of at least some of these lymphomas.

A number of occupational and environmental factors have been invoked as possible causes of NHL, although the data is often weak and often contradictory. An increased risk of disease has been found among persons employed in the agriculture, forestry, fishing, construction, metal working, hair care, painting, dry cleaning, and cosmetology industries (6,77). Some of the increased incidence of NHL among farmers may be accounted for by herbicide exposure (38). The environmental exposure that may be most closely linked to NHL is that of hair dyes (15). Other environmental factors associated with an increased incidence of NHL include exposure to benzene (both follicular and diffuse lymphomas), oils and greases (follicular), solvents other than benzene and formaldehyde (diffuse), chlorophenols, and phenoxyacetic acids (6,77). Low doses of radiation do not appear to be associated with NHL, although NHL does arise infrequently following high-dose, possibly near lethal, radiation treatments (10).

GRADING

The Working Formulation and the Kiel classification both use a grading system (Tables 5-2, 5-3). Low-grade lymphomas include the previously designated "favorable" lymphomas and the intermediate- and high-grade categories include the "unfavorable" lymphomas (69). In the Kiel classification, high grade encompasses all high-grade lymphomas and some intermediate-grade lymphomas of the Working Formulation. The management of patients with NHL is currently based on histologic grade in addition to clinical stage.

Low-grade lymphomas are uncommon in patients younger than 40 years. The median age of patients at the time of presentation is 55 to 66 years, with a slight male predominance. Low-grade lymphomas commonly present in advanced stage, with a high incidence of bone marrow involvement. They have an indolent biologic behavior and are responsive to therapeutic modalities but patients are rarely cured with currently available treatment regimens (70). Relapses occur linearly over time and the disease-free survival curve does not reach a plateau. In contrast, high-grade lymphomas occur over a wide age range, but are proportionately more common in childhood. They present evenly distributed over all stages, with less frequent bone marrow involvement. However, extranodal presentations are more common in high-grade lymphomas. A lower percentage of patients with high-grade lymphomas respond well to therapy, but the chance for cure is much greater than for low-grade lymphomas.

The grading system using the Working Formulation data base was derived from a statistical analysis of the survival of patients treated for lymphoma between 1971 and 1975. It is likely, therefore, that with current therapeutic modalities, the relative survival for patients with NHL might differ considerably. Also, there was little difference in survival between one histologic subtype and another according to the Working Formulation: 5-year survival for the least favorable low-grade lymphoma (follicular mixed) was 50 percent and 45 percent for the most favorable intermediate-grade lymphoma (follicular large cell) (39). Similarly, there was little difference in survival of patients with intermediate-grade lymphomas of the diffuse large cell type and high-grade immunoblastic lymphoma: 35 percent and 32 percent at 5 years, respectively. Moreover, a recent retrospective analysis of 85 carefully studied patients with diffuse large cell lymphoma at Stanford University revealed no significant difference in overall survival of patients subclassified as having intermediate-grade lymphoma of large cell type and high-grade immunoblastic lymphoma (51).

STAGING AND SPREAD

Although the Ann Arbor staging system (Table 5-5) was initially devised for the study of patients with Hodgkin's disease (72), it has also been used for NHL. In most instances, knowledge of the Ann Arbor stage is important in determining the appropriate initial therapy for patients with NHL (71). Clinical stage is limited to information derived from initial clinical staging and biopsy studies (including bone marrow biopsy) while pathologic stage includes information obtained from multiple biopsies obtained at the time of exploratory procedures such as laparotomy.

The Ann Arbor staging scheme is less useful for guiding treatment and predicting prognosis in NHL than Hodgkin's disease (40a,71). With the exception of the nodular lymphocyte predominance form of Hodgkin's disease, a form of con-

siderable controversy at this time, Hodgkin's disease is a relatively homogenous clinicopathologic entity, whereas NHL in all probability represents multiple disorders of the lymphoid system with diverse origins, pathogeneses, and clinical characteristics. A major shortcoming of the Ann Arbor system when applied to NHL is its failure to incorporate consideration for tumor bulk in the designation of stage. In addition, in contrast to Hodgkin's disease, patients with NHL generally do not present with localized disease and have a relatively high incidence of extranodal site involvement. Certain sites of involvement of intermediate- and high-grade lymphomas are associated with a poorer prognosis: bone marrow, gastrointestinal tract, liver, and central nervous system (39). Other clinical factors that are important in planning therapy and predicting outcome for NHL patients include age, bulk of disease, performance status, sex, and serum enzyme levels such as lactate dehydrogenase (LDH) (40a). Some studies have demonstrated declining response rates with increasing patient age with diffuse large cell lymphoma. In some instances, males are associated with a poorer outcome (39).

NHL of all subtypes usually presents in peripheral lymph nodes; this is especially true for small lymphocytic lymphoma and follicular lymphoma in which the lymph node is the initial site of biopsy in over 80 percent of patients (60). Extranodal sites are initially biopsied in up to 30 to 40 percent of cases of NHL, with mediastinal presentation particularly common in lymphoblastic lymphoma, and presentation in the gastrointestinal tract and Waldeyer's ring common in diffuse large cell lymphoma and small noncleaved cell lymphoma.

Comparative studies of the relationship of histology to site in NHL (18,32,48,73) and Hodgkin's disease (27,44,47) have demonstrated that the anatomic distribution of lesions differs considerably. Most significant is the high incidence of gastrointestinal tract, Waldeyer's ring, and mesenteric lymph node involvement by NHL, in contrast with the low incidence in Hodgkin's disease (60, 73). In past years, mesenteric lymph node involvement represented occult disease not demonstrable by lymphangiography (16); however, recently developed radiologic techniques such as computerized tomography (CT) and magnetic resonance imaging (MRI)

Table 5-5

ANN ARBOR STAGING CLASSIFICATION SYSTEM*

Stage I	Involvement of a single lymph node region (I) or a single extralymphatic organ or site (E)
Stage II	Involvement of two or more lymph node regions on the same side of the diaphragm (II) or localized involvement of an extralymphatic organ or site and one or more lymph node regions on the same side of the diaphragm (IIE)
Stage III	Involvement of lymph node regions on both sides of the diaphragm (III), which may also be accompanied by involvement of the spleen (IIIS) or by localized involvement of an extralymphatic organ or site (IIIE) or both (IIISE)
Stage IV	Diffuse or disseminated involvement of one or more extralymphatic organs or tissues, with or without associated lymph node involvement

*The presence or absence of the classic systemic symptoms (fever, night sweats, or unexplained loss of 10 percent or more of body weight) in the 6 months preceding admission is denoted by the letters B and A, respectively. Biopsy-documented involvement of stage IV sites is also denoted by letter suffixes: marrow = M+, lung = L+, liver = H+, pleura = P+, bone = O+, skin and subcutaneous tissue = D+.

have enabled clinicians to identify these sites of involvement. The incidence of splenic disease in NHL compares with that seen in Hodgkin's disease. Approximately 50 percent of affected spleens are of normal weight and size and may not be detected by clinical methods (39,48). However, NHL shows a greater tendency for dissemination to liver and bone marrow in untreated patients when compared with Hodgkin's disease, with an approximately 50 percent incidence of involvement of each site at presentation (18). Recognition of this high incidence of systemic involvement, along with the limited importance of precise staging in treatment decisions, has made laparotomy unnecessary in the staging of NHL. In contrast, the incidence of hilar/mediastinal involvement in patients with NHL is generally lower than that observed in Hodgkin's disease.

Follicular lymphomas show a particular tendency for widespread dissemination because they involve abdominal organs (spleen, liver, and abdominal lymph nodes: 72 percent) and the bone marrow (80 to 85 percent). Peripheral blood involvement by low-grade lymphomas was recognized many years ago by Rosenthal et al. (74) and Rappaport et al. (68) who identified the "notched-nucleus" cell in the peripheral blood of patients with follicular lymphomas. Currently, flow cytometry and genotyping are used to identify neoplastic cells in the peripheral blood that are undetected by morphologic examination (40,82).

Some subtypes of NHL overlap with leukemia because of their widespread involvement in the peripheral blood and bone marrow. Thus, B-lineage small lymphocytic lymphoma may represent a spectrum of the same biologic disease as B-cell chronic lymphocytic leukemia, although many clinicians continue to distinguish the two for clinical reasons. Similarly, T-cell lymphoblastic lymphoma shares many biologic similarities with T-cell acute lymphoblastic leukemia, with the arbitrary clinical distinction made on the relative degree of involvement of the peripheral blood and bone marrow.

There may be a greater variation in histologic and cytologic features in individual NHL patients at presentation or during the subsequent course of the disease (20). A variety of terms have been applied to changes in architectural pattern or cell type. Evolution or transformation implies progression from a low-grade to a higher grade lymphoma: small lymphocytic progressing to large cell lymphoma or follicular small cleaved to diffuse large cell type. Composite lymphomas comprise those that have two distinct architectural and cytologic lymphoma subtypes occurring at the same anatomic tissue or site at the same time (33,49). The term discordant has been applied to lymphomas that have divergent histologic features in different anatomic sites and this has been reported in 30 percent of patients who undergo multiple biopsies within a short period of time (see chapter 17) (29,56).

Although less frequently associated with NHL (2 percent) than with Hodgkin's disease (12 percent), isolated sarcoid-like granulomata can be observed in the spleen, liver, lymph nodes, and bone marrow of patients undergoing surgical staging procedures (43,48). Their presence has not influenced staging criteria or treatment decisions since these granulomata are not considered evidence of lymphomatous involvement of the respective organs in which they are identified. The nature of these granulomata has been the subject of much speculation; however, in patients with Hodgkin's disease, granulomata are associated with a better survival rate. They may represent an unusual "host response" to the neoplastic disorder (75). Similar studies have yet to be performed on patients with NHL. On the other hand, prominent epithelioid granulomas may mask an underlying NHL or may erroneously be interpreted as sarcoidosis (12).

A special section on extranodal lymphomas has not been included in this Fascicle. These are discussed in other tumor Fascicles according to the site of involvement. Nonetheless, appropriate references will be made to such lymphomas in the ensuing chapters.

REFERENCES

1. Acker B, Hoppe RT, Colby TV, Cox RS, Kaplan HS, Rosenberg SA. Histologic conversion in the non-Hodgkin lymphomas. J Clin Oncol 1983;1:11–6.
2. Agnarsson BA, Kadin ME. Ki-1 positive large cell lymphoma. A morphologic and immunologic study of 19 cases. Am J Surg Pathol 1988;12:264–74.
3. Bennett MH, Farrer-Brown G, Henry K, Jelliffe AM. Classification of non-Hodgkin's lymphomas. Lancet 1974;2:405–6.
4. Berard CW, Dorfman RF. Histopathology of malignant lymphomas. Clin Hematol 1974;3:39–76.
5. _____, O'Conor GT, Thomas LB, et al. Histopathological definition of Burkitt's tumor. Bulletin No. 40. Geneva: World Health Organization, 1969;40:601–7.
6. Blair A, Linos A, Stewart PA, et al. Comments on occupational and environmental factors in the origin of non-Hodgkin's lymphoma. Cancer Res 1992;52(19 Suppl):5501–2s.
7. Blayney DW, Jaffe ES, Blattner WA, et al. The human T-cell leukemia/lymphoma virus (HTLV) associated with American adult T-cell leukemia/lymphoma (ATL). Blood 1983;62:401–5.
8. _____, Jaffe ES, Fisher RI, et al. The human T-cell leukemia/lymphoma virus (HTLV), lymphoma, lytic bone lesions, and hypercalcemia. Ann Intern Med 1983;98:144–51.
9. Bloomfield CD, Goldman A, Dick F, Brunning RD, Kennedy BJ. Multivariate analysis of prognostic factors in the non-Hodgkin's malignant lymphoma. Cancer 1974;33:870–9.
10. Boice JD. Radiation and non-Hodgkin's lymphoma. Cancer Res 1992;52 (Suppl):5489–91s.
11. Boring CC, Squires TS, Tong T. Cancer statistics, 1993. CA Cancer J Clin 1993;43:7–26.
12. Braylan RC, Long JC, Jaffe ES, Greco FA, Orr SL, Berard CW. Malignant lymphoma obscured by concomitant extensive epithelioid granulomas: report of three cases with similar clinicopathologic features. Cancer 1977;39:1146–55.
13. Broder S, Bunn PA, Jaffe ES, Greco FA, Orr SL, Berard CW. T-cell lymphoproliferative syndrome associated with human T-cell leukemia/lymphoma virus. Ann Intern Med 1984;100:543–57.
14. Brown TC, Peters MV, Bergsagel DE, Reid J. A retrospective analysis of the clinical results in relation to the Rappaport histological classification. Br J Cancer 1975;31(Suppl 2):174–86.
15. Cantor KP, Blair A, Everett G, et al. Hair dye use and risk of leukemia and lymphoma. Am J Public Health 1988;78:570–1.
16. Castellino RA, Billingham M, Dorfman RF. Lymphographic accuracy in Hodgkin's disease and malignant lymphoma with a note on the reactive lymph node as a cause of most false-positive lymphograms. Invest Radiol 1974;9:155–65.
17. Catovsky D, Greaves MF, Rose M, et al. Adult T-cell lymphoma-leukemia in Blacks from the West Indies. Lancet 1982;1:639–43.
18. Chabner BA, Johnson RE, Young RC, et al. Sequential non-surgical and surgical staging of the non-Hodgkin's lymphomas. Ann Intern Med 1987;83:149–54.
19. Classification of non-Hodgkin's lymphomas: reproducibility of major classification systems. NCI Non-Hodgkin's Classification Project Writing Committee. Cancer 1985;55:91–5.
20. Cullen MH, Lister TA, Brearley RI, Shand WS, Stansfeld AG. Histopathologic transformation of non-Hodgkin's lymphoma: a prospective study. Cancer 1979;44:645–51.
21. Devesa SS, Fears T. Non-Hodgkin's lymphoma time trends: United States and International data. Cancer Res 1992;52(19 Suppl):5432–40s.
22. DeVita VT, Hubbard SM. The curative potential of chemotherapy in the treatment of Hodgkin's disease and non-Hodgkin's lymphomas. In: Rosenberg S, Kaplan HS, eds. Malignant lymphomas. Etiology, immunology, pathology, treatment. Bristol-Myers Cancer Symposia. New York: Academic Press, 1982:379–418.

23. _____, Rappaport H, Frei E. Announcement of formation of the Lymphoma Task Force and Pathology Reference Center. Cancer 1968;2:1087–8.

24. Dorfman RF. Classification of non-Hodgkin's lymphomas [Letter]. Lancet 1974;1:1295–6.

25. _____. Classification of non-Hodgkin's lymphomas [Letter]. Lancet 1974;2:961–2.

26. _____. The non-Hodgkin's lymphomas. In: Rebuck J, Berard CW, Abell MR, eds. The reticuloendothelial system. Baltimore: Williams & Wilkins, 1975:262–81. (International Academy of Pathology Vol 16.)

27. _____. Relationship of histology to site in Hodgkin's disease. Cancer Res 1971;31:1786–93.

28. Epstein MA, Achong BG, Barr YM. Virus particles in cultured lymphoblasts from Burkitt's lymphoma. Lancet 1964;1:702–3.

29. Fisher RI, Jones RB, DeVita VT Jr, et al. Natural history of malignant lymphomas with divergent histologies at staging evaluation. Cancer 1981;47:2022–5.

30. Frizzera G, Murphy SB. Follicular (nodular) lymphoma in childhood: a rare clinico-pathological entity. Report of eight cases from four cancer centers. Cancer 1979;44:2218–35.

31. Gerard-Marchant R, Hamlin I, Lennert K, Rilke F, Stansfeld AG, Van Unnik JAM. Classification of non-Hodgkin's lymphomas. Lancet 1974;2:406–8.

32. Goffinet DR, Warnke R, Dunnick NR, et al. Clinical and surgical (laparotomy) evaluation of patients with non-Hodgkin's lymphomas. Cancer Treat Rep 1977;61:981–92.

33. Gonzales C, Medeiros J, Jaffe ES. Composite lymphoma: a clinicopathologic analysis of nine patients with Hodgkin's disease and B-cell non-Hodgkin's lymphoma. Am J Clin Pathol 1991;96:81–9.

34. Hale S, Gatter KC, Heryet A, Mason DY. The value of immunocytochemistry in differentiating high-grade lymphoma from other anaplastic tumors: a study of anaplastic tumors from 1940-1960. Leuk Lymphoma 1989;1:59–63.

35. Harrington DS, Ye YL, Weisenburger DD, et al. Malignant lymphoma in Nebraska and Guangzhou, China: a comparative study. Hum Pathol 1987;18:924–8.

36. Harris NL, Jaffe ES, Stein H, et al. A revised European-American classification of lymphoid neoplasms: a proposal from the International Lymphoma Study Group. Blood 1994;84:1361–92.

37. Hastrup N, Hamilton-Dutoit S, Ralfkiaer E, Pallesen G. Peripheral T-cell lymphomas: an evaluation of reproducibility of the updated Kiel classification. Histopathology 1991;18:99–105.

38. Hoar SK, Blair A, Holmes FF, et al. Agricultural herbicide use and risk of lymphoma and soft tissue sarcoma. JAMA 1986;256:1141–7.

39. Hoppe RT. The non-Hodgkin's lymphomas: pathology, staging, treatment. Curr Probl Cancer 1987;11:363–447.

40. Horning SJ, Galili N, Cleary ML, Sklar J. Detection of non-Hodgkin's lymphoma in the peripheral blood by analysis of antigen receptor gene rearrangements: results of a prospective study. Blood 1990;75:1139–45.

40a. International Non-Hodgkin's Lymphoma Prognostic Factors Project: a predictive model for aggressive non-Hodgkin's lymphoma. N Engl J Med 1993;329:987–94.

41. Isaacson PJ. Lymphomas of mucosa-associated lymphoid tissue (MALT). Histopathology 1990;16:617–9.

42. Jones SE, Fuks Z, Bull M, et al. Non-Hodgkin's lymphomas. IV. Clinicopathologic correlation in 405 cases. Cancer 1973;31:806–23.

43. Kadin ME, Donaldson SS, Dorfman RF. Isolated granulomas in Hodgkin's disease. N Engl J Med 1970;283:859–61.

44. _____, Glatstein E, Dorfman RF. Clinicopathologic studies of 117 untreated patients subjected to laparotomy for the staging of Hodgkin's disease. Cancer 1971;27:1277–94.

45. _____, Sako D, Berliner N, et al. Childhood Ki-1 lymphoma presenting with skin lesions and peripheral lymphadenopathy. Blood 1986;68:1042–9.

46. Kant JA, Hubbard SM, Longo DL, Simon RM, DeVita VT Jr, Jaffe ES. The pathologic and clinical heterogeneity of lymphocyte-depleted Hodgkin's disease. J Clin Oncol 1986;4:284–94.

47. Kaplan HS, Dorfman RF, Nelson TS, Rosenberg SA. Staging laparotomy and splenectomy in Hodgkin's disease: analysis of indications and patterns of involvement in 285 consecutive, unselected patients. Natl Cancer Inst Monogr 1973;36:291–301.

48. Kim H, Dorfman RF. Morphological studies of 84 untreated patients subjected to laparotomy for the staging of non-Hodgkin's lymphomas. Cancer 1974;33:657–74.

49. _____, Hendrickson R, Dorfman RF. Composite lymphoma. Cancer 1977;40:959–76.

50. _____, Zelman RJ, Fox MA et al. Pathology panel for Lymphoma Clinical Studies: a comprehensive analysis of cases accumulated since its inception. JNCI 1982;68:43–67.

51. Kwak LW, Wilson M, Weiss LM, Horning SJ, Warnke RA, Dorfman RF. Clinical significance of morphologic subdivision in diffuse large cell lymphoma. Cancer 1991;68:1988–93.

52. Lenoir GM, Philip T, Sohier R. Burkitt-type lymphoma—EBV-association and cytogenetic markers in cases from various geographic locations. In: Magrath IT, O'Conor GT, Ramot B, eds. Pathogenesis of leukemias and lymphomas: environmental influences. New York: Raven Press, 1984:283–95.

53. Levine AM, Shibata D, Sullivan-Halley J, et al. Epidemiological and biological study of acquired immunodeficiency syndrome-related lymphoma in the county of Los Angeles: preliminary results. Cancer Res 1992;52(19 Suppl):5482–4s.

54. Lukes RJ, Collins RD. Immunological characterization of human malignant lymphomas. Cancer 1974;34(4 Suppl):1488–503.

55. Mathe G, Rappaport H, O'Conor GT, et al. Histological and cytological typing of neoplastic diseases of haematopoietic and lymphoid tissues. International Histological Classification of Tumors, No. 14. Geneva: World Health Organization, 1976.

56. Mead GM, Kushlan P, O'Neil M, Burke JS, Rosenberg SA. Clinical aspects of non-Hodgkin's lymphomas presenting with discordant histologic subtypes. Cancer 1983;52:1496–501.

57. Medeiros LJ, Jaffe ES, Chen YY, Weiss LM. Localization of Epstein-Barr viral genomes in angiocentric immunoproliferative lesions. Am J Surg Pathol 1992;16:439–47.

58. Molina A, Lombard C, Donlon T, Bangs CD, Dorfman RF. Immunohistochemical and cytogenetic studies indicate that malignant angioendotheliomatosis is a primary intravascular (angiotropic) lymphoma. Cancer 1990;66:474–9.

59. Nathwani BN, Kim H, Rappaport H. Malignant lymphoma, lymphoblastic. Cancer 1976;38:964–83.

60. National Cancer Institute sponsored study of classifications of non-Hodgkin's lymphomas: summary and description of a working formulation for clinical usage. The Non-Hodgkin's Lymphoma Pathologic Classification Project. Cancer 1982;49:2112–35.

61. Ng CS, Chan JK, Lo ST, Poon YF. Immunophenotypic analysis of non-Hodgkin's lymphomas in Chinese. A study of 765 cases in Hong Kong. Pathology 1986; 18:419–25.

62. Ngan BY, Warnke RA, Wilson M, Takagi K, Cleary ML, Dorfman RF. Monocytoid B-cell lymphoma: a study of 36 cases. Hum Pathol 1991;22:409–21.

63. Pinto A, Hutchison RE, Grant L, Trevenen CL, Berard CW. Follicular lymphomas in pediatric patients. Mod Pathol 1990;3:308–13.

64. Poiesz BJ, Ruscetti FW, Gazdar AF, Bunn PA, Minna JD, Gallo RC. Detection and isolation of type-C retrovirus particles from fresh and cultured lymphocytes of a patient with cutaneous T-cell lymphoma. Proc Natl Acad Sci USA 1980;77:7415–9.

65. Randhawa PS, Jaffe R, Demetris AJ, et al. The systemic distribution of Epstein-Barr virus genomes in fatal post-transplantation lymphoproliferative disorders. An in situ hybridization study. Am J Pathol 1991;138:1027–33.

66. Rappaport H. Tumors of the hematopoietic system. Atlas of Tumor Pathology, 1st Series, Fascicle 8. Washington, D.C.: Armed Forces Institute of Pathology, 1966:47–61.

67. _____, Braylan RC. Changing concepts in the classification of malignant neoplasms of the hematopoietic system. In: Rebuck J, Berard CW, Abell MR, eds. The reticuloendothelial system. Baltimore: Williams & Wilkins, 1975:1–19. (International Academy of Pathology, Vol. 16.)

68. _____, Winter WJ, Hicks EB. Follicular lymphoma. A re-evaluation of its position in the scheme of malignant lymphoma, based on a survey of 253 cases. Cancer 1956;9:792–821.

69. Rosenberg SA. Current concepts in cancer: non-Hodgkin's lymphoma—selection of treatment on the basis of histologic type. N Engl J Med 1979;301:924–8.

70. _____. Karnovsky Memorial Lecture. The low-grade non-Hodgkin's lymphoma: challenges and opportunities. J Clin Oncol 1985;3:299–310.

71. _____. Validity of the Ann Arbor staging classification for the non-Hodgkin's lymphomas. Cancer Treat Rep 1977;61:1023–87.

72. _____, Boiron M, DeVita VT Jr, et al. Report of the Committee on Hodgkin's Disease Staging Procedures. Cancer Res 1971;31:1862–3.

73. _____, Dorfman RF, Kaplan HS. A summary of the results of a review of 405 patients with non-Hodgkin's lymphoma at Stanford University. Br J Cancer 1975; 31:168–73.

74. Rosenthal N, Dreskin OH, Vural IL, Zak FG. The significance of hematogones in blood, bone marrow and lymph node aspiration in giant follicular lymphoblastoma. Acta Hematol 1952;8:368–77.

75. Sacks EL, Donaldson SS, Gordon J, Dorfman RF. Epithelioid granulomas associated with Hodgkin's disease: clinical correlations in 55 previously untreated patients. Cancer 1978;41:562–7.

76. Schein PS, Chabner BA, Canellos GP, Young RC, Berard C, DeVita VT. Potential for prolonged disease-free survival following combination chemotherapy of non-Hodgkin's lymphoma. Blood 1974;43:181–9.

77. Scherr PA, Hutchison GB, Neiman RS. Non-Hodgkin's lymphoma an occupational exposure. Cancer Res 1992;52(19 Suppl):5503–9s.

78. Sheibani K, Battifora H, Winberg CD, et al. Further evidence that malignant angioendotheliomatosis is an angiotrophic large cell lymphoma. N Engl J Med 1986;314:943–8.

79. _____, Sohn CC, Burke JS, Winberg CD, Wu AM, Rappaport H. Monocytoid B-cell lymphoma: a novel B-cell neoplasm. Am J Pathol 1986;124:310–8.

80. Silverberg E, Lubera J. Cancer statistics, 1987. CA Cancer J Clin 1987;37:2–19.

81. Simon R, Durrleman S, Hoppe RT, et al. The Non-Hodgkin's Lymphoma Pathologic Classification Project. Long-term follow-up of 1153 patients with non-Hodgkin's lymphomas. Ann Intern Med 1988; 109:939–45.

82. Smith BR, Weinberg DS, Robert NJ, et al. Circulating monoclonal B lymphocytes in non-Hodgkin's lymphoma. N Engl J Med 1984;311:1476–81.

83. Stansfeld AG, Diebold J, Kapanci Y, et al. Updated Kiel classification [Letter]. Lancet 1988;1:292–3.

84. Suchi T, Lennert K, Tu LY, et al. Histopathology and immunohistochemistry of peripheral T-cell lymphomas: a proposal for their classification. J Clin Pathol 1987;40:995–1015.

85. Tucker MA, Coleman CN, Cox RS, Vorghese A, Rosenberg SA. Risk of second cancers after treatment for Hodgkin's disease. N Engl J Med 1988;318:76–81.

86. Uchiyama T, Yodoi J, Sagawa K, Takatsuki K, Uchino H. Adult T-cell leukemia: clinical and hematologic features of 16 cases. Blood 1977;50:481–92.

87. Warnke RA. Tumor progression in malignant lymphomas. Bull Cancer (Paris) 1991;78:181–6.

88. _____, Gatter KC, Falini B, et al. Diagnosis of human lymphoma with monoclonal antileukocyte antibodies. N Engl J Med 1983;309:1275–81.

89. Weiss LM, Gaffey MJ, Chen YY, Frierson HF Jr. Frequency of Epstein-Barr viral DNA in Western sino-nasal and Waldeyer's ring lymphomas. Am J Surg Pathol 1992;16:156–62.

90. Winberg CD, Nathwani BN, Bearman RN, Rappaport H. Follicular (nodular) lymphoma during the first two decades of life: a clinicopathologic study of 12 cases. Cancer 1981;48:2233–35.

91. Ziegler JL, Beckstead JA, Volberding PA, et al. Non-Hodgkin's lymphoma in 90 homosexual men: relationship to generalized lymphadenopathy and acquired immunodeficiency syndrome (AIDS). N Engl J Med 1984;311:565–70.

6

MALIGNANT LYMPHOMA, FOLLICULAR
(SMALL CLEAVED, MIXED, AND LARGE CELL; CENTROBLASTIC-CENTROCYTIC AND CENTROBLASTIC)

Definition. Follicular lymphoma is a B-cell neoplasm that recapitulates both the architectural and cytologic features of the normal secondary lymphoid follicle. It is composed of a variable admixture of small cleaved cells (centrocytes) and large cleaved/noncleaved cells (centroblasts) (66,105,117,130,148,219,237). In the Rappaport classification, follicular lymphoma is known as *nodular lymphoma*. In the Working Formulation (48,176), there are three categories of follicular lymphoma: *predominantly small cleaved cell; mixed small cleaved and large cell;* and *predominantly large cell*. The first two categories are sometimes grouped under the umbrella term *low-grade follicular lymphoma*. Follicular lymphoma of predominantly large cell type is considered *intermediate grade* because of its more aggressive behavior (94,144, 188). In the updated Kiel classification, most cases are classified as centroblastic-centrocytic; others are placed in the centroblastic category (129,130,218).

Incidence. There are geographic differences in the frequency and absolute incidence of follicular lymphoma, and the disease is more common in whites (89,176). In the United States, the percentage of follicular lymphomas among non-Hodgkin lymphomas ranges from 20 to 40 percent (79,89,171,176); in Britain and Germany, it is approximately 20 percent (60,130,171); in Asia and Africa it is only about 10 percent (33,46,79, 107,138,169,171,182,212).

Natural History and Clinical Features. Follicular lymphoma is predominantly a disease of adults, and the median age of patients at the time of presentation is 55 years (89). There is an approximately equal sex incidence or slight female predominance (130,176).

Patients usually present with lymphadenopathy, which typically involves multiple sites. The enlarged lymph nodes are often painless and of insidious onset. There may be a history of waxing and waning enlargement of the nodes. Approximately 20 percent of patients have systemic symptoms (5). Some patients also have splenomegaly. Less than 10 percent of patients have extranodal presentation in the absence of nodal involvement (145). Rarely, patients present with lymphocytosis, but physical examination almost always reveals significant lymphadenopathy (218).

Follicular lymphoma is essentially a disseminated disease. Patients usually present with high-stage disease: over 80 percent are stage III to IV (28,71). Surgical staging shows abdominal organ involvement in more than 70 percent of patients, including spleen (25 to 55 percent), splenic hilar and para-aortic lymph nodes (greater than 50 percent), and mesenteric lymph nodes (68 percent) (27,71,89,111). Morphologic assessment shows bone marrow involvement in 40 percent of cases (40,176,203), and peripheral blood involvement is common.

Follicular lymphoma has an indolent natural history, characterized by stability of disease, slow progression, continuous and repeated relapses despite achievement of complete remission with treatment, tendency to undergo spontaneous remission, and response to immune manipulation (5,93,204). The overall spontaneous regression rate is 23 percent, with an even higher rate (30 percent) in patients with the small cleaved cell subtype (93,194). The duration of spontaneous regression is usually longer than 1 year and may be indefinite, although the tumor eventually relapses in most cases.

There is a strong tendency for follicular lymphoma to progress to large B-cell lymphoma, irrespective of whether or not treatment is given. At 5 to 10 years after diagnosis, lymph node biopsies from as many as 50 percent of patients undergoing a second biopsy procedure show evidence of transformation to a more aggressive histologic subtype (204). It is estimated that 60 to 80 percent of cases transform during the clinical course (44,64,199). Moreover, in those patients with follicular lymphoma who die of their disease, the lymphoma only rarely retains the initial follicular pattern (64). An undetected "composite lymphoma" at disease onset should be considered in those patients whose tumors undergo histologic transformation (114). Conversely, diffuse large cell lymphomas sometimes relapse as follicular lymphoma after therapy (86,152).

Follicular lymphomas in children have the following characteristics, in contrast to the more common adult form: presentation with localized (stage I to II) disease; frequent involvement of the head and neck or inguinal region; a mixed cell or large cell histologic composition; and a favorable outcome (59,191,242,243).

Follicular lymphomas occurring in the second decade of life have a biologic behavior similar to that in adults (242).

Microscopic Findings. *Architectural Features.* In the prototypic case, a lymph node involved by follicular lymphoma shows a uniform nodularity with little variation in the size and shape of the follicles. There is a back-to-back arrangement of follicles; these follicles are less well-defined than reactive germinal centers because they possess a limited mantle zone or lack a mantle zone altogether (figs. 6-1, 6-2). There may be peripheral fading and coalescence of follicles (fig. 6-3). The intervening lymphoid stroma, including venules and reticulin fibers, is compressed between the expanding follicles, a feature best demonstrated by silver impregnation (fig. 6-4). Because of the marked crowding, the density of the follicles (frequently more than 40 follicles per 40X magnification field, with a median of 47) is statistically higher than that seen in reactive follicular hyperplasia (median, 30 follicles) (168). Infiltration of the nodal capsule and perinodal blood vessels by lymphoma cells is not uncommon, and neoplastic follicles can be formed in the perinodal adipose tissue (fig. 6-5).

In other cases, the histologic architecture deviates from that described above. In such cases, a diagnosis of lymphoma is based on assessment of all histologic features, and may require support by ancillary studies. The neoplastic follicles can vary significantly in size and shape, including formation of large, irregularly shaped or serrated follicles (figs. 6-5, top; 6-6). The follicles are sometimes not crowded, and are instead separated by an appreciable amount of interfollicular lymphoid tissue (fig. 6-7). Some follicles have

well-defined or even thick mantle zones (figs. 6-7, right; 6-8–6-10). There may even be incomplete involvement of a lymph node, with reactive follicles and patent sinuses still identifiable in some areas of the node (fig. 6-11) (46,47,198).

Cytologic Composition. The germinal center of a reactive follicle often shows cellular polarization: the pale-staining area ("pale zone") beneath the eccentric mantle cap is composed predominantly of small cleaved cells (centrocytes), and the darker-staining area ("dark zone") opposite the lymphoid cap is composed mainly of large noncleaved cells (centroblasts) (fig. 6-12). This phenomenon is readily observed in lymphoid follicles of the tonsil, but can be difficult to appreciate in lymph nodes. Cellular polarization is almost never seen in follicular lymphoma, although it is present in rare cases of follicular mixed cell lymphoma, in which the larger cells may aggregate at one pole of the follicle (fig. 6-13).

The germinal centers of reactive follicles are typically composed of a mixture of small cleaved cells (centrocytes) and large noncleaved cells (centroblasts), with the latter often outnumbering the former, especially in the florid follicles (fig. 6-14). Mitotic figures are readily identified. In follicular lymphoma, the cellular composition is variable depending on the subtype (fig. 6-15). The predominantly small cleaved cell subtype comprises a monomorphous population of small cleaved cells (centrocytes) with few large lymphoid cells (fig. 6-16). The predominantly large cell subtype comprises large lymphoid cells (centroblasts) forming a monotonous population or intermingled with small cleaved cells (centrocytes) (fig. 6-17). Mitotic count is often low, except for the large cell subtype.

Within the neoplastic follicles are scattered small T lymphocytes and follicular dendritic cells. The small T lymphocytes have round or slightly irregular nuclei, and do not show the often elongated contours of small cleaved cells; the reactive T lymphocytes sometimes have an activated appearance. The follicular dendritic cells, which form discrete meshworks in the follicles, are best visualized by immunohistochemical staining. However, they can also be recognized histologically by their round to ovoid empty-looking nuclei, delicate and violaceous-staining nuclear membrane, small central nucleolus, indistinct cell borders, and occasional

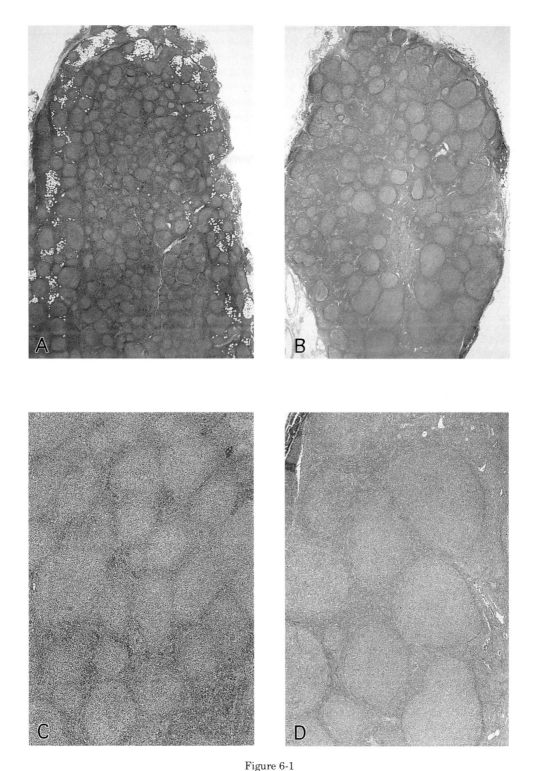

Figure 6-1
FOLLICULAR LYMPHOMA: LYMPH NODE SHOWING PROTOTYPIC HISTOLOGIC FEATURES
A: This case shows a uniform nodularity throughout the lymph node with little variation in size and shape of the follicles which show a back-to-back arrangement. Follicles are also seen in the perinodal adipose tissue.
B: Another example showing tightly packed, fairly uniform follicles distributed throughout the nodal parenchyma.
C,D: Poorly defined follicles show a back-to-back arrangement, lack of cellular polarization, and absence of tingible body macrophages. There is more variation in the size of the follicles in D.

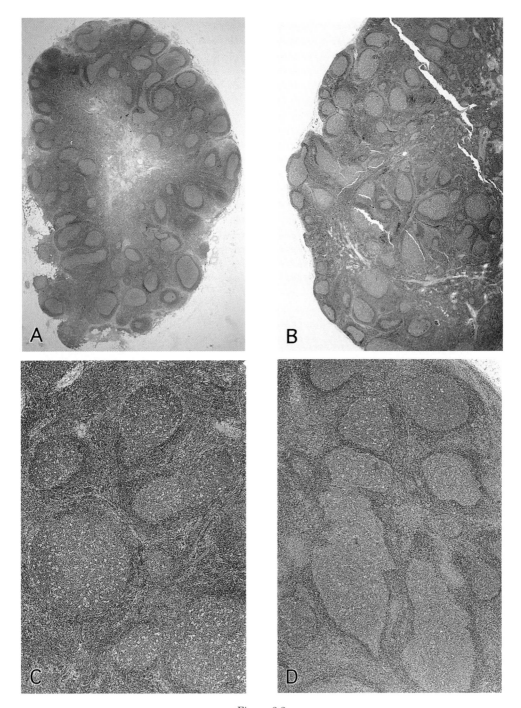

Figure 6-2
REACTIVE FOLLICULAR HYPERPLASIA: LYMPH NODE

A: Discrete follicles, which are well separated by interfollicular tissue, are disposed predominantly in the cortex. Since the follicles are not crowded, there are fewer follicles per unit area compared with figure 6-1A. In this example, the follicles are mostly round or ovoid.

B: Another typical example, showing marked variation in size of the reactive follicles, which are well delimited by mantles and separated by an appreciable amount of interfollicular tissue. In this case, the follicles are distributed throughout the entire node. Again there are fewer follicles per unit area compared with figure 6-1B.

C: The germinal centers are surrounded by mantles and show cellular polarization, i.e., aggregation of large follicular center cells and tingible body macrophages opposite the eccentric lymphoid (mantle) cap.

D: Reactive follicles are frequently irregular and surrounded by discrete mantles. Note the "starry-sky" appearance of the follicles imparted by the tingible body macrophages.

Table 6-1

**REPORTED CLINICAL SIGNIFICANCE OF THE PRESENCE
OF DIFFUSE AREAS IN FOLLICULAR LYMPHOMAS**

Report	Impact of Presence of Diffuse Areas on Prognosis
Warnke 1977 (236)	FSCL and FML: no influence on prognosis for up to 50 percent diffuse areas
Colby et al. 1980 (39)	FSCL: geater than 25 percent diffuse areas associated with worse prognosis compared with purely follicular tumors FML, FLCL: insufficient cases for statistical analysis
Hu et al. 1985 (96)	FML: worse prognosis only with 50 percent or more diffuse areas
Ezdinli et al. 1987 (53)	FSCL, FML: worse prognosis if greater than 25 percent diffuse areas (median survival 39.6 months, versus 68.2 months for purely follicular tumors)
Weisenburger et al. 1991 (238)	FSCL: no effect FML, FLCL: worse prognosis if greater than 40 percent diffuse areas
Bastion et al. 1991 (11)	No influence
Bartlett et al. 1994 (9)	FLCL: increasing areas of diffuse histology associated with worse prognosis compared with purely follicular tumors

FSCL = follicular small cleaved cell lymphoma; FML = follicular mixed small cleaved and large cell lymphoma; FLCL = follicular large cell lymphoma.

binucleation (figs. 6-16, 6-18). There can be scattered polykaryocytes (115). Plasma cells are rarely seen in neoplastic follicles.

In contrast to reactive follicles, the follicles of follicular lymphoma usually exhibit a conspicuous absence of tingible body macrophages (fig. 6-19). Consistent absence of these macrophages in all follicles is a feature strongly favoring a diagnosis of follicular lymphoma over reactive follicular hyperplasia, although occasional cases of follicular lymphoma, especially the large cell subtype, do exhibit these macrophages (fig. 6-20). In patients who have received steroid therapy prior to lymph node biopsy, the follicles may also show a striking starry-sky pattern, reflecting phagocytosis of degenerating nuclear material by tingible body macrophages. In some instances, the neoplastic follicles contain epithelioid histiocytes with or without formation of granulomas; the significance of this is not clear (111).

In some cases of follicular lymphoma, atypical lymphoid cells with cleaved nuclei (neoplastic cells) can be identified in the interfollicular lymphoid stroma and this occurrence is readily highlighted by immunostaining with B-lineage markers (fig. 6-21). This contrasts with reactive lymphoid hyperplasia, in which the paracortical and interfollicular zones are occupied by normal-appearing small lymphocytes (predominated by T-lineage cells).

Diffuse Component in Follicular Lymphoma. In many cases, a diffuse pattern of infiltration accompanies the follicular component. The presence of any degree of follicular architecture identifies a lymphoma as follicular lymphoma. When a diffuse component is present, the qualifying term "follicular, with diffuse areas" or "follicular and diffuse" is often applied, although the terms have not been precisely defined. The following terminology has recently been proposed by Harris and Ferry (83): follicular, more than 75 percent follicular; follicular and diffuse, 25 to 75 percent follicular; and focally follicular, less than 25 percent follicular.

The presence of atypical, presumably neoplastic, lymphoid cells in the narrow interfollicular zones alone does not qualify as a diffuse component, which is defined by the occurrence of microscopic fields of diffuse lymphomatous infiltration (with cytologic features of follicular center cells) that lack interspersed neoplastic follicles (fig. 6-22). The diffuse areas commonly show sclerosis and an increased infiltrate of reactive small T lymphocytes.

In follicular lymphoma, the diffuse component tends to increase over time (104,144). A number of studies have addressed the prognostic implications of diffuse areas in various subtypes of follicular lymphoma (Table 6-1). The results are conflicting, probably because of difficulties in

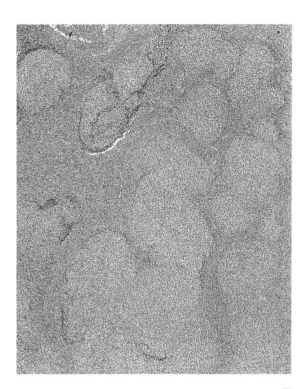

Figure 6-3
FOLLICULAR LYMPHOMA: LYMPH NODE
Ill-defined follicles show peripheral fading and coalescence, a phenomenon that is more striking in the right figure.

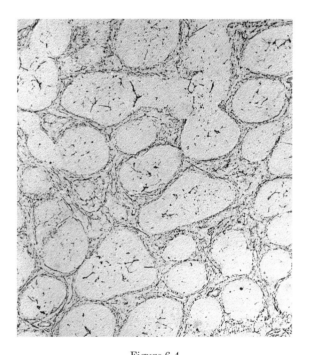

Figure 6-4
FOLLICULAR LYMPHOMA: LYMPH NODE
Silver impregnated section demonstrates compression of reticulin fibers and venules between the follicles.

quantitation of the diffuse component, sampling problems, poor reproducibility in the subclassification of follicular lymphomas, and different therapies used. Nonetheless, most studies do show at least a trend towards a better survival for the purely follicular tumors versus those with a diffuse component, although the difference may not be statistically significant (9,11,18,39,68,76, 96,176,188,236,238). It appears that for follicular small cleaved cell lymphoma and mixed cell lymphoma, the prognosis is worsened only if the diffuse areas contribute at least 25 to 50 percent of the tumor (39,53,96,238); however, for follicular large cell lymphoma, even a minor diffuse component may worsen the prognosis (Table 6-1) (9).

Histologic Transformation to a Diffuse Large Cell Lymphoma. Diffuse foci in a follicular lymphoma must be distinguished from transformation to a diffuse large cell lymphoma, which is associated with a markedly worse prognosis. Histologic transformation is evidenced by a significant increase in large lymphoid cells, which often form solid clusters and sheets. These large cells usually have the cytologic features of large noncleaved

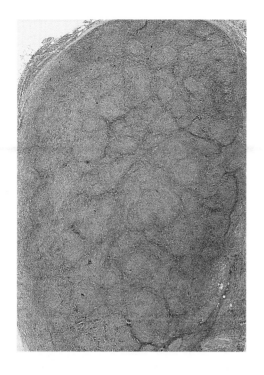

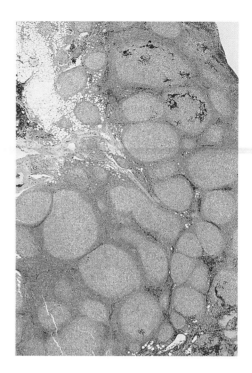

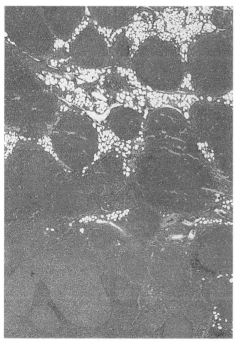

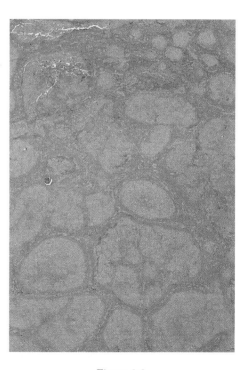

Figure 6-5
FOLLICULAR LYMPHOMA: LYMPH NODE

Top: The follicles are vague and show peripheral fading/coalescence. Capsular infiltration (not in the form of follicles) is seen in the left upper field.

Bottom: In this case, neoplastic follicles have breached the capsule and are found in the perinodal adipose tissue, a feature strongly favoring a diagnosis of follicular lymphoma over reactive follicular hyperplasia.

Figure 6-6
FOLLICULAR LYMPHOMA: LYMPH NODE

Top: The follicles vary considerably in size, and lack well-defined mantle zones. Neoplastic follicles are also seen in the surrounding adipose tissue (left upper field).

Bottom: The follicles vary markedly in size and shape. They are surrounded by thin mantles in this example. Tingible body macrophages are not evident.

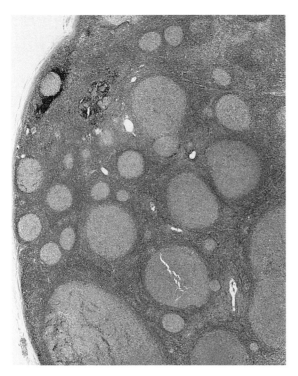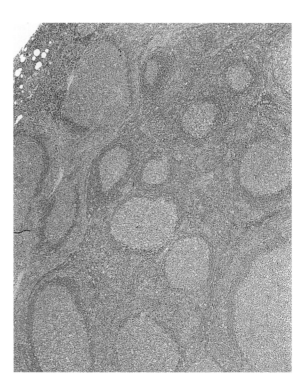

Figure 6-7
FOLLICULAR LYMPHOMA WITH BROAD INTERFOLLICULAR ZONES

Left: The follicles are separated by an appreciable amount of interfollicular lymphoid stroma. The lack of cellular polarization and absence of tingible body macrophages suggest that this represents follicular lymphoma rather than reactive follicular hyperplasia. The cellular monotony seen at high magnification (not shown) provides further support for such an interpretation.

Right: This case of follicular lymphoma is difficult to diagnose from architectural features. The follicles are surrounded by well-defined mantles and are separated by a considerable amount of interfollicular tissue, features that favor a diagnosis of reactive follicular hyperplasia. Clues to the neoplastic nature of the process are the spillage of the lymphoid infiltrate into the perinodal tissue (left upper field) and the cellular monotony evident on higher magnification (not shown). Ancillary techniques may be required to confirm the diagnosis.

Table 6-2

SUBCLASSIFICATION OF FOLLICULAR LYMPHOMA: COMPARISON OF THE WORKING FORMULATION AND THE UPDATED KIEL CLASSIFICATION

Working Formulation	Updated Kiel Classification
Predominantly small cleaved cell	Centroblastic-centrocytic
Mixed small cleaved and large cell	Centroblastic-centrocytic
Predominantly large cell	Centroblastic

cells (centroblasts) or immunoblasts, but sometimes of anaplastic large cells (fig. 6-23). The process represents evolution of the original neoplastic clone to a more rapidly proliferating cell type (83). Histologic transformation can occur either at the time of presentation (composite lymphoma) or at relapse; in some cases, a gradual increase in large cells can be documented on repeated biopsies.

Subclassification of the Follicular Lymphomas. The Working Formulation identifies three subtypes of follicular lymphoma according to the cellular composition: predominantly small cleaved cell, mixed small cleaved and large cell, and predominantly large cell. Equivalent terms in the updated Kiel classification are shown in Table 6-2 (219).

Criteria for Subclassification. There is continuing debate regarding the precise methods for morphologically subclassifying follicular lymphomas.

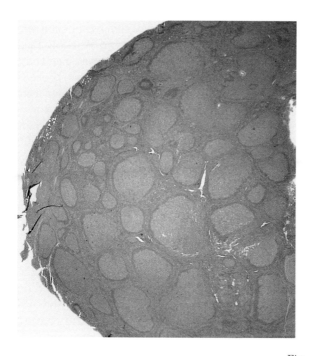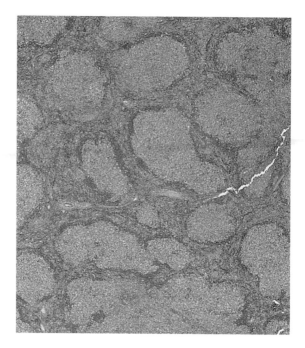

Figure 6-8
FOLLICULAR LYMPHOMA WITH LYMPHOCYTIC MANTLES AROUND THE FOLLICLES
Left: The follicles are surrounded by thin mantles, but their neoplastic nature is betrayed by the uniform staining of all the germinal centers, reflecting monotony of cell composition and lack of tingible body macrophages.
Right: The follicles have discrete thin mantles, and many have serrated outlines. Clues to the neoplastic nature of the process are the crowding of the follicles and the cellular monotony evident on higher magnification (not shown).

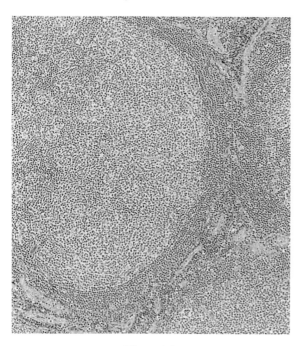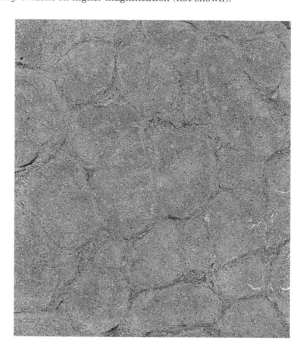

Figure 6-9
FOLLICULAR LYMPHOMA WITH LYMPHOCYTIC
MANTLES AROUND THE FOLLICLES

The follicles are surrounded by mantles composed of a monotonous population of small cleaved cells with no cellular polarization or interspersed tingible body macrophages.

Figure 6-10
FOLLICULAR LYMPHOMA WITH THICK
MANTLES AROUND THE FOLLICLES

An unusual example with very thick mantles surrounding the neoplastic follicles. Such cases may be difficult to distinguish from mantle cell lymphoma.

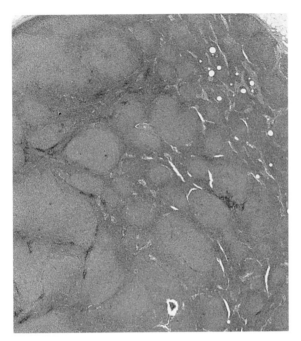

Figure 6-11
FOLLICULAR LYMPHOMA WITH INCOMPLETE
EFFACEMENT OF NODAL ARCHITECTURE

Closely packed, ill-defined follicles are distributed throughout the node, but residual sinusoids can still be seen on the right.

The dividing lines are drawn somewhat arbitrarily (144). Both the Rappaport and Working Formulation classifications include a mixed cell category to encompass those cases in which there is no clear preponderance of one cell type over another (176,197). Visual estimation of the percentage of large noncleaved cells is often used for subclassification: less than 25 percent, 25 to 50 percent, and more than 50 percent, respectively, for each subtype. The reproducibility of this estimation method, however, is limited (161).

In 1983, Mann and Berard (151) proposed an alternative method, which has been analyzed and recommended for use by Nathwani et al. (165, 166). This method is based on averaged counts of large noncleaved cells (centroblasts) per high-power field (HPF) within the follicles, based on counting 20 HPFs using a 40X objective and 10X eyepiece. Problems arise from the arbitrary nature of the cut-off points, differences in magnification from one microscope to another (see Table 6-3 for the adjusted cut-off points), the nonstandardized thickness of the sections, the varying quality of the sections examined, and the reproducibility of this counting method. There are also cells with

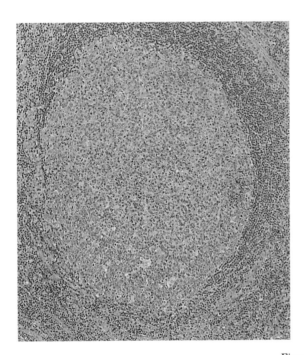

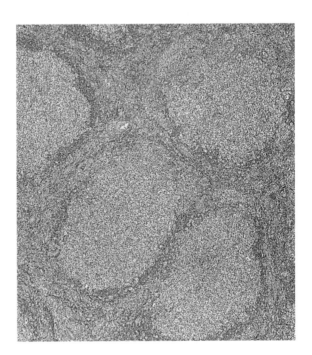

Figure 6-12
HYPERPLASTIC LYMPHOID FOLLICLE CONTRASTED WITH NEOPLASTIC FOLLICLES

Left: A hyperplastic follicle with cellular polarization: an eccentric mantle cap, a pale zone, and a dark zone (from top to bottom). Some tingible body macrophages are evident even at this magnification, and they are more prominent in the dark zone.
Right: Although these neoplastic follicles have thin mantles, they lack cellular polarization and tingible body macrophages.

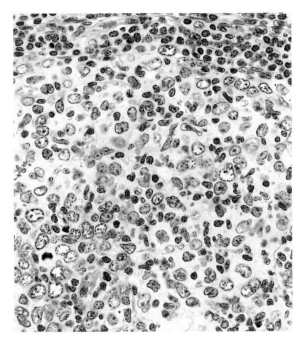

Figure 6-13
FOLLICULAR MIXED CELL
LYMPHOMA: LYMPH NODE

In this follicle, the large cells are aggregated focally, simulating cellular polarization.

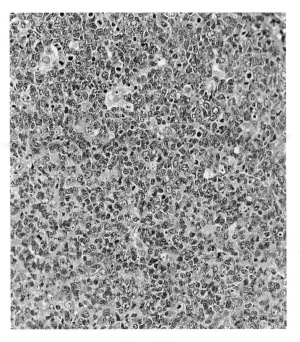

Figure 6-14
REACTIVE FOLLICULAR HYPERPLASIA:
CELLULAR COMPOSITION OF
A HYPERPLASTIC FOLLICLE

This field shows a germinal center, with the dark zone located on the top and the pale zone on the bottom. The dark zone is dominated by large noncleaved cells (centroblasts) with round vesicular nuclei, multiple membrane-bound nucleoli, and a thin rim of basophilic cytoplasm. Mitotic figures are easily identified, and there are interspersed tingible body macrophages. In the pale zone, small cleaved cells (centrocytes) predominate; they have irregular angulated nuclei and scanty cytoplasm.

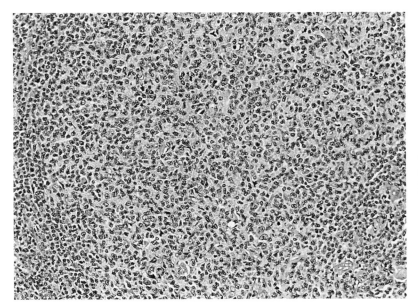

Figure 6-15
FOLLICULAR LYMPHOMA:
CELLULAR COMPOSITION OF
A NEOPLASTIC FOLLICLE

This field depicts a neoplastic follicle, which lacks cellular polarization and shows a fairly monotonous population of small cleaved cells. Note the absence of tingible body macrophages.

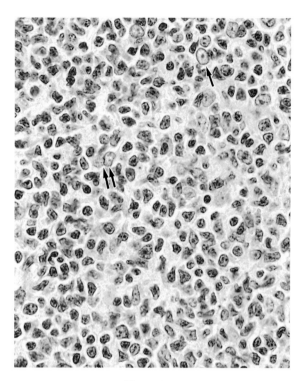

Figure 6-16
FOLLICULAR SMALL CLEAVED CELL
LYMPHOMA: LYMPH NODE

The neoplastic follicle is populated almost exclusively by small cleaved cells with angulated nuclear membranes and scanty cytoplasm. The interspersed follicular dendritic cells, which have an indistinct cellular outline, empty chromatin, and a small distinct nucleolus, are indicated by arrows (including a binucleated form indicated by two arrows).

cytologic features intermediate between small cleaved cells and large noncleaved cells, and these are difficult to classify reproducibly. Interspersed follicular dendritic cells (with ill-defined cell borders) can also be mistaken for large noncleaved cells. Jaffe et al. (104) consider the high cut-off point of 15 large cells per HPF to be too low, resulting in too many cases categorized as follicular large cell lymphoma.

In the updated Kiel classification, follicular centroblastic lymphoma is distinguished from follicular centroblastic-centrocytic lymphoma by the presence of solid foci of centroblasts (130). Harris and Ferry (83) have proposed considering both large noncleaved cells and large cleaved cells (large centrocytes) as large cells in the subclassification of follicular lymphoma into grades 1, 2, and 3.

Although most studies show that subclassification of follicular lymphoma has clinical relevance, in some studies the percentage of large cells does not influence the outcome (11). More objective and reproducible methods for subclassification are needed to separate patients into favorable and unfavorable prognostic groups. Because of the poor reproducibility of the currently used subclassification systems and differences in criteria that have been applied, reports on the differences in the various subtypes of follicular lymphoma have to be taken with some skepticism.

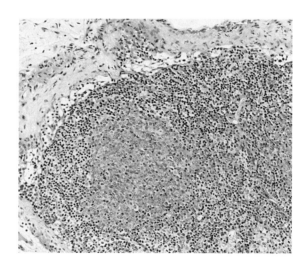 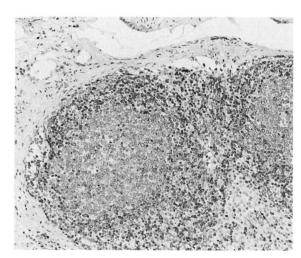

Figure 6-17
FOLLICULAR LARGE CELL LYMPHOMA: LYMPH NODE
Left: The two follicles in this field show a fairly monotonous population of large cells, but lack tingible body macrophages.
Right: The neoplastic nature of these follicles is supported by positive immunostaining for *bcl*-2 protein (brown). Note that the mantle zone and interfollicular lymphocytes are also *bcl*-2 positive, which is the normal staining pattern of these cell types.

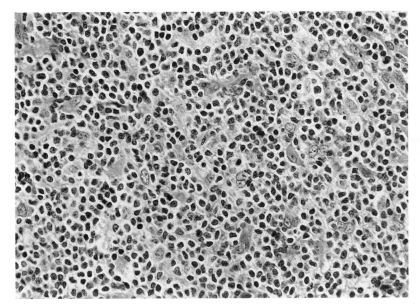

Figure 6-18
FOLLICULAR SMALL CLEAVED
CELL LYMPHOMA WITH
CONSPICUOUS FOLLICULAR
DENDRITIC CELLS
In this case, the small cleaved cells (centrocytes) are unusual in that the nuclei do not show prominent cleaving and many appear round. In this field, practically all the larger cells are follicular dendritic cells, which have indistinct cell boundaries, delicate nuclear membranes, empty nucleoplasms, and small distinct nucleoli. Some of the follicular dendritic cells are binucleated.

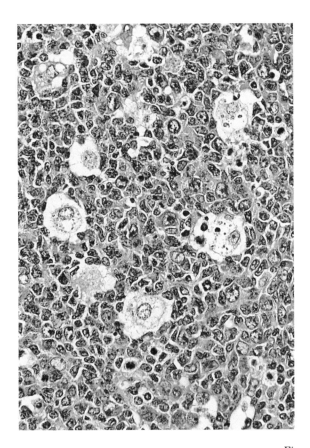

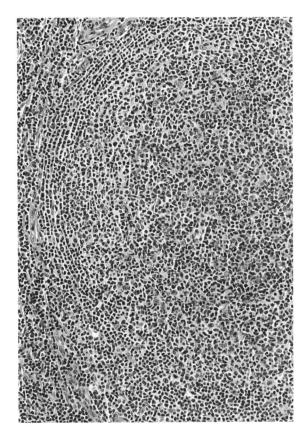

Figure 6-19
HYPERPLASTIC FOLLICLE CONTRASTED WITH NEOPLASTIC FOLLICLE
Left: In reactive lymphoid hyperplasia, the follicles are often rich in tingible body macrophages that have phagocytosed cellular debris. The macrophages impart a starry-sky appearance to the follicles. Note the admixture of small cleaved cells and large noncleaved cells comprising the main population of the follicle.
Right: The neoplastic follicle in follicular lymphoma is usually devoid of tingible body macrophages.

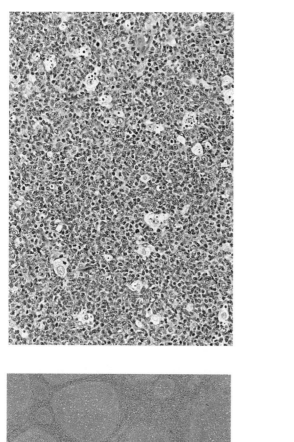

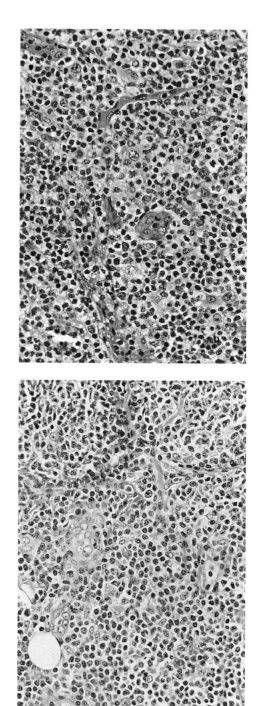

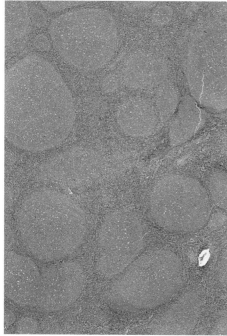

Figure 6-20
FOLLICULAR LYMPHOMA WITH
TINGIBLE BODY MACROPHAGES

Top: This example of follicular lymphoma is rich in tingible body macrophages. Distinction from reactive follicular hyperplasia is practically impossible based on this field alone.

Bottom: The neoplastic nature of the process is best appreciated on low magnification, wherein the follicles are crowded and lack well-defined mantles.

Figure 6-21
FOLLICULAR LYMPHOMA: INTERFOLLICULAR ZONE

Top: In this case, the interfollicular zone (which is rich in high endothelial venules) contains small cleaved cells in addition to small lymphocytes, consistent with infiltration by lymphoma.

Bottom: In this case, the interfollicular zone (middle and lower fields) is populated only by small lymphocytes with round or at most slightly irregular nuclei. The cytology is different from that of the neoplastic cells within the follicles (upper field). Thus this case does not show interfollicular involvement.

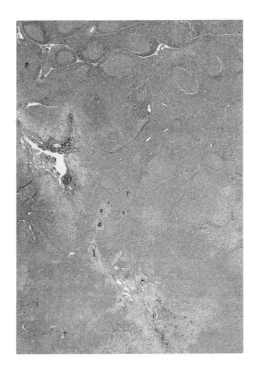

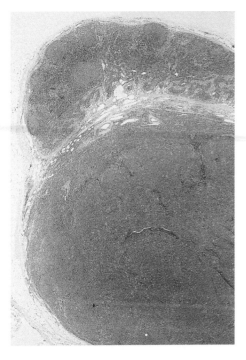

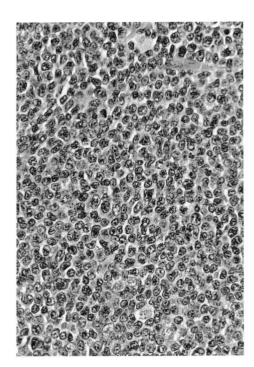

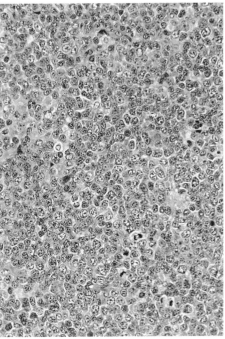

Figure 6-22
FOLLICULAR LYMPHOMA WITH DIFFUSE AREAS

Top: Follicular growth pattern (upper field) merges into diffuse areas (middle and lower fields). The latter is associated with some degree of sclerosis.

Bottom: The diffuse foci comprise small cleaved cells similar to those seen in the follicles.

Figure 6-23
FOLLICULAR LYMPHOMA WITH HISTOLOGIC
TRANSFORMATION AT INITIAL PRESENTATION
("COMPOSITE LYMPHOMA")

Top: The lymph node in the upper field shows involvement by follicular lymphoma. In the other lymph node, there is diffuse growth of large lymphoid cells.

Bottom: The large lymphoid cells have the cytologic features of large noncleaved cells (centroblasts) and are mitotically active.

Table 6-3

**ADJUSTED LARGE NONCLEAVED CELL COUNT FOR
DIFFERENT MICROSCOPES WHEN THE MANN-BERARD CRITERIA
ARE USED FOR SUBCLASSIFICATION OF FOLLICULAR LYMPHOMA**

Microscope	Objective	Eyepiece	HPF* Area (mm^2)	Low Cut-Off Count (per HPF)	High Cut-Off Count (per HPF)
American optical	40X	WF 10X	0.117	5	15
		WF 15X	0.096	4	12
Olympus	40X	WF 10X	0.159	7	20
		WF 15X	0.071	3	9
Nikon	40X	WF 10X	0.159	7	20
		WF 15X	0.096	4	12

*HPF = high-power field; WF = wide field.

Table 6-4

**CLINICAL FEATURES OF THE HISTOLOGIC SUBTYPES OF FOLLICULAR LYMPHOMA
ACCORDING TO THE DATA FROM THE NCI-SPONSORED STUDY ***

	Follicular Small Cleaved Cell Lymphoma	Follicular Mixed Cell Lymphoma	Follicular Large Cell Lymphoma
Relative frequency	66%	23%	11%
Median age	54.3 yrs	56.1 yrs	55.4 yrs
Stage			
I to II	18%	27%	27%
III to IV	82%	73%	73%
Bone marrow involvement	51%	30%	34%
Survival			
Median	7.2 yrs	5.1 yrs	3.0 yrs
5-year	70%	50%	45%
Complete remission rate	73%	65%	61%
Median time to relapse	5.0 yrs	5.2 yrs	>8.0 yrs

*National Cancer Institute–sponsored study; from reference 176.

Malignant Lymphoma, Follicular, Predominantly Small Cleaved Cell Type (Centroblastic-Centrocytic [Small], Follicular). This category is often termed *follicular small cleaved cell lymphoma* (Table 6-4). The follicles comprise a monotonous population of small lymphoid cells with nuclei that are slightly larger than those of normal lymphocytes and nuclear membranes that are irregular with prominent indentations, angulations, and linear cleavage planes; these cells are termed small cleaved cells (centrocytes) (fig. 6-24). The cells can appear remarkably elongated in some cases (fig. 6-24B); in other cases, the nuclei appear rounder and show minimal cleaving (fig. 6-18). The chromatin is relatively coarse, and nucleoli are small or inconspicuous. Cytoplasm is typically scanty. Mitoses are rare or absent, as are tingible body macrophages (fig. 6-15). Large noncleaved cells with basophilic cytoplasm, round nuclei, vesicular chromatin, and one to three membrane-bound nucleoli (centroblasts) are present in small numbers (less than 25 percent of the neoplastic population or fewer than 5 per HPF), but can be difficult to find (fig. 6-24C).

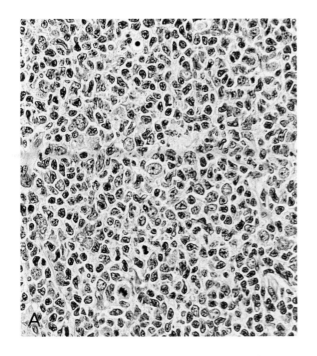

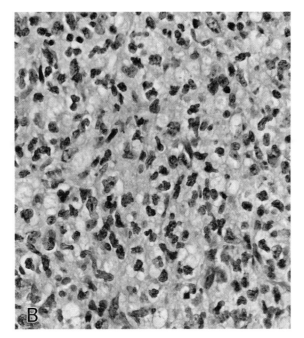

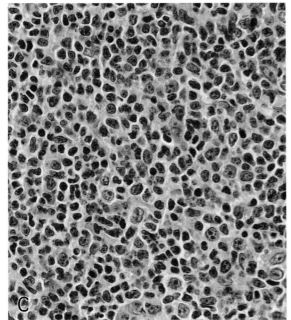

Figure 6-24
FOLLICULAR SMALL CLEAVED CELL LYMPHOMA
A: The neoplastic follicle is composed almost entirely of small cleaved cells with indented, angulated nuclear membranes and linear cleavage planes. These cells possess little if any discernible cytoplasm. There are interspersed follicular dendritic cells appearing as "naked" nuclei. Few mitotic figures are seen.
B: Many of the small cleaved cells in this case appear "dysplastic," with strikingly elongated nuclei.
C: In this case, large noncleaved cells are easier to find among a majority of small cleaved cells. Note the absence of tingible body macrophages.

Malignant Lymphoma, Follicular Mixed Small Cleaved and Large Cell Type (Centroblastic/Centrocytic [Small], Follicular). This category (often termed *follicular mixed cell lymphoma*) encompasses follicular lymphomas that have an obvious admixture of small cleaved cells (centrocytes) and large noncleaved cells (centroblasts) (fig. 6-25). Large cleaved cells with inconspicuous nucleoli and scanty cytoplasm can also be present. The large noncleaved cells should comprise 25 to 50 percent of the cellular population, or 5 to 15 cells per HPF. Mitoses may be evident. Small and large cells are usually admixed in a disorderly fashion, and lack the cellular polarization of reactive follicular hyperplasia. Rarely, aggregates of large cells may simulate polarization (fig. 6-13).

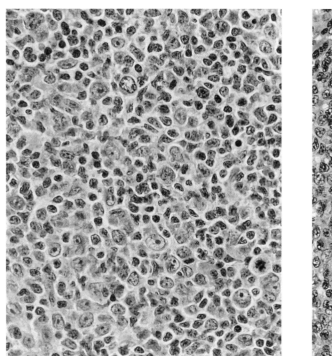 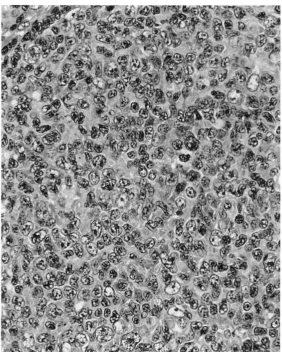

Figure 6-25
FOLLICULAR MIXED CELL LYMPHOMA

Left: There is an intimate admixture of small cleaved cells (centrocytes) and large noncleaved cells (centroblasts) with no cellular polarization. Tingible body macrophages are lacking.

Right: In this case, there is an admixture of small and large cells, but there are also cells with intermediate features that are not easy to classify.

Malignant Lymphoma, Follicular, Predominantly Large Cell Type (Centroblastic/Centrocytic [Large] and Centroblastic, Follicular). This category is often termed *follicular large cell lymphoma*. The majority of cells within the follicles are large cleaved or large noncleaved cells, although the latter usually predominate and should comprise more than 50 percent of the cellular population or more than 15 cells per HPF. Although the large noncleaved cells typically have round nuclei, they can have irregular nuclear foldings (fig. 6-26). There can be intermingled pleomorphic cells or multinucleated forms resembling Reed-Sternberg cells. Those cases with a significant number of immunoblasts are referred to as the *polymorphic centroblastic type* in the updated Kiel classification (130). Mitoses are usually numerous. Tingible body macrophages may be observed. Follicular large cell lymphoma is more likely than the other subtypes to have a diffuse component.

Cellular Heterogeneity of Neoplastic Follicles. Often, there are variations in cellular composition from follicle to follicle in the same lymph node. The grading of such cases of follicular lymphoma is difficult, but generally the lymphoma is subclassified according to the "worst" areas present. If there is apparent focal evolution to follicular large cell lymphoma, a descriptive report mentioning all components present is helpful.

Although we previously reported a consistency of histologic features at multiple sites after surgical staging procedures at Stanford University Medical Center (111), we have recently observed less consistency of morphologic features from one lymph node biopsy to another in sequential lymph node biopsies performed within a short period of time in order to obtain additional tissue for anti-idiotype studies and antibody therapy. In some patients initially diagnosed with follicular large cell lymphoma, a subsequent lymph node biopsy demonstrated the features of follicular

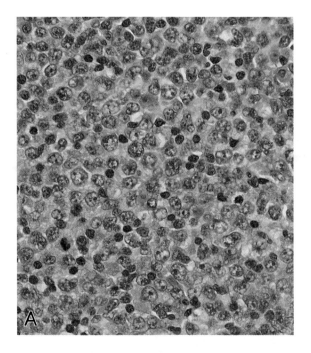

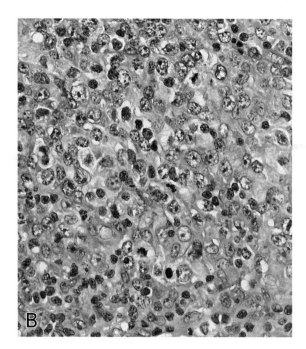

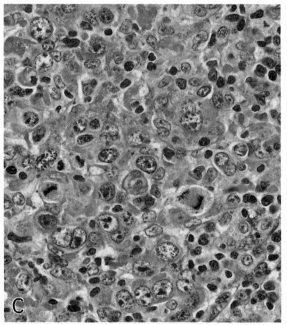

Figure 6-26
FOLLICULAR LARGE CELL LYMPHOMA
A: This follicle is composed predominantly of large non-cleaved cells mixed with a few small cleaved cells, giving a "monotonous" appearance. Note absence of tingible body macrophages.
B: This case is also predominated by large noncleaved cells which vary in size. Note the mitotic figures.
C: In this case, highly pleomorphic ("dysplastic") cells are present. The nuclei vary significantly in size and shape, and nucleoli are prominent.

small cleaved cell type. We have also observed evolution to a higher grade lymphoma at other sites, either at the same point in time, or in biopsies performed within a short period. This implies that, despite their indolent biologic behavior, follicular lymphomas comprise a dynamic process of cellular differentiation or transformation that may vary from one lymph node to another in the same patient. Such observations compound the problem of subclassification, grading, and treatment of follicular lymphoma.

Morphologic Variants of Follicular Lymphoma. *Sclerosis.* Sclerosis is a common phenomenon in follicular lymphoma, and the term *nodular sclerotic lymphosarcoma* has previously been applied (12,13,235). Sclerosis can take the

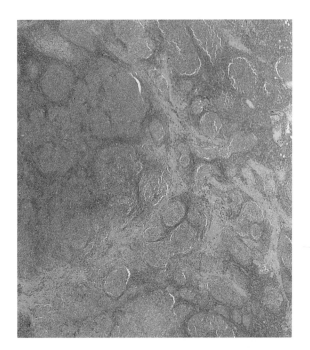
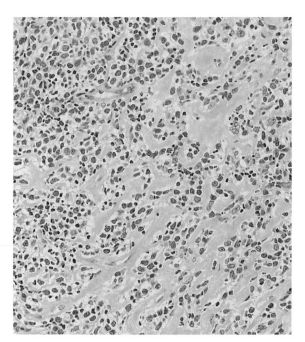

Figure 6-27
FOLLICULAR LYMPHOMA WITH SCLEROSIS: LYMPH NODE
Left: Neoplastic follicles are traversed by collagenous bands.
Right: Fine compartmentalizing sclerosis, entrapping clusters of lymphoma cells.

form of broad collagenous bands subdividing the lymphoma into irregular nodules and extending into perinodal soft tissues, or a fine compartmentalization around clusters of lymphoma cells (fig. 6-27). Immunohistochemical and ultrastructural studies suggest that the extracellular fibrotic material is composed predominantly of fibronectin, in addition to type I, III, and IV collagen, probably produced by fibroblasts and myofibroblasts (155). Although previously considered to be a favorable prognostic factor, sclerosis has not been shown to be an independent prognostic factor by multivariate analysis (176).

Amorphous Extracellular Material. Amorphous periodic acid–schiff (PAS)-positive eosinophilic extracellular material, which may be seen within the germinal centers of reactive follicles, occurs in some follicular lymphomas (202). The extracellular "proteinaceous precipitate" may be sparse or so abundant as to mask the underlying lymphoma (fig. 6-28). It has been shown by ultrastructural studies to comprise membranous structures, membrane-bound vesicles, and electron-dense bodies (fig. 6-29), similar to those seen in signet ring cell lymphomas (35,47).

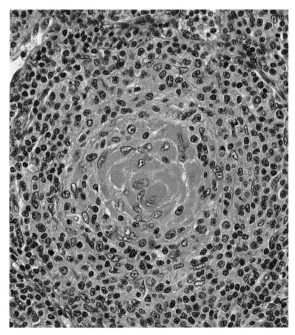

Figure 6-28
FOLLICULAR LYMPHOMA WITH AMORPHOUS
EXTRACELLULAR MATERIAL
Abundant extracellular amorphous material is deposited in the neoplastic follicles.

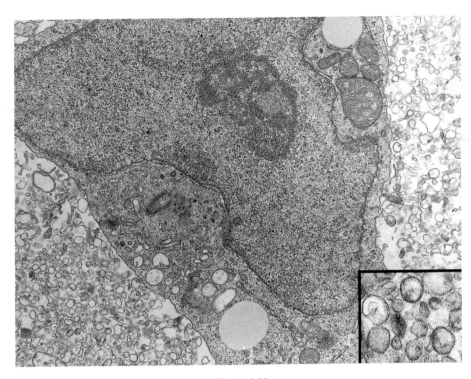

Figure 6-29
FOLLICULAR LYMPHOMA WITH AMORPHOUS EXTRACELLULAR MATERIAL
Electron micrograph shows the amorphous extracellular material to be composed of membranous profiles (inset).

Total Infarction of Lymph Node. Lymph node involved by lymphoma can undergo spontaneous total infarction. Among the various lymphoma types that show a propensity for infarction, follicular lymphoma constitutes an important group (130,154). Thus, further biopsies and follow-up are essential to clarify the diagnosis.

Follicular Signet Ring Cell Lymphoma. The neoplastic cells of follicular lymphomas occasionally contain clear cytoplasmic vacuoles (fig. 6-30) or Russell body–type cytoplasmic inclusions (fig. 6-31), which compress the moon-shaped nucleus toward one pole of the cell to impart a signet ring appearance (fig. 6-32) (80,112,216). Most of the signet ring cells are small cleaved cells (centrocytes), usually confined to the neoplastic follicles, but sometimes also seen in the interfollicular areas.

Immunohistochemical studies have demonstrated monoclonal IgG in cells with clear cytoplasmic vacuoles. Ultrastructurally, the vacuoles contain evenly sized microspherules which commonly accumulate at the periphery (fig. 6-33); the vacuole may represent a giant multivesicular body resulting from the coalescence of smaller multivesicular

bodies (51). It has been hypothesized that these structures are either dilated Golgi vesicles or cell membrane–derived endocytic vesicles. The immunoglobulin demonstrated in the vacuoles is probably associated with the cell membrane rather than immunoglobulin stored within the vacuole.

The Russell body–type inclusions usually stain for monotypic IgM. Ultrastructurally they comprise membrane-bound, homogeneous, electron-dense material, consistent with intracisternal accumulation of immunoglobulin (232).

Multilobated Nuclei in Follicular Lymphoma. In some follicular lymphomas, particularly the predominantly large cell type, cells with multilobated nuclei constitute a conspicuous proportion of the neoplastic cells (31,233).

Cerebriform Nuclei in Follicular Lymphoma. Cells with cerebriform nuclear contours, although traditionally considered to be characteristic of mycosis fungoides, occur in approximately 1.5 percent of follicular lymphomas (fig. 6-34) (167).

Plasmacytic Differentiation in Follicular Lymphoma. In a review of 198 cases of follicular lymphoma, Keith et al. (109) identified large

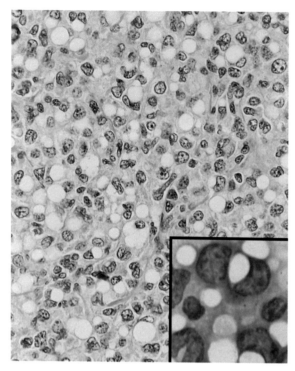

Figure 6-30
FOLLICULAR LYMPHOMA WITH SIGNET RING
CELLS (CLEAR VACUOLE TYPE): LYMPH NODE
Numerous signet ring cells are seen in the follicles. These
cells possess clear cytoplasmic vacuoles compressing the
moon-shaped nucleus toward one pole of the cell. Inset:
Signet ring cells are seen in this Giemsa-stained touch
imprint. Note indentation of the nucleus.

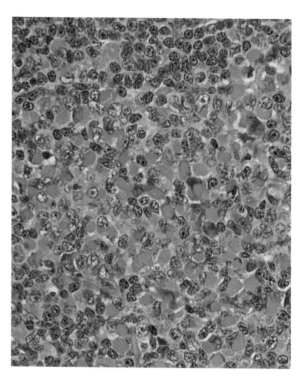

Figure 6-31
FOLLICULAR LYMPHOMA WITH SIGNET RING
CELLS (RUSSELL BODY TYPE): LYMPH NODE
Many cells in the neoplastic follicles contain a homogenous,
eosinophilic globule that displaces and compresses the nucleus.

numbers of plasma cells in 17 (8.6 percent). The
plasma cells were polytypic in 10 cases and
monotypic in 7 cases (3.5 percent). The phenomenon of plasmacytic differentiation in follicular
lymphomas is not unexpected given the ability
of reactive germinal centers to produce plasma
cell precursors after antigen stimulation (57,
109,132,230). The plasma cells usually occur in
an interfollicular, but sometimes intrafollicular,
location (fig. 6-35). When the latter is striking,
the term *follicular plasmacytoma* is sometimes
applied (207). The plasma cells can contain Russell or Dutcher bodies. There can be serum paraprotein identical to the immunoglobulin type
demonstrated in the plasma cell population (230).

Rosette Formation in Follicular Lymphoma.
Frizzera et al. (58) were the first to describe
Homer-Wright–type rosettes (traditionally considered to be the hallmark of neuroblastic tumors) in follicular lymphoma (58). The rosettes

are composed of lymphoma cells surrounding a
central area of eosinophilic fibrillary material
(fig. 6-36). Ultrastructural studies show a central aggregate of narrow cytoplasmic processes
derived from the lymphoma cells (fig. 6-37). The
eosinophilic fibrillary material expresses the same
surface antigens as the lymphoma, as expected
from its ultrastructural composition (fig. 6-38).

*Floral Variant of Follicular Lymphoma (Vari-
ant Mimicking Progressive Transformation of
Germinal Centers).* Osborne and Butler (184)
first drew attention to follicular lymphomas that
morphologically mimic progressive transformation of germinal centers (floral variant). The
lymphomatous nodules are uniformly surrounded and invaded by the mantle zone small
lymphocytes, resulting in a serrated, amoeboid,
or floral configuration (fig. 6-39) (69). Although
the neoplastic nature of this lesion was debated
(153,206), recent immunologic and genotypic
data provide clear support for its interpretation
as a variant of follicular lymphoma (69,186),

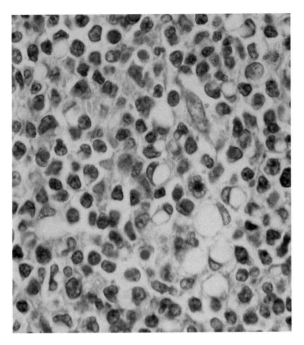

Figure 6-32
SIGNET RING CELL FOLLICULAR
LYMPH NODE

This periodic acid–Schiff (PAS) stain demonstrates both clear vacuoles and PAS-positive Russell body–type cytoplasmic inclusions.

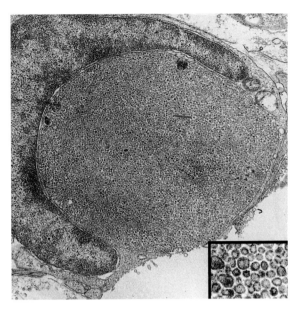

Figure 6-33
SIGNET RING CELL FOLLICULAR
LYMPHOMA: LYMPH NODE

This electron micrograph of a signet ring cell (clear vacuole type) shows even-sized microspherules and microvesicles (inset), ultrastructurally similar to the membranous profiles of the extracellular amorphous material seen in some follicular lymphomas (see figure 6-29). In most other cells, the microspherules accumulate only at the rim, and the center is empty.

including light chain restriction, immunoglobulin gene rearrangements, and overexpression of *bcl*-2 protein. The small lymphocytes that invade the neoplastic follicles are a mixture of B and T cells (69). Although most cases show predominance of large cells, the follicular lymphoma can have a mixed cell or predominantly small cleaved cell composition.

The floral variant of follicular lymphoma does not differ clinically from the usual cases of follicular lymphoma. The importance of recognizing this variant lies in its being potentially mistaken for progressive transformation of germinal centers and nodular lymphocyte predominance Hodgkin's disease (24,193).

Follicular Lymphoma with Hyaline-Vascular Follicles. Rare examples of follicular lymphoma comprise neoplastic follicles showing a concentric arrangement of lymphoid cells and penetration by hyalinized venules, mimicking hyaline-vascular Castleman's disease (fig. 6-40). The diagnosis of lymphoma is confirmed by demonstration of light chain restriction or by genotypic analysis.

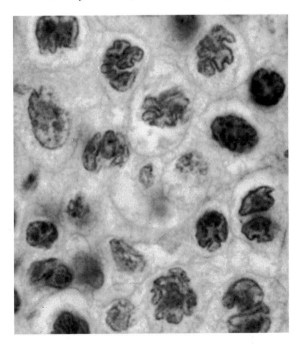

Figure 6-34
FOLLICULAR LYMPHOMA WITH
CEREBRIFORM NUCLEI: LYMPH NODE

The nuclear membranes have many indentations, imparting cerebriform nuclear contours. (Courtesy of Dr. Bharat Nathwani, Los Angeles, CA.)

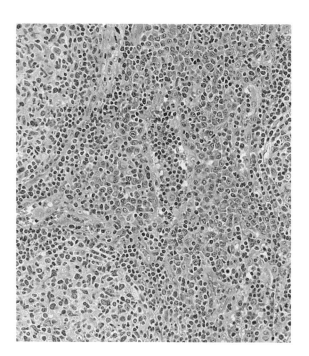
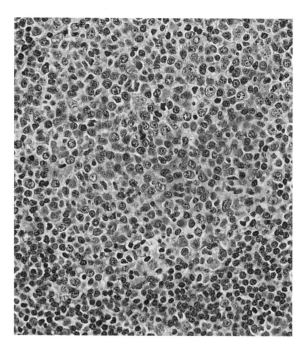

Figure 6-35
FOLLICULAR LYMPHOMA WITH PLASMA CELL DIFFERENTIATION
Left: The interfollicular zones are rich in mature-looking plasma cells, which are shown on immunohistochemical studies to be monotypic.
Right: An example showing marked plasmacytic differentiation in the neoplastic follicles.

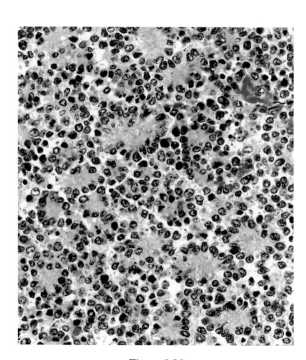

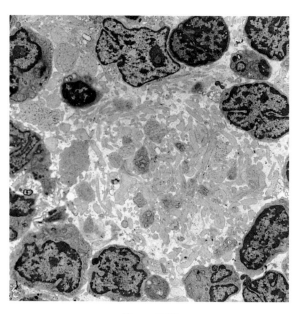

Figure 6-37
FOLLICULAR LYMPHOMA WITH
ROSETTE FORMATION: LYMPH NODE
Electron micrograph demonstrates central aggregates of narrow cytoplasmic processes surrounded by atypical lymphoid cells with indented and angulated nuclear membranes. (Fig. 3A from Frizzera G, Gajl-Peczalska K, Sibley RK, Rosai J, Cerhwitz D, Hurd DD. Rosette formation in malignant lymphoma. Am J Pathol 1985;119:351–6.)

Figure 6-36
FOLLICULAR LYMPHOMA WITH ROSETTE
FORMATION: LYMPH NODE
Lymphoma cells surround central areas of tangled fibrillary materials, simulating Homer-Wright rosettes.

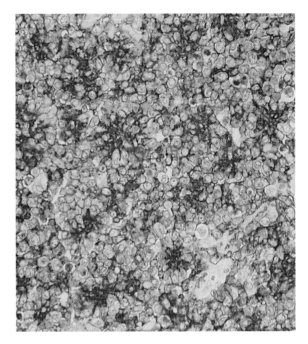

Figure 6-38
FOLLICULAR LYMPHOMA WITH ROSETTE
FORMATION: LYMPH NODE
Immunohistochemical staining demonstrates that both the lymphoid cells and the fibrillary material that they surround express CD20 (L26).

"Reverse" Variant of Follicular Lymphoma. In most cases of follicular lymphoma, the neoplastic follicles appear as pale-staining nodules surrounded by dark-staining mantles or interfollicular tissues. Rarely, the neoplastic follicles have dark-staining centers and pale-staining cuffs, the reverse of the usual pattern (fig. 6-41). These *reverse* or *inverse follicles* are attributed to the concentration of small cleaved cells (centrocytes) in the centers of the follicles, and lighter staining large noncleaved cells (centroblasts) in the periphery (30,165). This variant of follicular lymphoma does not appear to have prognostic significance, but its unusual appearance may lead to confusion with mantle cell lymphoma, monocytoid B-cell lymphoma, or even nodular lymphocyte predominance Hodgkin's disease.

Follicular Lymphoma Showing Monocytoid B-Cell Differentiation. Some follicular lymphomas are associated with a component of neoplastic monocytoid B cells (*"composite lymphomas"*). The monocytoid B cells often form pale collars of variable widths around the neoplastic follicles; this can also create a "reverse" appearance to the follicles (fig. 6-42). They are recognized by their

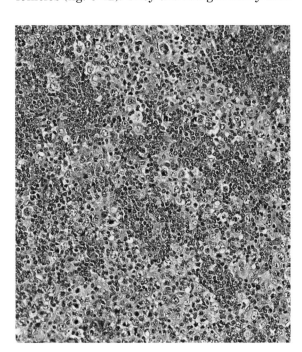

Figure 6-39
FOLLICULAR LYMPHOMA, FLORAL VARIANT: LYMPH NODE
Left: The large neoplastic follicles, which have serrated contours, show invaginations of the mantles into the centers, resulting in a floral configuration.
Right: Irregular islands of dark-staining small lymphocytes extend into the neoplastic follicles, which are composed mostly of large cells.

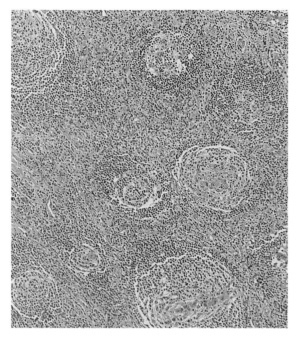

Figure 6-40
FOLLICULAR LYMPHOMA WITH
HYALINE-VASCULAR NEOPLASTIC FOLLICLES
The penetration of the neoplastic follicles by venules and the concentric arrangement of cells resemble hyaline-vascular Castleman's disease. Immunoglobulin light chain restriction was demonstrated in this case (results not shown).

medium-sized nuclei, relatively fine chromatin, small nucleoli, and moderate amount of pale cytoplasm (fig. 6-42, right). They appear to be derived from the same clone as the follicular lymphoma. Genotypic studies have demonstrated *bcl*-2 gene rearrangement in such cases (163,214).

Follicular Immunoblastic/Plasmablastic Lymphoma. Rare follicular lymphomas are composed of large cells with cytologic features of immunoblasts or plasmablasts: prominent central nucleolus and an appreciable amount of plasmacytoid (basophilic) cytoplasm (fig. 6-43) (19,29). There are too few cases for any conclusion to be made on the behavior of this variant.

Follicular Small Lymphocytic Lymphoma. Rare cases of follicular lymphoma exhibit the cellular composition of small lymphocytic lymphoma, that is, small lymphocytes with round nuclei and condensed chromatin, which may be admixed with occasional larger cells with features of prolymphocytes and paraimmunoblasts (fig. 6-44) (32). The demonstration of *bcl*-2 gene rearrangement in most cases studied suggests that this tumor is biologically a follicular rather than small lymphocytic lymphoma. Further

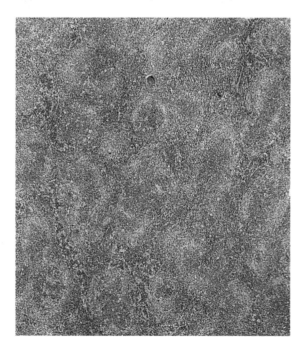

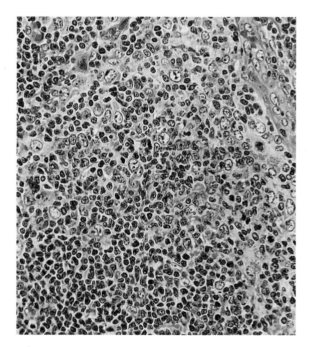

Figure 6-41
FOLLICULAR LYMPHOMA, REVERSE VARIANT: LYMPH NODE
Left: The neoplastic follicles have dark-staining centers and pale-staining cuffs, the reverse of the usual pattern.
Right: Higher magnification shows concentration of small cleaved cells in the centers of the neoplastic follicles and accumulation of large noncleaved cells in the periphery.

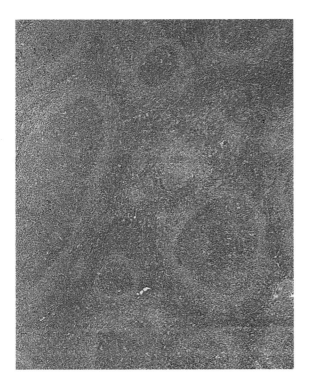 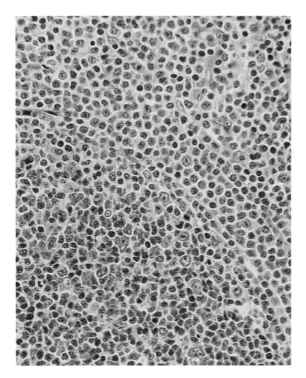

Figure 6-42
FOLLICULAR LYMPHOMA WITH MONOCYTOID B-CELL DIFFERENTIATION
Top: Pale-staining collars surround the neoplastic follicles in this follicular lymphoma. The pattern closely simulates that seen in figure 6-41, left.
Right: The collars are formed by medium-sized monocytoid B cells with clear cytoplasm (upper field). Contrast these cells with the follicular center cells in the lower field, which appear more crowded because of less cytoplasm.

proof that this is indeed a follicular lymphoma will require demonstration of follicular dendritic cell meshworks in the follicles.

"Blastic" Variant of Follicular Lymphoma. A blastic (lymphoblastic) form of follicular lymphoma was described by Come et al. (41), but was subsequently reinterpreted as the blastoid variant of mantle cell lymphoma (124). Transformation of follicular lymphoma to a lymphoma with small noncleaved cells has also been reported (fig. 6-45) (44,211,240,245).

Composite Lymphoma. A significant proportion of composite lymphomas comprise low-grade follicular lymphomas in various combinations with higher-grade follicular or diffuse lymphomas (114). Of those cases comprising both Hodgkin's disease and non-Hodgkin's lymphoma, most of the latter are follicular lymphomas (72,77). The significance of this phenomenon and possible interrelationships between these non-Hodgkin lymphomas and Hodgkin's disease are discussed in greater detail in chapter 17.

Clinical and Histologic Characteristics of Follicular Lymphoma Occurring in Selected Extranodal Sites. *Bone Marrow Involvement.* Biopsy is preferred to marrow clot sections and aspirate smears for evaluating bone marrow for the presence of follicular lymphoma (106). The incidence of bone marrow involvement with follicular mixed cell or large cell lymphoma is lower than with follicular small cleaved cell lymphoma (Table 6-4) (150,176).

Although extensive infiltration may be seen in some cases, the characteristic pattern of involvement comprises focal paratrabecular infiltrates of lymphoid cells (fig. 6-46), frequently associated with an increase in reticulin fibers (40). This pattern is particularly characteristic of the follicular small cleaved cell type (40,203). In some cases, the paratrabecular lymphoid infiltrates show less cytologic atypia than that seen in lymph nodes and some nodules may be more centrally located, making the distinction from benign lymphoid aggregates difficult.

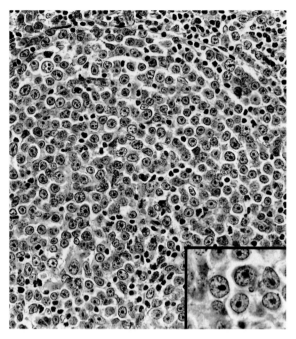

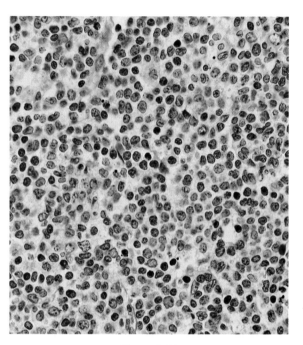

Figure 6-43
FOLLICULAR LYMPHOMA, IMMUNOBLASTIC TYPE
    The neoplastic cells that make up the follicles have the cytologic features of immunoblasts, i.e., large cells with centrally placed prominent nucleoli (inset).

Figure 6-44
FOLLICULAR SMALL LYMPHOCYTIC LYMPHOMA
    The neoplastic follicles comprise mostly small lymphocytes with dark, round or minimally irregular nuclei.

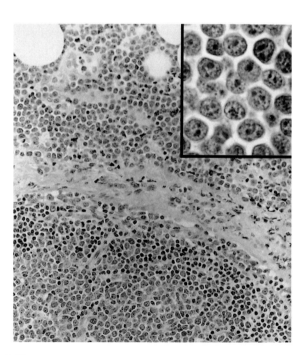

Figure 6-45
FOLLICULAR LYMPHOMA, BLASTIC VARIANT: LYMPH NODE
    Left: This follicle is composed predominantly of small cleaved cells.
    Right: This follicle (lower field), in the same lymph node, contains "blast cells" (small noncleaved cells, inset) which have infiltrated the surrounding adipose tissue (upper field).

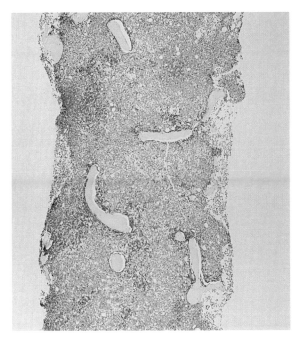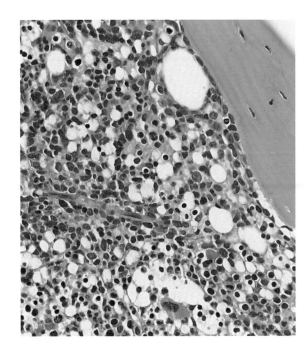

Figure 6-46
FOLLICULAR LYMPHOMA: BONE MARROW INVOLVEMENT
Left: Bone marrow involvement by follicular lymphoma is characterized by focal paratrabecular infiltrates, well highlighted in this immunohistochemical preparation using L26 (CD20). Although the neoplastic infiltrate is also seen in the intertrabecular regions (brown), there is selective concentration of tumor cells around the bony trabeculae.
Right: Small cleaved cells with elongated angulated nuclei are seen predominantly adjacent to the surface of the bony trabeculae. Normal bone marrow cells are seen in the left lower field.

After intensive chemotherapy, the involved areas may become "hypocellular paratrabecular foci," characterized by loosely arranged reticulin fibers sparsely populated by cells. There may or may not be residual lymphoma cells in these foci. The finding of hypocellular paratrabecular foci is an indication to examine the specimen by deeper sectioning to determine whether there is residual lymphoma in the bone marrow (185).

Patients with a long history of disease and those who have undergone extensive chemotherapy may have bone marrow infiltrates showing a marked degree of cellular pleomorphism, with cells resembling Reed-Sternberg cells (156).

Although bone marrow infiltrates may be cytologically similar to the lymphoma in the initial lymph node biopsy, discordant cytologic patterns are also seen (55,116,157): patients with follicular large cell lymphoma in lymph nodes may have bone marrow infiltrates composed predominantly of small cleaved cells (centrocytes). When the histologic subtypes are discordant, initial therapy should be directed at the more aggressive component (157).

See chapter 9 for the discordant finding of follicular lymphoma in the bone marrow of patients presenting with diffuse large B-cell lymphoma.

Peripheral Blood Involvement. Many patients with follicular lymphoma have circulating lymphoma cells that comprise a low to high percentage of the total leukocyte count (which may be elevated or normal). The term *lymphosarcoma cell leukemia* denotes the leukemic phase of follicular lymphoma (160,198,208). The lymphoma cells characteristically have scanty cytoplasm that stains pale blue in Romanowsky stain. The nucleus may be partially or completely divided by a characteristic cleft ("notched nucleus" or "buttock" cell). The chromatin stains intensely and is compactly clumped (fig. 6-47). Often, bulbous projections or pseudolobules distort the nuclear outlines.

Even if there are no recognizable atypical lymphoid cells in the peripheral blood, immunogenetic studies can identify clonal populations in a significant proportion of cases (14,92,95,123,215).

Splenic Involvement. Follicular lymphoma frequently involves the spleen, although affected

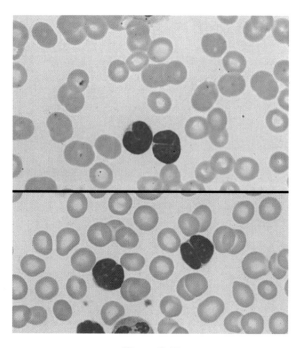

Figure 6-47

FOLLICULAR LYMPHOMA: PERIPHERAL BLOOD

Several "notched nucleus" cells are seen in the peripheral smear. The nuclei are partially or completely divided by a characteristic cleft. The chromatin stains intensely and is compactly clumped. (Romanowsky stain)

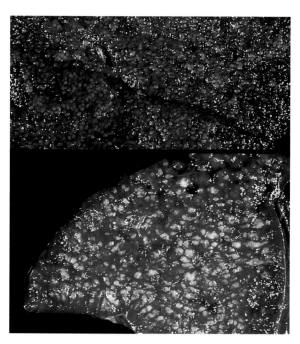

Figure 6-48

FOLLICULAR LYMPHOMA: SPLEEN

Follicular lymphomas of predominantly small cleaved cell and mixed cell types are characterized by a uniform distribution of small nodules throughout the spleen.

spleens may not be enlarged. Studies based on staging laparotomies have demonstrated involvement of the spleen in 25 to 55 percent of patients (27,28,71,111). On occasion, massive splenomegaly may be the initial manifestation of the disease (143).

Follicular lymphomas of predominantly small cleaved cell and mixed cell types characteristically show a uniform distribution of well-defined nodules throughout the spleen, with little variation in size and shape (fig. 6-48) (111). For the most part, these nodules are located in expanded Malpighian corpuscles. The corpuscles can be entirely replaced by neoplastic cells or there may still be a rim of residual normal-appearing lymphocytes (mantle and marginal zones; see chapter 20). On occasion, the spleen is less extensively involved, with only scattered tumor nodules. Such lesions must be distinguished from localized reactive lymphoid hyperplasia of the spleen, characterized by closely apposed germinal centers surrounded by mantles of small lymphocytes (23).

The splenic lesions of follicular large cell lymphoma are usually composed of large irregular

nodules varying considerably in size and shape, and scattered in an irregular fashion throughout the spleen; there is no discernible relationship to Malpighian corpuscles (fig. 6-49).

Hepatic Involvement. Hepatic involvement is more common with follicular small cleaved cell lymphoma than with the other two subtypes of follicular lymphoma (113). The lymphoma primarily involves the portal triads, often encroaching upon limiting plates or peripheral portions of the lobule (fig. 6-50). Rarely, follicular lymphoma may extensively involve the liver, obliterating large areas of the hepatic parenchyma (fig. 6-51).

Cutaneous Involvement. Cutaneous follicular lymphoma is identified by histologic criteria similar to that used in lymph nodes, based on the distinctive pattern of nodularity (fig. 6-52) and by the characteristic cytologic features (22,45). As with other non-Hodgkin's lymphomas involving skin, there is a predilection for the scalp and forehead. Primary cutaneous follicular lymphomas are uncommon (63). Patients with disease confined to the skin have a significantly longer relapse-free survival period than those with extracutaneous disseminated lymphoma (22).

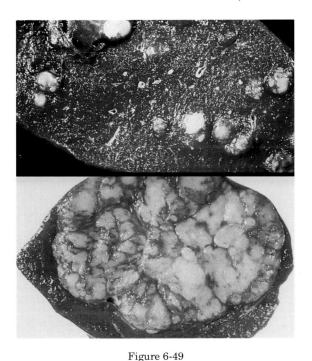

Figure 6-49
FOLLICULAR LYMPHOMA: SPLEEN
Splenic lesions of follicular large cell lymphoma comprise large, irregular tumor masses varying in shape and size.

Figure 6-50
FOLLICULAR LYMPHOMA INVOLVING LIVER
The portal tracts of the liver show heavy lymphoid cell infiltration, with encroachment on the limiting plates.

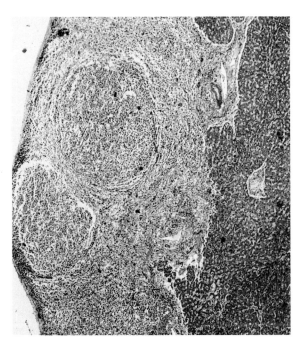

Figure 6-51
FOLLICULAR LYMPHOMA INVOLVING LIVER
There is subcapsular involvement of the liver, with recognizable follicles.

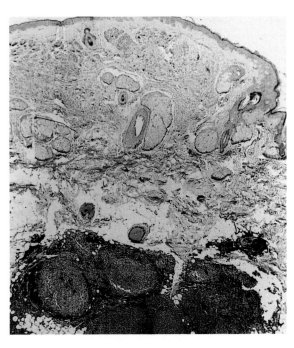

Figure 6-52
FOLLICULAR LYMPHOMA: SUBCUTANEOUS TISSUE
The lymphomatous infiltrate in the subcutis comprises closely packed follicles, in a pattern similar to that observed in nodal follicular lymphoma.

Gastrointestinal Involvement. Follicular lymphoma can involve the gastrointestinal tract, sometimes as the primary site of disease, albeit rarely (fig. 6-53) (125,136). Primary follicular lymphoma of the gastrointestinal tract most commonly involves the small intestines (especially the terminal ileum), and usually presents with obstruction. Follicular small cleaved cell and mixed cell lymphomas are the most commonly encountered subtypes. The lymphoma can affect both the lamina propria and the intestinal wall, and may be associated with extensive sclerosis. Polypoid lesions may be seen and may be multiple throughout the colon or small intestine, producing the picture of multiple lymphomatous polyposis which is more commonly caused by mantle cell lymphoma (42,100,179).

Immunologic Findings. The neoplastic cells of follicular lymphomas are of B lineage and monoclonal (105,135,225). Moreover, all components of the normal germinal center, i.e., follicular center B cells, small T cells, macrophages, and follicular dendritic cells, can be identified within the neoplastic follicles (17,62,81–84,88,117,131,133,174).

B-Cell Markers. The neoplastic cells express pan-B antigens, such as CD19, CD20, CD22, and CD79a, in addition to HLA-DR, CDw75 (LN1), and CD74 (LN2) (fig. 6-54). They usually express surface or cytoplasmic immunoglobulins with light chain restriction (45). Immunoglobulin heavy chain class switching occurs with greater frequency in follicular lymphomas than in other low-grade lymphomas, consistent with observations made in normal germinal centers. The usual immunoglobulin isotype is IgM, but sometimes a second isotype is expressed (IgD, IgG, or infrequently, IgA) on the cell surface (237). In approximately 10 percent of follicular lymphomas, particularly the large cell type, there is no detectable immunoglobulin (174). The mantle cell lymphocytes that surround the neoplastic follicles, if present, are often polytypic and are presumably reactive in nature. However, at least in some cases, they express the same immunoglobulin light chain as the neoplastic follicles and thus represent part of the neoplastic clone (82,237).

CD10 (CALLA) has been identified in approximately 60 percent of cases. CD5 and CD43 are typically lacking. Staining for CD23 is often, but not invariably, negative (130).

Bcl-2 Protein. Approximately 85 percent of follicular lymphomas stain for *bcl*-2 protein

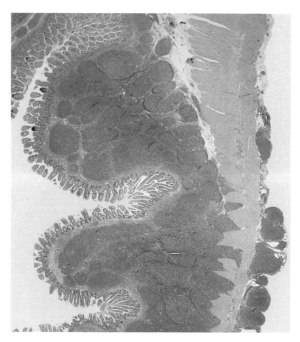

Figure 6-53
FOLLICULAR LYMPHOMA: SMALL INTESTINE
Lymphomatous follicles involve the submucosa, muscularis, and serosa of the small intestine.

(small cleaved cell type, 100 percent; mixed cell type, 85 percent; large cell type, 75 percent) (fig. 6-55) (65,172,190,229). Therefore, immunohistologic detection of *bcl*-2 is an important tool for distinguishing follicular lymphoma from follicular hyperplasia, because the follicular center cells of reactive follicles do not stain for *bcl*-2 (fig. 6-56) (7,128,229). However, this does not apply to detection of *bcl*-2 mRNA in situ, since the *bcl*-2 gene is transcribed in both neoplastic and reactive follicular center cells; the latter do not express *bcl*-2 protein, presumably by regulating translation of *bcl*-2 mRNA (36). Immunostaining for *bcl*-2 is of no value for distinguishing follicular lymphoma from other types of lymphoma, because immunoreactive *bcl*-2 protein is also present in a wide variety of B- and T-cell lymphomas lacking t(14;18), normal B and T lymphocytes, normal hematopoietic precursors, and many nonhematopoietic cells and tumors (36,119,190,251).

In the rare cases of Hodgkin's disease that supervene in patients with a prior history of follicular lymphoma, the Reed-Sternberg cells express bcl-2 protein, suggesting a possible histogenetic relationship between the two lymphomas under these circumstances (72,126).

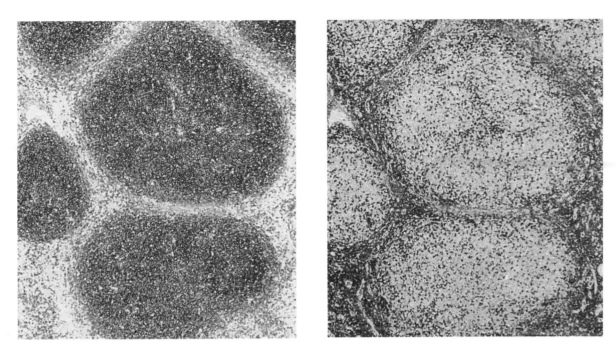

Figure 6-54
FOLLICULAR LYMPHOMA: IMMUNOHISTOCHEMICAL STAINING OF LYMPH NODE
Left: The neoplastic follicles stain intensely for CD20 (L26).
Right: Staining with Leu-22 (CD43) shows significant numbers of T cells within the neoplastic follicles in addition to the surrounding compressed lymphoid stroma.

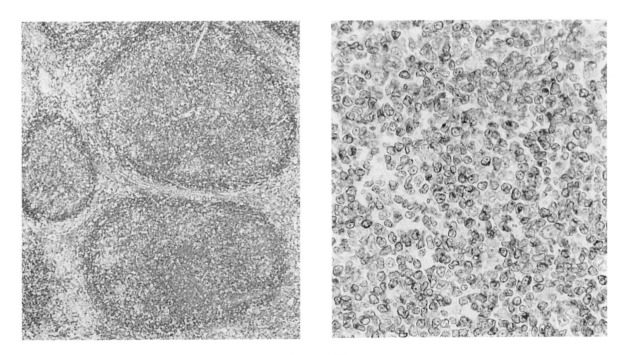

Figure 6-55
FOLLICULAR LYMPHOMA: IMMUNOSTAINING FOR *bcl*-2 PROTEIN IN LYMPH NODE
Left: Neoplastic cells within the follicles show strong staining for *bcl*-2. The lymphocytes in the thin mantles and the interfollicular regions also show *bcl*-2 reactivity.
Right: The neoplastic cells show cytoplasmic staining for *bcl*-2. The staining is accentuated in the perinuclear space and Golgi zone.

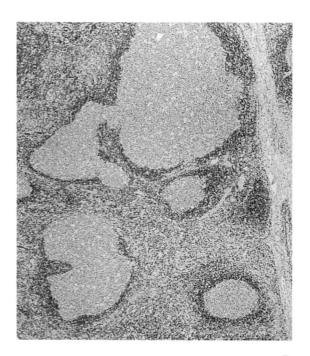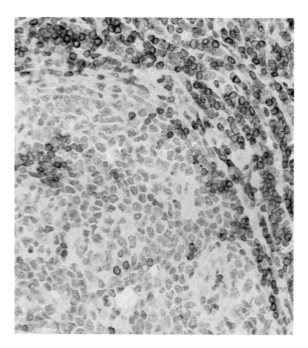

Figure 6-56

REACTIVE FOLLICULAR HYPERPLASIA: IMMUNOSTAINING FOR *bcl*-2 PROTEIN IN LYMPH NODE

Left: The germinal centers are *bcl*-2 negative, contrasting with the positive cells in the mantles and interfollicular regions.
Right: Higher magnification showing that the majority of cells in the germinal center are *bcl*-2 negative; the few positive cells are small lymphocytes. The mantle zone small lymphocytes (right upper field) stain for *bcl*-2.

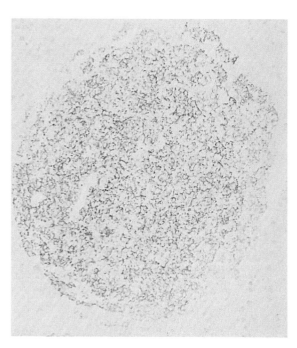

Figure 6-57

FOLLICULAR LYMPHOMA: IMMUNOSTAINED FOR FOLLICULAR DENDRITIC CELLS

In the neoplastic follicle, there is a tight meshwork of follicular dendritic cells, as demonstrated by immunostaining with CD35 (To5).

Other Cellular Constituents. Monoclonal antibodies directed against follicular dendritic cells (such as CD21, CD35, KiM4, R4/23) demonstrate a well-organized, concentric dendritic cell meshwork in each follicle (fig. 6-57) (84,209). When the growth pattern becomes diffuse, the follicular dendritic cell meshwork becomes sparse or is lost (130).

Many immunoregulatory T cells are demonstrable within the neoplastic follicles, with CD4-positive cells predominating over CD8-positive cells (fig. 6-54, right) (81,223). Some of the T cells have an activated appearance (16). T cells can be so abundant that the lymphoma may be mistaken to be of T lineage on flow cytometric immunologic analysis (103). In addition, occasional CD57 (Leu-7)-positive cells are present both within and between the neoplastic follicles (162,222).

CD30-positive large cells are frequently identified at the edge of the neoplastic follicles. They appear to be B cells, but it is still unclear whether they are part of the malignant process (192). The interfollicular zones are often rich in T cells (fig. 6-54, right), but they may contain an appreciable number of monoclonal B cells in cases showing involvement of the interfollicular zones (130,223).

Molecular and Cytogenetic Findings. *Immunoglobulin Gene Rearrangements.* Rearrangements of immunoglobulin heavy and light chain genes are seen in virtually all cases, as expected from the B lineage of follicular lymphoma, including those that do not express surface immunoglobulin (158,174). Like the physiologic cells of the germinal centers, somatic hypermutations are commonly detected in the variable regions (VH) of the immunoglobulin gene (98). The occasional occurrence of more than two clonal immunoglobulin rearrangements or varying patterns of clonally rearranged genes in different biopsies from the same patient reflects the unique capacity of follicular lymphoma cells to actively mutate and class switch their immunoglobulin genes; this is analogous to normal germinal center B cells involved in maturation of the secondary immune response (134).

t(14;18) Translocation and bcl-2 Gene Rearrangement. Cytogenetic analyses have shown that more than 85 percent of follicular lymphomas contain a characteristic translocation involving the long arms of chromosomes 14 and 18, i.e., t(14;18)(q32;q21) (248). Molecular studies have shown that a gene designated *bcl*-2 (B-cell lymphoma/leukemia) is translocated from its normal position on chromosome 18 to chromosome 14, in juxtaposition with the J-region of the immunoglobulin heavy chain gene (see fig. 3-9) (37,227,228). The breakpoints on chromosome 18 are primarily clustered into two relatively narrow regions in a noncoding part of the *bcl*-2 gene, known as the major breakpoint region (mbr) and minor cluster region (mcr) (158). The breakpoints are clustered within the mbr in 50 to 60 percent of follicular lymphomas, and within the mcr in 25 percent. Other minor regions lying 3' or 5' of the gene are involved in less than 20 percent of cases. For unexplained reasons, the frequency of *bcl*-2 gene rearrangement in Asians and Europeans is lower (27 to 57 percent) than in Americans (3,33,137,142,189). Somatic mutations are also frequently found in the translocated *bcl*-2 gene, presumably occurring as a part of the immunoglobulin gene somatic hypermutation process in germinal center B cells (224).

The *bcl*-2 gene product is an integral membrane protein localized to the inner mitochondrial membrane; it normally prevents programmed cell death (apoptosis) of B cells and extends their survival (34,87,234). Unlike the normal germinal cen-

ters, which switch off *bcl*-2 protein synthesis to promote cell turnover, the neoplastic cells in follicular lymphoma persistently overexpress *bcl*-2 protein as a result of the chromosomal translocation, resulting in "accumulation" of cells and lack of involution like the normal germinal centers. Thus *bcl*-2 constitutes a novel category of oncoprotein, one associated with cell survival as opposed to proliferation, and these biologic properties are consistent with the indolent behavior of follicular lymphoma.

Although a t(14;18) or *bcl*-2 gene rearrangement is characteristic of follicular lymphoma, this abnormality can also be found in approximately 30 percent of diffuse large B-cell lymphomas in whites (21,180,226,241,248). In Asians, *bcl*-2 gene rearrangement is uncommon among diffuse B-cell lymphomas (less than 5 percent) (33,137,142).

DNA probes have been used to detect *bcl*-2 rearrangements as a molecular adjunct to routine cytogenetic detection of the t(14;18) translocation (241). Furthermore, since the translocation breakpoint sites on both chromosomes 14 and 18 tend to occur in restricted locations, polymerase chain reaction (PCR) methods have been devised to amplify t(14;18) breakpoint junctional sequences (127,173). These approaches have been used to detect occult disease (residual tumor) in the blood or bone marrow of patients before and after therapy for follicular lymphoma, and to assess the efficiency of bone marrow purging in patients treated by autologous bone marrow transplantation (54,74,94,173,195). Such studies have produced confusing results, but the following findings appear to be common. In patients with high-stage disease, t(14;18)-positive cells can frequently be detected in the blood or bone marrow despite the absence of morphologic evidence of marrow involvement (15,73,74,220). t(14;18)-positive cells are often detectable in the blood or bone marrow of patients with stage I to II disease, suggesting that even cases of apparently localized disease are in fact disseminated (15,123). For patients treated by conventional chemotherapy, t(14;18)-positive cells often persist in the blood/bone marrow despite apparently successful treatment (74). Such cells have even been detected in patients in long-term (more than 10 years) clinical remission (195). On the other hand, occasional patients with clinical evidence of disease may not have a positive PCR reaction

(122). Thus PCR detection of t(14;18)-positive cells may not be useful for monitoring patients for evidence of remission or early relapse (122). It appears that chemotherapy cannot totally eradicate the disease, or that the t(14;18)-positive cells detected by PCR may not represent lymphoma cells but rather cells carrying the translocation but lacking additional cellular changes for malignant transformation (73). For patients treated by autologous bone marrow transplantation with immunologically purged marrow or by allogenic marrow transplantation, at least some achieve apparent cure as evidenced by a negative t(14;18) assay in blood/bone marrow, suggesting that bone marrow transplantation may be "curative" in some patients with follicular lymphoma (73,75,159). Persistence or reappearance of t(14;18)-positive cells in the bone marrow usually indicates impending relapse.

In spite of the excellent results with PCR-based diagnostic methods, PCR applied to t(14;18) has several limitations. It is not able to detect all t(14;18) breakpoints, since current approaches only identify breakpoints occurring in the two "hot spots" flanking the *bcl*-2 gene (43,121). Interestingly, PCR examination of reactive lymphoid tissues from normal individuals has shown that up to half of the tissues contain rare cells that carry the t(14;18), perhaps underscoring the frequency of aberrant gene rearrangement events and suggesting that *bcl*-2 translocations are necessary but not sufficient for the development of follicular lymphoma (6,139). This apparently ubiquitous, low-level presence of cells with t(14;18) translocations may pose a practical limit to the application of PCR for longitudinal assessment of minimal residual disease in follicular lymphoma patients, although a recent study shows that standard PCR assay (single-run, two-primer, non-nested assay) does not detect t(14;18) in reactive lymphoid hyperplasia; this implies that t(14;18) detected by the standard non-enhanced PCR technique is probably significant and indicative of disease (181,210). No single method (i.e., cytogenetics, Southern blot, or PCR) can detect the genetic lesions underlying deregulated *bcl*-2 expression in all cases of follicular lymphoma and each approach has its relative merits and limitations (250).

Other Genetic Changes. Follicular lymphomas with a t(14;18) translocation behave no differently from those lacking this chromosomal translocation (226). The t(14;18) with associated *bcl*-2 deregulation probably constitutes a major determinant of the follicular architectural pattern of these lymphomas but does not determine biologic aggressiveness and clinical behavior of follicular lymphoma subtypes. Rather, additional genomic events appear to account for histopathologic subtypes of follicular lymphoma, their clinical course, and response to treatment (247). Those with t(14;18) as a single defect usually have a follicular small cleaved cell morphology and an indolent course. Additional genomic defects such as deletion 13q32; deletion 6q; trisomy 2, 3, 7, 12, 18, or 21; or duplication 2p are associated with a mixed cell or large cell composition or a more aggressive clinical course (247, 248). A recent study shows 6q23-26 and 17p abnormalities to be associated with a shorter survival and higher frequency of transformation (226).

Rare cases of follicular lymphoma showing t(8;14)(q24;q32) have been reported; the breakpoints seem to fall outside of the commonly affected sites seen in the t(8;14) of high-grade non-Hodgkin's lymphoma, and the clinical course of these cases is not aggressive (120). A small proportion of follicular lymphomas (6 to 13 percent) show rearrangement of *bcl*-6 gene (3q27); the significance of this is currently unclear (see chapter 9 for details).

Histologic Transformation. Secondary c-myc gene translocations account for only a small fraction of cases (8 percent) with histologic conversion of low-grade follicular lymphoma to diffuse large cell lymphoma (141,245). It is possible that bcl-3 gene (17q22) rearrangement, acquired during the indolent follicular phase of the disease, may contribute to histologic progression in a small percentage (8 percent) of cases (246). By far, acquisition of p53 gene mutations is most frequently (25 to 30 percent of cases) associated with histologic transformation of follicular lymphoma (141,205).

Differential Diagnosis. *Florid Reactive Follicular Hyperplasia, including Rheumatoid Lymphadenopathy, Luetic Lymphadenitis, Toxoplasmic Lymphadenitis, and Plasma Cell Variant of Castleman's Disease.* Florid reactive follicular hyperplasia of lymph node can occur as an idiopathic condition, or in association with well-defined diseases such as rheumatoid lymphadenopathy, luetic lymphadenitis (syphilis), toxoplasmic

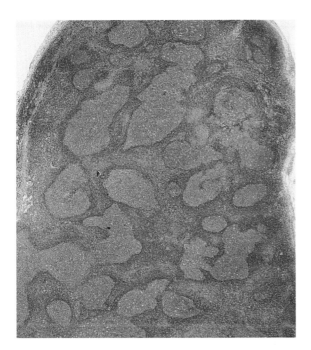 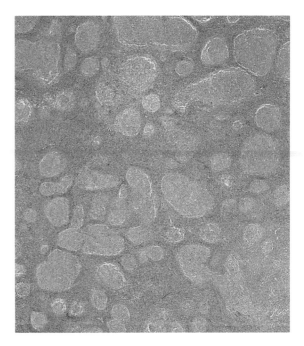

Figure 6-58

REACTIVE FOLLICULAR HYPERPLASIA CONTRASTED WITH FOLLICULAR LYMPHOMA

Left: In this case of reactive follicular hyperplasia, the follicles are irregular shaped, as commonly observed in this condition. The follicles are surrounded by well-defined mantles, albeit thin in areas. A starry-sky pattern (due to the presence of interspersed tingible body macrophages) can be observed in the follicles. There is still an appreciable amount of interfollicular tissue.

Right: Although this example of follicular lymphoma displays irregular-shaped follicles, they are tightly packed and lack well-defined mantles or a starry-sky pattern. There are obviously more nodules per unit area compared with the figure on the left, a characteristic feature of follicular lymphoma.

lymphadenitis, and plasma cell variant of Castleman's disease (52,70,85,118,164,178,217). The idiopathic form typically occurs in young adults, and usually affects a solitary lymph node in the submandibular or cervical region (168, 183,187). The lymphoid follicles are well separated and predominantly distributed in the cortex, contrasting with the tightly packed follicles that extend throughout the entire node in most cases of follicular lymphoma. The follicles often vary in size and shape (sometimes dumbbell or serpentine shaped), and have well-defined mantles (figs. 6-2, 6-58). They contain a heterogeneous population of follicular center cells (large cells often predominating over small cells) that are mitotically active and interspersed with tingible body macrophages (fig. 6-14). Cellular polarization (with dark zone and light zone) can usually be observed in at least some follicles, although this feature may be difficult to appreciate (figs. 6-2; 6-12, left; 6-59). Some cases may be accompanied by a significant component of monocytoid B cells in the perifollicular zones and sinusoids (fig. 6-60).

The specific types of lymphadenopathy often show specific histologic changes in addition to the component of reactive follicular hyperplasia. In rheumatoid lymphadenopathy, interfollicular plasmacytosis is often prominent, and neutrophils can usually be identified in the sinuses (fig. 6-61). In luetic lymphadenitis, the capsule of the lymph node is often thickened and inflamed, plasmacytosis is common, venulitis is often present, and granulomas are sometimes found (fig. 6-62). In toxoplasmic lymphadenitis, monocytoid B cells are prominent, and there are scattered or small aggregates of epithelioid histiocytes, some of which encroach on the germinal centers (fig. 6-63). In the plasma cell variant of Castleman's disease, reactive follicles (which often contain PAS-positive eosinophilic material) are separated by prominent infiltrates of plasma cells, which extend all the way to the cortical region (fig. 6-64). Nonetheless, distinction of these various entities requires clinicopathologic correlation and sometimes special investigations.

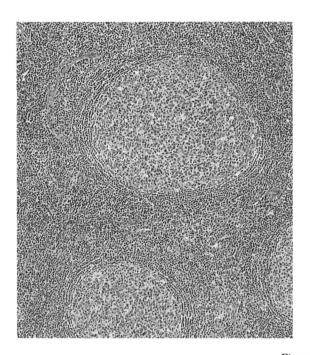 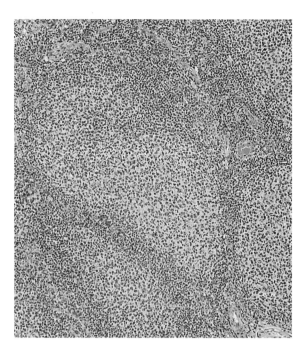

Figure 6-59
REACTIVE FOLLICULAR HYPERPLASIA CONTRASTED WITH FOLLICULAR LYMPHOMA

Left: In this example of reactive follicular hyperplasia, the two follicles are completely surrounded by mantles and separated by abundant interfollicular tissue. The cellular composition appears to be mixed. However, cellular polarization is not evident and tingible body macrophages are few. Immunohistochemical staining may be required for distinction from follicular lymphoma.

Right: In follicular lymphoma, the follicles often give an impression of cellular monotony. In contrast to the left, the follicles are poorly defined and crowded.

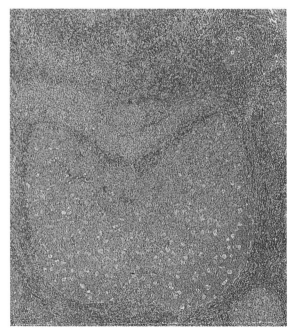 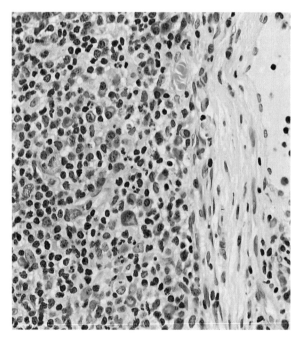

Figure 6-60
REACTIVE FOLLICULAR HYPERPLASIA WITH MONOCYTOID B-CELL REACTION: LYMPH NODE

The top of this hyperplastic follicle shows cellular polarization and is surrounded by an arc of pale-staining monocytoid B cells.

Figure 6-61
REACTIVE LYMPHADENOPATHY OF RHEUMATOID ARTHRITIS

Some neutrophils are seen in the subcapsular sinus. Plasma cells are also evident in this field.

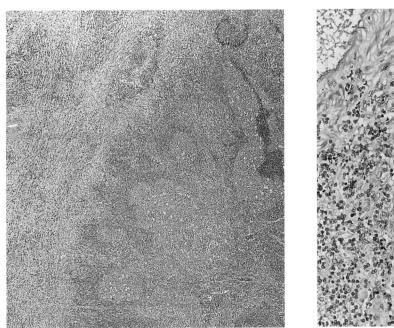
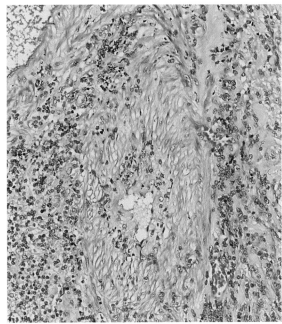

Figure 6-62
LUETIC (SYPHILITIC) LYMPHADENOPATHY

Left: The lymph node shows florid reactive follicles with irregular contours and many tingible body macrophages (right field). The capsule (left field) is thickened and infiltrated by mononuclear cells.

Right: Venulitis is evident in a capsular blood vessel.

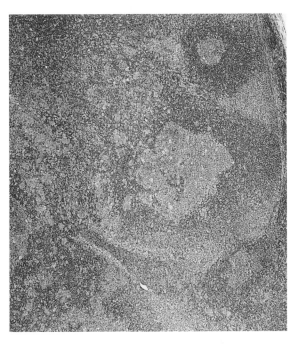
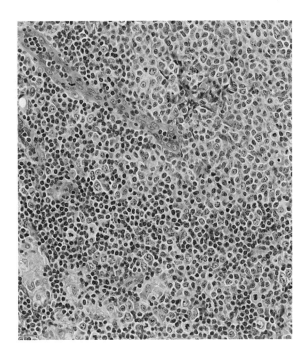

Figure 6-63
TOXOPLASMIC LYMPHADENITIS

Left: This illustration depicts the characteristic triad of toxoplasmic lymphadenitis: reactive follicular hyperplasia, monocytoid B-cell reaction, and epithelioid histiocytic aggregates. Monocytoid B cells form pale-staining arcs around the follicles and in the sinusoids. Scattered in the paracortex are small pink clusters of epithelioid histiocytes; some of these histiocytes extend into the germinal centers.

Right: Higher magnification showing monocytoid B cells in the upper right field; these cells are medium sized and have a moderate amount of pale cytoplasm. Small clusters of epithelioid histiocytes are seen in the left lower field.

Table 6-5

HISTOPATHOLOGIC CRITERIA FOR DIFFERENTIATING
FOLLICULAR LYMPHOMA FROM REACTIVE FOLLICULAR HYPERPLASIA*

Major criterion
  Closely packed follicles distributed throughout the lymph node and separated by scanty interfollicular tissues

Minor criteria
  Consistent absence of tingible body macrophages in the follicles
  Monotony of cellular composition: almost pure population of small cleaved cells (centrocytes)
  Consistent absence of cellular polarization in the follicles
  Follicular mantles absent or thin/incomplete
  Presence of follicles in perinodal tissues
  Dysplastic follicular center cells, e.g., cells with extremely elongated nuclei, bizarre cells, signet ring
    cells, many multilobated cells
  Presence of atypical cells (follicular center cells) in the interfollicular regions

* Diagnosis of follicular lymphoma can be made in the presence of the single major criterion (provided that the follicles are confirmed on higher magnification to be composed of follicular center cells), or two or more minor criteria. If in doubt, apply ancillary techniques for confirmation of diagnosis (see Table 6-6).

Morphologic Criteria. Distinction between follicular lymphoma and florid reactive follicular hyperplasia can be difficult. The single most important criterion is the low-magnification architectural arrangement of the follicles. A pattern of back-to-back follicles disposed throughout the nodal parenchyma, producing a sieve-like pattern, is diagnostic of follicular lymphoma, as long as the cellular composition is confirmed to be of follicular center cell type on higher magnification. This pattern is evident in 85 percent of all cases of follicular lymphoma (figs. 6-1; 6-3; 6-6; 6-58, right) (151,168).

If the above-mentioned prototypic histologic pattern is not seen, two or more of the minor criteria listed in Table 6-5 must be present to diagnose follicular lymphoma (figs. 6-7–6-10, 6-20, 6-65, 6-66). Nonetheless, some caveats have to be mentioned. Although neoplastic follicles are characteristically deficient in the mantles, some cases of follicular lymphoma can have remarkably thick mantles. On the other hand, reactive lymphoid follicles can be deficient in mantles, in particular in florid reactive hyperplasia in childhood and human immunodeficiency virus–associated lymphadenopathy (fig. 6-67) (217). Some cases of follicular lymphoma can be rich in tingible body macrophages (fig. 6-20). It is also evident from Table 6-5 that it is easiest to diagnose follicular small cleaved cell

lymphoma because of the monotony of the cellular composition (fig. 6-24), but more difficult in those cases with a mixed cell or predominantly large cell population because of the resemblance to the cellular composition of the reactive follicles (figs. 6-25, 6-26). In rheumatoid lymphadenopathy, reactive follicle centers can be paradoxically predominated by small cleaved cells (centrocytes), with few mitotic figures and few tingible body macrophages (118). Interfollicular tissues should be carefully assessed for atypical cells to support a diagnosis of follicular lymphoma. Even in reactive conditions, the interfollicular small lymphocytes exhibit a mild degree of nuclear irregularity. The interfollicular lymphoid cells must be larger than the small round lymphocytes and have obviously angulated nuclei to be considered indicative of infiltration by lymphoma (fig. 6-21).

The various histologic features have to be analyzed in well-preserved portions of the specimen. In suboptimally fixed tissues (especially from the central portion), even reactive follicles may appear worrisome because cellular polarization, lymphocytic mantles, and tingible body macrophages often become inapparent, and the cellular shrinkage may give an erroneous impression of small cleaved cell predominance.

Besides histologic features, age is also an important consideration. Since follicular lymphoma is extremely rare below the age of 20

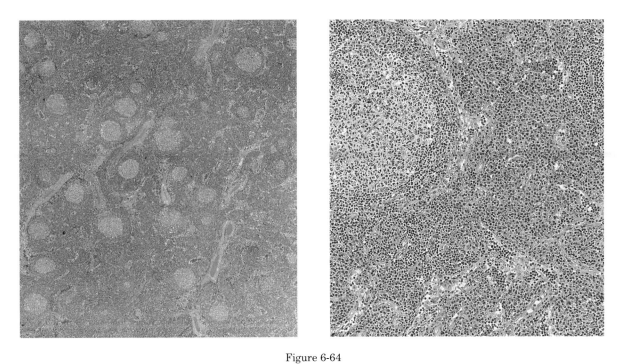

Figure 6-64
CASTLEMAN'S DISEASE, PLASMA CELL TYPE: LYMPH NODE
Left: Reactive follicles are separated by an appreciable amount of violaceous-staining interfollicular tissue.
Right: The interfollicular tissue comprises predominantly sheets of plasma cells.

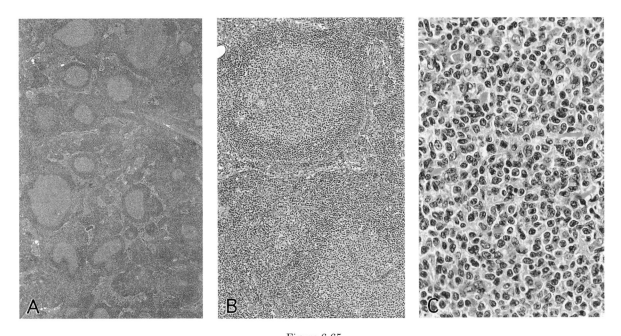

Figure 6-65
FOLLICULAR LYMPHOMA IN LYMPH NODE: DIFFICULT CASE
A: On low magnification, the follicles possess well-defined mantles and are widely spaced, and the sinuses are well preserved. These features resemble those of reactive follicular hyperplasia.
B: Consistent lack of cellular polarization and tingible body macrophages should strongly raise a suspicion of follicular lymphoma.
C: Since the follicles show a monotonous population of small cleaved cells, a diagnosis of follicular lymphoma becomes fully tenable.

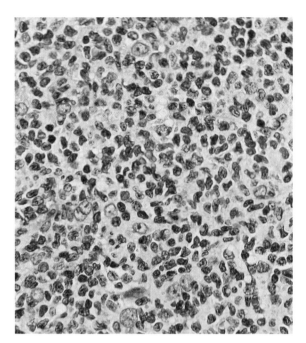

Figure 6-66
FOLLICULAR LYMPHOMA WITH
DYSPLASTIC FOLLICULAR CENTER CELLS

This follicle is predominated by small cleaved cells, many of which have elongated nuclei. There are occasional "dysplastic" cells (cells with clear cytoplasmic vacuoles [signet ring cells]) which are not seen in the germinal centers of reactive follicles.

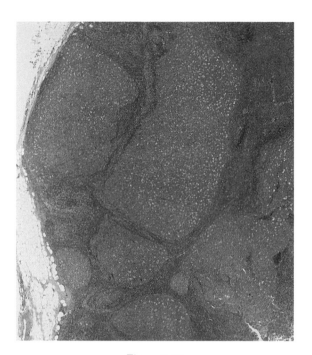

Figure 6-67
FLORID REACTIVE FOLLICULAR HYPERPLASIA
WITH DEFICIENT MANTLES (LYMPH NODE),
OCCURRING IN A 6-YEAR-OLD CHILD

The follicles are quite closely packed and lack well-defined lymphocytic mantles, features that are observed in florid reactive follicular hyperplasia in children. Features supporting a "benign" interpretation of this worrisome picture are the presence of numerous tingible body macrophages and a suggestion of cellular polarization (presence of pale and dark zones) in the follicles. In such a young patient, follicular lymphoma should be diagnosed only if supported by immunohistochemical or genotypic studies.

years, this diagnosis should be made with utmost caution and only with support by ancillary techniques in that age group (130).

Ancillary Techniques. Should there be any uncertainty about the diagnosis, the ancillary techniques shown in Table 6-6 are extremely helpful for confirming a diagnosis of follicular lymphoma versus reactive follicular hyperplasia.

AIDS-Related Lymphadenopathy. The explosive follicular hyperplasia in this syndrome is particularly likely to be mistaken for follicular lymphoma. This lesion is characterized by hyperplastic follicles, many of which have "naked" germinal centers that are deficient in mantles; follicle lysis (disruption of the follicular dendritic cell network and hemorrhage into germinal centers); polykaryocytes within or outside germinal centers; and prominent monocytoid B cells (fig. 6-68) (25). Although the mantles of the follicles are often deficient, the reactive nature of the follicles can be clearly recognized by the presence of cellular polarization and the abundance of tingible body macrophages.

Castleman's Disease, Hyaline-Vascular Type. Castleman's disease of the hyaline-vascular type is a reactive condition characterized by follicles that possess a broad mantle zone with an "onionskin" pattern surrounding relatively small germinal centers (with a predominance of follicular dendritic cells and a decrease in follicular center B cells); the germinal centers contain hyalinized vessels, which often transfix the broadened mantle zone (fig. 6-69). In some cases, the follicles are large and formed mostly by small lymphocytes, but are punctuated by multiple small germinal centers (fig. 6-70) (49,56,110).

In rare cases of follicular lymphoma, the neoplastic follicles can be penetrated by hyalinized venules (fig. 6-40). Such cases can be distinguished from Castleman's disease by a richer component of follicular center B cells in the follicle centers, and the presence in other areas of more typical histologic features of follicular lymphoma. In problematic

Table 6-6

ANCILLARY TECHNIQUES FOR DIAGNOSIS OF FOLLICULAR LYMPHOMA VERSUS REACTIVE FOLLICULAR HYPERPLASIA

Immunohistochemical staining
    Staining of the follicular center cells for *bcl*-2 protein (most helpful) (7,128,244)
    Immunoglobulin light chain restriction (very helpful; can be performed on either fresh/frozen or
        paraffin-embedded tissues, but the staining is more reliable in the former; the results can sometimes
        be difficult to interpret because of interstitial staining)
    Staining of the follicular center cells for MT2 (CD45RA) (positive in approximately 50 percent of cases)
        (21,128,170,177)

Genotypic studies (Southern blot or polymerase chain reaction)
    Immunoglobulin gene rearrangement
    Bcl-2 gene rearrangement

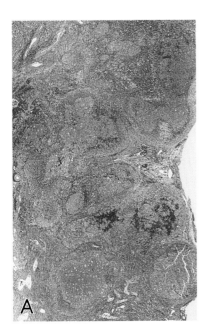 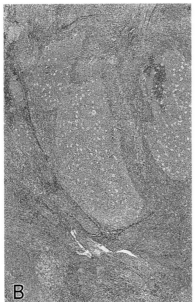 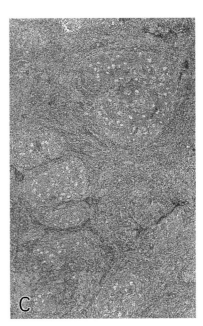

Figure 6-68

AIDS-RELATED LYMPHADENOPATHY WITH FLORID FOLLICULAR HYPERPLASIA

A, B: These figures are characterized by large, bizarre-shaped follicles that still maintain lymphocytic mantles. Note hemorrhage and intrusion of dark-staining small lymphocytes into the follicles as a manifestation of follicle lysis; bleeding probably occurred into the weakened follicles (with partially disrupted follicular dendritic cell networks) during the biopsy procedure. The follicles are clearly reactive by virtue of the cellular polarization and numerous tingible body macrophages.

C: In this example, the reactive follicles are totally devoid of lymphocytic mantles. In contrast to follicular lymphoma, tingible body macrophages are abundant and polarization is seen in the follicles. Follicle lysis is also evidenced by multiple small foci of invagination of small lymphocytes into the follicle centers.

cases, immunostaining for *bcl*-2 protein and immunoglobulin light chain is helpful for distinction.

Progressive Transformation of Germinal Centers (PTGC). PTGC is a benign condition of unknown etiology, but occasional cases may presage the development of Hodgkin's disease, especially the nodular lymphocyte predominance type (24,78,193,231). Histologically, it is characterized by the presence

of scattered large expansile "transformed" follicles in a background of usual-looking reactive follicles (fig. 6-71, left). The transformed follicles are formed mostly by small lymphocytes, but they do contain scattered follicular center B cells, which may be isolated or form irregular small clusters (fig. 6-71, right). Meshworks of follicular dendritic cells are present in these follicles.

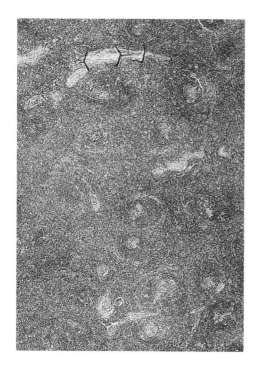

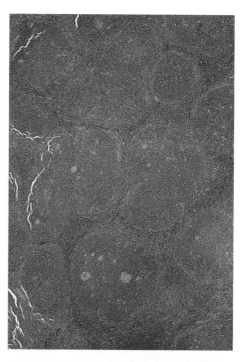

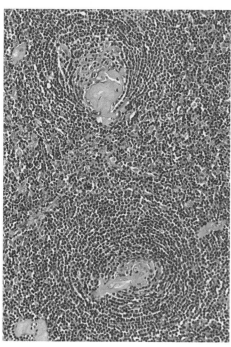

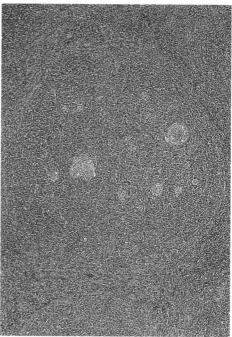

Figure 6-69
CASTLEMAN'S DISEASE,
HYALINE-VASCULAR TYPE: LYMPH NODE

Top: This lesion is characterized by multiple nodules of lymphoid tissue with abnormal germinal centers that are separated by hypervascular interfollicular tissue.

Bottom: The lymphoid nodules show concentric arrangement of small lymphocytes, small germinal centers depleted of follicular center B cells, and penetration by hyalinized venules.

Figure 6-70
CASTLEMAN'S DISEASE,
HYALINE-VASCULAR TYPE: LYMPH NODE

Top: In this case, the lymphoid nodules are much larger compared with those of figure 6-69. They are also separated by hypervascular interfollicular tissue, but appear to contain multiple small germinal centers, a feature, which if present, is practically diagnostic of hyaline-vascular Castleman's disease.

Bottom: A nodule with multiple abnormal, small germinal centers. Note the increased venules both in the nodule and interfollicular tissue.

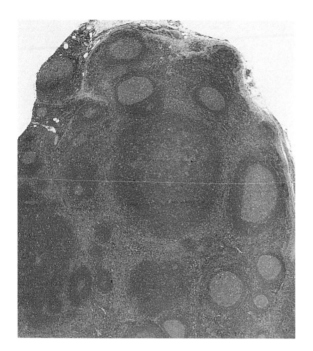 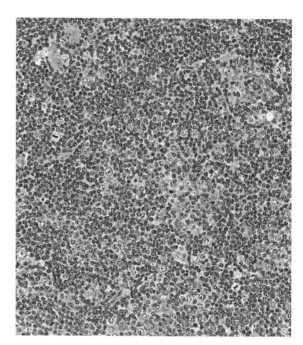

Figure 6-71
PROGRESSIVE TRANSFORMATION OF GERMINAL CENTERS: LYMPH NODE

Left: Several large, expansile, dark-staining lymphoid nodules are evident amid clearly reactive lymphoid follicles. These large nodules (progressed transformed germinal centers) lack discrete light-staining germinal centers.

Right: The nodules are formed mostly by small lymphocytes, with some interspersed larger and paler-staining cells, which represent follicular center B cells and follicular dendritic cells.

The floral variant of follicular lymphoma mimics PTGC by virtue of the thick mantles and ingrowth of small lymphocytes into the neoplastic follicles. In contrast to PTGC, all the follicles (nodules) are abnormal and there are no reactive follicles in the background. There is usually predominance of large follicular center cells, which may show dysplastic features. Atypical lymphoid cells between the follicles and in the perinodal tissues also supports a diagnosis of lymphoma over PTGC.

Nodular Lymphocyte Predominance Hodgkin's Disease. The nodules of nodular lymphocyte predominance Hodgkin's disease, which are composed predominantly of small lymphocytes, may contain cohesive aggregates of lymphocytic and histiocytic (L&H) cells, resembling follicular lymphoma, including the floral variant (figs. 6-39, 6-72). L&H cells ("popcorn cells") may at times resemble large noncleaved follicular center cells, thus compounding the diagnostic dilemma (24, 193,221). The lymphoid nodules of nodular lymphocyte predominance Hodgkin's disease are generally larger than those of follicular lymphoma. The presence of a significant component

of small cleaved cells (centrocytes) in or between the nodules strongly favors a diagnosis of follicular lymphoma over nodular lymphocyte predominance Hodgkin's disease. Immunoperoxidase studies may be necessary for diagnosis. Both L&H cells and large follicular center cells react with B-cell markers but the L&H cells are also often positive for epithelial membrane antigen and are characteristically surrounded by a wreath of Leu-7–positive T cells (see chapter 15).

Mantle Cell Lymphoma. Some cases of mantle cell lymphoma have a vague or prominent nodular architecture due to centripetal effacement of the germinal centers, mimicking follicular lymphoma (fig. 6-73) (8,196). Identification of a mantle zone growth pattern in areas and total absence of large noncleaved cells (centroblasts) favor a diagnosis of mantle cell lymphoma over follicular lymphoma (fig. 6-74); immunohistochemical studies may still be required for the distinction. The neoplastic cells of follicular lymphoma lack CD5 and CD43, often lack IgD, may express IgG, and are often CD10 positive. The tumor cells of mantle cell lymphoma express IgM/IgD, CD5, and CD43 and usually lack

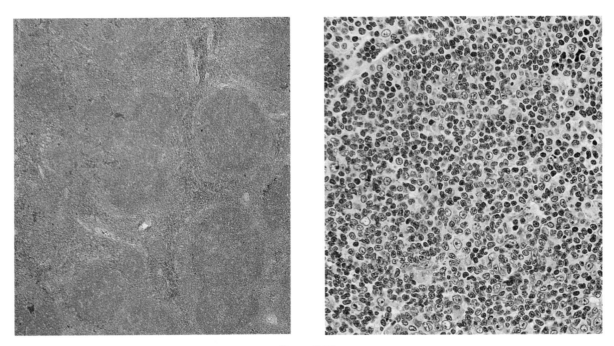

Figure 6-72
FOLLICULAR LYMPHOMA HISTOLOGICALLY SIMULATING NLPHD

Left: This follicular lymphoma comprises large, discrete, dark-staining nodules, mimicking the architectural pattern of nodular lymphocyte predominance Hodgkin's disease (NLPHD) and does not belong to the floral variant.

Right: In the nodules (follicles), the small cleaved cells (demonstrated by immunohistochemical staining to express monotypic immunoglobulin) are admixed with many small lymphocytes. L&H cells are not seen.

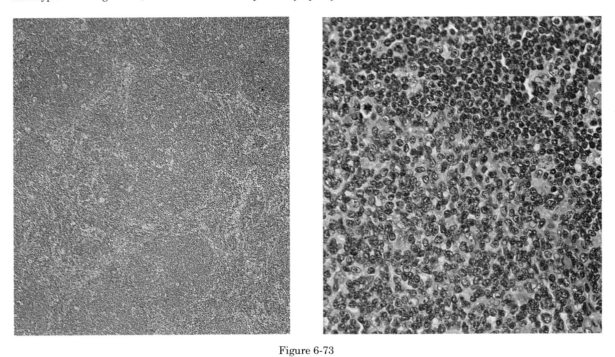

Figure 6-73
MANTLE CELL LYMPHOMA WITH A PROMINENT NODULAR GROWTH PATTERN: LYMPH NODE

Left: The lymphoma displays a nodular growth pattern.

Right: Compared with the interfollicular small lymphocytes (upper field), the lymphoma cells have larger and more irregular nuclei, and less condensed chromatin. These cells cannot be reliably distinguished from the small cleaved cells (centrocytes) of follicular lymphoma. In contrast to follicular lymphoma, there are no interspersed large noncleaved cells. (Figures 6-73 and 6-74 are from the same case.)

CD10. In contrast to follicular lymphoma, mantle cell lymphomas are associated with a disrupted, disorganized meshwork of follicular dendritic cells.

Low-Grade B-Cell Lymphoma of Mucosa-Associated Lymphoid Tissue with Follicular Colonization. Low-grade B-cell lymphoma of mucosa-associated lymphoid tissue (MALT) can show remarkable colonization of the scattered reactive lymphoid follicles, producing a nodular pattern that is very difficult to distinguish from follicular lymphoma (fig. 6-75) (101,102). In fact, at least some of the cases of follicular or follicular/diffuse lymphomas reported in various extranodal sites might represent this entity. Features favoring a diagnosis of low-grade B-cell lymphoma of MALT over follicular lymphoma are: 1) presence of lymphoepithelial lesions; 2) perifollicular growth pattern in areas; 3) confinement of the follicles to areas where reactive follicles commonly occur (e.g., mucosa and submucosa but not the muscularis of the gastrointestinal tract); 4) more cytoplasm in the centrocyte-like cells compared with the small cleaved cells (centrocytes) of follicular lymphoma;

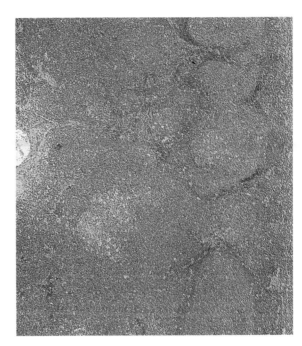

Figure 6-74
MANTLE CELL LYMPHOMA: LYMPH NODE

In some areas, a mantle zone growth pattern is evident. Broad rims of dark-staining lymphoid cells surround the residual reactive germinal centers.

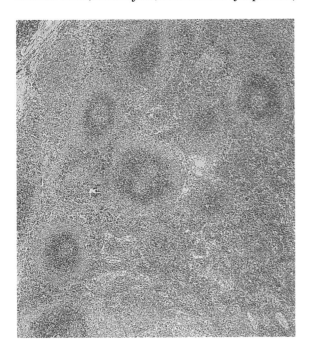

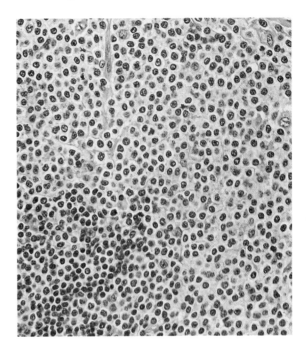

Figure 6-75
LOW-GRADE B-CELL LYMPHOMA OF MUCOSA-ASSOCIATED LYMPHOID TISSUE (FROM STOMACH)

Left: A nodular growth pattern is seen in this perigastric lymph node draining a gastric low-grade B-cell lymphoma of MALT. The nodular pattern is created by pale-staining lymphoid cells proliferating around and replacing the preexisting lymphoid follicles, a so-called perifollicular or marginal zone pattern.

Right: Higher magnification of one of the nodules shows overgrowth of cells with clear cytoplasm; residual small lymphoid cells of the preexisting follicle are seen in the left lower field.

5) frequent occurrence of plasma cell differentiation; 6) lack of CD10 immunoreactivity; and 7) lack of *bcl*-2 gene rearrangement (fig. 6-75).

Small Lymphocytic Lymphoma/Chronic Lymphocytic Leukemia with Prominent Pseudofollicles (Proliferation Centers). See chapter 7.

Lymphoblastic Lymphoma with a Lobular Pattern. In lymphoblastic lymphoma affecting lymph nodes, the lymphoblasts sometimes grow in nodular aggregates, imparting a "pseudonodular" or lobular pattern, superficially resembling a follicular lymphoma (99). The cytologic features of the lymphoblasts, which have fine chromatin and inconspicuous nucleoli associated with numerous mitoses, differ significantly from those of follicular center cells. Appropriate immunoperoxidase studies help with the distinction. Lymphoblastic lymphoma is terminal deoxynucleotidyl transferase (TdT) positive, whereas follicular lymphoma is not. Demonstration of T lineage on the neoplastic cells (most cases of lymphoblastic lymphoma) also excludes follicular lymphoma.

Other Conditions that May Have a Nodular Growth Pattern. Mast cell disease can exhibit a vague nodular pattern due to replacement of preexisting reactive follicles (see chapter 19). Even post-thymic T-cell lymphoma can occasionally involve lymph node in a nodular pattern (149,175).

Treatment and Prognosis. Commonly used treatment modalities include radiation therapy and chemotherapy; anti-idiotypic antibody therapy and bone marrow transplantation are promising treatment possibilities (20,200,249). Radiation therapy may consist of palliative radiation only to sites of active disease, extended-field radiotherapy, or even total lymphoid irradiation in some circumstances (8 9). Chemotherapeutic regimes are generally mild, consisting of either a single-drug such as chlorambucil or cyclophosphamide or, more commonly, a relatively nontoxic combination such as cyclophosphamide-vincristine-prednisone (CVP) or cyclophosphamide-adriamycin-oncovin-prednisone (CHOP), although some investigators have used highly aggressive, multiple chemotherapeutic agents (204).

Despite the indolent biologic behavior of low-grade follicular lymphoma (median survival, 7 years), the disease is rarely cured using currently available treatment programs, except in the small proportion of patients with stage I disease (89,93,96,194). Patients with stage I disease are treated by radiation therapy, with or without chemotherapy, with a curative intent, and the prognosis is excellent (5). For higher stage disease, the main strategy of treatment is symptomatic control rather than cure, thus the use of single agent chemotherapy or "mild" combination chemotherapy. The importance of managing selected asymptomatic patients without initial therapy ("watch and wait" policy) is also now well recognized, since spontaneous remission sometimes occurs (93,194). This treatment approach does not apparently compromise the overall survival: the median survival is 11 years, and the actuarial survival at 15 years is 40 percent (5,93). It should be noted, however, that most of these patients eventually require therapy due to progression of disease; approximately 50 percent are treated by the third year of observation (204). Some studies have suggested that follicular mixed cell lymphoma may be cured by intensive chemotherapy, but only long-term follow-up will clarify this debatable issue (1,60,67,145,146). There is also evidence that patients with follicular mixed cell lymphoma treated by combination chemotherapy have more durable remissions and even longer overall survival rates than those with follicular small cleaved cell lymphoma (60,239).

Because follicular large cell lymphomas tend to be aggressive (213), intensive chemotherapy regimens (including adriamycin or doxorubicin) are usually used (5). Observation without therapy is generally not recommended (9). Remissions, once achieved, are more durable than for low-grade follicular lymphoma. Treated in this way, the reported 10-year survival is at least 50 percent, which is superior to that reported in the original Working Formulation study (10-year survival, 30 percent) (176,213). The survival curve reaches a plateau, suggesting that follicular large cell lymphoma may be curable, a contention that is still debated (1,4,5,9,68,94,108, 188). Patients with discordant lymphoma (low-grade follicular lymphoma in other sites or in a second biopsy in addition to follicular large cell lymphoma) show a greater tendency to relapse and a lower overall survival compared with those having pure follicular large cell lymphoma (9).

Paradoxically, when transformation to a diffuse large cell lymphoma occurs (which is associated with a poor prognosis and a survival of usually less than 1 year if untreated), the disease becomes potentially curable by aggressive chemotherapy, presumably because of the high proliferative fraction. Approximately one third of cases have lasting remissions (91,97,145). Some patients relapse with diffuse large cell lymphoma or follicular lymphoma (86,152).

Prognostic Factors. Table 6-7 lists the various prognostic factors that have been reported to have an influence on the overall survival or relapse-free survival (1,9,10,26,38,60,61,76,201,213). The more important factors are discussed below.

Stage. Stage I disease is associated with a much better prognosis than stage II to IV disease, with a reported 14-year survival of 70 percent in the former and 30 percent in the latter (213).

Histologic Subclassification. Follicular lymphomas with predominantly small cleaved cell or mixed cell composition have been shown in many studies to have a significantly better prognosis than those with a predominance of large cells (176,213).

Degree of Nodularity. It is well known that follicular lymphoma has a much better prognosis than diffuse lymphoma of comparable histology (90,176,236). There is also evidence that follicular lymphomas with a significant diffuse component have a worse prognosis than those that are predominantly follicular.

Age. Some studies have shown an age of under 40 years is associated with a better prognosis (1,60,140).

Histologic Transformation to a Diffuse Large Cell Lymphoma. This is associated with a poor prognosis, the median survival being 10 months following diagnosis of the transformation (60). However, aggressive chemotherapy can result in complete remission in about one third of cases and some remissions are long lasting.

Large Tumor Bulk. Presence of splenomegaly, hepatomegaly, abnormal liver function tests, bulky tumor (more than 5 cm), and B symptoms correlate with a less favorable prognosis (1,60).

Genetic Alterations. Described above.

Complete Response on First Treatment. This is associated with a more favorable survival (1,60).

Risk models, including the International Prognostic Index designed for aggressive lymphomas, that stratify patients into different risk groups, have been successfully applied to follicular lymphomas (9,10,38,147,201). However, since only a small proportion of patients fall into

Table 6-7

REPORTED UNFAVORABLE PROGNOSTIC FACTORS IN FOLLICULAR LYMPHOMA

	Parameters Associated with Earlier Failure, Decreased Progression-Free Survival, or Decreased Overall Survival
Clinical features	Male sex Age (over 40 years) Bulky tumor (greater than 5 cm) More than one extranodal site Hepatosplenomegaly Advanced stage Poor performance status Systemic symptoms Bone marrow involvement
Laboratory findings	Increased LDH level Increased ß2-microglobulin level (greater than 3 mg/L) Anemia Abnormal liver function tests
Histologic features	High percent of large cells High percent of diffuse areas (more than 25 percent) High mitotic count (more than 50/10 HPF), although one study has not shown the mitotic count to be of independent prognostic value (50) Transformation to diffuse large cell lymphoma
Special studies	High proliferation fraction (S+G2 more than or equal to 18 percent) DNA aneuploidy
Genetic findings	Additional genomic changes, e.g., deletion 13q32; 6q abnormality trisomy 2, 3, 7, 12, 18, 21; duplication 2p; 17p abnormality
Treatment characteristics	Failure to achieve complete remission on first treatment

the high risk group, these prognostic indices are not yet ideal for treatment purposes (10).

Several factors are associated with an increased risk of histologic transformation (10, 38,226): 1) failure to achieve complete remission with initial therapy; 2) more than one extranodal site of disease; 3) bone marrow involvement; 4) high beta-2-microglobulin level; 5) overexpression or mutation of the p53 gene; and 6) 6q23-26 or 17p chromosomal abnormality.

REFERENCES

1. Aisenberg AC. Malignant lymphoma: biology, natural history, and treatment. Philadelphia: Lea & Febiger, 1991.

2. _____, Wilkes BM, Jacobson JO. The bcl-2 gene is rearranged in many diffuse B-cell lymphomas. Blood 1988;71:969–72.

3. Amakawa R, Fukuhara S, Ohno H, et al. Involvement of bcl-2 gene in Japanese follicular lymphoma. Blood 1989;73:787–91.

4. Anderson JR, Vose JM, Bierman PJ, et al. Clinical features and prognosis of follicular large cell lymphoma: a report from the Nebraska Lymphoma Study Group. J Clin Oncol 1993;11:218–24.

5. Armitage JO. Non-Hodgkin's lymphoma. In: Handin RI, Lux SE, Stossel TP, eds. Blood: principles and practice of hematology. Philadelphia: J.B. Lippincott, 1995:813–50.

6. Aster JC, Kobayashi Y, Shiota M, Mori S, Sklar J. Detection of the t(14;18) at similar frequencies in hyperplastic lymphoid tissues from American and Japanese patients. Am J Pathol 1992;141:291–9.

7. Banks PM. When is a new diagnostic method established? [Editorial] Hum Pathol 1993;24:1153–4.

8. _____, Chan J, Cleary ML, et al. Mantle cell lymphoma: a proposal for unification of morphologic, immunologic and molecular data. Am J Surg Pathol 1992;16:637–40.

9. Bartlett NL, Rizeq M, Dorfman RF, Halpern J, Horning SJ. Follicular large cell lymphoma: intermediate or low grade? J Clin Oncol 1994;12:1349–57.

10. Bastion Y, Coiffier B. Is the international prognostic index for aggressive lymphoma patients useful for follicular lymphoma patients? [Editorial] J Clin Oncol 1994;12:1340–2.

11. _____, Berger F, Bryon PA, Felman P, Ffreuch M, Coiffier B. Follicular lymphomas: assessment of prognostic factors in 127 patients followed for 10 years. Ann Oncol 1991;2(Suppl 2):123–9.

12. Bennett MH. Sclerosis in non-Hodgkin's lymphomata. Br J Cancer 1975;31 (Suppl 2):44–52.

13. _____, Millett Y. Nodular sclerotic lymphosarcoma: a possible new clinicopathological entity. Clin Radiol 1969;20:339–43.

14. Berliner N, Ault KA, Martin P, Weinberg S. Detection of clonal excess in lymphoproliferative disease by kappa/gamma analysis: correlation with immunoglobulin gene DNA rearrangement. Blood 1986;67:80–5.

15. Berinstein NL, Reis MD, Ngan BY, Sawka CA, Jamal HH, Kuzniar B. Detection of occult lymphoma in peripheral blood and bone marrow of patients with untreated early-stage and advanced-stage follicular lymphoma. J Clin Oncol 1993;11:1344–52.

16. Bonar MJ, Hurtubise PE, Swerdlow SH. T-cell morphology in nodular follicular center cell lymphomas. Diagn Clin Immunol 1987;5:14–9.

17. Braziel RM, Sussman E, Jaffe, ES, Nekcers LM, Cossman J. Induction of immunoglobulin secretion in follicular non-Hodgkin's lymphomas: role of immunoregulatory T-cells. Blood 1985;66:128–34.

18. Brittinger G, Bartels H, Common H, et al. Clinical and prognostic relevance of the Kiel classification of non-Hodgkin's lymphomas: results of a prospective multicenter study by the Kiel Lymphoma Study Group. Hematol Oncol 1984;2:269–306.

19. Brown RW, Pugh WC, Butler JJ. Follicular lymphoma of immunoblastic/plasmablastic type [Abstract]. Mod Pathol 1991;4:68A.

20. Brown SL, Miller RA, Horning SJ, et. al. Treatment of B-cell lymphomas with anti-idiotype antibodies alone and in combination with alpha-interferon. Blood 1989; 73:651–61.

21. Browne G, Tobin B, Carney DN, Dervan PA. Aberrant MT2 positivity distinguishes follicular lymphoma from reactive follicular hyperplasia in B5 and formalin-fixed paraffin sections. Am J Clin Pathol 1991;96:90–4.

22. Burke JS, Hoppe RT, Cibull ML, Dorfman RF. Cutaneous malignant lymphoma: a pathologic study of 50 cases with clinical analysis of 37. Cancer 1981;47:300–10.

23. _____, Osborne BM. Localized reactive lymphoid hyperplasia of the spleen simulating malignant lymphoma. A report of seven cases. Am J Surg Pathol 1983;7:373–80.

24. Burns BF, Colby TV, Dorfman RF. Differential diagnostic features of nodular L&H Hodgkin's disease including progressive transformation of germinal centers. Am J Surg Pathol 1984;8:253–61.

25. _____, Wood GS, Dorfman RF. The varied histopathology of lymphadenopathy in the homosexual male. Am J Surg Pathol 1985;9:287–97.

26. Cameron DA, Leonard RCF, Mao JH, et al. Identification of prognostic groups in follicular lymphoma. The Scotland and Newcastle Lymphoma Group Therapy Working Party. Leuk Lymphoma 1993;10:89–99.

27. Castellani R, Bonadonna G, Spinelli P, Bajetta E, Galante E, Rilke F. Sequential pathologic staging of untreated non-Hodgkin's lymphomas by laparoscopy and laparotomy combined with marrow biopsy. Cancer 1977;40:2322–8.

28. Chabner BA, Johnson RE, Young RC, et al. Sequential nonsurgical and surgical staging of non-Hodgkin's lymphoma. Cancer 1978;42:922–25.

29. Chan JK, Hui PK, Ng CS. Follicular immunoblastic lymphoma: neoplastic counterpart of the intrafollicular immunoblast? Pathology 1990;22:103–5.

30. _____, Ng CS, Hui PK. An unusual morphological variant of follicular lymphoma. Report of two cases. Histopathology 1988;12:649–58.

31. _____, Ng CS, Tung S. Multilobated B cell lymphoma, a variant of centroblastic lymphoma. Report of four cases. Histopathology 1986;10:601–12.

32. Chang KL, Arber DA, Shibata D, Rappaport H, Weiss LM. Follicular small lymphocytic lymphoma. Am J Surg Pathol 1994;18:999–1009.

33. Chen PM, Lin SH, Seto M, et al. Rearrangements of bcl-2 genes in malignant lymphomas in Chinese patients. Cancer 1993;72:3701–6.

34. Chen-Levy Z, Nourse J, Cleary ML. The bcl-2 candidate proto-oncogene product is a 24-kilodalton integral-membrane protein highly expressed in lymphoid cell lines and lymphomas carrying the t(14;18) translocation. Mol Cell Biol 1989;9:701–10.

35. Chittal SM, Caveriviere P, Voigt JJ, et al. Follicular lymphoma with abundant PAS positive extracellular material: immunohistochemical and ultrastructural observations. Am J Surg Pathol 1987;11:618–24.

36. Chleq-Deschamps CM, LeBrun DP, Huie P, et al. Topographical dissociation of bcl-2 messenger RNA and protein expression in human lymphoid tissues. Blood 1993;81:293–8.

37. Cleary ML, Sklar J. Nucleotide sequence of a t(14;18) chromosomal breakpoint in follicular lymphoma and demonstration of a breakpoint-cluster region near a transcriptionally active locus on chromosome 18. Proc Natl Acad Sci USA 1985;82:7439–43.

38. Coiffier B, Bastion Y, Berger F, Felman P, Bryon PA. Prognostic factors in follicular lymphomas. Semin Oncol 1993;20(Suppl 5):89–95.

39. Colby TV, Hoppe RT, Burke JS. Nodular lymphoma: clinicopathologic correlations of parafollicular small lymphocytes and degree of nodularity. Cancer 1980;45:2364–67.

40. Coller BS, Chabner BA, Gralnick HR. Frequencies and patterns of bone marrow involvement in non-Hodgkin's lymphomas: observations of the value of bilateral biopsies. Am J Hematol 1977;3:105–19.

41. Come SE, Jaffe ES, Andersen JC, et al. Non-Hodgkin's lymphomas in leukemic phase: clinicopathologic correlations. Am J Med 1980;69:667–74.

42. Cornes JS. Multiple lymphomatous polyposis of the gastrointestinal tract. Cancer 1961;14:249–57.

43. Crisan D, Anstett MJ. Bcl-2 gene rearrangements in follicular lymphomas. Lab Med 1993;24:579–88.

44. Cullen MH, Lister TA, Brearley RL, Shand WS, Stansfeld AG. Histological transformation of non-Hodgkin's lymphoma: a prospective study. Cancer 1979;44:645–51.

45. Dabski K, Banks PM, Winkelmann RK. Clinicopathologic spectrum of cutaneous manifestations in systemic follicular lymphoma. A study of 11 patients. Cancer 1989;64:1480–5.

46. Dorfman RF. Follicular (nodular) lymphoma in South Africa: a study of 94 cases. In: Symposium on lymphoid tumours in Africa. Paris: S Karger, 1964:211–28.

47. _____. Classical concepts of nodular (follicular) lymphomas. In: Berard CW, Bennett JM, Ishikawa E, eds. Malignant diseases of the hematopoietic system. Baltimore: University Park Press, 1973;15:177–88. (GANN Monograph on Cancer Research, No. 15.)

48. _____, Burke J, Berard CW. A working formulation of non-Hodgkin's lymphomas: background, recommendations, histologic criteria and relationship to other classifications. In: Rosenberg SA, Kaplan HS, eds. Malignant lymphomas: etiology, immunology, pathology, treatment. New York: Academic Press, 1980: 351–68. (Bristol-Meyers Cancer Symposia, Vol. 3.)

49. _____, Warnke R. Lymphadenopathy simulating the malignant lymphomas. Hum Pathol 1974;5:519–50.

50. Ellison DJ, Nathwani BN, Metter GE, et al. Mitotic counts in follicular lymphomas. Hum Pathol 1987;18:502–5.

51. Erlandson RA. Diagnostic transmission electron microscopy of tumors: with clinicopatholoical, immunohistochemical, and cytogenetic correlations. New York: Raven Press, 1994:497.

52. Evans N. Lymphadenitis of secondary syphilis: its resemblance to giant follicular lymphadenopathy. Arch Pathol 1944;37:175–9.

53. Ezdinli EZ, Costello WG, Kucuk O, Berard CW. Effect of the degree of nodularity on the survival of patients with nodular lymphomas. J Clin Oncol 1987;5:413–18.

54. Finke J, Slanina J, Lange W, Dolken G. Persistence of circulating t(14;18)+ cells in long-term remission after radiation therapy for localized-stage follicular lymphoma. J Clin Oncol 1993;11:1668–73.

55. Fisher RI, Jones RB, DeVita VT, et al. Natural history of malignant lymphomas with divergent histologies at staging evaluation. Cancer 1981;47:2022–55.

56. Frizzera G. Castleman's disease and related disorders. Semin Diagn Pathol 1988;5:346–64.

57. _____, Anaya JS, Banks PM. Neoplastic plasma cells in follicular lymphomas. Clinical and pathologic findings in six cases. Virchows Arch [A] 1986;409:149–62.

58. _____, Gajl-Peczalska K, Sibley RK, Rosai J, Cerhwitz D, Hurd DD. Rosette formation in malignant lymphoma. Am J Pathol 1985;119:351–6.

59. _____, Murphy SB. Follicular (nodular) lymphoma in childhood: a rare clinical-pathological entity. Report of eight cases from four cancer centers. Cancer 1979;44:2218–35.

60. Gallagher CJ, Gregory WM, Jones AE, et al. Follicular lymphoma: prognostic factors for response and survival. J Clin Oncol 1986;4:1470–80.

61. _____, Lister TA. Follicular non-Hodgkin's lymphomas. Clin Haematol 1987;1:141–55.

62. Garcia CF, Warnke RA, Weiss LM. Follicular large cell lymphoma: an immunophenotype study. Am J Pathol 1986;123:425–31.

63. _____, Weiss LM, Warnke RA, Wood GS. Cutaneous follicular lymphoma. Am J Surg Pathol 1986;10:454–63.

64. Garvin AJ, Simon RM, Osborne CK, Merrill J, Young RC, Berard CW. An autopsy study of histologic progression in non-Hodgkin's lymphomas: 192 cases from the National Cancer Institute. Cancer 1983;52:393–8.

65. Gaulard P, d'Agay MF, Peuchmaur M, et al. Expression of the bcl-2 gene product in follicular lymphoma. Am J Pathol 1992;140:1089–95.

66. Gerard-Marchant R, Hamlin I, Lennert K, Rilke F, Stansfeld AG, van Unnik JA. Classification of non-Hodgkin's lymphomas [Letter]. Lancet 1974;2:406–8.

67. Glick JH, Barnes JM, Ezdinli EZ, et al. Nodular mixed lymphoma: results of a randomized trial failing to confirm prolonged disease-free survival with COPP chemotherapy. Blood 1981;58:920–5.

68. _____, McFadden E, Costello W, et al. Nodular histiocytic lymphoma: factors influencing prognosis and implication for aggressive chemotherapy. Cancer 1982;49:840–5.

69. Goates JJ, Kamel OW, LeBrun DP, Benharroch D, Dorfman RF. The floral variant of follicular lymphoma, immunologic and molecular studies support a neoplastic process. Am J Surg Pathol 1994;18:37–47.

70. Goffinet DR, Hoyt C, Eltringham JR. Secondary syphilis misdiagnosed as a lymphoma. Calif Med 1970;112:22–3.

71. _____, Warnke R, Dunnick NR, et al. Clinical and surgical (laparotomy) evaluation of patients with non-Hodgkin's lymphomas. Cancer Treat Rep 1977;61:981–92.

72. Gonzalez CL, Medeiros J, Jaffe ES. Composite lymphoma: a clinical pathologic analysis of nine patients with Hodgkin's disease and B-cell non-Hodgkin's lymphoma Am J Clin Pathol 1991;96:81–9.

73. Gribben JG. Attainment of molecular remission: a worthwhile goal? J Clin Oncol 1994;12:1532–4.

74. _____, Freedman AS, Woo SD. All advanced stage non-Hodgkin's lymphomas with a polymerase chain reaction amplifiable breakpoint of bcl-2 have residual cells containing the bcl-2 rearrangement at evaluation and after treatment. Blood 1991;78:3275–80.

75. _____, Nadler LM. Monitoring minimal residual disease. Semin Oncol 1993;20(Suppl 5):143–55.

76. Griffin NR, Howard MR, Quirke P, O'Brien CJ, Child JA, Bird CC. Prognostic indicators in centroblastic-centrocytic lymphoma. J Clin Pathol 1988;41:866–70.

77. Hansmann ML, Fellbaum C, Hui PK, Lennert K. Morphological and immunohistochemical investigation of non-Hodgkin's lymphoma combined with Hodgkin's disease. Histopathology 1989;15:35–48.

78. _____, Fellbaum C, Hui PK, Moubayed P. Progressive transformation of germinal centers with and without association to Hodgkin's disease. Am J Clin Pathol 1990;93:219–26.

79. Harrington DS, Ye Y, Weisenburger DD, et al. Malignant lymphoma in Nebraska and Guangzhou, China: a comparative study. Hum Pathol 1987;18:924–8.

80. Harris M, Eyden B, Reed G. Signet ring lymphomas: a rare variant of follicular lymphoma. J Clin Pathol 1981;34:884–91.

81. Harris NL, Bhan AK. Distribution of T-cell subsets in follicular and diffuse lymphomas of B-cell type. Am J Pathol 1983;113:172–80.

82. _____, Date RE. The distribution of neoplastic and normal B-lymphoid cells in nodular lymphomas: use of an immunoperoxidase technique on frozen section. Hum Pathol 1982;13:610–7.

83. _____, Ferry JA. Follicular lymphoma and related disorders (germinal center lymphomas). In: Knowles DM, ed. Neoplastic hematopathology. Baltimore: Williams & Wilkins, 1992:645–74.

84. _____, Nadler LM, Bhan AK. Immunohistological characterization of two malignant lymphomas of germinal center type (centroblastic/centrocytic and centrocytic) with monoclonal antibodies, follicular and diffuse lymphomas of small cleaved cell are related but distinct entities. Am J Pathol 1984;117:262–72.

85. Hartsock RJ, Halling LW, King FM. Luetic lymphadenitis: a clinical and histologic study of 20 cases. Am J Clin Pathol 1970;53:304–14.

86. Head DR, Avakian J, Kjeldsberg CR, Cerezo L. Relapse of intermediate or high grade (unfavorable) non-Hodgkin's lymphoma as a low grade (favorable) non-Hodgkin's lymphoma. Report of four cases. Am J Clin Pathology 1988;89:106–8.

87. Hockenbery D, Nunez G, Milliman C, Schreiber RD, Korsmeyer SJ. Bcl-2 is an inner mitochondrial protein that blocks programmed cell death. Nature 1990;348:334.

88. Hollema H, Poppema S. Immunophenotypes of malignant lymphoma centroblastic-centrocytic and malignant lymphoma centrocytic: an immunohistologic study indicating a derivation from different stages of B-cell differentiation. Hum Pathol 1988;19:1053–9.

89. Hoppe RT. The non-Hodgkin's lymphomas: pathology, staging, treatment. Curr Probl Cancer 1987;11:363–447.

90. _____. A Working Formulation of non-Hodgkin's lymphomas for clinical use: clinicopathological and prognostic correlations. In: Rosenberg SA, Kaplan HS, eds. Malignant lymphomas: etiology, immunology, pathology, treatment. Bristol-Myers Cancer Symposium. New York: Academic Press, 1982:469–83.

91. Horning SJ. Natural history of and therapy for the indolent non-Hodgkin's lymphomas. Semin Oncol 1993;20(Suppl 5):75–88.

92. _____, Galili N, Cleary ML, Sklar J. Detection of non-Hodgkin's lymphoma in the peripheral blood by analysis of antigen receptor gene rearrangements: results of a prospective study. Blood 1990;75:1139–45.

93. _____, Rosenberg SA. The natural history of initially untreated low grade non-Hodgkin's lymphomas. N Engl J Med 1984;311:1471–5.

94. _____, Weiss LM, Nevitt JB, Warnke RA. Clinical and pathologic features of follicular large cell (nodular histiocytic) lymphoma. Cancer 1987;59:1470–4.

95. Hu E, Trela M, Thompson J, et al. Detection of B-cell lymphoma in peripheral blood by DNA hybridization. Lancet 1985;2:1092–5.

96. _____, Weiss LM, Hoppe RT, Horning SJ. Follicular and diffuse mixed small cleaved and large cell lymphoma—a clinicopathologic study. J Clin Oncol 1985;3:1183–7.

97. Hubbard SM, Chabner BA, DeVita VT Jr, et al. Histologic progression in non-Hodgkin's lymphoma. Blood 1982;59:258–64.

98. Hummel M, Tamaru JI, Kalvelage B, Stein H. Mantle cell (previously centrocytic) lymphomas express VH genes with no or very little somatic mutations like the physiologic cells of the follicle mantle. Blood 1994;184:403–7.

99. Ioachim HL, Finbeiner JA. Pseudonodular pattern of T-cell lymphoma. Cancer 1980;45:1370–8.

100. Isaacson PG, Maclennan KA, Subbuswamy SG. Multiple lymphomatous polyposis of the gastrointestinal tract. Histopathology 1984;8:641–56.

101. _____, Norton AJ. Extranodal lymphomas. Edinburgh: Churchill Livingstone, 1994.

102. _____, Wotherspoon AC, Diss T, Pan L. Follicular colonization in B-cell lymphoma of mucosa-associated lymphoid tissue. Am J Surg Pathol 1991;15:819–28.

103. Jaffe ES, Longo DL, Cossman J, et al. Diffuse B cell lymphomas with T cell predominance in patients with follicular lymphoma or "pseudo-T-cell lymphoma" [Abstract]. Lab Invest 1984;50:27A–8A.

104. _____, Raffeld M, Medeiros LJ. Histopathologic subtypes of indolent lymphomas: caricatures of the mature B-cell system. Semin Oncol 1993;20(Suppl 5):3–30.

105. _____, Shevach EM, Frank MM, Berard CW, Green I. Nodular lymphoma: evidence for origin from follicular B-lymphocytes. N Engl J Med 1974;290:813–9.

106. Juneja SK, Wolf MM, Cooper IA. Value of bilateral bone marrow biopsy specimens in non-Hodgkin's lymphoma. J Clin Pathol 1990;43:630–2.

107. Kadin ME, Berard CW, Nanba K, Wakasa H. Lymphoproliferative diseases in Japan and Western countries. Proceedings of the United States-Japan seminar, September 6 and 7, 1982, in Seattle, Washington. Hum Pathol 1983;14:745–72.

108. Kantarjian HM, McLaughlin P, Fuller LM, et al. Follicular large cell lymphoma: analysis and prognostic factors in 62 patients. J Clin Oncol 1984;2:811–9.

109. Keith TA, Cousar JB, Glick AD, Vogler LB, Collins RD. Plasmacytic differentiation in follicular center cell (FCC) lymphomas. Am J Clin Pathol 1985;84:283–90.

110. Keller AR, Hochholzer L, Castleman B. Hyaline-vascular and plasma-cell types of giant lymph node hyperplasia of the mediastinum and other locations. Cancer 1972;29:670–83.

111. Kim H, Dorfman RF. Morphological studies of 84 untreated patients subjected to laparotomy for the staging of non-Hodgkin's lymphomas. Cancer 1974;33:657–74.

112. _____, Dorfman RF, Rappaport H. Signet-ring lymphoma: a rare morphologic and functional expression of nodular (follicular) lymphoma. Am J Surg Pathol 1978;2:119–32.

113. Kim H, Dorfman RF, Rosenberg SA. Pathology of malignant lymphomas in the liver: application in staging. In: Popper H, Schaffner H, eds. Progress in liver diseases. New York: Grune and Stratton, 1976:683–98.

114. _____, Hendrickson MR, Dorfman RF. Composite lymphoma. Cancer 1977;40:959–76.

115. Kjeldsberg CR, Kim H. Polykaryocytes resembling Warthin-Finkeldey giant cells in reactive and neoplastic lymphoid disorders. Hum Pathol 1981;12:267–72.

116. Kluin PM, van Krieken JH, Kleiverda K, Kluin-Nelemans HC. Discordant morphologic characteristics of B-cell lymphomas in bone marrow and lymph node biopsies. Am J Clin Pathol 1990;94:59–66.

117. Kojima M. A concept of follicular lymphoma. A proposal for existence of a neoplasm originating from the germinal center. In: Berard CW, Bennett JM, Ishikawa E, eds. Malignant diseases of the hematopoietic system. Baltimore: University Park Press, 1973;15:195–207. (GANN Monograph on Cancer Research, No. 15.)

118. Kondratowicz GM, Symmons DP, Bacon PA, Mageed RA, Jones EL. Rheumatoid lymphadenopathy: morphological and immunohistochemical study. J Clin Pathol 1990;43:106–11.

119. Korsmeyer SJ. Bcl-2 initiates a new category of oncogenes: regulators of cell death [Review]. Blood 1992;80:879–86.

120. Ladanyi M, Offit K, Parsa NZ, et al. Follicular lymphoma with t(8;14)(q24;q32): a distinct clinical and molecular subset of t(8;14)-bearing lymphomas. Blood 1992;79:2124–30.

121. _____, Wang S. Detection of rearrangements of the bcl-2 major breakpoint region in follicular lymphomas. Correlation of polymerase chain reaction results with Southern blot analysis. Diagn Mol Pathol 1992;1:31–5.

122. Lambrechts AC, Hupkes PE, Dorssers LC, Van't Veer MB. Clinical significance of t(14;18)-positive cells in the circulation of patients with stage III or IV follicular non-Hodgkin's lymphoma during first remission. J Clin Oncol 1994;12:1541–6.

123. _____, Hupkes PE, Dorssers LC, Van't Veer MB. Translocation t(14;18)-positive cells are present in the circulation of the majority of patients with localized (stage I and II) follicular non-Hodgkin's lymphoma. Blood 1993;82:2510–6.

124. Lardelli P, Bookman MA, Sundeen J, Longo DL, Jaffe ES. Lymphocytic lymphoma of intermediate differentiation: morphologic and immunophenotypic spectrum and clinical correlations. Am J Surg Pathol 1990;14:752–63.

125. LeBrun DP, Kamel OW, Cleary ML, Dorfman RF, Warnke RA. Follicular lymphomas of the gastrointestinal tract. Pathologic features in 31 cases and bcl-2 oncogene protein expression. Am J Pathol 1992;140:1327–35.

126. _____, Ngan BY, Weiss LM, Huie P, Warnke RA, Cleary ML. The bcl-2 oncogene in Hodgkin's disease arising in the setting of follicular non-Hodgkin's lymphoma. Blood 1994;83:223–30.

127. Lee MS, Chang KS, Cabanillas F, Freireich EJ, Trujillo JM, Stass SA. Detection of minimal residual cells carrying the t(14;18) by DNA sequence amplification. Science 1987;237:175–8.

128. Lee Wood B, Bacchi MM, Bacchi CE, Kidd P, Gown AM. Immunocytochemical differentiation of reactive hyperplasia from follicular lymphoma using monoclonal antibodies to cell surface and proliferation-related markers. Appli Immunohistochem 1994;2:48–53.

129. Lennert K. Malignant lymphomas other than Hodgkin's disease. Histology, cytology, ultrastructure, immunology. New York, Springer-Verlag, 1978:244–7, 338–45.

130. _____, Feller AC. Histopathology of non-Hodgkin's lymphomas. (Based on the updated Kiel classification). 2nd ed. Berlin: Springer-Verlag, 1992.

131. _____, Niedorf HR. Reticulum cells with desmosomal connections in follicular lymphoma. Virchows Arch [B] Cell Pathol 1969;4:148–50.

132. _____, Stein H. The germinal centre: morphology, histochemistry and immunohistology. In: Joos M, Christopher E, eds. Lymphoproliferative diseases of the skin. Berlin: Springer-Verlag, 1982:3–15.

133. Levine GD, Dorfman RF. Nodular lymphoma: an ultrastructural study of its relationship to germinal centers and a correlation of light and electron microscopic findings. Cancer 1975;35:148–64.

134. Levy R, Levy S, Cleary ML, et al. Somatic mutation in human B cell tumors. Immunol Rev 1987;96:43–58.

135. _____, Warnke R, Dorfman RF, Haimovich J. The monoclonality of B-cell lymphomas. J Exp Med 1977; 145:1014–28.

136. Lewin KJ, Ranchod M, Dorfman RF. Lymphomas of the gastrointestinal tract: a study of 117 cases presenting with gastrointestinal disease. Cancer 1978;42:693–707.

137. Liang R, Chan V, Chan TK, Chiu E, Todd D. Rearrangement of immunoglobulin, T-cell receptor, and bcl-2 genes in malignant lymphomas in Hong Kong. Cancer 1990;66:1743–7.

138. _____, Loke SL, Ho FC, Chiu E, Chan TK, Todd D. Histologic subtypes and survival of Chinese patients with non-Hodgkin's lymphomas. Cancer 1990;66:1850–5.

139. Limpens J, de Jong D, van Krieken JH, et al. Bcl-2/JH rearrangements in benign lymphoid tissues with follicular hyperplasia. Oncogene 1991;6:2271–6.

140. Lister TA. The management of follicular lymphoma. Ann Oncol 1991;2(Suppl 2):131–5.

141. Lo Coco F, Gaidano G, Louie DC, Offit K, Chaganti RSK, Dalla-Favera R. p53 mutations are associated with histologic transformation of follicular lymphoma. Blood 1993;82:2289–95.

142. Loke SL, Pittaluga S, Srivastava G, Raffeld M, Ho FCS. Translocation of bcl-2 gene in non-Hodgkin lymphomas in Hong Kong Chinese. Br J Haematol 1990;76:65–9.

143. Long JC, Aisenberg AC. Malignant lymphoma diagnosed at splenectomy and idiopathic splenomegaly. A clinicopathologic comparison. Cancer 1974;33:1054–61.

144. Longo DL. What's the deal with follicular lymphoma? [Editorial] Blood 1993;11:202–8.

145. _____, Wilson W. Follicular lymphomas. In: Magrath IT, ed. The non-Hodgkin's lymphomas. Baltimore: Williams & Wilkins, 1990:29–30.

146. _____, Young RC, Hubbard SM, et al. Prolonged initial remission in patients with nodular mixed lymphoma. Ann Intern Med 1984;100:651–6.

147. Lopez-Guillermo A, Montserrat E, Bosch F, Terol MJ, Campo E, Rozman C. Applicability of the International Index for aggressive lymphomas to patients with low-grade lymphoma. J Clin Oncol 1994;12:1343–8.

148. Lukes RJ, Collins RD. New observations on follicular lymphoma. In: Berard CW, Bennett JM, Ishikawa E, eds. Malignant diseases of the hematopoietic system. Baltimore: University Park Press, 1973;15:209–15. (GANN Monograph on Cancer Research, No. 15.)

149. Macon WR, Williams ME, Greer JP, Cousar JB. Paracortical nodular T-cell lymphoma. Identification of an unusual variant of peripheral T-cell lymphoma Am J Surg Pathol 1995;19:297–303.

150. Mann RB. Follicular lymphoma and lymphocytic lymphoma of intermediate differentiation. In: Jaffe ES, ed. Surgical pathology of the lymph nodes and related organs. Major problems in pathology, vol. 16, Philadelphia: WB Saunders, 1985:165–202.

151. _____, Berard CW. Criteria for the cytologic subclassification of follicular lymphomas: a proposed alternative method. Hematol Oncol 1983;1:187–92.

152. Marazuela M, Yebra M, Giron JA. Late relapse with nodular lymphoma after treatment for diffuse non-Hodgkin's lymphoma. Cancer 1991;67:1950–3.

153. Martin JM. Premature article—follicular lymphoma [Letter]. Am J Clin Pathol 1988;90:519–20.

154. Maurer R, Schmid U, Davies JD, Mahy NJ, Stansfeld AG, Lukes RJ. Lymph node infarction and malignant lymphoma: a multicentre survey of European, English and American cases. Histopathology 1986;10:571–88.

155. McCurley TL, Gay RE, Gay S, Glick AD, Haralson MA, Collins RD. The extracellular matrix in sclerosing follicular center cell lymphomas: an immunohistochemical and ultrastructural study. Hum Pathol 1986;17:930–8.

156. McKenna RW, Brunning RD. Reed-Sternberg-like cells in nodular lymphoma involving the bone marrow. Am J Clin Pathol 1975;63:779–85.

157. Mead GM, Kushlan P, O'Neil M, Burke JS, Rosenberg SA. Clinical aspects of non-Hodgkin's lymphomas presenting with discordant histologic subtypes. Cancer 1983;52:1496–501.

158. Medeiros LJ, Bagg A, Cossman J. Application of molecular genetics to the diagnosis of hematopoietic neoplasms. In: Knowles DM, ed. Neoplastic hematopathology. Baltimore: Williams & Wilkins, 1992:263–98.

159. Meijerink JP, Goverde GJ, Smetsers TF, et al. Quantitation of follicular non-Hodgkin lymphoma cells carrying t(14;18) in a patient before and after allogeneic bone marrow transplantation. Ann Oncol 1994;5(Suppl 1):S43–5.

160. Melo JV, Robinson DS, De Oliveria MP, et al. Morphology and immunology of circulating cells in leukaemic phase of follicular lymphoma. J Clin Pathol 1988;41:951–9.

161. Metter GE, Nathwani BN, Burke JS, et al. Morphologic subclassification of follicular lymphoma: variability of diagnosis among hematopathologists, a collaborative study between the Repository Center and Pathology Panel for Lymphoma Clinical Studies. J Clin Oncol 1985;3:25–38.

162. Miller ML, Tubbs RR, Fishleder AJ, Savage RA, Sebek BA, Weick JK. Immunoregulatory Leu-7+ and T8+ lymphocytes in B-cell follicular lymphomas. Hum Pathol 1984;15:810–7.

163. Mollejo M, Menarguez J, Cristobal E, et al. Monocytoid B cells, a comparative clinical pathological study of their distribution in different types of low grade lymphomas. Am J Surg Pathol 1994;18:1131–39.

164. Motulsky AG, Weinberg S, Saphar O, Rosenberg E. Lymph nodes in rheumatoid arthritis. Arch Intern Med 1952;90:660–76.

165. Nathwani BN. Diagnostic significance of morphologic patterns in lymph node proliferations. In: Knowles DM, ed. Neoplastic hematopathology. Baltimore: Williams & Wilkins, 1992:407–25.

166. _____, Metter GE, Miller TP, et al. What should be the morphologic criteria for the subdivision of follicular lymphomas? Blood 1986;68:837–45.

167. _____, Sheibani K, Winberg CD, Burke JS, Rappaport H. Neoplastic B cells with cerebriform nuclei in follicular lymphomas. Hum Pathol 1985;16:173–80.

168. _____, Winberg C, Diamond LW, Bearman RW, Kim H. Morphologic criteria for the differentiation of follicular lymphoma from florid reactive hyperplasia: a study of 80 cases. Cancer 1981;48:1794–806.

169. Ng CS, Chan JK. Malignant lymphomas in Chinese: what is the East-West difference? [Letter] Hum Pathol 1988;19:614–5.

170. _____, Chan JK, Hui PK, Lo ST. Monoclonal antibodies reactive with normal and neoplastic T-cells in paraffin sections. Hum Pathol 1988;19:295–303.

171. _____, Chan JK, Lo ST, Poon YF. Immunophenotypic analysis of non-Hodgkin's lymphomas in Chinese. A study of 75 cases in Hong Kong. Pathology 1986;18:419–25.

172. Ngan BY, Chen-Levy Z, Weiss LM, Warnke RA, Cleary ML. Expression in non-Hodgkin's lymphoma of the bcl-2 protein associated with the t(14;18) chromosomal translocation. N Engl J Med 1988;318:1638–44.

173. _____, Nourse J, Cleary ML. Detection of chromosomal translocation t(14;18) within the minor cluster region of bcl-2 by polymerase chain reaction and direct genomic sequencing of the enzymatically amplified DNA in follicular lymphomas. Blood 1989;73:1759–62.

174. _____, Warnke RA, Cleary ML. Variability of immunoglobulin expression in follicular lymphoma; an immunohistologic and molecular genetic study. Am J Pathol 1989;135:1139–44.

175. Nguyen DT, Diamond LW, Lorenzen J, Zhao M, Hansmann ML, Fischer R. An unusual pattern of lymph node involvement in mycosis fungoides simulating neoplastic follicles. Arch Pathol Lab Med 1994;118:749–51.

176. Non-Hodgkin's Lymphoma Pathologic Classification Project. National Cancer Institute sponsored study of classifications of non-Hodgkin's lymphomas: summary and description of a working formulation for clinical usage. Cancer 1982;49:2112–35.

177. Norton AJ, Rivas C, Isaacson PG. A comparison between monoclonal antibody MT2 and immunoglobulin staining in the differential diagnosis of follicular lymphoid proliferation in routinely fixed wax-embedded biopsies. Am J Pathol 1989;134:63–70.

178. Nosanchuk JS, Schnitzer B. Follicular hyperplasia in lymph nodes from patients with rheumatoid arthritis. Cancer 1969;24:243–54.

179. O'Briain DS, Kennedy MJ, Daly PA, et al. Multiple lymphomatous polyposis of the gastrointestinal tract. A clinicopathologically distinctive form of non-Hodgkin lymphoma of B-cell centrocytic type. Am J Surg Pathol 1989;13:691–9.

180. Offit K, Koduru PR, Hollis R, et al. 18q21 rearrangement in diffuse large cell lymphoma: incidence and clinical significance. Br J Haematol 1989;72:178–83.

181. O'Leary TJ, Stetler-Stevenson M. Diagnosis of t(14;18) by polymerase chain reaction. The natural evolution of a laboratory test [Editorial]. Arch Pathol Lab Med 1994;118:789–90.

182. Okpala IE, Akang EE, Okpala UJ. Lymphomas in University College Hospital, Ibandan, Nigeria. Cancer 1991;68:1356–60.

183. Osborne BM, Butler JJ. Clinical implications of nodal reactive follicular hyperplasia in the elderly patients with enlarged lymph nodes. Mod Pathol 1991;4:24–30.

184. _____, Butler JJ. Follicular lymphoma mimicking progressive transformation of germinal centers. Am J Clin Pathol 1987;88:264–9.

185. _____, Butler JJ. Hypocellular paratrabecular foci of treated small cleaved cell lymphoma in bone marrow biopsies. Am J Surg Pathol 1989;13:382–8.

186. _____, Butler JJ, Pugh WC, Luthra R, Ordonez NG. Follicular lymphoma variant mimicking progressive transformation of germinal centers: immunophenotypic, genotypic and clinical findings in 7 patients [Abstract]. Mod Pathol 1994;7:118A.

187. _____, Butler JJ, Variakojis D, Kott M. Reactive lymph node hyperplasia with giant follicles. Am J Clin Pathol 1982;78:493–9.

188. Osborne CK, Norton L, Young RC, et al. Nodular histiocytic lymphoma: an aggressive nodular lymphoma with potential for prolonged disease-free survival. Blood 1980;56:98–103.

189. Pezzella F, Ralfkiaer E, Gatter KC, Mason DY. The 14;18 translocation in European cases of follicular lymphoma: comparison of Southern blotting and the polymerase chain reaction. Br J Haematol 1990;76:58–64.

190. _____, Tse AG, Cordell JL, Pulford KA, Gatter DC, Mason DY. Expression of the bcl-2 oncogene protein is not specific for the 14;18 chromosomal translocation. Am J Pathol 1990;137:225–32.

191. Pinto A, Hutchison RE, Grant LH, Trevenen CL, Berard CW. Follicular lymphomas in pediatric patients. Mod Pathol 1990;3:308–13.

192. Piris M, Gatter KC, Mason DY. CD30 expression in follicular lymphoma. Histopathology 1991;18:25–9.

193. Poppema S, Kaiserling E, Lennert K. Hodgkin's disease with lymphocyte predominance, nodular type (nodular paragranuloma) and progressively transformed germinal centres—a cytohistological study. Histopathology 1979;3:295–308.

194. Portlock CS, Rosenberg SA. No initial therapy for stage III and IV non-Hodgkin lymphomas of favorable histologic types. Ann Intern Med 1979;90:10–3.

195. Price CG, Meerabux J, Murtagh S, et al. The significance of circulating cells carrying t(14;18) in long term remission from follicular lymphoma. J Clin Oncol 1991;9:1527–32.

196. Pugh WC, Majlis A, Rodriguez J, Cabanillas F. Mantle cell lymphoma with a nodular configuration simulating follicular center lymphoma: pathological and clinical correlates in 12 cases [Abstract]. Mod Pathol 1994;7:119A.

197. Rappaport H. Tumors of the hematopoietic system. Atlas of Tumor Pathology, 1st series, Fascicle 8. Washington, D.C.: Armed Forces Institute of Pathology, 1966.

198. _____, Winter WJ, Hicks ED. Follicular lymphoma: a re-evaluation of its position in the scheme of malignant lymphoma based on a survey of 253 cases. Cancer 1956;9:792–821.

199. Risdall R, Hoppe RT, Warnke R. Non-Hodgkin's lymphoma, a study of the evolution of the disease based upon 92 autopsied cases. Cancer 1979;44:529–42.

200. Rohatiner AZS, Lister TA. New approaches to the treatment of follicular lymphoma. Br J Haematol 1991;79:349–54.

201. Romaguera JE, McLaughlin P, North L, et al. Multivariate analysis of prognostic factors in stage IV follicular low-grade lymphomas: a risk model. J Clin Oncol 1991;9:762–9.

202. Rosas-Uribe A, Variakojis D, Rappaport H. Proteinaceous precipitate in nodular (follicular) lymphomas. Cancer 1973;31:534–42.

203. Rosenberg SA. Bone marrow involvement in the non-Hodgkin's lymphomata. Br J Cancer 1975;31(Suppl): 261–9.

204. _____. The low-grade non-Hodgkin's lymphomas: challenges and opportunities. J Clin Oncol 1985;3:299–310.

205. Sander CA, Yano T, Clark HM, et al. p53 mutation is associated with progression in follicular lymphomas. Blood 1993;82:1994–2004.

206. Sandhaus LM, Voelkerding K, Raska K. Follicular lymphoma mimicking progressive transformation of germinal centers: immunologic analysis of a case. [Letter]. Am J Clin Pathol 1988;90:518–9.

207. Schmid U, Karow J, Lennert K. Follicular malignant non-Hodgkin's lymphoma with pronounced plasmacytic differentiation: a plasmacytoma-like lymphoma. Virchows Arch [A] 1985;405:473–81.

208. Schnitzer B, Loesel LS, Reed RE. Lymphosarcoma cell leukemia: a clinicopathologic study. Cancer 26:1970; 1082–96.

209. Scoazec JY, Berg F, Magaud JP, Brochier J, Coiffier B, Bryon PA. The dendritic reticulum cell pattern in B cell lymphomas of the small cleaved, mixed and large cell types: an immunohistochemical study of 48 cases. Hum Pathol 1989;20:124–31.

210. Segal GH, Scott M, Jorgensen T, Braylan RC. Standard polymerase chain reaction analysis does not detect t(14;18) in reactive lymphoid hyperplasia. Arch Pathol Lab Med 1994;118:791–4.

211. Sham RL, Phatak P, Carignan J, Janas J, Olson JP. Progression of follicular large cell lymphoma to Burkitt's lymphoma. Cancer 1989;63:700–2.

212. Shih LY, Liang DC. Non-Hodgkin's lymphomas in Asia. Hematol Oncol Clin N Am 1991;5:983–99.

213. Simon R, Durrleman S, Hoppe RT, et al. The Non-Hodgkin's Lymphoma Pathologic Classification Project. Long-term follow up of 1153 patients with non-Hodgkin's lymphomas. Ann Intern Med 1988;109:939–45.

214. Slovak ML, Weiss LM, Nathwani BN, Bernstein L, Levine AM. Cytogenetic studies of composite lymphomas: monocytoid B-cell lymphoma and other B-cell non-Hodgkin's lymphomas. Hum Pathol 1993;24:1086–94.

215. Smith BR, Weinberg DS, Robert NJ, et al. Circulating monoclonal B lymphocytes in non-Hodgkin's lymphoma. N Engl J Med 1984;311:1476–81.

216. Spagnolo DV, Papadimitriou JM, Matz LR, Walters MN. Nodular lymphomas with intracellular immunoglobulin inclusions: report of three cases and a review. Pathology 1982;14:415–27.

217. Stansfeld AG. Inflammatory and reactive diseases. In: Stansfeld AG, d'Ardenne AJ, eds. Lymph node biopsy interpretation. 2nd ed. Edinburgh: Churchill Livingstone, 1992:55–115.

218. _____. Low grade B cell lymphomas. In: Stansfeld AG, d'Ardenne AJ, eds. Lymph node biopsy interpretation. 2nd ed. Edinburgh: Churchill Livingstone, 1992:229–83.

219. _____, Diebold J, Kapanci Y, et al. Updated Kiel classification. Lancet 1988;1:292–3.

220. Stetler-Stevenson M, Raffeld M, Cohen P, Cossman J. Detection of occult follicular lymphoma by specific DNA amplification. Blood 1988;72:1822–5.

221. Sundeen JT, Cossman J, Jaffe ES. Lymphocyte predominant Hodgkin's disease nodular subtype with coexistent large cell lymphoma. Histological progression or composite malignancy? Am J Surg Pathol 1988;12:599–606.

222. Swerdlow SH, Murray LJ. Natural killer (Leu 7+) cells in reactive lymphoid tissues and malignant lymphomas. Am J Clin Pathol 1984;81:459–63.

223. _____, Murray LJ, Habeshaw JA, Stansfeld AG. B- and T-cell subsets in follicular centroblastic/centrocytic (cleaved follicular center cell) lymphoma: an immunohistologic analysis of 26 lymph nodes and three spleens. Hum Pathol 1985;16:339–52.

224. Tanaka S, Louie DC, Kant JA, Reed JC. Frequent incidence of somatic mutations in translocated BCL 2 oncogenes of non-Hodgkin's lymphomas. Blood 1992;79:229–37.

225. Taylor CR. An immunohistological study of follicular lymphoma, reticulum cell sarcoma and Hodgkin's disease. Eur J Cancer 1986;12:61–75.

226. Tilly H, Rossi A, Stamatoullas A, et al. Prognostic value of chromosomal abnormalities in follicular lymphoma. Blood 1994;84:1043–9.

227. Tsujimoto Y, Cossman J, Jaffe E, Croce CM. Involvement of the bcl-2 gene in human follicular lymphoma. Science 1985;228:1440–3.

228. _____, Finger LR, Yunis J, Nowell PC, Croce CM. Cloning of the chromosome breakpoint of neoplastic B-cells with the t(14;18) chromosome translocation. Science 1984;226:1097–9.

229. Utz GL, Swerdlow SH. Distinction of follicular hyperplasia from follicular lymphoma in B5-fixed tissues: comparison of MT2 and bcl-2 antibodies. Hum Pathol 1993;24:1155–8.

230. Vago JF, Hurtubise PE, Redden-Borowski MN, Martelo OJ, Swerdlow SH. Follicular center-cell lymphoma with plasmacytic differentiation, monoclonal paraprotein, and peripheral blood involvement. Recapitulation of normal B-cell development. Am J Surg Pathol 1985;9:764–70.

231. van den Oord JJ, De Wolf-Peeters C, Desmet VJ. Immunohistochemical analysis of progressively transformed follicular centers. Am J Clin Pathol 1985; 83:560–4.

232. van den Tweel JG, Taylor CR, Parker JW, Lukes RJ. Immunoglobulin inclusions in non-Hodgkin's lymphomas. Am J Clin Pathol 1978;69:306–13.

233. van der Putte SC, Schuurman HJ, Rademakers LH, Kluin P, van Unnik JA. Malignant lymphoma of follicular center cell with marked nuclear lobation. Virchows Arch [Cell Pathol] 1984;46:91–107.

234. Vaux DL, Cory S, Adams JM. Bcl-2 gene promotes hematopoietic cell survival and cooperates with c-myc to immortalize pre-B cells. Nature 1988;335:440–2.

235. Waldron JA Jr, Newcomer LN, Katz ME, Cadman E. Sclerosing variants of follicular center cell lymphomas presenting in the retroperitoneum. Cancer 1983;52:712–20.

236. Warnke RA, Kim H, Fuks Z, Dorfman RF. The co-existence of nodular and diffuse patterns in nodular non-Hodgkin's lymphomas: significance and clinicopathologic correlation. Cancer 1977;40:1229–33.

237. _____, Levy R. Immunopathology of follicular lymphomas. A model of B-lymphocyte homing. N Engl J Med 1978;298:481–6.

238. Weisenburger D, Bast M, Armitage J. When does a diffuse component in composite follicular and diffuse non-Hodgkin's lymphoma affect prognosis? [Abstract] Mod Pathol 1991;4:85A.

239. _____, Chan WC. Lymphomas of follicles. Mantle cell and follicular center cell lymphomas. Am J Clin Pathol 1993;99:409–20.

240. Weiss LM, Warnke RA. Follicular lymphoma with blastic conversion: a report of two cases with confirmation by immunoperoxidase studies on bone marrow sections. Am J Clin Pathol 1985;83:681–6.

241. _____, Warnke RA, Sklar J, Cleary ML. Molecular analysis of the t(14;18) chromosomal translocation in malignant lymphomas. N Engl J Med 1987;317:1185–9.

242. Winberg CD, Nathwani BN, Bearman RM, Rappaport H. Follicular (nodular) lymphoma during the first two decades of life: a clinicopathological study of 12 patients. Cancer 1985;48:2223–35.

243. Wright DH, Isaacson PG. Follicular center cell lymphoma of childhood: a report of 3 cases and a discussion of its relationship to Burkitt's lymphoma. Cancer 1981;47:915–25.

244. Wood BL, Bacchi MM, Bacchi CE, Kidd P, Gown AM. Immunocytochemical differentiation of reactive hyperplasia from follicular lymphoma using monoclonal antibodies to cell surface and proliferation-related markers. Diagn Immunohistochem 1994;2:48–53.

245. Yano T, Jaffe ES, Longo DL, Raffeld M. MYC rearrangements in histologically progressed follicular lymphomas. Blood 1992;80:758–67.

246. _____, Sander CA, Andrade RE, et al. Molecular analysis of the BCL-3 locus at chromosome 17q22 in B-cell neoplasms. Blood 1993;82:1813–9.

247. Yunis JJ, Frizzera G, Okon MM, McKenna J, Theologides A, Arneson M. Multiple recurrent genomic defects in follicular lymphoma. A possible model for cancer. N Engl J Med 1987;316:79–84.

248. _____, Oken MM, Kaplan ME, Ensrud KM, Howe RR, Theologides A. Distinctive chromosomal abnormalities in histologic subtypes of non-Hodgkin's lymphoma. N Engl J Med 1982;307:1231–6.

249. Zelenetz AD, Campbell MJ, Bahler DW, et al. Follicular lymphoma: a model of lymphoid tumor progression in man. Ann Oncol 1991;2(Suppl 2):115–22.

250. _____, Chu G, Galili N, et al. Enhanced detection of the t(14;18) translocation in malignant lymphoma using pulsed-field gel electrophoresis. Blood 1991;78:1552–60.

251. Zutter M, Hockenbery D, Silverman GA, Korsmeyer SJ. Immunolocalization of the bcl-2 protein within hematopoietic neoplasms. Blood 1991;78:1062–8.

✧✧✧

7
MALIGNANT LYMPHOMA, SMALL LYMPHOCYTIC AND DIFFUSE SMALL CLEAVED CELL (CENTROCYTIC)

Diffuse lymphomas of small lymphoid cells consist of a heterogeneous group of generally indolent lymphomas and include: 1) small lymphocytic lymphoma (morphologically indistinguishable from chronic lymphocytic leukemia); 2) mantle cell lymphoma, which includes both the diffuse and mantle zone patterns of lymphomas composed of so-called intermediately differentiated lymphocytes (these lymphomas comprise most of those designated centrocytic in the Kiel classification and diffuse small cleaved cell in the Working Formulation); 3) low-grade B-cell lymphoma of mucosa-associated lymphoid tissue (MALT); 4) monocytoid B-cell lymphoma (both monocytoid B-cell lymphoma and mucosa-associated low-grade lymphoma appear to be related to marginal zone B cells); and 5) small lymphocytic lymphoma with plasmacytoid features (lymphoplasmacytoid/lymphoplasmacytic immunocytoma in the Kiel classification). Current morphologic, immunologic, and molecular parameters cannot clearly separate some of these entities. Furthermore, since some of these entities have only been described recently, data on prevalence, clinical behavior, incidence of transformation, and prognosis are incomplete. Newer immunophenotypic and molecular markers may more clearly delineate their defining characteristics.

SMALL LYMPHOCYTIC LYMPHOMA

Definition. Malignant lymphoma, small lymphocytic type, is a neoplasm composed of lymphocytes that have the cytologic appearance of the unstimulated lymphocytes normally residing in the primary follicles or the mantle zone of secondary follicles of lymphoid tissue.

Incidence. Small lymphocytic lymphomas accounted for approximately 5 percent of non-Hodgkin's lymphomas in the National Cancer Institute (NCI)–sponsored study (71), but their incidence may be 15 to 20 percent if chronic lymphocytic leukemia (CLL) or related entities are included (8). Lymphocytic lymphoma comprises a higher percentage of lymphomas in the Kiel classification but 75 percent of these patients have either a peripheral blood lymphocyte count over 4,000/mm^3 or a total peripheral blood leukocyte count over 11,000/mm^3 (52). In a recent review of nonfollicular small B-cell lymphomas, approximately one third were small lymphocytic, one fourth were mantle cell, and one fourth were mucosa associated (8).

These lymphomas occur at a median age of approximately 60 years and rarely present in patients before the age of 30 (71). Men and women are equally affected.

Natural History and Clinical Features. A diagnosis is made by lymph node biopsy in approximately 80 percent of patients (71). Pathologic stage IV disease can be documented in approximately 80 percent of patients and is usually due to bone marrow involvement (71). A significant number of patients give a history of waxing and waning adenopathy. Spontaneous regression occurs in 15 percent of untreated patients (38); this suggests a dynamic interplay between tumor cells and immunoregulatory mechanisms. The risk of histologic transformation increases with time but is significantly lower (approximately 10 to 20 percent) than in patients with low-grade follicular lymphoma (8,38). Rarely, follow-up biopsies show histologic and phenotypic features of Hodgkin's disease (32,101). These patients have a less fulminant clinical course than those whose tumors transform to large cell lymphoma (Richter's syndrome) (11). Patients whose biopsies show features of small lymphocytic lymphoma but who have an absolute lymphocytosis (greater than 5,000/mm^3) are generally regarded as having CLL (see below).

T-lineage lymphomas composed of cytologically benign small lymphocytes are rare and their natural history and clinical features are not well defined.

Microscopic Findings. When the normal architecture of a lymph node is effaced by a monotonous proliferation of small lymphocytes with round nuclear contours and scant cytoplasm, the diagnosis is either small lymphocytic lymphoma

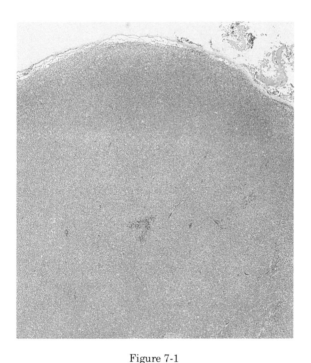

Figure 7-1
SMALL LYMPHOCYTIC LYMPHOMA
The normal architecture of this lymph node is effaced by an infiltrate of small lymphocytes.

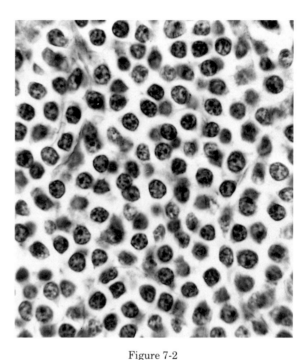

Figure 7-2
SMALL LYMPHOCYTIC LYMPHOMA
The lymphoma cells in this case are indistinguishable from the lymphocytes that normally inhabit the primary follicles and mantle zones of secondary follicles of lymphoid tissue.

or CLL (figs. 7-1, 7-2). The nuclear chromatin of the proliferating cells is clumped and nucleoli are either inconspicuous or small. Nuclei may show slight irregularities, particularly if tissue is fixed in a metal-based fixative. Mitotic figures are usually infrequent. In approximately one third of cases, the lymphoma extensively involves the perinodal adipose tissue (6). About 75 percent of cases show complete effacement of normal nodal architecture. When intact normal structures such as secondary follicles with germinal centers, paracortical zones, or sinuses are present, special immunologic or molecular studies can confirm the diagnosis. Infrequently, residual follicles are numerous and such cases have been termed *interfollicular small lymphocytic lymphoma* (fig. 7-3) (27). A rare example of small lymphocytic lymphoma selectively involving lymph node B zones has also been described (14).

At low magnification, 40 percent of small lymphocytic lymphomas have pale staining areas with a vague nodular pattern (fig. 7-4) (6); this increases to over 80 percent if cases with CLL are included (53). This pseudofollicular pattern is more common than a diffuse pattern in CLL (52).

Because these pale areas do not represent true follicles, the terms pseudofollicles, proliferation centers, or growth centers have been used to describe these indistinct nodules. They contain varying numbers of medium to large (15 to 30 μm) lymphoid cells with prominent central nucleoli (small and large prolymphocytes) admixed with more loosely packed small lymphocytes (fig. 7-5). Occasionally, the larger cells have multiple small nucleoli (fig. 7-5). Giemsa stains distinguish smaller cells with less basophilic cytoplasm (prolymphocytes) (fig. 7-5) from larger paraimmunoblasts (52,53). A clinically more aggressive paraimmunoblastic variant of small lymphocytic lymphoma/leukemia has been described (79). A tumor-forming subtype that has a propensity to infiltrate veins and may be associated with a worse prognosis was described by Lennert (52). Prolymphocytes are numerous in this subtype. These pseudofollicules are often smaller and less well defined than the neoplastic follicles of a follicular lymphoma and never have remnants of residual normal mantle zones. Their cellular composition of small lymphocytes,

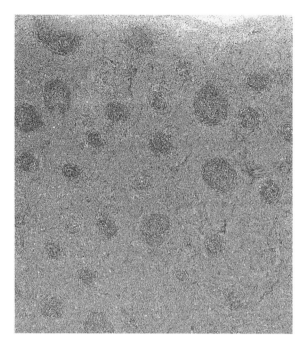

Figure 7-3
INTERFOLLICULAR SMALL
LYMPHOCYTIC LYMPHOMA

Numerous darkly stained follicles (many with Castleman-like features) are scattered throughout this section of small lymphocytic lymphoma. Frozen section immunohistochemical studies confirmed a lambda-expressing interfollicular lymphocytic proliferation and demonstrated a normal pattern of dendritic and cellular immunoglobulin staining in the follicles.

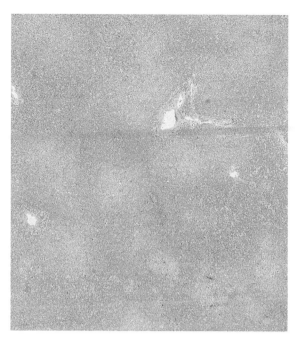

Figure 7-4
SMALL LYMPHOCYTIC LYMPHOMA
WITH PROLIFERATION CENTERS

Note the vague pale-staining nodules in this section of a cervical lymph node.

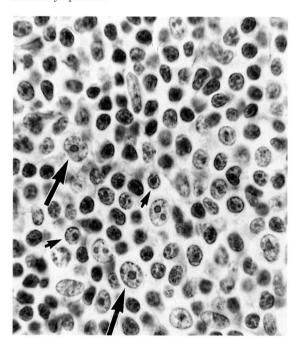

Figure 7-5
SMALL LYMPHOCYTIC LYMPHOMA
WITH PROLIFERATION CENTERS

Admixed with small lymphocytes in one of the proliferation centers are prolymphocytes (small arrows) and paraimmunoblasts (large arrows) as well as occasional large cells with multiple small nucleoli.

prolymphocytes, and paraimmunoblasts distinguishes them from the small cleaved and large (cleaved and noncleaved) lymphoid cells of follicular lymphomas (66). A diffuse admixture of small lymphocytes and prolymphocytes should not be confused with a more aggressive diffuse mixed small and large cell lymphoma. Rarely, small lymphocytic lymphomas may be associated with extensive epithelioid granulomas, which may obscure the underlying lymphoma (fig. 7-6) (10).

Infrequent cases of small lymphocytic lymphoma and CLL contain multilobated or multinucleated cells of the type seen in lymphocyte predominance or other subtypes of Hodgkin's disease (23). These pleomorphic large cells may express the same immunoglobulin light chain as the small lymphocytes (19,88) or may have many of the phenotypic features of Hodgkin cells (32,101), including the expression of Epstein-Barr virus (EBV) (see chapter 17) (61).

Figure 7-6
SMALL LYMPHOCYTIC LYMPHOMA OBSCURED
BY EPITHELIOID HISTIOCYTES
This B-cell small lymphocytic lymphoma (confirmed by the identification of lambda light chain monotypia in frozen sections) is associated with numerous epithelioid histiocytes simulating Lennert's lymphoma.

SMALL LYMPHOCYTIC LYMPHOMA WITH PLASMACYTOID FEATURES (LYMPHOPLASMACYTOID/LYMPHO-PLASMACYTIC IMMUNOCYTOMA)

Definition. Malignant lymphoma, small lymphocytic with plasmacytoid features, is a neoplasm composed of small lymphocytes that show maturation toward plasma cells without demonstrating features of other low-grade lymphoma subtypes (many lymphomas occasionally show differentiation to plasma cells including CLL, mantle cell lymphoma, monocytoid B-cell lymphoma, MALT lymphoma, and follicular lymphoma).

Incidence. Lymphoplasmacytoid lymphomas accounted for approximately 5 percent of the lymphomas in the NCI-sponsored study when classified according to the Kiel criteria (71). However, the incidence of this subtype may be significantly lower if only those lymphomas that lack features of other diffuse small cell types are included.

Natural History and Clinical Features. Many clinical features are similar to those of small lymphocytic lymphoma. In addition, most patients whose lymphomas have prominent plasmacytoid features or who have widespread disease have a monoclonal immunoglobulin in the serum or urine (usually IgM but occasionally IgG or IgA) and may have the clinical manifestations of Waldenström's macroglobulinemia. Probably less than 10 percent of cases of small lymphocytic lymphoma or CLL without plasmacytoid features have a monoclonal serum or urine protein. Small lymphocytic lymphomas with plasmacytoid features involve extranodal sites other than bone marrow, spleen, and liver more commonly than their nonplasmacytoid counterparts. Common sites of involvement include skin, orbital soft tissue, gastrointestinal tract, and Waldeyer's ring (52) although some of these lymphomas may be low-grade lymphomas of MALT in which plasmacytoid features are prominent. In some series, patients do not have a peripheral blood lymphocytosis (34); however, Lennert reports lymphocytosis in approximately 30 percent of patients (52). About 10 percent of patients develop a localized or generalized lymphoma composed of large lymphoid cells (often immunoblastic with plasmacytoid features).

Microscopic Findings. Plasmacytoid lymphocytes typically have the nuclei of lymphocytes but the amphophilic or basophilic cytoplasm of plasma cells (fig. 7-7). The incidence of small lymphocytic lymphomas with plasmacytoid features may vary considerably and depends not only on how carefully a case is scrutinized for plasmacytoid features but also on the availability of stains that highlight this feature, such as Giemsa or methyl-green pyronin (MGP). Eosinophilic cytoplasmic inclusions (Russell bodies) or inclusions resulting from invaginations into the nucleus (Dutcher bodies) (fig. 7-8, 7-9) are indicators of immunoglobulin-secreting cells. Dutcher bodies are typically associated with monoclonal proteins (57). A variety of crystalline forms of immunoglobulins have been described in lymphoproliferative disorders (fig. 7-10). If the monoclonal protein has a high content of hexose, typically IgM, the inclusions will stain with periodic acid–Schiff (PAS) (fig. 7-9). The occurrence of various inclusions may be an indication of abnormal production of immunoglobulins or faulty storage or secretion. When crystalline forms occur, they may be released into the tissues or circulation and taken up by macrophages. Extracellular proteinaceous precipitates may also be

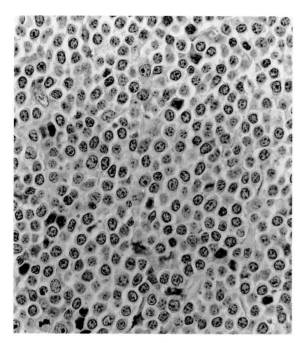

Figure 7-7
SMALL LYMPHOCYTIC LYMPHOMA
WITH PLASMACYTOID FEATURES
(LYMPHOPLASMACYTOID IMMUNOCYTOMA)

Many of the cells in this lymphoma have the nuclear features of small lymphocytes but with moderate to large amounts of cytoplasm which is often eccentric.

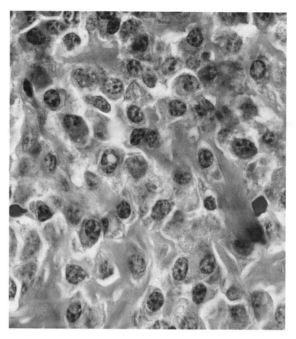

Figure 7-8
SMALL LYMPHOCYTIC LYMPHOMA WITH
PLASMACYTIC FEATURES

Many of the cells in this lymphoma have nuclear and cytoplasmic features of plasma cells. Note a Dutcher body to the left of center.

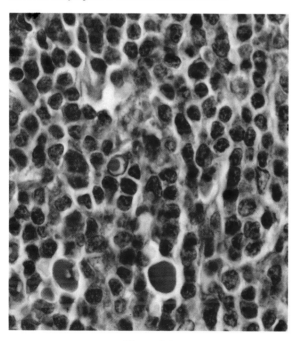

Figure 7-9
INTRANUCLEAR INCLUSION (DUTCHER
BODY) IN PLASMACYTOID LYMPHOMA

PAS stain highlights cytoplasmic immunoglobulin inclusions and their extensions into the nucleus in this small lymphocytic lymphoma with plasmacytoid features.

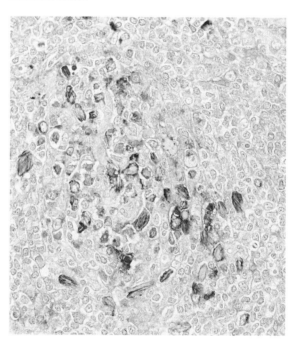

Figure 7-10
CRYSTALLINE IMMUNOGLOBULIN INCLUSIONS
IN PLASMACYTOID LYMPHOMA (MALT LYMPHOMA)

The inclusions in these lymphoma cells are highlighted by the dark cytoplasmic kappa staining (immunoperoxidase with hematoxylin counterstain). The lymphoma cells appear to largely replace a germinal center (follicular colonization).

seen. Typical plasma cells can also be seen and in some cases paraffin section stains for immunoglobulin light chains may help determine whether the plasma cells are a component of the neoplasm.

Small lymphocytic lymphomas with plasmacytoid features that have a small to moderate number of plasmacytoid lymphocytes or plasma cells conform to lymphoplasmacytoid lymphoma in the Kiel classification (fig. 7-7). When plasmacytoid lymphocytes, and especially plasma cells, are more frequent the cases are designated *lymphoplasmacytic type* and correspond best to the lesions described in macroglobulinemia of Waldenström (fig. 7-8) (52). A pseudofollicular pattern is infrequent. Mast cells may be prominent and hemosiderosis is often present as a consequence of autoimmune hemolytic anemia or transfusions. In the original Kiel classification (deleted in the updated version) the polymorphic subtype of immunocytoma refers to cases dominated by small lymphocytes but with an admixture of immunoblasts, large noncleaved cells, and small cleaved cells (52). Epithelioid histiocytes (fig. 7-6) occasionally are sufficiently numerous to mimic "Lennert's lymphoma," which is usually of T lineage (74). This polymorphic subtype accounted for approximately 20 percent of cases of immunocytoma in the NCI study (71), and was classified as intermediate-grade diffuse mixed small and large cell lymphoma in the Working Formulation; recent data on this subtype (now designated large cell–rich immunocytoma) suggests a more aggressive clinical behavior than other subtypes (8).

MANTLE CELL (INTERMEDIATE LYMPHOCYTIC/MANTLE ZONE/CENTROCYTIC/DIFFUSE SMALL CLEAVED CELL) LYMPHOMA

Definition. Malignant lymphoma, mantle cell type, is a neoplasm composed of small to medium-sized lymphocytes that in most cases have irregular nuclei, inconspicuous nucleoli, and scant cytoplasm. This lymphoma lacks proliferation centers; large lymphoid cells are rare (4).

Incidence. Mantle cell (centrocytic) lymphoma accounted for approximately 12 percent of cases in the NCI classification study (71). However, a recent study suggests an incidence of approximately 6 percent (8).

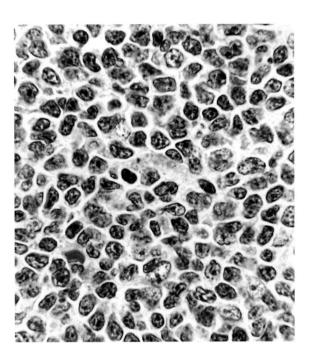

Figure 7-11
MANTLE CELL LYMPHOMA
Most cells show nuclear irregularities of mild to moderate degree. The clumped nuclear chromatin and relatively low mitotic activity are typical of this lymphoma. (Figures 7-11 and 7-14 are from the same case.)

Natural History and Clinical Features. The clinical features are similar to those of small lymphocytic lymphoma. There is a higher incidence of splenic, Waldeyer's ring, and gastrointestinal involvement (8) which may manifest as lymphomatous polyposis. As much as 35 percent of patients with mantle cell lymphomas have an absolute lymphocytosis at the time of diagnosis (26,76,98). Progression or transformation in this lymphoma typically manifests as a "blastic" or "blastoid" rather than large cell subtype (9,50).

Microscopic Findings. Mantle cell lymphoma was initially termed intermediate lymphocytic lymphoma and referred to those cases that could not be easily assigned to the small lymphocytic or small cleaved cell categories (7). The predominant cell shows irregularities or indentations of the nuclear membrane (fig. 7-11). These nuclear irregularities are more pronounced after fixation in a metal-based fixative (fig. 7-12). According to Weisenburger (99), these lymphomas are generally composed of an admixture of small round lymphocytes and small cleaved

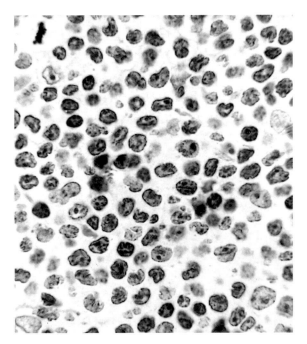

Figure 7-12
MANTLE CELL LYMPHOMA
The degree of nuclear irregularity is accentuated by fixation in a metal-based fixative, in this instance B5.

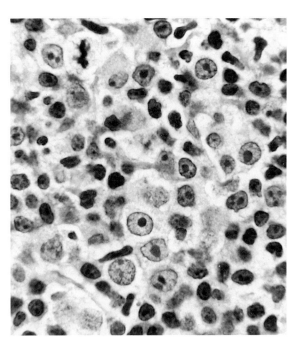

Figure 7-13
SMALL LYMPHOCYTIC LYMPHOMA WITH
PROLIFERATION CENTERS SIMULATING
MANTLE CELL LYMPHOMA
Note the nuclear irregularities in the small lymphoid cells and the many prolymphocytes and paraimmunoblasts in this proliferation center (see text).

cells, with neither more than 30 percent of the total population. Analogous to small lymphocytic lymphomas, the nuclei of the lymphoma cells show clumped chromatin and variable mitotic activity, often low but sometimes high (see below). Approximately 50 percent of cases contain lymphocytes with alkaline phosphatase activity, a finding that is not specific for this variant but tends to distinguish these cases from small lymphocytic lymphoma and CLL and links the intermediate lymphocytic cell to primary follicles or mantle zones of secondary follicles . However, alkaline phosphatase activity has also been described as a feature of marginal zone B cells and their related lymphomas (97). Based on recent studies demonstrating a more favorable survival in cases with proliferation centers, it is recommended that these cases be included in the small lymphocytic category and not in the mantle cell category (fig. 7-13) (76,98). Many mantle cell lymphomas contain scattered nonphagocytic histiocytes with pale eosinophilic cytoplasm (see fig. 7-21). Lennert (53) emphasized the presence of hyaline deposits around small capillaries but not postcapillary venules in the analogous centrocytic lymphomas.

Up to half of the cases have follicles in which the mantle zones are expanded by atypical cells that appear to compress residual germinal centers (fig. 7-14). These cases have been referred to as *mantle zone lymphoma*. The focal presence of a mantle zone pattern in some diffuse cases led Weisenburger (26,100) to suggest that mantle zone lymphoma is a follicular variant of intermediate lymphocytic lymphoma. Initial biopsies may show frequent germinal centers with expanded mantle zones while subsequent biopsies may show a diffuse pattern. In some cases, the cellular composition may be dominated by cells with round or, conversely, highly irregular nuclear contours or plasmacytoid features (33,77). Nevertheless, plasmacytoid features appear to be less common in mantle cell lymphoma than in the other diffuse small cell types. In occasional cases, the preservation of normal germinal centers may be focal and the nodular pattern sufficiently pronounced to make the distinction from follicular lymphoma difficult (fig. 7-15). However, the cytologic features described above, in

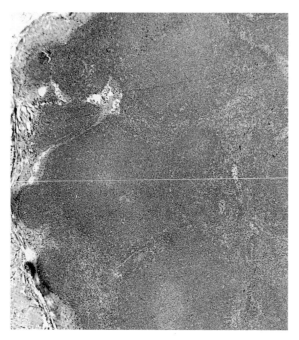

Figure 7-14
MANTLE CELL LYMPHOMA,
MANTLE ZONE PATTERN
Note the expanded mantle zones and normal or compressed germinal centers. An adjacent lymph node showed a diffuse pattern.

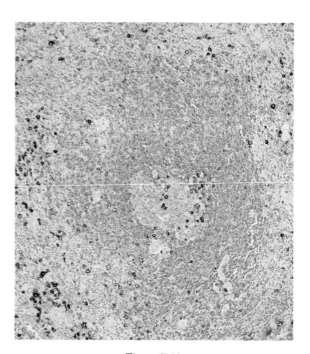

Figure 7-16
MANTLE CELL LYMPHOMA, MANTLE ZONE PATTERN
Mantle zone cells stain for lambda light chains in this paraffin section. (Immunoperoxidase with hematoxylin counterstain) (Figures 7-16–7-20 are from the same case.)

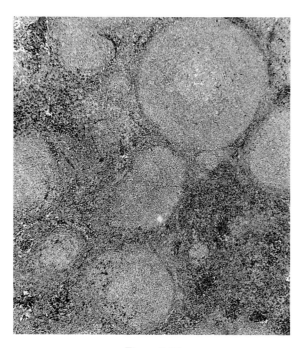

Figure 7-15
MANTLE CELL LYMPHOMA WITH
PRONOUNCED MANTLE ZONE PATTERN
Note the single residual germinal center in the nodule at upper right. This pattern closely simulates that of follicular lymphoma.

addition to the phenotypic (figs. 7-16–7-20) and molecular features described below help distinguish the two. A blastic/blastoid appearance of the cells, i.e., analogous to lymphoblasts rather than large lymphoid cells (fig. 7-21) indicates histologic progression/transformation (9,50). Scattered eosinophilic histiocytes, some of which contain cellular debris, may be unusually prominent in these "blastoid" cases (fig. 7-21, left). Transformation to large cell lymphoma is rare.

MONOCYTOID B-CELL LYMPHOMA

Definition. Malignant lymphoma, monocytoid B-cell type, is a neoplasm composed of small to medium-sized lymphocytes with round or slightly indented nuclei and relatively abundant, clear cytoplasm. These cells resemble the lymphocytes that populate the marginal zones of the spleen and may be admixed with small numbers of large lymphoid cells. Plasmacytoid lymphocytes and plasma cells may also be present.

Incidence. This lymphoma is less common than other types of diffuse small cell lymphoma, particularly if the definition is restricted to nodal

Figure 7-17
MANTLE CELL LYMPHOMA, MANTLE ZONE PATTERN

Mantle zone cells do not stain for kappa whereas rare plasma cells do stain darkly. (Immunoperoxidase with hematoxylin counterstain)

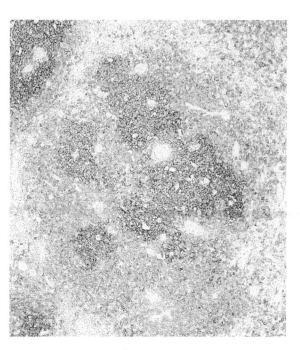

Figure 7-18
MANTLE CELL LYMPHOMA (CD20+)

Most of the small cells in this paraffin section stain for L26 (CD20). Residual germinal center cells are darkly stained. (Immunoperoxidase with hematoxylin counterstain)

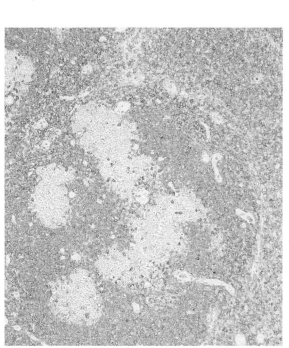

Figure 7-19
MANTLE CELL LYMPHOMA (CD43+)

The same small lymphoma cells show anomalous staining for the T-associated marker Leu-22 (CD43) supporting a diagnosis of lymphoma; the residual germinal centers do not stain. (Immunoperoxidase with hematoxylin counterstain)

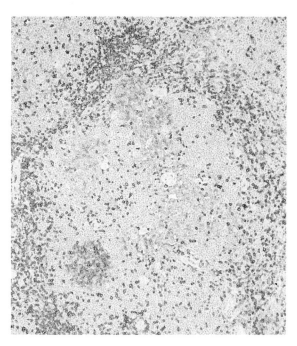

Figure 7-20
MANTLE CELL LYMPHOMA (CD45RO-)

In contrast to the extensive staining with Leu-22, only scattered T cells are labeled by A6 (CD45RO). (Immunoperoxidase with hematoxylin counterstain)

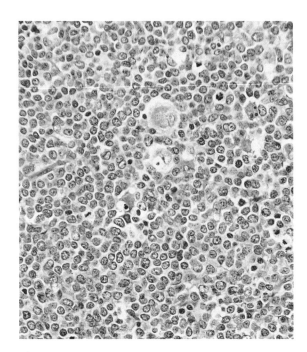 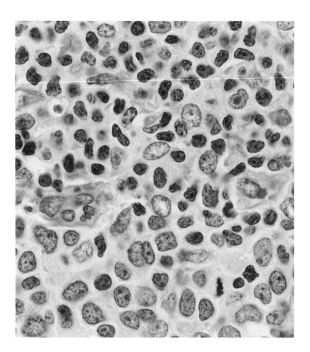

Figure 7-21
BLASTIC/BLASTOID VARIANT OF MANTLE CELL LYMPHOMA

Left: The lymphoma cells have medium-sized nuclei with rather fine nuclear chromatin. Mitotic figures are more numerous than in the usual case of mantle cell lymphoma. Interspersed histiocytes with abundant cytoplasm are common both in the usual type and the blastic variant. The lymphoma cells in this case stained for mμ, delta, and lambda chains as well as for CD5.

Right: In a different case with the same phenotype, typical mantle cell lymphoma cells at top are smaller and have more angulated nuclei with clumped chromatin when compared to the "blastoid" cells at the bottom. A previous biopsy from this patient did not show "blastic" features.

presentations (8). In contrast to other diffuse small cell lymphomas, monocytoid B-cell lymphoma occurs 2 to 5 times more frequently in women (70,86).

Natural History and Clinical Features. In contrast to patients with small lymphocytic lymphoma, with or without plasmacytoid features, and mantle cell lymphoma, those with monocytoid B-cell lymphoma more often have localized rather than generalized lymphadenopathy. This lymphoma, particularly if it involves extranodal sites, shows significant overlap with lymphoma of MALT (43). One report of 21 cases of monocytoid B-cell lymphoma documented involvement of a mucosal site in five patients at presentation and in an additional two during the course of disease (18).

Some patients have the clinical findings of autoimmune disorders such as Sjögren's syndrome (55,70,84,86). Some present with salivary gland lesions which were misinterpreted in the past as benign lymphoepithelial lesions (myoepithelial sialadenitis). Histologic or immunologic findings may support low-grade lymphoma in some cases; in other cases clonal populations

of B cells are seen by gene rearrangement analysis but whose significance is uncertain (29). Nevertheless, patients with Sjögren's syndrome have an increased incidence of malignant lymphoma (46) and patients whose biopsies contain clonal populations of B cells may have early low-grade lymphoma or are at risk for developing overt lymphoma. Bone marrow and peripheral blood involvement is uncommon (13) but may be associated with a worse prognosis (95).

Histologic transformation to large cell lymphoma may be seen in monocytoid B-cell lymphoma and appears to be associated with a worse prognosis (70). Several cases have shown an unexplained association with other low-grade lymphomas, including follicular lymphoma (70). They do not appear to represent follicular colonization (see below) since a t(14;18) translocation or *bcl*-2 expression is seen (70). They may represent unusual examples of follicular lymphoma with differentiation toward plasma cells that manifest prominent monocytoid features (see chapter 17).

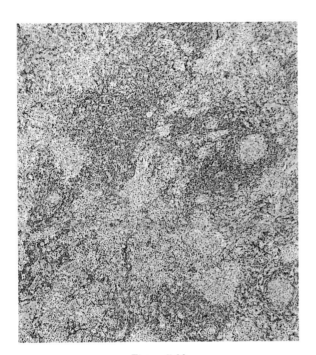

Figure 7-22
MONOCYTOID B-CELL LYMPHOMA
Note the patchy perifollicular infiltrate of pale cells.

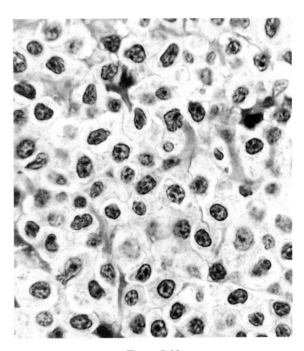

Figure 7-23
MONOCYTOID B-CELL LYMPHOMA
Note the small round or slightly indented nuclei, abundant clear cytoplasm, and distinct cell margins.

Microscopic Findings. Monocytoid B-cell lymphomas are composed of cells with small or medium-sized, round or slightly indented nuclei containing clumped chromatin and cytoplasm that is relatively abundant and clear (figs. 7-22, 7-23) (86,87). Thus, the cells resemble the reactive monocytoid cells seen in the sinuses of lymph nodes in conditions such as toxoplasmic lymphadenitis. These lymphomas have also been reported as arising from parafollicular B lymphocytes (21), resembling hairy cell leukemia (3), or being related to marginal zones (78). The majority of cases demonstrate a predominant sinusoidal pattern that may resemble florid examples of monocytoid B-cell hyperplasia; other cases have an interfollicular, marginal zone, or diffuse pattern (86). Plasmacytoid features may be prominent in some cases (65). When these lymphomas involve extranodal sites such as salivary glands, the monocytoid cells typically surround and involve epimyoepithelial islands (fig. 7-24) (70). At these sites, they are identical to lymphomas of MALT (43). Follicular colonization may be seen and may occasionally simulate progression to large cell lymphoma (44).

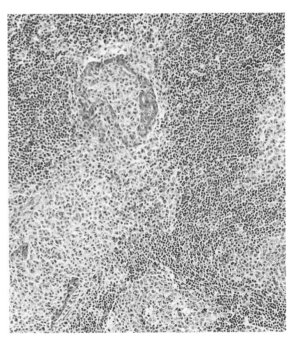

Figure 7-24
MONOCYTOID B-CELL LYMPHOMA
An epimyoepithelial island near the top is surrounded and infiltrated (lymphoepithelial lesion) by the monocytoid cells. A secondary follicle is present near the bottom. This intraparotid lymph node was removed from a 35-year-old woman who had been successfully treated for nodular sclerosing Hodgkin's disease 10 years before.

Monocytoid B-cell lymphoma cells closely resemble those of hairy cell leukemia and mastocytosis; however, the clinical features of these disorders do not overlap. Frequent eosinophilia is seen in mastocytosis, and special histochemical and immunologic studies can distinguish problematic cases. Extramedullary infiltrates of monocytic leukemia have nuclei with fine chromatin and are associated with greater mitotic activity than monocytoid B-cell lymphoma.

LOW-GRADE LYMPHOMA OF MUCOSA-ASSOCIATED LYMPHOID TISSUE

Definition. Low-grade lymphoma of mucosa-associated lymphoid tissue (MALT) is a neoplasm in which the small cell composition may vary and includes small lymphocytes, monocytoid B-cells, cells with slightly irregular nuclei (centrocyte-like), plasmacytoid cells, and plasma cells. Occasional large lymphoid cells are seen.

Incidence. In a recent review, this subtype comprised one fourth of nonfollicular small B-cell lymphomas (8). Similar to monocytoid B-cell lymphoma, a female predominance is observed.

Natural History and Clinical Features. This lymphoma may present in a variety of extranodal sites including stomach, intestine, salivary gland, lung, thyroid, lacrimal gland, conjunctiva, bladder, kidney, skin, and soft tissue (42,45,75). It may remain localized for significant periods of time and has a propensity to relapse in the same or other extranodal sites. Many diffuse lymphocytic infiltrates in these extranodal sites that were labeled pseudolymphoma in the past may represent low-grade lymphomas of MALT (48). Patients may have a variety of associated conditions including Sjögren's syndrome, Hashimoto's thyroiditis, and *Helicobacter* gastritis typically preceding the development of this lymphoma. In one patient, a clonal relationship was shown between a gastric low-grade MALT lymphoma and a lip infiltrate sampled 11 years later when the patient developed Sjögren's syndrome (24). Some gastric lymphomas may regress with anti-*Helicobacter* therapy (105). Transformation to large cell lymphoma may occur; in one series, nearly 20 percent of gastric lymphomas showed coexistence of low-grade and intermediate/high-grade components (15).

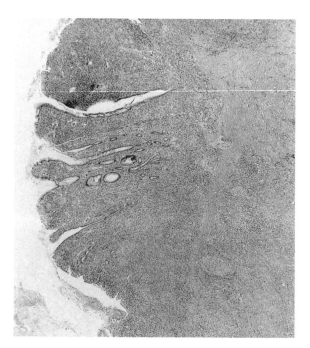

Figure 7-25
LOW-GRADE LYMPHOMA OF MUCOSA-ASSOCIATED LYMPHOID TISSUE (STOMACH)
Note the infiltration of the lamina propria of the stomach with loss of glands. The vague nodules were interpreted as colonization of preexisting follicles (see figure 7-10).

Microscopic Findings. There may be a diffuse, perifollicular (marginal zone), interfollicular, or rarely, a follicular pattern. Reactive follicles are consistently present and typically surrounded by a tumor cell infiltrate consisting of small to medium-sized lymphoid cells whose central feature is an irregular nuclear contour (centrocyte-like) (figs. 7-23, 7-25, 7-26). At one end of the spectrum, these cells closely resemble small lymphocytes, while at the other end they may contain abundant pale-staining cytoplasm, imparting a monocytoid appearance (figs. 7-23, 7-26). The centrocyte-like cells selectively invade epithelial structures to form characteristic lymphoepithelial lesions (figs. 7-24, 7-26) and may show plasma cell differentiation (fig. 7-27). The neoplastic component is often most prevalent adjacent to the epithelium. The follicles, which are typically reactive, can in some instances be selectively colonized by lymphoma cells (figs. 7-10, 7-25) (44). Usually, only occasional large lymphoid cells are present, but colonized follicles may contain a predominance of large cells, a finding that does not imply progression and a worse prognosis.

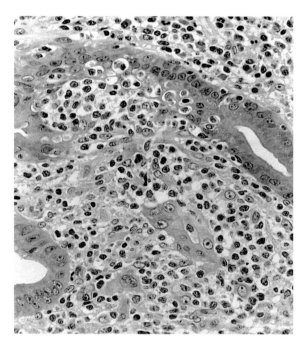

Figure 7-26
LOW-GRADE LYMPHOMA OF MUCOSA-
ASSOCIATED LYMPHOID TISSUE (STOMACH)
There is a proliferation of centrocyte-like cells with pale
to clear cytoplasm. These cells infiltrate and expand the
gastric glands, forming lymphoepithelial lesions.

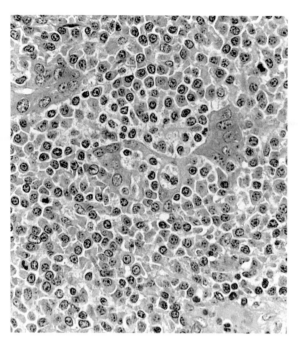

Figure 7-27
LOW-GRADE LYMPHOMA OF MUCOSA-
ASSOCIATED LYMPHOID TISSUE (STOMACH)
This example shows prominent plasma cell differentiation
in areas. A few centrocyte-like cells are seen invading a gland.

Immunologic Findings. With rare exceptions (fig. 7-28), small lymphocytic lymphomas and related entities are B-lineage neoplasms which express immunoglobulin of a single light chain type (figs. 7-16, 7-17). The immunologic features of small lymphocytic lymphoma and the related entities of CLL, lymphoplasmacytoid lymphoma, mantle cell lymphoma, and low-grade MALT lymphoma/monocytoid B-cell lymphoma show certain phenotypic differences but few if any markers that absolutely categorize an individual case of lymphoma. Furthermore, lymphoid cells comprising neoplastic disorders such as CLL were initially thought to be frozen at a particular stage of B-cell differentiation, but in vitro studies have shown that CLL cells can be induced to differentiate into immunoglobulin-secreting plasma cells (94). As a corollary, some small lymphocytic lymphomas show plasmacytoid or monocytoid features in different areas of the same biopsy or in biopsies obtained from different sites or at different times; variation in immunologic features may also be seen in such cases. Low level expression of surface immunoglobulin has been

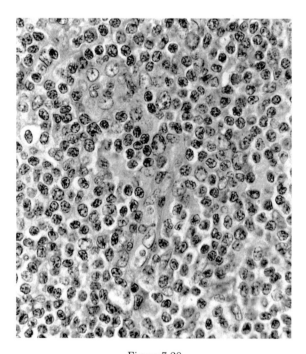

Figure 7-28
SMALL LYMPHOCYTIC LYMPHOMA (T LINEAGE)
Note the foldings and protrusions ("knobs") of the nuclei
and the prominent high endothelial venules. This lymphoma
was CD4 positive.

Table 7-1

DIFFERENTIAL EXPRESSION OF SELECTED IMMUNOLOGIC MARKERS IN SMALL LYMPHOCYTIC LYMPHOMA AND RELATED ENTITIES*

	Small Lymphocytic Lymphoma (percent)	Chronic Lymphocytic Leukemia (percent)	Plasmacytoid Small Lymphocytic Lymphoma (percent)	Mantle Cell Lymphoma (percent)	Monocytoid B-Cell/MALT Lymphoma (percent)
Immunoglobulin					
kappa	55	75	75	45	75
mμ	40	10	45	25	75
mμ + delta	25	75	20	75	0
mμ + gamma	20	10	35	5	0
gamma	20	10	15	0	25
CD5	75	100	40	80	0
CD11c	15	15	20	?	15-85
CD23	90	90	15	15	15
CD25	30	50	70	30	0
CD43	80	75	60	60	30

*From references 25,30,31,33,50,59,69,70,78,86,87,89–92,109.
Approximate percent of cases stained based on a compilation of the studies cited.

Figure 7-29
SMALL LYMPHOCYTIC LYMPHOMA (CD5+)

The lymphoma cells stain less intensely for Leu-1 (CD5) than the few darkly stained T-cells in this frozen section. (Immunoperoxidase with methylene blue counterstain)

used by some investigators to differentiate small lymphocytic lymphoma or CLL from related entities but this finding may not be reliable in an individual case. In addition, CLL cells typically display receptors for mouse erythrocytes but other B-cell neoplasms, such as small lymphocytic lymphoma, may also display these receptors, though often to a lesser degree (5,36). Expression of one or more types of complement receptors and Fc receptors is also commonly seen.

Table 7-1 summarizes many of the phenotypic markers whose expression varies significantly among the small lymphocytic lymphomas and related entities. For example, CD23 is frequently expressed in small lymphocytic lymphoma/CLL but seldom expressed in the other types of lymphoma (25,109). Monocytoid B-cell lymphomas and mucosa-associated lymphomas rarely express CD5 and CD25 but more frequently express CD11c than the other groups. Many of the mantle cell lymphomas express the normal T-cell markers CD5 and CD43 (figs. 7-19, 7-29), which distinguish them from the occasional follicular lymphomas with which they may be confused (20,69). Frequent expression of cross-reactive idiotypes associated with IgM autoantibodies is seen in various CD5-expressing lymphoproliferative disorders, including CLL and small lymphocytic lymphoma, with or without plasmacytoid features or a gammopathy (47). Lack of CD5 expression has been associated with extranodal presentation in small lymphocytic and mantle cell lymphoma but not in small lymphocytic lymphoma with plasmacytoid features (93).

Although there is some controversy regarding the phenotype of cells in the "proliferation centers" of these lymphomas, a proliferation marker such as Ki-67 typically demonstrates a somewhat higher percentage of labeled cells in these centers compared to adjacent areas and compared to the 5 to 10 percent labeling seen in small lymphocytic lymphomas. These proliferation centers also typically express transferrin receptors and about 50 percent of cases also express interleukin 2 receptors (59). Faint staining of small numbers of follicular dendritic cells by complement receptor antibodies has been described in proliferation centers (59). A recent study confirmed this observation and also reported a lesser number of *bcl*-2 stained cells, providing an additional link to reactive follicles; these authors speculated that proliferation centers may be sites of antigen driven proliferation (85). In contrast, the vague nodules of mantle cell lymphoma often demonstrate ill-defined, expanded clusters of follicular dendritic cells (FDCs); these loose meshworks of FDCs may be useful in differential diagnosis. In an effort to find markers that might explain the difference in peripheral blood involvement between small lymphocytic lymphoma and CLL, Inghirami et al. (41) reported differential expression of the lymphocyte function-associated antigen 1 (LFA-1) molecules in these disorders, but this observation has not been confirmed.

Coexpression of a B marker such as CD20 and the T-associated marker CD43 in paraffin sections aids in the immunodiagnosis of these lymphomas (see figs. 7-18–7-20) (20,69), particularly since paraffin section staining for kappa and lambda light chains may not be successful in nonplasmacytoid lymphomas. However, CD20 staining may be weak or occasionally absent and this, together with CD43 staining, might erroneously suggest a T-lineage lymphoma. A paraffin-reactive B-restricted marker like CD79 (mb-1) or a B-associated marker like CD45RA can be used as an alternative to CD20 but should be carefully compared to a paraffin-reactive T-restricted marker such as polyclonal CD3 or a T-associated marker like CD45RO since a subset of T-cells stains with CD45RA (see chapter 2).

Molecular and Cytogenetic Findings. Since most small lymphocytic lymphomas are B-lineage neoplasms that express immunoglobulin of a single light chain type, molecular analyses of immunoglobulin gene configurations invariably demonstrate rearranged heavy and light chain genes (17,35). Although molecular studies are generally not necessary for the routine diagnosis of small lymphocytic lymphoma, they help demonstrate monoclonal B-cell populations, particularly in small lymphocytic proliferations at extranodal sites and in many lesions with the features of "pseudolymphoma" (22,67). Clonal immunoglobulin gene rearrangements may not be as diagnostic of clinically malignant disease at some extranodal sites as they have been for lymphocytic lesions of the salivary gland, with benign morphologic and polyclonal immunophenotypic features, only some of which progress to overt lymphoma (29). Immunoglobulin gene rearrangement configurations are not helpful in distinguishing among the related entities of CLL, lymphoplasmacytoid lymphoma, mantle cell lymphoma, and monocytoid B-cell lymphoma since these are also mature B-lineage malignancies with productively rearranged immunoglobulin genes.

Small lymphocytic lymphomas and their related entities are cytogenetically heterogeneous (83). They tend to be pseudodiploid (54) and share some of the cytogenetic features of their leukemic counterpart, CLL. Trisomy of chromosome 12 has been reported in up to 40 percent of small lymphocytic lymphomas (compared to 50 percent of CLL) in one series (56); however, it has also been observed in virtually every lymphoma subtype and therefore cannot be considered specific for small lymphocytic proliferations.

The t(11;14)(q13;q32) translocation has been reported in small lymphocytic and mantle cell lymphomas in addition to CLL, and less frequently in prolymphocytic leukemia, multiple myeloma, and other lymphomas (49,83). The t(11;14) abnormality results in deregulation and relocalization of the *bcl*-1 proto-oncogene (also called PRAD1) into the proximity of the immunoglobulin heavy chain gene (96). Breakpoints

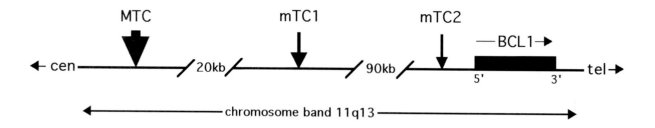

Figure 7-30
DISTRIBUTION OF BREAKPOINT CLUSTER REGIONS FLANKING THE *bcl*-1 GENE ON CHROMOSOME 11Q13
Schematic diagram of chromosome 11q13 DNA flanking the *bcl*-1 gene and locations of breakpoint cluster regions. The solid box denotes the *bcl*-1 gene. TEL, telomere; CEN, centromere; MTC, major translocation cluster region containing majority of t(11;14) breakpoints; mTC1 and mTC2, minor translocation cluster regions containing a minority of breakpoints.

occur over a large distance flanking the *bcl*-1 gene (fig. 7-30); many occur near or within a restricted region known as the major translocation cluster (MTC) (60,80,81,96). The *bcl*-1 gene codes for a new member of the cyclin family of proteins that regulate progression through the cell cycle (63,102). Molecular cytogenetic studies using currently available 11q13 DNA probes have demonstrated that up to 50 percent of intermediate lymphocytic and centrocytic lymphomas have *bcl*-1 rearrangements (81,82,102,107), supporting the view that these lymphoma subtypes constitute a unique histopathologic entity, now called mantle cell lymphoma (4). However, *bcl*-1 DNA rearrangements and the t(11;14) translocation are not specific for this entity. Studies of the prevalence of *bcl*-1 involvement in lymphoma subtypes are currently hampered by the fact that the 11q13 DNA probes employed do not detect rearrangements in all lymphomas and leukemias with t(11;14) cytogenetic abnormalities. Antibodies directed against *bcl*-1 would assist these efforts and likely prove diagnostically useful. In small lymphocytic lymphomas, t(11;14) has been associated with a propensity to develop into diffuse large cell lymphoma; in intermediate lymphocytic lymphomas, *bcl*-1 rearrangements are associated with an unfavorable prognosis (40,108). These rearrangements are not a feature of lymphomas of MALT, consistent with a separate pathogenesis for these disorders (107).

A rare but recurrent translocation in small lymphocytic lymphoma/CLL is the t(14;19) (q32;q13) which molecular studies have shown results in the juxtaposition of the *bcl*-3 gene with immunoglobulin heavy chain gene (56). A t(9;14)(p13;q32) abnormality has been seen in some cases of small lymphocytic lymphoma with plasmacytoid features (72). The t(14;18) has been reported occasionally in small lymphocytic lymphomas but not with the consistency observed in follicular lymphomas (83), although recent reports of *bcl*-2 translocations with immunoglobulin light chain genes in CLL (2) should prompt studies of similar molecular cytogenetic abnormalities in small lymphocytic lymphomas and related entities. The *bcl*-2 gene rearrangement, the molecular hallmark of t(14;18), is not a feature of monocytoid B-cell lymphomas or lymphomas of MALT (70,107); however, trisomy 3 has recently been associated with these MALT lymphomas (106). Translocations and deletions of 14q22-24 and 11q have also been reported in small lymphocytic lymphomas and other subtypes but their molecular consequences are currently unknown (54).

Differential Diagnosis. *Chronic Lymphocytic Leukemia (CLL).* No histologic criteria exist to distinguish small lymphocytic lymphoma from CLL; the Kiel classification does not distinguish the two. The criteria for CLL recommended by a National Cancer Institute–sponsored working group include greater than $5,000/mm^3$ circulating lymphocytes and greater than 30 percent lymphocytes in the bone marrow (16). Reports in the literature commonly use the degree of lymphocytosis to segregate cases into small lymphocytic lymphoma or CLL: the arbitrary degree of lymphocytosis used for a diagnosis of CLL varies from $4,000/mm^3$ to $15,000/mm^3$. Many studies of

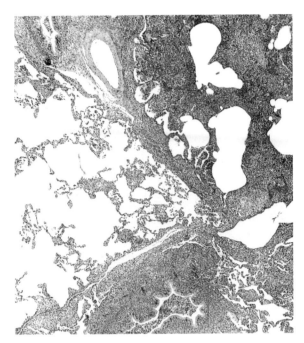

Figure 7-31
LYMPHOID HYPERPLASIA OF THE LUNG
The extent of this lymphoid infiltrate and its pattern of involvement of lymphatic routes (bronchoarterial rays, veins, septa, and pleura) suggested a diagnosis of lymphoma. (Figures 7-31 and 7-32 are from same case.)

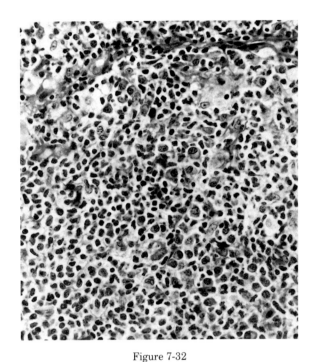

Figure 7-32
LYMPHOID HYPERPLASIA OF THE LUNG
The nuclear irregularities in many of the lymphoid cells also suggested a diagnosis of lymphoma but plasma cells were focally abundant and immunohistochemical findings did not support lymphoma. This patient presented with interstitial infiltrates and was known to be HIV positive.

small lymphocytic lymphoma and its variants include patients with peripheral lymphocytosis. In the past, some hematopathologists maintained that all patients with small lymphocytic lymphoma (without lymphocytosis) would progress to CLL; however, Pangalis et al. (73) noted that only 6 of 41 patients with small lymphocytic lymphoma developed a lymphocytosis in a follow-up period ranging from 24 to 150 months. In a more recent study, 10 of 54 patients with small lymphocytic lymphoma developed a marked lymphocytosis consistent with CLL; these 10 patients had a significantly higher median initial lymphocyte count ($2,790/mm^3$) than those patients who did not develop CLL ($1,580/mm^3$) (62). The development of CLL in this subset of patients did not adversely affect their survival. The lymph node findings in patients with CLL have been well described (6,23).

Lymphocyte Predominance Hodgkin's Disease (LPHD). The most common and least controversial form of LPHD is the nodular form, comprising large nodules forming a mass lesion in lymph nodes. These architectural features and the presence of lymphocytic and histiocytic (L&H) cells or "popcorn" cells in a background rich in lymphocytes and histiocytes should allow differentiation from small lymphocytic lymphoma and its variants. The less common and more controversial diffuse lymphocytic and histiocytic types include vaguely nodular LPHD (confirmed by phenotypic studies), mixed cellularity Hodgkin's disease, B-cell lymphoma, and T-cell lymphoma (68). Immunophenotypic or molecular studies may be necessary for diagnosis. Small lymphocytic lymphomas are rare in young patients, and LPHD should be considered first since it is more common in this age group.

Extranodal Lymphoid Hyperplasia (figs. 7-31, 7-32). Many extranodal lymphocytic infiltrates in sites such as the orbital soft tissue, stomach, salivary gland, and lung, which were termed lymphoid hyperplasia, pseudolymphoma, or benign lymphoepithelial lesion in the past, are really low-grade lymphomas (12). Before the availability of immunologic and molecular methods of diagnosis, it was not appreciated that many low-grade lymphomas could be associated with histologic features that previously suggested a benign, reactive process. These include reactive follicles, preserved normal glandular structures, and associated non-neoplastic cells such as plasma cells and epithelioid histiocytes resulting in a polymorphous infiltrate (as in polymorphous immunocytoma). When infiltrates are extensive and destructive or associated with lymphoepithelial lesions, when they lack reactive follicles, or when significant numbers of cells appear cytologically abnormal a firm diagnosis of malignant lymphoma can often be made. However, when both reactive and neoplastic features are present, when either the small size or cellular distortion in a biopsy compromises diagnosis, or when cytologic features are ambiguous, a variety of ancillary studies can be performed to aid in diagnosis. Since benign and malignant infiltrates can coexist in the same lesion, potential sampling problems can compromise the accuracy of diagnosis. Patients with apparently benign lymphoid infiltrates should be clinically observed for unsuspected lymphoma and the subsequent development of overt lymphoma. It is not uncommon for reactive lymphoid infiltrates in the skin to be present in the superficial dermis overlying deeper infiltrates of lymphoma (103). In addition, clonal populations of B cells, which can only be detected by molecular methods, may precede the development of histologically apparent lymphoma composed of the same clonal population (104). Thus, many of the architectural and cellular features that are used for the diagnosis of small lymphocytic lymphoma and related entities in lymph nodes can be applied to extranodal sites; when the histologic features are not diagnostic, special studies can be performed on paraffin-embedded or fresh tissue.

Lymphoblastic Lymphoma. Suboptimally prepared biopsies of lymphoblastic lymphoma with nuclear chromatin clumping may result in an erroneous diagnosis of small lymphocytic lymphoma. Most lymphoblastic lymphomas occur in young patients and a high mitotic rate is common, in contrast to the older age incidence and low mitotic rate typical of small lymphocytic lymphoma and its variants. Identification of the blastic/blastoid variant of mantle cell lymphoma may require correlation with previous biopsy findings or phenotypic, cytogenetic, or molecular studies.

Diffuse Small Cleaved Cell (Centrocytic) Lymphoma. If diagnostic criteria include the same degree of nuclear irregularities as for follicular small cleaved cell lymphoma and if lymphoblastic lymphomas are excluded, diffuse small cleaved cell lymphomas are rare. Many cases formerly designated as "diffuse small cleaved cell" or "centrocytic" lymphoma would today be designated mantle cell (intermediate/mantle zone) lymphoma (1). Nevertheless, a recent study of 33 cases of diffuse small cleaved cell lymphoma identified 4 as T-cell, 9 with a prior history of follicular lymphoma, and only a few with phenotypic features typical of mantle cell lymphoma (51).

Diffuse Mixed Small and Large Cell Lymphoma. When prolymphocytes and paraimmunoblasts are interspersed with small lymphocytes in small lymphocytic lymphoma, a diagnosis of diffuse mixed lymphoma may be considered. However, the background small lymphocytes of diffuse mixed lymphomas of T-cell type and diffuse mixed lymphomas that represent progression from follicular lymphomas characteristically have irregular nuclear outlines. In addition, many cases designated as diffuse mixed lymphoma represent large cell B-cell lymphomas rich in T cells and require immunologic studies for identification.

Follicular Lymphoma. Cases of small lymphocytic lymphoma with many pseudofollicles may be mistaken for follicular lymphoma. As previously discussed, the cellular composition of the follicles of follicular lymphoma differs from the pseudofollicles of small lymphocytic lymphoma and its variants (fig. 7-5) and retained mantle zones are not typical of small lymphocytic lymphomas. A pronounced mantle zone pattern may simulate follicular lymphoma but the cellular composition is different and occasional residual germinal centers can be identified in the nodules of the mantle zone lymphoma (fig. 7-15). Expression of CD5 (fig. 7-29) and lack of expression of CD10 by small lymphocytic lymphoma and its variants may be helpful in this distinction.

Treatment. Patients with small lymphocytic lymphoma and related disorders are generally responsive to a variety of therapies including single drug chemotherapy, combination chemotherapy, and irradiation (37). Despite a high complete response rate, there is often a continuous pattern of relapses. Since patients with advanced stage small lymphocytic lymphoma are seldom cured by conventional therapy, live relatively long periods with recurrent disease, and are often elderly and asymptomatic, it is now common practice to defer treatment of these patients until it is necessitated by disease progression. In a group of patients at Stanford who received no initial treatment, the median time to the institution of therapy was 6 years (38). Whereas differences in clinical stage at presentation do not translate into differences in survival, a small group of patients with limited stage small lymphocytic lymphoma showed prolonged freedom from relapse: 80 percent of stage I and 60 percent of stage II patients at 10 years following irradiation (62).

MALT lymphomas have been managed by surgical excision alone or with additional radiotherapy or chemotherapy, but tumor regression has recently been described in gastric MALT lymphoma patients following anti-*Helicobacter* therapy (105). The rationale for this approach is provided by studies demonstrating that in vitro growth of lymphoma cells from a given patient depends on the presence of a particular strain of *Helicobacter* as well as T cells (39). However, a recent study of 43 patients with diverse lymphomas of MALT reported a relapse rate similar to that for patients with small lymphocytic/lymphoplasmacytoid lymphomas (8).

Prognosis. Small lymphocytic lymphoma has an indolent natural history, with 60 percent of patients alive at 5 years and a median survival of approximately 6 years (71). Similar median survival periods have been published for CLL, small lymphocytic lymphoma with plasmacytoid features, monocytoid B-cell lymphoma, and mantle cell lymphoma with a nodular/mantle zone pattern. Median survival times in diffuse forms of mantle cell lymphoma vary from 2.5 to more than 5 years (9,58,98). A recent report of nonfollicular small B-cell lymphoma found significantly shorter median survivals in large cell–rich immuno-

cytoma (4.5 years) and mantle cell lymphoma (4.3 years) in contrast to small lymphocytic lymphoma with or without plasmacytoid features (10 years) and lymphomas of MALT (8 years) (8).

Attempts to correlate survival with histologic, immunologic, or other parameters have met with variable results. Whereas initial studies did not report that increased numbers of large lymphoid cells adversely affected survival in patients with CLL/small lymphocytic lymphoma (23,28), a recent large study determined that large cell grades II and III (defined in this study as cases with aggregates [grade II] or admixed large cells [grade III]) adversely affected survival but only in the leukemic patients (6). In contrast, another study reported that 87 percent of small lymphocytic lymphoma patients whose biopsies showed a pseudofollicular pattern were alive at 10 years versus 47 percent of patients whose biopsies showed a diffuse pattern (62). Other parameters that have shown an adverse effect on survival in some studies are advanced age, presence of B symptoms (62), presence of anemia, and lack of complete response to treatment (6) as well as factors associated with poor prognosis in other lymphoma subtypes: advanced clinical stage, poor performance status, tumor bulk, and high lactate dehydrogenase or beta-2-microglobulin levels (8).

A morphologic study by Evans et al. (28) identified decreased survival in a small number of cases of CLL/small lymphocytic lymphoma with a mitotic rate of 30 or more per 20 high-power fields. A recent study confirmed this observation by identifying an adverse effect of increased numbers of proliferating cells in diffuse small cell lymphomas as assessed by the Ki-67 antibody and also suggested that a low number of associated CD4-positive T-helper cells adversely affected survival (58). Increased numbers of proliferating cells (often associated with blastic morphology) have also been associated with shorter median survival periods in mantle cell lymphoma (9).

REFERENCES

1. Abe M, Ono N, Tominaga K, et al. Histogenesis of diffuse small cleaved cell lymphoma. An immunohistochemical and molecular genetic (bcl-2 gene) study with comparison to follicular small cleaved cell lymphoma and mantle zone lymphoma. Cancer 1992;70:821–9.
2. Adachi M, Cossman J, Longo D, Croce CM, Tsujimoto Y. Variant translocation of the bcl-2 gene to immunoglobu-

lin lambda light chain gene in chronic lymphocytic leukemia. Proc Natl Acad Sci USA 1989;86:2771–4.
3. Agnarsson BA, Kadin ME. An unusual B-cell lymphoma simulating hairy cell leukemia. Am J Clin Pathol 1987;88:752–9.

4. Banks PM, Chan J, Cleary ML, et al. Mantle cell lymphoma. A proposal for unification of morphologic, immunologic, and molecular data. Am J Surg Pathol 1992;16:637–40.

5. Batata A, Shen B. Relationship between chronic lymphocytic leukemia and small lymphocytic lymphoma. A comparative study of membrane phenotypes in 270 cases. Cancer 1992;70:625–32.

6. Ben-Ezra J, Burke JS, Swartz WG, et al. Small lymphocytic lymphoma: a clinicopathologic analysis of 268 cases. Blood 1989;73:579–87.

7. Berard CW. Reticuloendothelial system: an overview of neoplasia. In: Rebuck JW, Berard CW, Abell MR, eds. The reticuloendothelial system. (Vol. 16) Baltimore: Williams & Wilkins, 1975:306–7. (International Academy of Pathology)

8. Berger F, Felman P, Sonet A, et al. Nonfollicular small B-cell lymphomas: a heterogeneous group of patients with distinct clinical features and outcome. Blood 1994;83:2829–35.

9. Bookman MA, Lardelli P, Jaffe ES, Duffey PL, Longo DL. Lymphocytic lymphoma of intermediate differentiation: morphologic, immunophenotypic, and prognostic factors. JNCI 1990;82:742–8.

10. Braylan RC, Long JC, Jaffe ES, Greco FA, Orr SL, Berard CW. Malignant lymphoma obscured by concomitant extensive epithelioid granulomas: report of 3 cases with similar clinicopathologic features. Cancer 1977;39:1146–55.

11. Brecher M, Banks PM. Hodgkin's disease variant of Richter's syndrome. Report of eight cases. Am J Clin Pathol 1990;93:333–9.

12. Burke JS. Histologic criteria for distinguishing between benign and malignant extranodal lymphoid infiltrates. Semin Diagn Pathol 1985;2:152–62.

13. Carbone A, Gloghini A, Pinto A, Attadia V, Zagonel V, Volpe R. Monocytoid B-cell lymphoma with bone marrow and peripheral blood involvement at presentation. Am J Clin Pathol 1989;92:228–36.

14. _____, Pinto A, Gloghini A, Volpe R, Zagonel V. B-zone small lymphocytic lymphoma: a morphologic, immunophenotypic, and clinical study with comparison to well-differentiated lymphocytic disorders. Hum Pathol 1992;23:438–48

15. Chan JK, Ng CS, Isaacson PG. Relationship between high-grade lymphoma and low-grade B-cell mucosa-associated lymphoid tissue lymphoma (MALToma) of the stomach. Am J Pathol 1990;136:1153–64.

16. Cheson BD, Bennett JM, Rai KR, et al. Guidelines for clinical protocols for chronic lymphocytic leukemia: recommendations of the National Cancer Institute-sponsored working group. Am J Hematol 1988;29:152–63.

17. Cleary ML, Chao J, Warnke R, Sklar J. Immunoglobulin gene rearrangement as a diagnostic criterion of B-cell lymphoma. Proc Natl Acad Sci USA 1984;81:593–7.

18. Cogliatti SB, Lennert K, Hansmann ML, Zwingers TL. Monocytoid B cell lymphoma: clinical and prognostic features of 21 patients. J Clin Pathol 1990;43:619–25.

19. Colby TV, Warnke RA, Burke JS, Dorfman RF. Differentiation of chronic lymphocytic leukemia from Hodgkin's disease using immunologic marker studies. Am J Surg Pathol 1981;5:707–10.

20. Contos M, Kornstein M, Innes D, Ben-Ezra J. The utility of CD20 and CD43 in subclassification of low-grade B-cell lymphoma on paraffin sections. Mod Pathol 1992;5:631–3.

21. Cousar JB, McGinn DL, Glick AD, List AF, Collins RD. Report of an unusual lymphoma arising from parafollicular B-lymphocytes (PBLs) or so-called monocytoid lymphocytes. Am J Clin Pathol 1987;87:121–8.

22. Davis RE, Warnke RA, Dorfman RF, Cleary ML. Utility of molecular genetic analysis for the diagnosis of neoplasia in morphologically and immunophenotypically equivocal hematolymphoid lesions. Cancer 1991;67:2890–9.

23. Dick F, Maca RD. The lymph node in chronic lymphocytic leukemia. Cancer 1978;41:283–92.

24. Diss TC, Peng H, Wotherspoon AC, Pan L, Speight PM, Isaacson PG. Brief report: a single neoplastic clone in sequential biopsy specimens from a patient with primary gastric mucosa-associated lymphoid-tissue lymphoma and Sjögren's syndrome. N Engl J Med 1993;329:172–5.

25. Dorfman DM, Pinkus GS. Distinction between small lymphocytic and mantle cell lymphoma by immunoreactivity for CD23. Mod Pathol 1994;7:326–31.

26. Duggan MJ, Weisenburger DD, Ye YL, et al. Mantle zone lymphoma. A clinicopathologic study of 22 cases. Cancer 1990;66:522–9.

27. Ellison DJ, Nathwani BN, Cho SY, Martin SE. Interfollicular small lymphocytic lymphoma: the diagnostic significance of pseudofollicles. Hum Pathol 1989;20: 1108–18.

28. Evans HL, Butler JJ, Youness EL. Malignant lymphoma, small lymphocytic type: a clinicopathologic study of 84 cases with suggested criteria for intermediate lymphocytic lymphoma. Cancer 1978;41:1440–55.

29. Fishleder A, Tubbs R, Hesse B, Levine H. Uniform detection of immunoglobulin-gene rearrangement in benign lymphoepithelial lesions. N Engl J Med 1987;316:1118–21.

30. Gelb AB, Rouse RV, Dorfman RF, Warnke RA. Detection of immunophenotypic abnormalities in paraffin-embedded B-lineage non-Hodgkin's lymphomas. Am J Clin Pathol. 1994;102:825–34.

31. Hall PA, D'Ardenne AJ, Richards MA, Stansfeld AG. Lymphoplasmacytoid lymphoma: an immunohistological study. J Pathol 1987;153:213–23.

32. Hansmann ML, Fellbaum C, Hui PK, Lennert K. Morphological and immunohistochemical investigation of non-Hodgkin's lymphoma combined with Hodgkin's disease. Histopathology 1989;15:35–48.

33. Harris NL, Bhan AK. B-cell neoplasms of the lymphocytic, lymphoplasmacytoid, and plasma cell types: immunohistologic analysis and clinical correlation. Hum Pathol 1985;16:829–37.

34. _____, Bhan AK. Mantle-zone lymphoma. A pattern produced by lymphomas of more than one cell type. Am J Surg Pathol 1985;9:872–82.

35. Henni T, Gaulard P, Divine M, et al. Comparison of genetic probe with immunophenotype analysis in lymphoproliferative disorders: a study of 87 cases. Blood 1988;72:1937–43.

36. Hicks MJ, Grogan TM, Fielder K, Spier CM. Differentiation of chronic lymphocytic leukemia from other well to intermediate differentiated lymphoproliferative disorders by the mouse rosette assay. Diagn Immunol 1986;4:31–6.

37. Horning SJ. Diffuse small cell lymphomas. In: Magrath IT, ed. The non-Hodgkin's lymphomas. London: Williams & Wilkins, 1990: 309–16.

38. _____, Rosenberg SA. The natural history of initially untreated low-grade non-Hodgkin's lymphomas. N Engl J Med 1984;311:1471–5.

39. Hussell T, Isaacson PG, Crabtree JE, Spencer J. The response of cells from low-grade B-cell gastric lymphomas of mucosa-associated lymphoid tissue to Helicobacter pylori. Lancet 1993;342:571–4.

40. Ince C, Blick M, Lee M, et al. Bcl-1 gene rearrangements in B cell lymphoma. Leukemia 1988;2:343–6.

41. Inghirami G, Wieczorek R, Zhu BY, Silber R, Dalla-Favera R, Knowles DM. Differential expression of LFA-1 molecules in non-Hodgkin's lymphoma and lymphoid leukemia. Blood 1988;72:1431–4

42. Isaacson PG. Lymphomas of mucosa-associated lymphoid tissue (MALT). Histopathology 1990;16:617–9.

43. _____, Spencer J. Monocytoid B-cell lymphomas. Am J Surg Pathol 1990;14:888–91.

44. _____, Wotherspoon AC, Diss T, Pan LX. Follicular colonization in B-cell lymphoma of mucosa-associated lymphoid tissue. Am J Surg Pathol 1991;15:819–28.

45. _____, Wright DH. Malignant lymphoma of mucosa-associated lymphoid tissue. Cancer 1983;52:1410–6.

46. Kassan SS, Thomas TL, Moutsopoulos HM, et al. Increased risk of lymphoma in sicca syndrome. Ann Intern Med 1978;89:888–92.

47. Kipps TJ, Robbins BA, Tefferi A, Meisenholder G, Banks PM, Carson DA. CD5-positive B-cell malignancies frequently express cross-reactive idiotypes associated with IgM autoantibodies. Am J Pathol 1990;136:809–16.

48. Knowles DM II, Halper JP, Jakobiec FA. The immunologic characterization of 40 extranodal lymphoid infiltrates. Usefulness in distinguishing between benign pseudolymphoma and malignant lymphoma. Cancer 1982;49:2321–35.

49. Koduru PR, Filippa DA, Richardson ME, et al. Cytogenetic and histologic correlations in malignant lymphoma. Blood 1987;69:97–102.

50. Lardelli P, Bookman MA, Sundeen J, Longo DL, Jaffe ES. Lymphocytic lymphoma of intermediate differentiation. Morphologic and immunophenotypic spectrum and clinical correlations. Am J Surg Pathol 1990;14:752–63.

51. Leith CP, Spier CM, Grogan TM, et al. Diffuse small cleaved-cell lymphoma: a heterogeneous disease with distinct immunobiologic subsets. J Clin Oncol 1992;10:1259–65.

52. Lennert K. Malignant lymphomas other than Hodgkin's disease. Histology. Cytology. Ultrastructure. Immunology. Berlin: Springer-Verlag, 1978:116.

53. _____, Feller AC. Histopathology of non-Hodgkin's lymphomas (based on the updated Kiel classification). 2nd ed. Berlin: Springer-Verlag, 1992.

54. Levine EG, Arthur DC, Frizzera G, Peterson BA, Hurd DD, Bloomfield CD. There are differences in cytogenetic abnormalities among histologic subtypes of the non-Hodgkin's lymphomas. Blood 1985;66:1414–22.

55. McCurley TL, Collins D, Ball E, Collins RD. Nodal and extranodal lymphoproliferative disorders in Sjögren's syndrome: a clinical and immunopathologic study. Hum Pathol 1990;21:482–92.

56. McKeithan TW, Rowley JD, Shows TB, Diaz MO. Cloning of the chromosome translocation breakpoint junction of the t(14;19) in chronic lymphocytic leukemia. Proc Natl Acad Sci USA 1987;84:9257–60.

57. Medeiros LJ, Harris NL. Immunohistologic analysis of small lymphocytic infiltrates of the orbit and conjunctiva. Hum Pathol 1990;21:1126–31.

58. _____, Picker LJ, Gelb AB, et al. Numbers of host helper T cells and proliferating cells predict survival in diffuse small-cell lymphomas. J Clin Oncol 1989;7:1009–17.

59. _____, Strickler JG, Picker LJ, Gelb AB, Weiss LM, Warnke RA. Well-differentiated lymphocytic neoplasms. Immunologic findings correlated with clinical presentation and morphologic features. Am J Pathol 1987;129:523–35.

60. Meeker TC, Grimaldi JC, O'Rourke R, Louie E, Juliusson G, Einhorn S. An additional breakpoint region in the BCL-1 locus associated with the t(11;14)(q13;q32) translocation of B-lymphocytic malignancy. Blood 1989;74:1801–6.

61. Momose H, Jaffe ES, Shin SS, Chen YY, Weiss LM. Chronic lymphocytic leukemia/small lymphocytic lymphoma with Reed-Sternberg-like cells and possible transformation to Hodgkin's disease. Mediation by Epstein-Barr virus. Am J Surg Pathol 1992;16:859–67.

62. Morrison WH, Hoppe RT, Weiss LM, Picozzi VJ Jr, Horning SJ. Small lymphocytic lymphoma. J Clin Oncol 1989;7:598–606.

63. Motokura T, Bloom T, Kim HG, et al. A novel cyclin encoded by a bcl1-linked candidate oncogene. Nature 1991;350:512–5.

64. Nanba K, Jaffe ES, Braylan RC, Soban EJ, Berard CW. Alkaline phosphatase-positive malignant lymphoma. A subtype of B-cell lymphoma. Am J Clin Pathol 1977;68:535–42.

65. Nathwani BN, Mohrmann RL, Brynes RK, Taylor CR, Hansmann ML, Sheibani K. Monocytoid B-cell lymphomas: an assessment of diagnostic criteria and a perspective on histogenesis. Hum Pathol 1992;23:1061–71.

66. _____, Winberg CD. Malignant lymphomas. In: Sommers SC, Rosen PP, ed. Norwalk: Appleton-Century-Crofts, 1983:22–64.

67. Neri A, Jakobiec FA, Pelicci PG, Dalla-Favera R, Knowles DM II. Immunoglobulin and T cell receptor beta chain gene rearrangement analysis of ocular adnexal lymphoid neoplasms: clinical and biologic implications. Blood 1987;70:1519–29.

68. Nicholas DS, Harris S, Wright DH. Lymphocyte predominance Hodgkin's disease—an immunohistochemical study. Histopathology 1990;16:157–65.

69. Ngan BY, Picker LJ, Medeiros LJ, Warnke RA. Immunophenotypic diagnosis of non-Hodgkin's lymphoma in paraffin sections. Co-expression of L60 (Leu-22) and L26 antigens correlates with malignant histologic findings. Am J Clin Pathol 1989;91:579–83.

70. _____, Warnke RA, Wilson M, Takagi K, Cleary ML, Dorfman RF. Monocytoid B-cell lymphoma: a study of 36 cases. Hum Pathol 1991;22:409–21.

71. Non-Hodgkin's Lymphoma Pathologic Classification Project. The National Cancer Institute sponsored study of classifications of non-Hodgkin's lymphomas: summary and description of a working formulation for clinical usage. Cancer 1982;49:2112–35.

72. Offit K, Parsa NZ, Filippa D, Jhanwar SC, Chaganti RS. t(9;14)(p13;q32) denotes a subset of low-grade non-Hodgkin's lymphoma with plasmacytoid differentiation. Blood 1992;80:2594–9.

73. Pangalis GA, Nathwani BN, Rappaport H. Malignant lymphoma, well differentiated lymphocytic: its relationship with chronic lymphocytic leukemia and macroglobulinemia of Waldenström. Cancer 1977;39:999–1010.

74. Patsouris E, Noel H, Lennert K. Histological and immunohistological findings in lymphoepithelioid cell lymphoma (Lennert's lymphoma). Am J Surg Pathol 1988;12:341–50.

75. Pelstring RJ, Essell JH, Kurtin PJ, Cohen AR, Banks PM. Diversity of organ site involvement among malignant lymphomas of mucosa-associated tissues. Am J Clin Pathol 1991;96:738–45.

76. Perry DA, Bast MA, Armitage JO, Weisenburger DD. Diffuse intermediate lymphocytic lymphoma. A clinicopathologic study and comparison with small lymphocytic lymphoma and diffuse small cleaved cell lymphoma. Cancer 1990;66:1995–2000.

77. Pileri S, Rivano MT, Gobbi M, Taruscio D, Lennert K. Neoplastic and reactive follicles within B-cell malignant lymphomas. A morphological and immunological study of 30 cases. Hematol Oncol 1985;3:243–60.

78. Piris MA, Rivas C, Morente M, Cruz MA, Rubio C, Oliva H. Monocytoid B-cell lymphoma, a tumour related to the marginal zone. Histopathology 1988;12:383–92. [55,83]

79. Pugh WC, Manning JT, Butler JJ. Paraimmunoblastic variant of small lymphocytic lymphoma/leukemia. Am J Surg Pathol 1988;12:907–17.

80. Rabbitts PH, Douglas J, Fischer P, et al. Chromosome abnormalities at 11q13 in B cell tumors. Oncogene 1988;3:99–103.

81. Rimokh R, Berger F, Cornillet P, et al. Break in the BCL1 locus is closely associated with intermediate lymphocytic lymphoma subtype. Genes Chromosom Cancer 1990;2:223–6.

82. _____, Berger F, Delsol G, et al. Rearrangement and overexpression of the BCL-1/PRAD-1 gene in intermediate lymphocytic lymphomas and in t(11q13)-bearing leukemias. Blood 1993;81:3063–7.

83. Sandberg AA. The chromosomes in human cancer and leukemia. New York: Elsevier, 1990.

84. Schmid U, Helbron D, Lennert K. Development of malignant lymphoma in myoepithelial sialadenitis (Sjögren's syndrome). Virchows Arch [A] 1982;295:11–43.

85. Schmid C, Isaacson PG. Proliferation centres in B-cell malignant lymphoma, lymphocytic (B-CLL): an immunophenotypic study. Histopathol 1994;24:445–51.

86. Sheibani K, Burke JS, Swartz WG, Nademanee A, Winberg CD. Monocytoid B-cell lymphoma. Clinicopathologic study of 21 cases of a unique type of low-grade lymphoma. Cancer 1988;62:1531–8.

87. _____, Sohn CC, Burke JS, Winberg CD, Wu AM, Rappaport H. Monocytoid B-cell lymphoma. A novel B-cell neoplasm. Am J Pathol 1986;124:310–8.

88. Shin SS, Ben-Ezra J, Burke JS, Sheibani K, Rappaport H. Reed-Sternberg-like cells in low-grade lymphomas are transformed neoplastic cells of B-cell lineage. Am J Clin Pathol 1993;99:658–62.

89. Spier CM, Grogan TM, Fielder K, Richter L, Rangel C. Immunophenotypes in "well-differentiated" lymphoproliferative disorders, with emphasis on small lymphocytic lymphoma. Hum Pathol 1986;17:1126–36.

90. Stein H, Lennert K, Feller AC, Mason DY. Immunohistological analysis of human lymphoma: correlation of histological and immunological categories. Adv Cancer Res 1984;42:67–147.

91. Strickler JG, Medeiros LJ, Copenhaver CM, Weiss LM, Warnke RA. Intermediate lymphocytic lymphoma: an immunophenotypic study with comparison to small lymphocytic lymphoma and diffuse small cleaved cell lymphoma. Hum Pathol 1988;19:550–4.

92. Stross WP, Warnke RA, Flavell DJ, et al. Molecule detected in formalin fixed tissue by antibodies MT1, DF-T1, and L60 (Leu-22) corresponds to CD43 antigen. J Clin Pathol 1989;42:953–61.

93. Sundeen JT, Longo DL, Jaffe ES. CD5 expression in B-cell small lymphocytic malignancies. Correlations with clinical presentation and sites of disease. Am J Surg Pathol 1992;16:130–7.

94. Tötterman TH, Nilsson K, Sundström C. Phorbol ester-induced differentiation of chronic lymphocytic leukemia cells. Nature 1980;288:176–8.

95. Traweek ST, Sheibani K. Monocytoid B-cell lymphoma. The biologic and clinical implications of peripheral blood involvement. Am J Clin Pathol 1992;97:591–8.

96. Tsujimoto Y, Yunis J, Onorato-Showe L, Erikson J, Nowell PC, Croce CM. Molecular cloning of the chromosomal breakpoint of B-cell lymphomas and leukemias with the t(11;14) chromosome translocation. Science 1984;224:1403–6.

97. van Krieken JH, von Schilling C, Kluin PM, Lennert K. Splenic marginal zone lymphocytes and related cells in the lymph node: a morphologic and immunohistochemical study. Hum Pathol 1989;20:320–5.

98. Weisenburger DD, Duggan MJ, Perry DA, Sanger WG, Armitage JO. Non-Hodgkin's lymphomas of mantle zone origin. Pathol Annu 1991;1:139–58.

99. _____, Kim H, Rappaport H. Malignant lymphoma, intermediate lymphocytic type: a clinicopathologic study of 42 cases. Cancer 1981;48:1415–25.

100. _____, Kim H, Rappaport H. Mantle-zone lymphoma: a follicular variant of intermediate lymphocytic lymphoma. Cancer 1982;49:1429–38.

101. Williams J, Schned A, Cotelingam JD, Jaffe ES. Chronic lymphocytic leukemia with coexistent Hodgkin's disease. Implications for the origin of the Reed-Sternberg cell. Am J Surg Pathol 1991;15:33–42.

102. Withers DA, Harvey RC, Faust JB, Melnyk O, Carey K, Meeker TC. Characterization of a candidate bcl-1 gene. Mol Cell Biol 1991;11:4846–53.

103. Wood GS, Burke JS, Horning S, Doggett RS, Levy R, Warnke RA. The immunologic and clinicopathologic heterogeneity of cutaneous lymphomas other than mycosis fungoides. Blood 1983;62:464–72.

104. _____, Ngan BY, Tung R, et al. Clonal rearrangements of immunoglobulin genes and progression to B cell lymphoma in cutaneous lymphoid hyperplasia. Am J Pathol 1989;135:13–9.

105. Wotherspoon AC, Doglioni C, Diss TC, et al. Regression of primary low-grade B-cell gastric lymphoma of mucosa-associated lymphoid tissue type after eradication of Helicobacter pylori. Lancet 1993;342:575–7.

106. _____, Finn T, Isaacson PG. Numerical abnormalities of chromosomes 3 and 7 in lymphomas of mucosa associated lymphoid tissue and the splenic marginal zone [Abstract]. Lab Invest 1994;7:124A.

107. _____, Pan LX, Diss TC, Isaacson PG. A genotypic study of low grade B-cell lymphomas, including lymphomas of mucosa associated lymphoid tissue (MALT). J Pathol 1990;162:135–40.

108. Yunis JJ. Clinical significance of high resolution chromosomes in the study of acute leukemias and non-Hodgkin's lymphomas. In: Fairbanks VF, ed. Current hematology, Vol. 3. New York: Wiley, 1984.

109. Zukerberg L, Medeiros L, Ferry J, Harris N. Diffuse low-grade B-cell lymphomas: four clinically distinct subtypes defined by a combination of morphologic and immunophenotypic features. Am J Clin Pathol 1993;100:373–85.

8

MALIGNANT LYMPHOMA, DIFFUSE, MIXED SMALL AND LARGE CELL

Definition. Malignant lymphoma, diffuse, mixed small and large cell, often called diffuse mixed cell lymphoma, is a non-Hodgkin's lymphoma characterized by diffuse growth and an intimate admixture of small and large lymphoid cells. It corresponds to the diffuse mixed lymphocytic-histiocytic lymphoma category in the Rappaport classification. The small lymphoid cell component is not required by definition to be neoplastic, and may in fact be entirely or predominantly reactive.

Diffuse mixed cell lymphoma is not a single biologic entity, but is the morphologic manifestation of a number of different lymphoma types (Table 8-1). Although it is convenient to make such a diagnosis on morphologic grounds alone, it is important, as far as possible, to subclassify the lymphoma with the aid of immunophenotypic or genotypic studies, because the subtypes appear to be associated with different prognoses.

Subtypes. Diffuse mixed cell lymphoma is a heterogeneous category that includes the following subtypes (Table 8-1):

1) *Diffuse mixed cell lymphoma of follicular center cell (FCC) type* corresponds to diffuse centroblastic-centrocytic lymphoma in the Kiel classification (fig. 8-1). This entity is rare in its pure form (33), and has been overdiagnosed in the past. In a reassessment of cases diagnosed as "diffuse centroblastic-centrocytic lymphoma," the European Lymphoma Club reinterpreted 80 percent as lymphoplasmacytic/lymphocytoid, centrocytic (mantle cell), and centrocytoid centroblastic (large cleaved cell) lymphomas (20). In a similar reappraisal, Stansfeld (29) found that several cases were clearly centrocytic (mantle cell) lymphomas containing occasional blast-type cells; some were from patients in whom previous biopsies had shown an obvious follicular lymphoma,

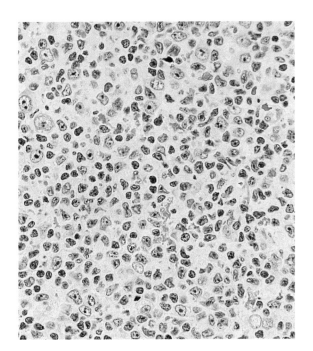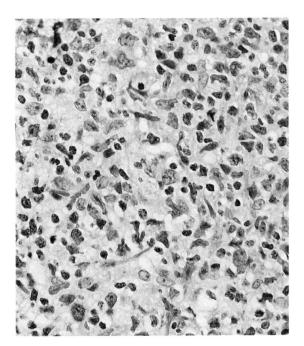

Figure 8-1
DIFFUSE MIXED CELL LYMPHOMA OF FOLLICULAR CENTER CELL TYPE
(DIFFUSE CENTROBLASTIC-CENTROCYTIC LYMPHOMA)

This type of lymphoma is characterized by an admixture of small lymphoid cells with angulated or cleaved nuclei and large lymphoid cells with distinct nucleoli. The small lymphoid cells in the right figure have more elongated and folded nuclei compared with those in the left figure.

Table 8-1

SUMMARY OF VARIOUS TYPES OF DIFFUSE MIXED CELL LYMPHOMA

Type	Lineage	Clinical Features	Histologic Features	Immunohisto-chemical Features	Behavior
Follicular center cell type (diffuse centroblastic-centrocytic) (4,6,9,14,18-20,25,33)	B	Adults, usually presenting with lymphadenopathy; may have a known history of follicular lymphoma or arising de novo; disease often at high stage at presentation; extranodal involvement is common	Small cells with angulated (cleaved) or elongated nuclei, fairly condensed chromatin, and scanty cytoplasm; large cells with round or folded nuclei, vesicular chromatin, and multiple distinct nucleoli; neoplastic follicles should be absent; sclerosis common	Pan-B+; CD5-; CD10+/-; CD23+/-; may have irregular loose meshworks of follicular dendritic cells	No reliable data in the literature on its behavior; some studies suggest that it is a low-grade neoplasm, but the prognosis is less favorable than for follicular lymphoma;
Post-thymic T-cell lymphoma	T	Usually adults; nodal or extranodal presentation; disease often at high stage at presentation	Prominent high endothelial venules; continuous spectrum of small, medium-sized, and large lymphoid cells; nuclear irregularities; chromatin pattern often granular; clear cytoplasm commonly seen in some cells; may show a rich component of inflammatory cells (such as eosinophils, histiocytes, and epithelioid cells)	Pan-T+ (often with loss of one or more pan-T antigens); usually CD4+, sometimes CD8+, CD4+CD8+ or CD4-CD8-	Generally an aggressive neoplasm
Lymphoplas-macytic/cytoid immuno-cytoma with increased blasts (polymorphic subtype) (3,4,18-20,33)	B	Usually older adults; nodal or extranodal presentation; may have monoclonal gammopathy (20-40 percent); disease often disseminated at presentation; occasional cases may have circulating lymphoma cells	Small lymphocytes; lymphoplasmacytoid cells; plasma cells; immunoblasts; rare follicular center cells; Dutcher bodies (nuclear pseudoinclusions of immunoglobulin) may be found; specific lymphoma types should be excluded (e.g. follicular lymphoma, low-grade B-cell lymphoma of MALT)	Pan B+; CD5-; CD10-; CD23-; sIg+, cIg+ (usually IgM type)	Low-grade neoplasm, but the prognosis is worse than that of B-SLL/CLL or conventional LP immunocytoma; median survival 55 months; may rarely transform to a diffuse large cell lymphoma
T-cell–rich large B-cell lymphoma	B	Older adults, usually presenting with lymphadenopathy; disease often disseminated at presentation	Small lymphocytes with round or irregular nuclei; scattered atypical large cells with round to folded nuclei, distinct nucleoli, and amphophilic cytoplasm; may show rich vascularity and component of inflammatory cells	Large atypical cells: pan-B+; small cells: pan-T+	Aggressive neoplasm; prognosis probably similar to conventional diffuse large cell lymphoma
Low-grade B-cell lymphoma of mucosa-associated lymphoid tissue (MALT) (3,15,33)	B	Any age; tumor often localized to mucosal site and/or regional lymph nodes at presentation	Small lymphoid cells with round or irregular nuclei and pale to clear cytoplasm; scattered large blast cells with vesicular nuclei and distinct nucleoli; glandular invasion (lymphoepithelial lesions) common; plasma cells common	Pan-B+; CD5-; CD10-; CD23-	Low-grade neoplasm, with median survival of 8 years; may show late relapse locally or in other mucosal sites; may transform to a diffuse large cell lymphoma

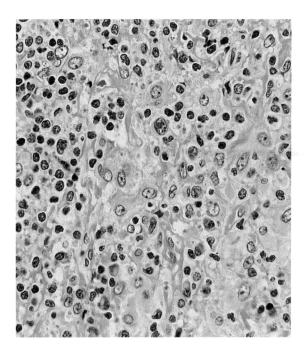

Figure 8-2
LYMPHOEPITHELIOID LYMPHOMA OF T LINEAGE (LENNERT'S LYMPHOMA)
Left: Numerous epithelioid histiocytes characteristically occur in coalescing small clusters without formation of discrete granulomas.
Right: Mildly atypical small and large lymphoid cells are present between the epithelioid histiocytes.

and most of the remainder had been misdiagnosed. Stansfeld concluded that diffuse centroblastic-centrocytic lymphoma unrelated to a follicle-forming tumor, in part or at some stage in the course of disease, is extremely rare.

2) *Post-thymic T-cell lymphoma showing a mixed cell composition* includes lymphoepithelioid (Lennert's) lymphoma (fig. 8-2), angioimmunoblastic lymphadenopathy (AILD)-like T-cell lymphoma (fig. 8-3), some pleomorphic T-cell lymphomas (fig. 8-4), and some angiocentric T-cell lymphomas (fig. 8-5) (see chapter 13).

3) *Lymphoplasmacytic/lymphoplasmacytoid immunocytoma of polymorphic subtype* in the original Kiel classification (fig. 8-6) and *lymphoplasmacytic immunocytoma with increased blasts* in the updated Kiel classification (20). In the Lukes-Collins classification, at least some cases of the polymorphic subtype of immunocytoma are considered a form of B-cell immunoblastic lymphoma (27). In a recent study, Berger et al. (3) designated such cases as *large cell–rich immunocytoma*, and found this tumor to be more aggressive (shorter time to treatment

failure and shorter survival time) than other nonfollicular small B-cell lymphomas other than mantle cell lymphoma.

4) *T-cell–rich large B-cell lymphoma.* It is controversial whether to classify this type of lymphoma in the "diffuse mixed cell" or "diffuse large cell" category in the Working Formulation. We prefer the large cell category because biologically only the large cell component is neoplastic (fig. 8-7) (see chapter 9).

5) Some examples of *low-grade B-cell lymphoma of mucosa-associated lymphoid tissue (MALT) with interspersed large cells* (fig. 8-8) (see chapter 7).

Some authors also include B-cell small lymphocytic lymphoma/chronic lymphocytic leukemia (B-SLL/CLL) with a moderate number of intermingled large cells (prolymphocytes and paraimmunoblasts) in the category of diffuse mixed cell lymphoma (12).

The reported percentage distribution of the above subtypes among diffuse mixed cell lymphoma is highly variable (Table 8-2), depending on the criteria of case selection (12,17,23,25,32).

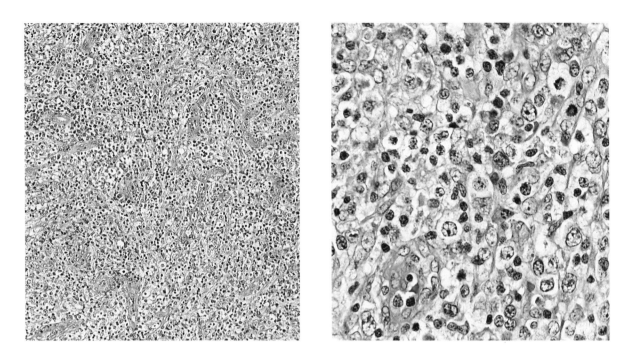

Figure 8-3
ANGIOIMMUNOBLASTIC LYMPHADENOPATHY–LIKE T-CELL LYMPHOMA

Left: Arborizing high endothelial venules are seen among the proliferated lymphoid cells.

Right: There is a mixture of small and large lymphoid cells. Many of the latter possess clear cytoplasm. There are intermingled plasma cells and eosinophils.

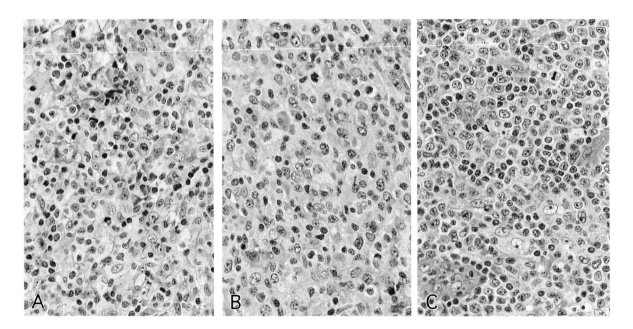

Figure 8-4
POST-THYMIC T-CELL LYMPHOMA OF LYMPH NODE

The examples depicted here show a continuous range of small, medium-sized, and large lymphoid cells. Some of the lymphoid cells have pale cytoplasm. The smaller cells, especially those seen in A, show irregular foldings of the nuclear membrane. The chromatin of the larger cells ranges from vesicular to granular.

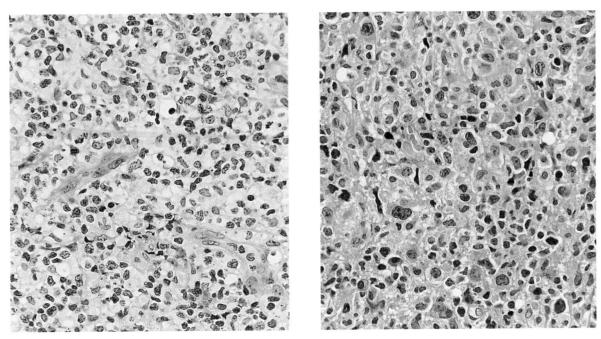

Figure 8-5
ANGIOCENTRIC T-CELL LYMPHOMA OF THE NASAL CAVITY WITH A MIXED CELL POPULATION
There is an intimate admixture of small and large lymphoid cells with irregularly folded nuclei. Many of the small cells have elongated angulated nuclei, simulating the small cleaved cells (centrocytes) seen in diffuse mixed cell lymphoma of follicular center cell type.

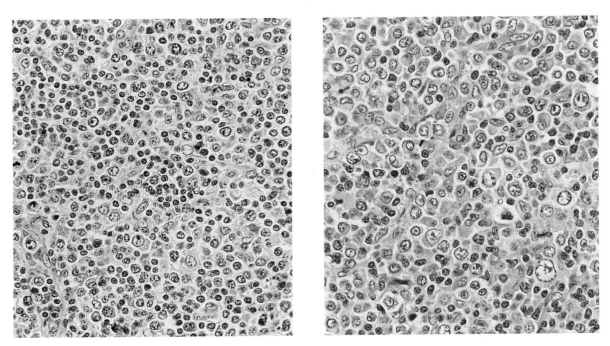

Figure 8-6
DIFFUSE MIXED CELL LYMPHOMA OF IMMUNOCYTOMA TYPE (POLYMORPHIC IMMUNOCYTOMA)
Left: There is a diffuse proliferation of small lymphocytes, lymphoplasmacytoid cells, plasma cells, and large lymphoid cells.
Right: The plasma cells appear immature and atypical.

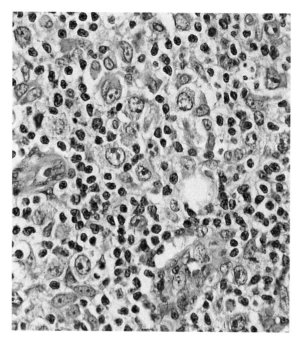

Figure 8-7
T-CELL–RICH LARGE B-CELL LYMPHOMA
Isolated, mildly atypical large lymphoid cells (shown to express monotypic immunoglobulin on immunostaining) are present in a background of small lymphocytes.

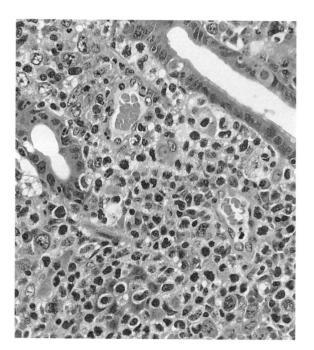

Figure 8-8
MUCOSA-ASSOCIATED LYMPHOID TISSUE LYMPHOMA OF THE STOMACH SHOWING A MIXED CELL POPULATION
There is a mixture of large nucleolated cells and small cells with irregular nuclei (centrocyte-like cells).

Table 8-2

SUMMARY OF STUDIES ATTEMPTING TO DELINEATE THE NATURE OF DIFFUSE MIXED CELL LYMPHOMA

Study	Technique	Entities	Significance or Conclusion
Nathwani et al. (62 cases) (25)	Morphologic	FCC type:16 (26%) Non-FCC, presumably T-lineage: 34 (55%) Unclassifiable: 4 (6%) Unresolved: 8 (13%)	FCC group better prognosis than non-FCC group; achievement of complete remission influences the survival of the non-FCC group but not the FCC group, suggesting that the former behaves like a high-grade lymphoma and the latter like a low-grade lymphoma
Foucar et al. (47 cases) (12)	Morphologic	FCC type: 20 (43%) Small lymphocytic or lymphoplasmacytoid lymphoma: 8 (17%) Immunoblastic-type, possibly including T-cell lymphomas: 12 (26%) Unclassified: 7 (15%)	Among the 3 groups, small lymphocytic or lymphoplasmacytoid lymphoma has best prognosis, and the "immunoblastic" group the worst
Winberg et al. (12 cases) (32)	Immunologic	B cell: 5 (42%) T cell: 7 (58%)	
Katzin et al. (13 cases) (17)	Immunologic and genotypic	All found to be of B-cell lineage	Most cases in this series correspond to T-cell–rich large B-cell lymphoma
Medeiros et al. (20 cases) (23)	Morphologic, immunologic, and genotypic	B-cell: 10 (50%) T-cell: 6 (30%) Uncertain: 4 (20%)	7 cases show *bcl*-2 gene rearrangement, suggesting FCC origin; prediction of lineage from morphology is very inaccurate

FCC = Follicular center cell.

 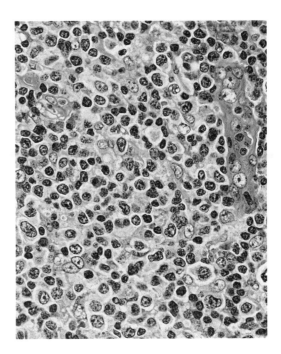

Figure 8-9
POST-THYMIC T-CELL LYMPHOMA OF T-ZONE TYPE
Left: The lymphoid infiltrate (pale staining) occurs predominantly between reactive lymphoid follicles.
Right: Most of the proliferated lymphoid cells possess round nuclei with a continuous range of sizes. A proportion of the lymphoid cells have clear cytoplasm.

Incidence, Natural History, and Clinical Features. Diffuse mixed cell lymphoma comprises 2 to 7 percent of all non-Hodgkin's lymphomas in Caucasians (12,25,31) and 11 to 33 percent in Asians and Hispanics (13,21,26,30). There are no distinctive clinical features, as expected from the heterogeneity of this entity. It occurs mostly in adults, with a median age of 58 years. There is no sex predilection (31). The presentation can be nodal or extranodal and 55 percent of patients have stage III or IV disease at presentation (31). The frequency of bone marrow involvement is 14 percent (28). Diffuse mixed cell lymphomas are aggressive, and usually treated as such (7,22,32). The complete remission rate is 69 percent (28). The median survival is 2.7 years, with a 5-year survival of 38 percent according to the National Cancer Institute–sponsored study (31). These figures are similar to those for diffuse large cell lymphoma (10,11,28,31). However, there are subtypes within this category that are more closely related to low-grade lymphomas, hence the importance of further delineation of the specific subtypes (Table 8-1).

Microscopic Findings. Tissues involved by diffuse mixed cell lymphoma show a diffuse infiltrate of small and large lymphoid cells which are intimately intermingled. The growth occasionally occurs between reactive lymphoid follicles (interfollicular or T-zone pattern) (fig. 8-9).

The proportion of large and small cells required for diagnosis has not been clearly defined (5), and there can be medium-sized cells that are difficult to categorize. Furthermore, it is difficult to distinguish, on morphologic grounds, whether the lymphoid cells (particularly the small ones) are neoplastic or reactive. Arbitrarily, when the small and large lymphoid cells are well mixed, the large cells do not outnumber the small cells, and the large cells do not form cohesive clusters, a morphologic diagnosis of diffuse mixed cell lymphoma is justified.

The cytologic features of the lymphoid cells differ from case to case (Table 8-1; figs. 8-1–8-9). Although small to medium-sized cells with elongated angulated nuclei are characteristic of FCC (centroblastic-centrocytic) lymphoma (fig. 8-1), similar cells can also be observed in some post-thymic T-cell lymphomas (fig. 8-5).

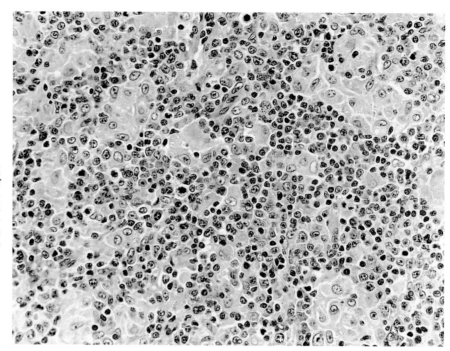

Figure 8-10
DIFFUSE MIXED CELL
LYMPHOMA OF
IMMUNOCYTOMA TYPE
(POLYMORPHIC
IMMUNOCYTOMA)

This example is associated
with a prominent component of
epithelioid histiocytes. Between the histiocytes, small
lymphocytes, lymphoplasmacytoid cells, and plasma cells
are intermingled with large
lymphoid cells.

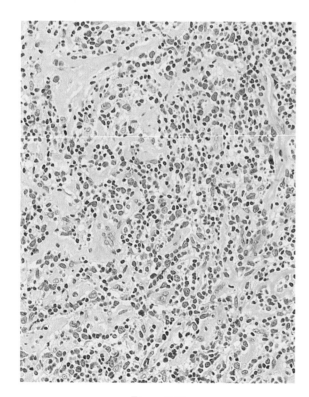

Figure 8-11
DIFFUSE MIXED CELL LYMPHOMA OF
FOLLICULAR CENTER CELL TYPE
(DIFFUSE CENTROBLASTIC-
CENTROCYTIC LYMPHOMA)

Sclerosis is common in this type of lymphoma.

There can be variable numbers of reactive cells, such as small lymphocytes, plasma cells, histiocytes, and eosinophils, intermingled with the neoplastic cells (figs. 8-3, 8-9). Coalescent small aggregates of epithelioid histiocytes are sometimes interspersed (so-called Lennert's lymphoma pattern), particularly in post-thymic T-cell lymphoma and lymphoplasmacytoid (LP) immunocytoma (fig. 8-10). Sclerosis may be present, and is often prominent in FCC lymphoma (fig. 8-11).

Immunohistologic Findings. Since prediction of lineage from histology is often inaccurate (16,23), immunohistochemical studies should always be performed to determine the lineage of diffuse mixed cell lymphoma, which encompasses several lymphoma types with different prognoses. Some cases stain for B-cell markers and some for T-cell markers, as expected from the heterogeneity of the category (Tables 8-1, 8-2) (32). Immunohistochemical staining should be interpreted cautiously: in the B-cell lymphomas, the neoplastic B-cells may be masked by large numbers of reactive T lymphocytes, giving a false impression of T-cell lymphoma. In such situations, the superior cytomorphologic correlation afforded by immunohistochemical studies on paraffin sections makes identification of markers expressed by the atypical cells easier.

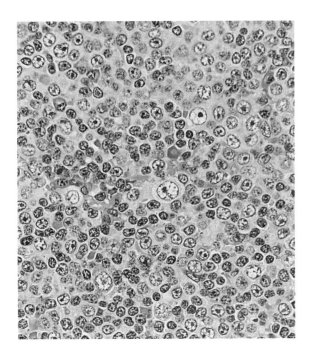 

Figure 8-12
B-CELL CHRONIC LYMPHOCYTIC LEUKEMIA INVOLVING LYMPH NODE
Left: Mixture of small lymphocytes and larger cells with central nucleoli (prolymphocytes and paraimmunoblasts). Note the round contour of the nuclei.
Right: The best clues to the diagnosis are the pale-staining proliferation centers.

The results of immunostaining may be equivocal or difficult to interpret in some cases, necessitating genotypic analysis to define the lineage (23).

Genotypic Findings. In one study, genotypic analysis confirmed that diffuse mixed cell lymphoma includes both T-lineage and B-lineage neoplasms, as demonstrated by rearrangements of the T-cell receptor and immunoglobulin genes, respectively (23). However, another study showed all cases to be of B lineage (Table 8-2) (17). The discrepancy can be explained by differences in the criteria of case selection. The demonstration of *bcl*-2 gene rearrangement in some cases suggests a relationship with follicular lymphoma in at least a proportion of cases.

Differential Diagnosis. *B-Cell Small Lymphocytic Lymphoma/Chronic Lymphocytic Leukemia (B-SLL/CLL).* Diffuse mixed cell lymphoma can be confused with B-SLL/CLL with a significant number of prolymphocytes and paraimmunoblasts, particularly when proliferation centers are inconspicuous and these larger cells are intimately intermingled with the small lymphocytes (fig. 8-12, left). It is important to

recognize B-SLL/CLL because it is a low-grade lymphoid neoplasm, with a reported median survival of 68 to 118 months (2,3), although cases showing an increased number of prolymphocytes and paraimmunoblasts have a slightly less favorable prognosis than those lacking this feature (2,8,18–20). B-SLL/CLL is recognized by the cytology of the small cells (small dark round nuclei, although slight irregularities in nuclear contour can sometimes occur), the centrally placed nucleoli and weak pyroninophilia of the large cells, and very importantly, the presence of proliferation centers (fig. 8-12, right). Distinction from the immunocytoma subtype of diffuse mixed cell lymphoma is by the absence of plasma cell differentiation, lack of Dutcher bodies, and by the cytology of the large cells (prolymphocytes and paraimmunoblasts) which are not as pyroninophilic as immunoblasts.

Rare cases of B-SLL/CLL with Reed-Sternberg–like cells may mimic T-cell–rich large B-cell lymphoma (24), but can be readily distinguished because the background small lymphocytes are monotypic B cells rather than T cells.

Diffuse Large Cell Lymphoma and Diffuse Small Cleaved Cell Lymphoma. The dividing lines between diffuse small cleaved cell (usually mantle cell lymphoma and low-grade B-cell lymphoma of MALT), diffuse mixed cell, and diffuse large cell lymphomas are not clear. The frequent presence of reactive small lymphoid cells, and occasional abundance of neoplastic medium-sized lymphoid cells, make it difficult to assess the actual percentages of neoplastic large cells and neoplastic small cells. We categorize a lymphoma as large cell type if either of the following features is present: large cells of more than 50 percent or tight clusters of large cells.

Diffuse mixed cell lymphoma is diagnosed instead of diffuse small cleaved cell lymphoma if more than a few large lymphoid cells are present in most high-magnification fields. Reactive histiocytes and follicular dendritic cells should not be counted as large cells.

Mantle Cell Lymphoma. Some cases of mantle cell lymphoma (pleomorphic or anaplastic type) may have interspersed larger cells among the small cells, giving an impression of diffuse mixed cell lymphoma. However, the large cells have a nuclear morphology similar to that of the small cells and scanty pale cytoplasm, features not seen in the large cells of diffuse mixed cell lymphoma (fig. 8-13), which often appear different from the surrounding small cells. Mantle cell lymphoma is often CD5+, CD10-, CD23- by immunophenotypic analysis (1).

Hodgkin's Disease. A mixed cellular population is a characteristic feature of Hodgkin's disease. However, Hodgkin's disease can be distinguished from diffuse mixed cell lymphoma by: large cells that often stand out in striking contrast to the nonactivated small cells in the background because of their large size and lack of transition with the background cells; large inclusion-like nucleolus in the large cells; the frequent presence of mixed inflammatory cells such as histiocytes, eosinophils, and plasma cells in the background; and the immunophenotype of the large cells (usually CD45-, CD15+, CD30+, in the absence of T- or B-lineage–specific markers).

Reactive Lymphoid Hyperplasia. Various types of lymphoid hyperplasia (including infectious mononucleosis) exhibiting a mixture of small and large lymphoid cells may mimic diffuse mixed cell lymphoma. The former diagnosis is

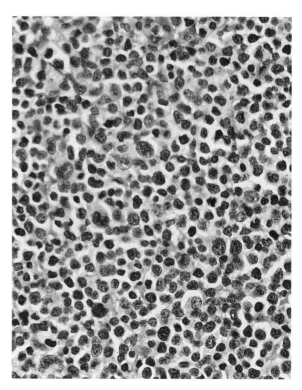

Figure 8-13
MANTLE CELL LYMPHOMA
WITH A MIXED CELL POPULATION
Interspersed among the irregular small lymphoid cells are larger cells with similar granular chromatin. These large cells do not have the vesicular nuclei and definite cytoplasmic rim characteristic of large noncleaved cells (centroblasts) in follicular center cell lymphoma.

favored when there is full or partial preservation of architecture (such as patent sinuses and reactive lymphoid follicles); lack of atypia in the lymphoid cells (the large cells have the appearance of reactive immunoblasts, although there may be binucleate forms mimicking Reed-Sternberg cells); and when the patient is young (figs. 8-14, 8-15). Lymphoma should be suspected if the architecture is totally effaced; the reactive follicles show destruction by the lymphoid proliferation; there are clear cells, lymphoid cells span a continuous range of cell sizes; or appreciable numbers of lymphoid cells show significant atypia (such as irregular nuclear foldings and coarse chromatin). In difficult cases, immunohistochemical studies (to look for light chain restriction in a B-cell proliferation and an aberrant phenotype in a T-cell proliferation) and genotypic studies are helpful.

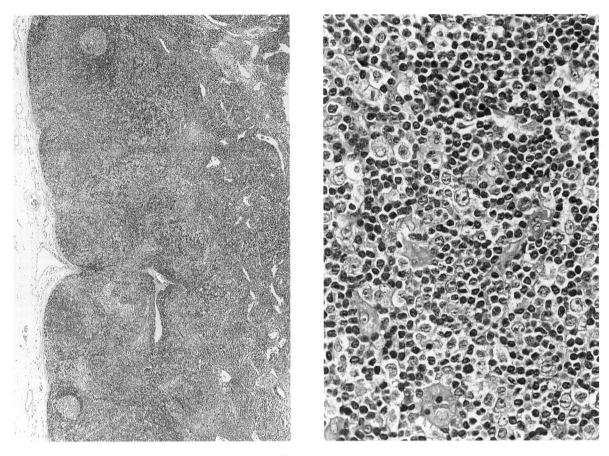

Figure 8-14
NONSPECIFIC PARACORTICAL HYPERPLASIA
Left: Low magnification showing the expanded paracortex; however, the architecture is preserved, with intact follicles and sinuses.
Right: In the paracortex, normal-looking immunoblasts are found among small lymphocytes.

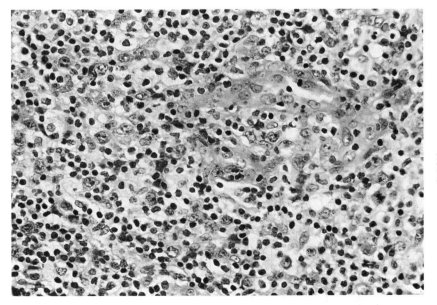

Figure 8-15
INFECTIOUS
MONONUCLEOSIS
INVOLVING LYMPH NODE
In this example, normal-looking immunoblasts occur among small lymphocytes. However, some degree of atypia can be seen in other cases.

REFERENCES

1. Banks PM, Chan J, Cleary ML, et al. Mantle cell lymphoma, a proposal for unification of morphologic, immunologic and molecular data. Am J Surg Pathol 1992;16:637–40.

2. Ben-Ezra J, Burke JS, Swartz WG, et al. Small lymphocytic lymphoma: a clinicopathologic analysis of 268 cases. Blood 1989;73:579–87.

3. Berger F, Felman P, Sonet A, et al. Nonfollicular small B-cell lymphomas: a heterogeneous group of patients with distinct clinical features and outcome. Blood 1994;83:2829–35.

4. Brittinger G, Bartels H, Common H, et al. Clinical and prognostic relevance of the Kiel classification of non-Hodgkin's lymphomas, results of a prospective multicenter study by the Kiel Lymphoma Study Group. Hematol Oncol 1984;2:269–306.

5. Burke JS. The histopathologic classification of non-Hodgkin's lymphomas: ambiguities in the Working Formulation and two newly reported categories. Semin Oncol 1990;17:3–10.

6. Colby TV, Hoppe RT, Burke JS. Nodular lymphoma, clinicopathologic correlations of parafollicular small lymphocytes and degree of nodularity. Cancer 1980;45:2364–7.

7. Cossman J, Jaffe ES, Fisher RI. Immunologic phenotype of diffuse, aggressive, non-Hodgkin's lymphomas. Correlation with clinical features. Cancer 1984;54:1310–7.

8. Dick FR, Maca RD. The lymph node in chronic lymphocytic leukemia. Cancer 1978;41:283–92.

9. Ezdinli EZ, Costello WG, Kucuk O, Berard CW. Effect of the degree of nodularity on the survival of patients with nodular lymphoma. J Clin Oncol 1987;5:413–8.

10. Fisher RI, Gaynor ER, Dahlberg S, et al. Comparison of a standard regimen (CHOP) with three intensive chemotherapy regimens for advanced non-Hodgkin's lymphoma. N Engl J Med 1993;328:1002–6.

11. _____, Hubbard SM, DeVita VT Jr, et al. Factors predicting long-term survival in diffuse mixed, histiocytic, or undifferentiated lymphoma. Blood 1981;58:45–51.

12. Foucar K, Armitage JO, Dick FR. Malignant lymphoma, diffuse mixed small and large cell. A clinicopathologic study of 47 cases. Cancer 1983;51:2090–9.

13. Harrington DS, Ye Y, Weisenburger DD, et al. Malignant lymphoma in Nebraska and Guangzhou, China: a comparative study. Hum Pathol 1987;18:924–8.

14. Hu E, Weiss LM, Hoppe RT, Horning SJ. Follicular and diffuse mixed small-cleaved and large-cell lymphoma — a clinicopathologic study. J Clin Oncol 1985;3:1183–7.

15. Isaacson PG. Gastrointestinal lymphomas and lymphoid hyperplasias. In: Knowles DM, ed. Neoplastic hematopathology. Baltimore: Williams & Wilkins, 1992:953–78.

16. Jaffe ES, Strauchen JA, Berard CW. Predictability of immunologic phenotype by morphologic criteria in diffuse aggressive non-Hodgkin's lymphomas. Am J Clin Pathol 1982;77:46–9.

17. Katzin WE, Linden MD, Fishleder AJ, Tubbs RR. Immunophenotypic and genotypic characterization of diffuse mixed non-Hodgkin's lymphomas. Am J Pathol 1989;135:615–21.

18. Lennert K. Malignant lymphomas other than Hodgkin's disease: histology, cytology, ultrastructure, immunology. Berlin: Springer-Verlag, 1978;209–63.

19. _____. Histopathology of non-Hodgkin's lymphomas (based on the Kiel classification). Berlin: Springer-Verlag, 1981;45–53.

20. _____, Feller AC. Histopathology of non-Hodgkin's lymphomas (based on the Updated Kiel Classification). 2nd ed. Berlin: Springer-Verlag, 1992:64-76,80–93.

22. Linch DC. Management of histologically aggressive non-Hodgkin's lymphomas. Br J Hematol 1994; 86:691–4.

21. Magrath I. The non-Hodgkin's lymphomas: an introduction. In: Magrath I, ed. The non-Hodgkin's lymphomas. Baltimore: Williams & Wilkins, 1990:1–14.

23. Medeiros LJ, Lardelli P, Stetler-Stevenson M, Longo DL, Jaffe ES. Genotypic analysis of diffuse mixed cell lymphomas. Comparison with morphologic and immunophenotypic findings. Am J Clin Pathol 1991;95:547–55.

24. Momose H, Jaffe ES, Shin SS, Chen YY, Weiss LM. Chronic lymphocytic leukemia/small lymphocytic lymphoma with Reed-Sternberg-like cells and possible transformation to Hodgkin's disease: mediation by Epstein-Barr virus. Am J Surg Pathol 1992;16:859–67.

25. Nathwani BN, Metter GE, Gams RA, et al. Malignant lymphoma, mixed cell type, diffuse. Blood 1983; 62:200–8.

31. Non-Hodgkin's Lymphoma Pathologic Classification Project. National Cancer Institute sponsored study of classifications of non-Hodgkin's lymphomas, summary and description of a working formulation for clinical usage. Cancer 1982;49:2112–35.

26. Ng CS, Chan JK, Lo ST, Poon YF. Immunophenotypic analysis of non-Hodgkin's lymphomas in Chinese, a study of 75 cases in Hong Kong. Pathology 1986;18:419–25.

27. Schneider DR, Taylor CR, Parker JW, Cramer AC, Meyer PR, Lukes RJ. Immunoblastic sarcoma of T- and B-cell types: morphologic description and comparison. Hum Pathol 1985;16:885–900.

28. Simon R, Durrleman S, Hoppe RT, et al. The Non-Hodgkin's Lymphoma Pathologic Classification Project. Long-term follow up of 1153 patients with non-Hodgkin's lymphoma. Ann Intern Med 1988;109:939–45.

29. Stansfeld AG. Low-grade B-cell lymphomas. In: Stansfeld AG, d'Ardenne AJ (eds). Lymph node biopsy interpretation. 2nd ed. Edinburgh: Churchill Livingstone, 1992:229–83.

30. Su IJ, Shih LY, Kadin ME, Dun P, Hsu SM. Pathologic and immunologic characterization of malignant lymphoma in Taiwan, with special reference to retrovirus-associated adult T-cell lymphoma/leukemia. Am J Clin Pathol 1985;84:715–23.

32. Winberg CD, Sheibani K, Burke JS, Wu A, Rappaport H. T-cell-rich lymphoproliferative disorders, morphologic and immunologic differential diagnoses. Cancer 1988;62:1539–55.

33. Zukerberg LR, Medeiros LJ, Ferry JA, Harris NL. Diffuse low-grade B-cell lymphomas: four clinically distinct subtypes defined by a combination of morphologic and immunophenotypic features. Am J Clin Pathol 1993;100:373–85.

9

MALIGNANT LYMPHOMA, DIFFUSE, LARGE CELL AND VARIANTS

DIFFUSE LARGE CELL LYMPHOMA

Definition. Malignant lymphoma, diffuse, large cell type, often termed *diffuse large cell lymphoma* in brief, is characterized by a diffuse proliferation of large neoplastic lymphoid cells whose nuclear size exceeds that of normal histiocytes. The lymphoma can be of B-cell or T-cell lineage; rarely, the lineage cannot be defined despite extensive immunohistochemical and genotypic analysis. In the Rappaport classification, it is equivalent to diffuse histiocytic lymphoma; in the Working Formulation, it includes malignant lymphoma, diffuse, large cell (cleaved or noncleaved) and malignant lymphoma, large cell immunoblastic; in the updated Kiel classification, it includes centroblastic lymphoma (diffuse), immunoblastic lymphoma (B- or T-cell type), pleomorphic T-cell lymphoma, medium-sized and large cell, and large cell anaplastic lymphoma.

General Features. Diffuse large cell lymphoma comprises 20 to 30 percent of all non-Hodgkin's lymphomas (59,104,105). Although it encompasses one intermediate-grade and one high-grade category in the Working Formulation, recent studies have shown no differences in clinical behavior between these two categories (1,40, 76,103,133). Therefore, for management purposes, it may be sufficient to give a diagnostic label of "diffuse large cell lymphoma," with additional information on immunophenotype if available. In fact, because of lack of reproducible criteria to distinguish between diffuse large cell and large cell immunoblastic lymphoma, the recently proposed Revised European-American Lymphoma Classification (60) simply lumps the two under one single category of diffuse large B-cell lymphoma for the B-lineage tumors, while the T-lineage tumors are classified separately.

Most cases of diffuse large cell lymphoma arise de novo (primary type). The secondary type is associated with: low-grade non-Hodgkin's lymphomas/leukemias of B-cell or T-cell lineage (follicular lymphoma, B-cell chronic lymphocytic leukemia [Richter's syndrome], lymphoplasmacytoid lymphoma, low-grade B-cell lymphoma of mucosa-associated lymphoid tissue, monocytoid B-cell lymphoma, mycosis fungoides, lymphoepithelioid [Lennert's] lymphoma), and Hodgkin's disease (either classic or nodular lymphocyte predominance) (19,58,77,139,140,166). It is estimated that 20 to 30 percent of diffuse large B-cell lymphomas evolve from follicular lymphoma. Diffuse large B-cell lymphoma associated with follicular lymphoma can manifest in several ways: 1) the large cell lymphoma can develop subsequent to the diagnosis of follicular lymphoma, sometimes after repeated relapses of the latter; 2) the large cell lymphoma can be diagnosed at the same time as the follicular lymphoma in the form of "composite" lymphoma or occult follicular lymphoma being discovered during staging procedures for the large cell lymphoma; and 3) a large cell lymphoma can relapse as pure follicular lymphoma, presumably with the latter being unmasked following eradication of the former component by treatment (17,29, 62,88,144).

In this chapter, the features of diffuse large cell lymphoma and its morphologic variants are discussed. Since diffuse large cell lymphoma is a morphologic diagnosis that includes B-cell and T-cell neoplasms, the discussion in this chapter overlaps with that of chapter 13 (post-thymic T-cell lymphomas). In this chapter greater emphasis is placed on the B-cell neoplasms.

Clinical Features. Although diffuse large cell lymphoma can occur at any age, it is predominantly a disease of adults and the elderly. There is an equal sex incidence or a slight male predominance (14,105).

The neoplasm generally grows rapidly, and presents as mass lesions. The presentation can be in nodal or extranodal sites, with the latter accounting for approximately 40 percent of all cases (1,47). Rarely, patients present with bone marrow disease in the absence of palpable lymphadenopathy (9,162). Approximately 30 percent of patients have B symptoms (fever, night sweats, or weight loss) (133). A small proportion of patients have hypergammaglobulinemia, which can be monoclonal or polyclonal; the latter is associated with post-thymic T-cell lymphomas (14,79,144).

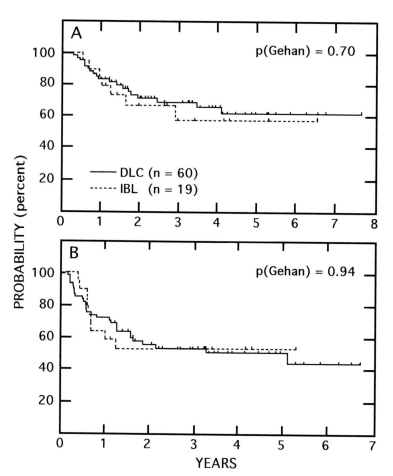

Figure 9-1
TYPICAL SURVIVAL CURVES OF
PATIENTS WITH DIFFUSE
LARGE CELL LYMPHOMA
Top: Actuarial survival of patients with
diffuse large cell (DLC) and immunoblastic
(IBL) subtypes.
Bottom: Actuarial freedom from progression of disease of patients with diffuse large cell
and immunoblastic subtypes. Data based on
patients treated at Stanford University Medical
Center, California. (Fig. 1 from Kwak LW, Wilson M, Weiss LM, Horning SJ, Warnke RA,
Dorfman RF. Clinical significance of morphologic subdivision in diffuse large cell lymphoma. Cancer 1991;68:1988–93.)

Occasionally, there is an underlying immunologic disorder such as systemic lupus erythematosus, Sjögren's syndrome, inherited immunodeficiency, acquired immunodeficiency, and iatrogenic immunosuppression (as in a transplant recipient). Epstein-Barr virus may play an etiologic role in a small fraction of cases, particularly those occurring in a setting of immunodeficiency (21,22,27,57,79,90,96,121,158).

Overall, the distribution of stage of disease at presentation is as follows: stage I, 18 percent; stage II, 30 percent; stage III, 12 percent; and stage IV, 40 percent (105,133). The frequency of bone marrow involvement is lower (10 to 30 percent) than in low-grade lymphomas (42,63, 105,133). Peripheral blood involvement is rare, and its occurrence usually presages a terminal phase of the disease.

The pattern of spread of diffuse large cell lymphoma is haphazard with respect to time and site. In general, dissemination occurs early in the course of disease. Although most patients die within 1 to 2 years if untreated, this tumor is potentially curable. Most patients achieving complete remission have a long disease-free survival, that is, cure, although some may relapse, usually within a few years (34). Patients who fail to achieve remission or have partial remission almost always die of the disease within a few years. This explains the characteristic biphasic survival curve of diffuse large cell lymphoma (fig. 9-1), with an initial steep downward slope (accounted for by early death of patients with partial or no remission) followed by a plateau (accounted for by patients achieving complete remission) (14,65).

Microscopic Findings. *Pattern of Involvement.* Irrespective of location, diffuse large cell lymphoma typically replaces the normal architecture with a diffuse, dense infiltrate of large lymphoid cells (fig. 9-2). However, the lymphoma occasionally exhibits a dispersed growth pattern in which the neoplastic cells are intimately intermingled

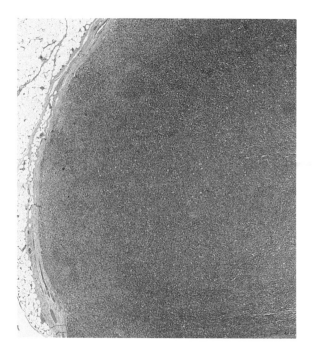

Figure 9-2
DIFFUSE LARGE CELL LYMPHOMA
INVOLVING LYMPH NODE
Note the diffuse growth and loss of the normal structures such as sinuses and lymphoid follicles.

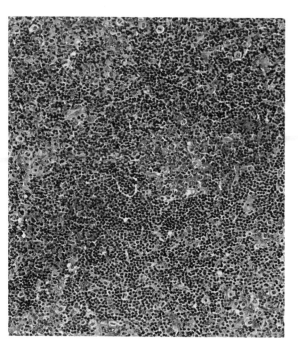

Figure 9-3
SUBTLE INVOLVEMENT OF LYMPH NODE
BY LARGE CELL LYMPHOMA
Isolated and small groups of large cells are dispersed among the normal lymphoid cells.

with the normal constituents of the tissues (fig. 9-3). In lymph nodes, infiltration of the perinodal tissues is common (fig. 9-4). At extranodal sites, there is usually permeative growth at the edges and frequent invasion of the blood vessel walls (fig. 9-5).

Nodal involvement can be complete, partial, sinusoidal, or interfollicular (figs. 9-2, 9-3). At times, the lymphoma may form discrete expansile nodules (fig. 9-6). These nodules differ from the follicles found in follicular lymphoma since they are focal, often large, and have a cytologic composition different from follicular center cells; follicular dendritic cell networks are not demonstrable. On rare occasions, a vague nodular (follicular) pattern may result from colonization of preexisting reactive follicles (fig. 9-7).

Subclassification. Diffuse large cell lymphoma can be of T-cell or B-cell lineage. Although the lineage can be suggested by certain histologic features (Table 9-1), prediction of lineage by morphologic criteria alone is highly unreliable (67, 97,103). Lineage can only be reliably determined by immunohistochemical or genotypic studies.

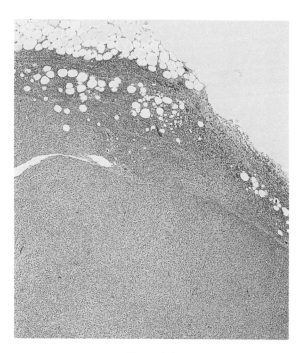

Figure 9-4
DIFFUSE LARGE CELL LYMPHOMA
INVOLVING LYMPH NODE
There is diffuse effacement of nodal architecture and prominent infiltration of the perinodal fat, which is a common feature.

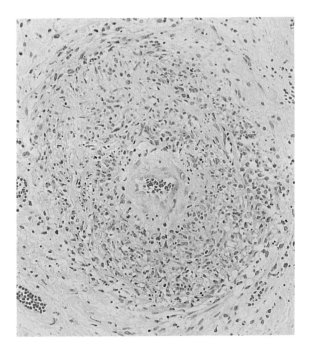

Figure 9-5
DIFFUSE LARGE B-CELL LYMPHOMA
INVOLVING SOFT TISSUES
In this example of large B-cell lymphoma, the blood vessel walls are extensively infiltrated by tumor cells. It should be noted that angiocentricity is not restricted to T-cell or natural killer cell lymphomas.

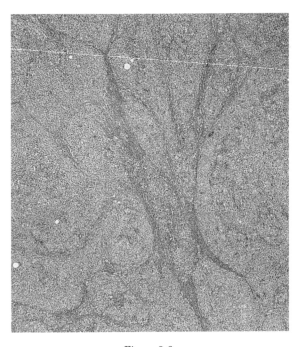

Figure 9-6
DIFFUSE LARGE B-CELL LYMPHOMA
INVOLVING LYMPH NODE
This case exhibits an unusual multinodular pattern.

Table 9-1

HISTOLOGIC FEATURES THAT MAY SUGGEST THE LINEAGE OF A DIFFUSE LARGE CELL LYMPHOMA*

B Cell	Basophilic (pyroninophilic) cytoplasm with pale Golgi zone
T Cell	Paracortical infiltrate with sparing of follicles
	Prominent high endothelial venules
	Continuous spectrum of lymphoid cell sizes
	Striking irregularities of nuclear contour
	Pale or clear cytoplasm
	Prominent inflammatory component, especially eosinophils
Histiocytic	Abundant eosinophilic cytoplasm

*From references 97,102,126,140. None of the features is entirely specific.

Subclassification of diffuse large cell lymphoma has been problematic because of lack of reproducible criteria. Although the large cell immunoblastic category of the Working Formulation (Table 9-2) is characterized by cells with large vesicular nuclei and prominent central nucleoli, many authors classify post-thymic T-cell lymphoma under this category ("polymorphous" subtype) despite the paucity of large cells and lack of cells with "immunoblastic" morphology (101,105).

According to the updated Kiel classification, the major categories of diffuse large cell lymphoma are centroblastic and immunoblastic lymphoma; the former is considered to be related to follicular center cells and the latter related to extrafollicular B lymphocytes. These have further been divided into several subtypes (Tables 9-3, 9-4) (66,77,139,141). The centrocytoid centroblastic lymphoma category is the most controversial: these lymphomas were formerly classified as large cell/anaplastic centrocytic (mantle cell) lymphomas, which appears to be more correct. The lymphoma cells are medium-sized rather than large (fig. 9-8). Recent immunohistochemical and genotypic data have confirmed that centrocytoid centroblastic lymphoma is biologically a mantle cell lymphoma (CD5+, *bcl*-1 gene rearrangement), albeit showing a relatively high proliferative fraction (112).

Table 9-2

SUBTYPES OF DIFFUSE LARGE CELL LYMPHOMA ACCORDING TO THE WORKING FORMULATION*

A. Diffuse, large cell: Large cleaved and/or large noncleaved cells; may have minor population of small cleaved cells.

    1. *Large cleaved cell type* — Cleaved nuclei; inconspicuous nucleoli; minimal cytoplasm. There should be less than 25 percent large noncleaved cells.

    2. *Large noncleaved cell type* —Oval vesicular nuclei; one or more distinct nucleoli, often apposed to the nuclear membrane; narrow rim of amphophilic or basophilic cytoplasm.

B. Large cell, immunoblastic: Large cells with round to oval vesicular nuclei and one or more prominent central nucleoli.

    1. *Plasmacytoid* —Eccentric nucleus; abundant amphophilic or basophilic cytoplasm.

    2. *Clear cell* —Central nucleus; abundant clear cytoplasm; chromatin often fine and evenly dispersed; nucleoli usually small and multiple.

    3. *Polymorphous* —Mixture of atypical small lymphoid cells (with twisted nuclei) and large clear cell immunoblasts. The latter may show pleomorphism, multinucleation, or hyperlobation.

    4. *Epithelioid cell component* —Polymorphous immunoblastic variant associated with prominent epithelioid cell component.

*From references 98,101,105.

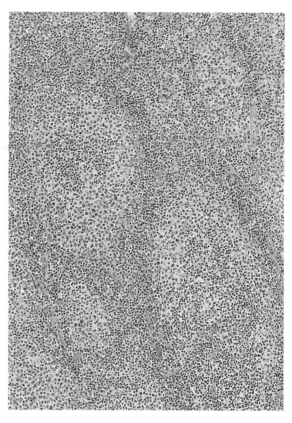

Figure 9-7
DIFFUSE LARGE B-CELL LYMPHOMA INVOLVING LYMPH NODE

This unusual example shows a vague nodular pattern, presumably due to colonization and replacement of the preexisting normal lymphoid follicles by lymphoma cells. Some residual follicular center cells can still be seen in some of these nodules.

Table 9-3

SUBTYPES OF CENTROBLASTIC LYMPHOMA ACCORDING TO THE UPDATED KIEL CLASSIFICATION*

I   **Monomorphic:** More than 60 percent typical centroblasts (medium-sized or large cells 10 to 14 μm, with fine chromatin, 2 to 4 small membrane-bound nucleoli, and scanty basophilic cytoplasm); less than 10 percent immunoblasts.

II   **Polymorphic:** More than 10 percent centroblasts (which can be typical, centrocytoid, or multilobated) are intermingled with more than 10 percent (10 to 90 percent) immunoblasts (large central nucleoli and abundant basophilic cytoplasm).

III   **Multilobated:** More than 10 to 20 percent large lymphoid cells with lobated nuclei (more than three lobes). The nuclei are often richer in chromatin than the typical centroblast, and nucleoli often appear less distinct. There can be admixed typical centroblasts and immunoblasts.

IV   **Centrocytoid:** Tumor cells show morphologic overlap between centrocyte and centroblast. The centrocytoid centroblasts are medium-sized cells (9 to 11 μm), with oval or elongated nuclei with an angulated outline; light-staining chromatin; multiple small nucleoli which are often located centrally; and scanty basophilic cytoplasm.

*From references 66,77,139,141.

Table 9-4

SUBTYPES OF IMMUNOBLASTIC LYMPHOMA ACCORDING TO THE UPDATED KIEL CLASSIFICATION*

A. Immunoblastic Lymphoma of B-Cell Type: Majority of cells are B immunoblasts, which can be mixed with plasma cells and lymphocytes. If present, centroblasts and centrocytes should comprise less than 10 percent of the tumor cell population.

   1. *B-immunoblastic lymphoma without plasmacytic differentiation:* Uniform population of large cells (12 to 15 μm) with round to oval nuclei, vesicular chromatin, a single centrally located nucleolus (occasionally multiple smaller, randomly located nucleoli), and an appreciable amount of basophilic cytoplasm. No plasmacytic differentiation.

   2. *B-immunoblastic lymphoma with plasmacytic differentiation:* The immunoblasts are usually smaller (10 to 13 μm), with round and eccentric nuclei, solitary or multiple central nucleoli, and intensely basophilic cytoplasm with a perinuclear pale Golgi zone. Admixed with plasma cells and plasmablasts.

   3. *B-immunoblastic lymphoma with a high content of lymphocytes:* Immunoblasts occur in groups or are dispersed in large numbers in a background of small lymphocytes and/or lymphoplasmacytoid cells. Many such cases appear to have arisen from chronic lymphocytic leukemia or lymphoplasmacytoid immunocytoma.

B. Immunoblastic Lymphoma of T-Cell Type: Fairly uniform large cells with round or oval nuclei, coarse chromatin, one large solitary nucleolus or several medium-sized nucleoli, and moderate amount of basophilic, amphophilic, or clear cytoplasm. By definition, the neoplastic cells express T-lineage markers.

* From references 66,77,139,141.

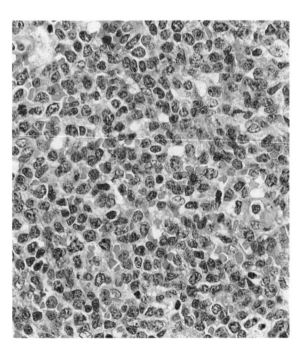

Figure 9-8
CENTROCYTOID CENTROBLASTIC
LYMPHOMA ACCORDING TO THE
UPDATED KIEL CLASSIFICATION
The lymph node is diffusely infiltrated by medium-sized cells with moderately irregular nuclei, fairly dense chromatin, and scant cytoplasm. Nucleoli are small. This lymphoma type is biologically a form of mantle cell lymphoma ("anaplastic" type). It is difficult to categorize this tumor in the Working Formulation.

Cytologic Appearances. The cytologic composition of diffuse large cell lymphoma is highly variable. The neoplastic cells are typically large, and the nuclei are larger than those of reactive histiocytes (figs. 9-9, 9-10). Occasionally, the nuclei are medium-sized (nuclear size comparable to that of a histiocyte), but they do not have the nuclear or cytoplasmic features of the common medium-sized cell lymphomas, such as lymphoblastic and small noncleaved cell lymphomas (fig. 9-11). The infiltrate can be monomorphous (fig. 9-9), or can exhibit considerable variation in the size of the tumor cells (fig. 9-12). Sometimes, neoplastic small cells with cleaved or irregular nuclei are admixed, but the large cells clearly predominate or form clusters.

The nuclei of the large lymphoma cells are round, oval, indented, elongated, cleaved, irregularly folded, or multilobated (77,105,139,143). The chromatin often shows clearing with condensation beneath the nuclear membrane, but it can be coarsely clumped or evenly dispersed. Nucleoli, which are multiple or solitary, are almost invariably conspicuous; they are centrally located, randomly distributed, or apposed to the nuclear membrane (figs. 9-9–9-18). There can be highly bizarre cells or multinucleated forms, some of which may mimic Reed-Sternberg cells (fig. 9-12, right). The cytoplasm varies in quantity, and can be clear, pale, eosinophilic, amphophilic, or basophilic (figs. 9-13, 9-19, 9-20).

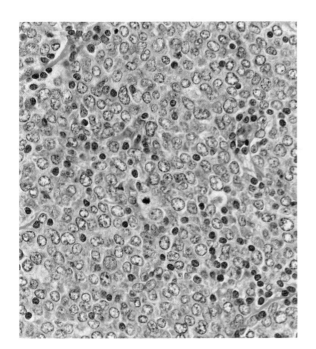 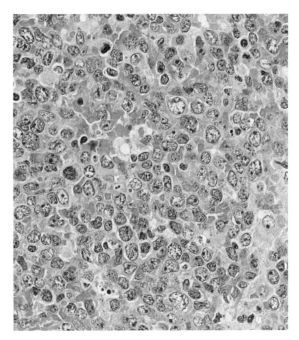

Figure 9-9
DIFFUSE LARGE B-CELL LYMPHOMA (CENTROBLASTIC LYMPHOMA, MONOMORPHIC SUBTYPE)
These two cases can be classified as large noncleaved cell lymphoma in the Working Formulation.
Left: The nuclei are mostly round, with vesicular chromatin and membrane-bound nucleoli.
Right: In this example, the chromatin is more dispersed. The nucleoli are mostly apposed to the nuclear membrane, as is characteristic of large noncleaved cells (centroblasts).

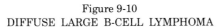

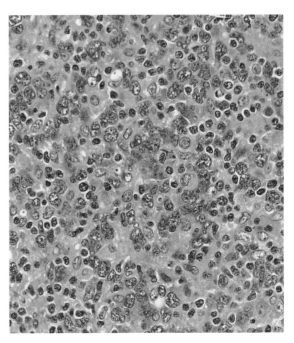

Figure 9-10
DIFFUSE LARGE B-CELL LYMPHOMA
Some of the large cells have membrane-bound nucleoli (large noncleaved cells or centroblasts), whereas others have central prominent nucleoli and a moderate amount of amphophilic cytoplasm (immunoblasts). It is difficult to categorize this case by the Working Formulation.

Figure 9-11
DIFFUSE LARGE B-CELL LYMPHOMA
In this example, the lymphoma cells are mostly of medium size, but do not look like the usual medium-sized cell lymphomas (lymphoblastic or Burkitt's). It is difficult to categorize this case either by the Working Formulation or updated Kiel classification.

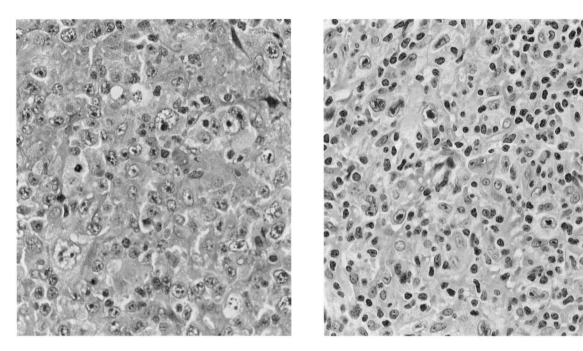

Figure 9-12
DIFFUSE LARGE B-CELL LYMPHOMA WITH PLEOMORPHIC CELLULAR COMPOSITION
There is significant variation in the sizes and shapes of the nuclei in these two cases. They can be classified as "large cell immunoblastic, polymorphous subtype" in the Working Formulation.

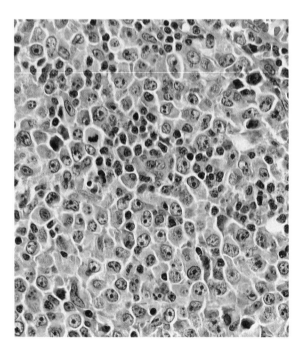

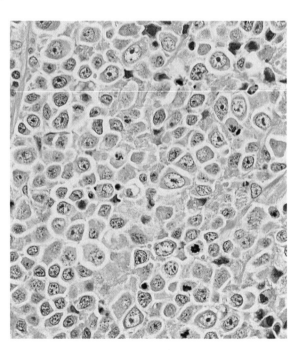

Figure 9-13
DIFFUSE LARGE B-CELL LYMPHOMA
(IMMUNOBLASTIC, PLASMACYTOID)

The lymphoma cells have large central nucleoli and plasmacytoid cytoplasm.

Figure 9-14
DIFFUSE LARGE B-CELL LYMPHOMA
(IMMUNOBLASTIC LYMPHOMA)

There is some variation in the size of the nuclei. Most nuclei have central nucleoli and the cells have an appreciable amount of amphophilic cytoplasm. Some nuclei have vesicular chromatin, whereas others have finely stippled chromatin.

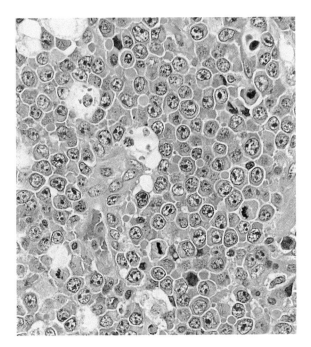

Figure 9-15
DIFFUSE LARGE B-CELL LYMPHOMA
(IMMUNOBLASTIC LYMPHOMA)
A monotonous population of large cells with central nucleoli and plasmacytoid cytoplasm is seen.

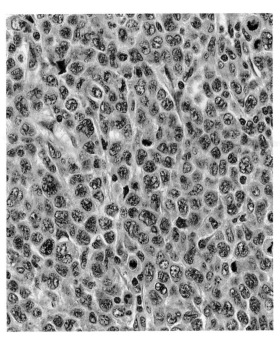

Figure 9-16
DIFFUSE LARGE CELL LYMPHOMA OF T LINEAGE
The nuclei show irregular folding and granular or coarse chromatin.

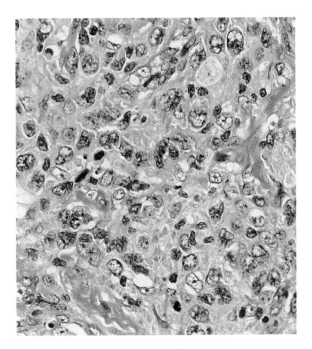

Figure 9-17
DIFFUSE LARGE B-CELL LYMPHOMA
The nuclei show variations in size and nuclear foldings.

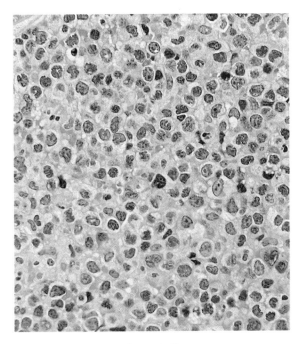

Figure 9-18
DIFFUSE LARGE CELL LYMPHOMA OF T LINEAGE
In this case, the nuclei exhibit a cerebriform configuration.

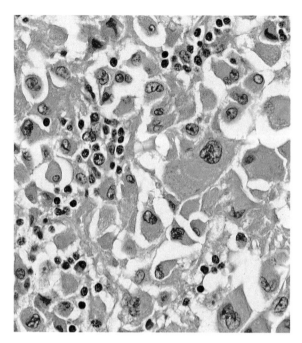

Figure 9-19
DIFFUSE LARGE B-CELL LYMPHOMA WITH
AN EPITHELIOID APPEARANCE

An unusual example of diffuse large B-cell lymphoma with abundant eosinophilic cytoplasm, resembling epithelioid histiocytes.

Mitotic figures, including atypical forms, are easily identified. Rarely, there is a component of neoplastic (monotypic) plasma cells expressing the same immunoglobulin light chain as the neoplastic large B cells (fig. 9-21).

Necrosis. Necrosis is common, taking the form of individual cell necrosis (apoptosis) or irregular foci of coagulative necrosis (fig. 9-22). Interspersed histiocytes containing phagocytosed nuclear debris can create a starry-sky pattern (fig. 9-23). Necrosis can be accompanied by the deposition of hematoxyphilic nuclear material on blood vessels (fig. 9-24). Sometimes total infarction of the lymph node, spontaneous or following fine needle aspiration, may mask the diagnosis of lymphoma (fig. 9-25); follow-up and further biopsies are therefore advisable for patients presenting with nodal infarction (24,89,145a).

Reactive Component. The lymphomatous infiltrate can be accompanied by a variable reactive component comprising small lymphocytes, plasma cells, eosinophils, and histiocytes (which may show hemophagocytosis, assume an epithelioid morphology, or form sarcoid-type granulomas) (figs. 9-26,

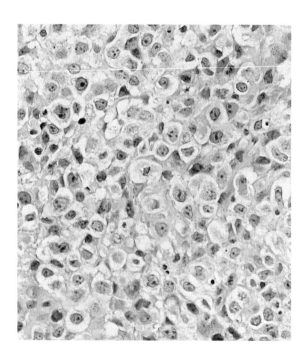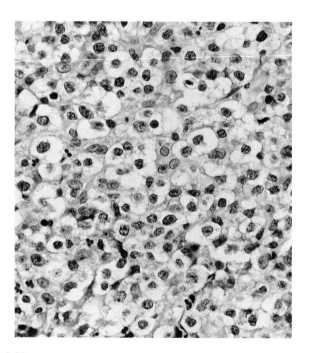

Figure 9-20
DIFFUSE LARGE CELL LYMPHOMA WITH CLEAR CELLS

Left: B-lineage large cell lymphoma with clear cytoplasm.
Right: T-lineage large cell lymphoma. The appearances are typical of those of so-called clear cell T immunoblasts, which have round nuclei, granular chromatin, multiple small nucleoli, and abundant clear cytoplasm. The nuclei are often medium-sized rather than large.

9-27). The reactive component is generally more prominent in T-cell than B-cell lymphomas.

Sclerosis. Sclerosis is a common finding. According to one study, it occurs in approximately half of the nodal cases (119). Several types of sclerosis have been described: 1) broad fibrous bands delineating the tumor into irregular or rounded large nodules; 2) compartmentalizing sclerosis dividing the tumor into small packets by narrow anastomosing bands of hyalinized stroma (fig. 9-28, left); and 3) diffuse sclerosis, characterized by delicate hyaline strands, frequently enveloping individual tumor cells (fig. 9-28, right). One study suggests that the compartmentalizing type of sclerosis is associated with a good prognosis, and the diffuse type a poor prognosis (119).

Low-Grade Component. In some cases, a component of low-grade lymphoma may be evident as a discrete component or intermingled with the large cell lymphoma. In large cell lymphoma arising from mycosis fungoides, the latter component may be evident as small lymphoid cells with cerebriform nuclei (fig. 9-29). A low-grade lymphoma of mucosa-associated lymphoid tissue type may be found on careful search in at

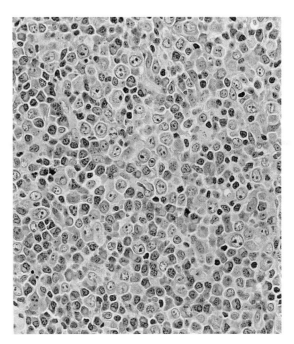

Figure 9-21
DIFFUSE LARGE B-CELL LYMPHOMA WITH PLASMA CELL DIFFERENTIATION
Admixed with the large lymphoma cells are plasma cells which are shown on immunohistochemical studies to express the same immunoglobulin light chain as the large cells.

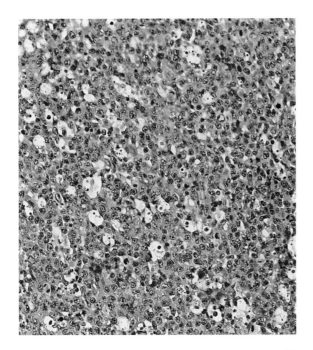

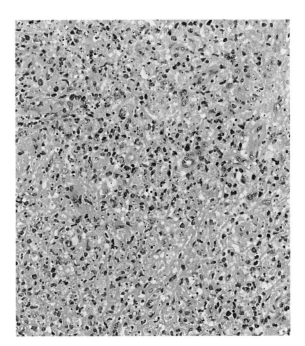

Figure 9-22
DIFFUSE LARGE B-CELL LYMPHOMA WITH PROMINENT KARYORRHEXIS
Left: Many apoptotic bodies are present in this large cell lymphoma.
Right: The presence of necrosis and abundant karyorrhectic debris may lead to an erroneous diagnosis of Kikuchi's lymphadenitis.

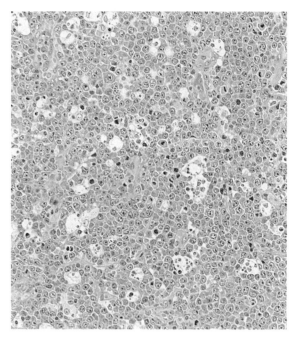

Figure 9-23
DIFFUSE LARGE CELL LYMPHOMA WITH
STARRY-SKY APPEARANCE
The starry-sky appearance is imparted by reactive histiocytes having phagocytosed nuclear debris.

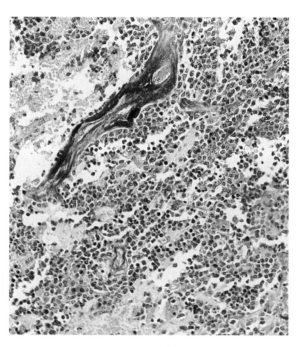

Figure 9-24
DIFFUSE LARGE CELL LYMPHOMA WITH
AZZOPARDI'S PHENOMENON
This lymphoma is highly necrotic. There is deposition of dark-staining nuclear material on the blood vessels, so-called Azzopardi's phenomenon.

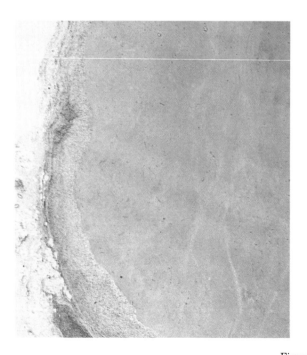

Figure 9-25
DIFFUSE LARGE CELL LYMPHOMA PRESENTING AS NODAL INFARCTION
Left: There is total coagulative necrosis.
Right: A rim of organizing tissue is seen in the upper field.

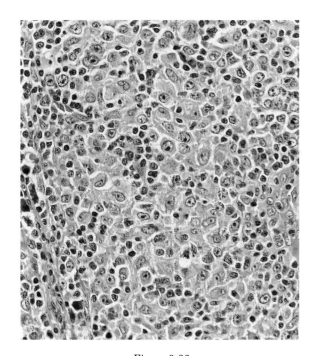

Figure 9-26
DIFFUSE LARGE CELL LYMPHOMA OF B LINEAGE
B-immunoblastic lymphoma with many intermingled small lymphocytes.

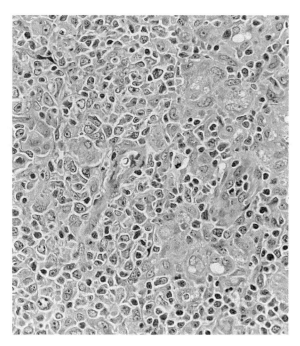

Figure 9-27
DIFFUSE LARGE CELL LYMPHOMA OF B LINEAGE
An example with many intermixed epithelioid histiocytes.

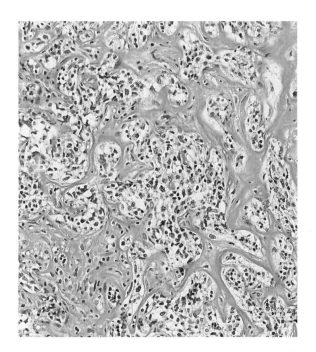

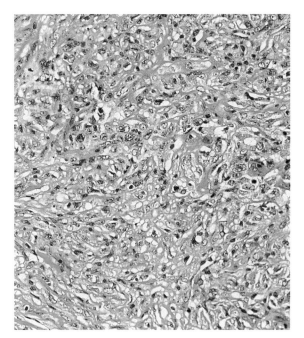

Figure 9-28
DIFFUSE LARGE CELL LYMPHOMA WITH SCLEROSIS
Left: The fibrous strands divide the tumor into packets (compartmentalization).
Right: Diffuse type of interstitial sclerosis.

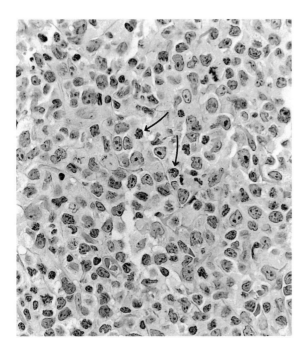

Figure 9-29
LARGE CELL LYMPHOMA (T LINEAGE)
ARISING FROM MYCOSIS FUNGOIDES
The large lymphoid cells possess nuclei with irregular foldings. Interspersed among them are small cells with cerebriform nuclei (arrows).

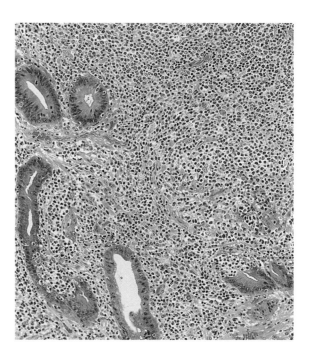

Figure 9-30
LARGE CELL LYMPHOMA (B LINEAGE)
ARISING FROM LOW-GRADE LYMPHOMA
OF MUCOSA-ASSOCIATED LYMPHOID TISSUE
In the lower field, the low-grade component is composed of centrocyte-like cells with invasion of the gastric glands. Large cells predominate in the upper field.

least some cases of mucosal large cell lymphoma (fig. 9-30) (19). Richter's syndrome can be recognized by the monotony of the small lymphocytes that occur in the background of the large cells (fig. 9-31) (58).

Spleen and Bone Marrow Involvement. The pattern of splenic involvement by diffuse large cell lymphoma is highly variable (see chapter 20). Bone marrow involvement can manifest as extensive diffuse infiltrates, haphazardly distributed tumor clusters, or isolated cells dispersed among the hemopoietic cells. The infiltrate is often accompanied by an increase in reticulin fibers. There can be morphologic discordance between the diagnostic biopsy and the bone marrow biopsy: 50 to 70 percent of cases with bone marrow involvement show a small cell lymphoma (often with features of follicular center cell lymphoma with paratrabecular distribution) instead in the bone marrow (29,72). The implication is that while involvement of bone marrow by large cell lymphoma (concordant marrow involvement) is an unfavorable prognostic factor, involvement of

marrow by small cleaved cell lymphoma has the same prognosis as those cases without marrow involvement (29,42,63,120). However, there is an increased risk of late relapse after complete remission in these cases, often in the form of low-grade lymphoma (17,120).

Immunologic Findings. Approximately 65 to 85 percent of diffuse large cell lymphomas are of B lineage and 15 to 35 percent are of T lineage (30,37,75,104,138,147). A few exhibit lineage markers of both, or fail to express lineage-specific markers ("null" cell). In the pediatric age group, the distribution of cellular lineage is as follows: T cell, 27 percent; B cell, 33 percent; null cell, 40 percent. There is a high frequency of CD30 expression (40 percent) (124).

This section will only cover B-lineage lymphomas; T-cell lymphomas are covered in chapter 13. Diffuse large B-cell lymphomas express various pan-B markers such as CD19, CD20, CD22, and CD79a, but there can be an "aberrant" lack of staining with one or more of these (114). Staining for surface or cytoplasmic immunoglobulin

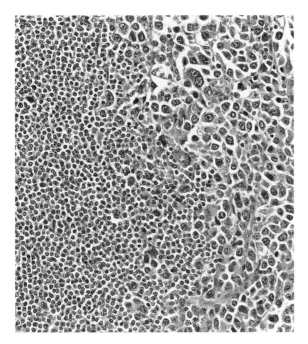

Figure 9-31
RICHTER'S SYNDROME

The large cell lymphoma (B lineage) is seen in the right field. Note the monotonous infiltrate of small lymphocytes in the left field, representing a preexisting B-cell chronic lymphocytic leukemic infiltration.

(usually IgM, sometimes IgG or other heavy chain types) can be demonstrated in 50 to 75 percent of cases; some are immunoglobulin negative (114,136,138). Cytoplasmic immunoglobulin is more commonly demonstrated in cases exhibiting plasmacytoid differentiation (141). The lymphomas are often HLA-DR positive, and show variable expression of activation and proliferative markers such as CD25 and CD30, as well as CD38 (T10), CD70, and CD71 (transferrin receptor) (134,141,157). Positive staining with anti-Leu-8 is common (92). A proportion of cases expresses CD5 (10 percent), CD9, CD10 (25 to 50 percent), CD21, or CD24 (13,77,114,134,156). Immunoreactive p53 protein can be detected in the lymphoma cells in some cases; since this occurs more frequently in large cell lymphomas than in low-grade lymphomas, p53 gene mutations may play a role in progression from the latter to the former (137). For cases related to follicular center cells, there may be small numbers of interspersed follicular dendritic cells (141). The proliferating fraction, as detected by Ki-67 staining, is usually high (greater than 40 percent).

When only paraffin-embedded tissues are available, the lineage of a diffuse large cell lymphoma can also be reliably determined by a panel of paraffin section–reactive antibodies such as CD20 (L26), CD79a (mb-1), CD3, CD43, and CD45RO (fig. 9-32) (see chapter 3).

Genotypic Findings. The genotypic findings are varied, as expected from the heterogeneity of the entity. Cases with a B-cell immunophenotype usually exhibit rearrangements of the immunoglobulin heavy and light chain genes, while the T-cell receptor genes are in a germline configuration (3,8,25,26,91,161). Rearrangements of the immunoglobulin gene may involve one or both alleles. T-cell lymphomas usually show rearrangements of the beta and gamma chain T-cell receptor genes, whereas the immunoglobulin genes are usually in the germline configuration (12,46,53,113,154). However, rarely, T-cell receptor gene rearrangement may be accompanied by rearrangements of the immunoglobulin heavy chain but not light chain genes. Sometimes no rearrangements of either the T-cell receptor or immunoglobulin genes are seen. Further details are covered in chapter 13.

Chromosomal translocation implicating the *bcl*-2 gene, i.e., t(14;18), a hallmark of follicular lymphoma, occurs in 20 to 30 percent of diffuse large B-cell lymphomas, suggesting a probable relationship with or evolution from follicular lymphoma (which may be occult) in these cases (2, 84,91,159). Patients with diffuse large cell lymphoma exhibiting *bcl*-2 rearrangement are approximately 11 years older than those lacking this feature (107,111). The *bcl*-2 gene is rarely rearranged in primary diffuse large cell lymphoma of the gastrointestinal tract or mucosal sites (less than 5 percent), suggesting no histogenetic relationship with follicular lymphoma for extranodal large cell lymphomas (118,152).

Ten to 12 percent of diffuse large cell lymphomas show reciprocal chromosomal translocation between the 3q27 region and various other chromosomal partners including, but not limited to, those carrying the immunoglobulin gene loci (14q32, 2p12, 22q11). The candidate proto-oncogene located at the breakpoint on 3q27, *bcl*-6 (also known as *LAZ3* or incorrectly as *bcl*-5), encodes an 89 kD zinc finger–type transcription factor normally expressed in mature B cells. Molecular analysis has shown that *bcl*-6 rearrangement

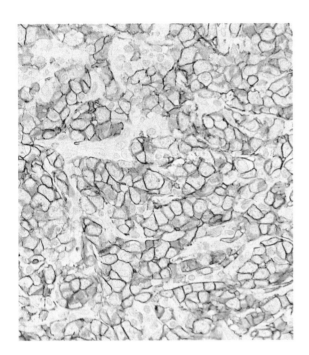 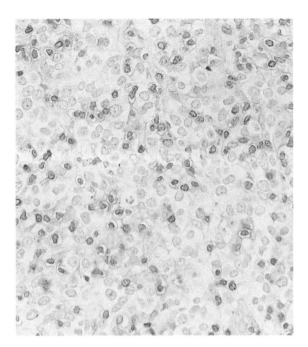

Figure 9-32
DIFFUSE LARGE B-CELL LYMPHOMA: IMMUNOHISTOCHEMICAL STUDIES
Left: In paraffin sections, the large cells show cell membrane immunoreactivity for CD20 (L26).
Right: Only isolated small lymphocytes are immunoreactive with CD3; the large cells are negative.

occurs in approximately one third of cases of diffuse large B-cell lymphoma, suggesting that there are instances of submicroscopic chromosomal alteration (10,11,31,70,71,87,93,108,110, 163,164). The breakpoints in *bcl*-6 usually occur in a 10-kb region around the first (untranslated) exon. *Bcl*-6 is rarely rearranged in other lymphoma types except for a small proportion (6 to 13 percent) of follicular lymphomas. The presence of *bcl*-6 rearrangement in diffuse large cell lymphoma is strongly correlated with extranodal involvement (110). *Bcl*-6 and *bcl*-2 rearrangements are practically mutually exclusive in diffuse large B-cell lymphomas, suggesting that *bcl*-6 rearrangement is an important mechanism underlying the de novo genesis of diffuse large B-cell lymphoma, especially at extranodal sites (31,71). A recent study indicates that 76 percent of all diffuse large B-cell lymphomas exhibit alterations (point mutation or small deletions) of the first exon of the *bcl*-6 gene, irrespective of whether the *bcl*-6 gene is rearranged, suggesting an even more important role of *bcl*-6 alterations in the genesis of this lymphoma type (92a).

Ten to 20 percent of diffuse large cell lymphomas show translocation of the oncogene c-*myc*, and a similar proportion show inactivation of the *Rb* gene (48,107). Presence of c-*myc* translocation does not have prognostic importance (110). A particularly high incidence of c-*myc* rearrangements (50 percent) has been reported in gastric large cell lymphoma, but the c-*myc* rearrangement does not comigrate with the immunoglobulin heavy chain gene rearrangement, suggesting lack of t(8;14) chromosomal translocation (151). Thus the molecular genetic findings suggest that mucosal large cell lymphoma may be histogenetically different from nodal large cell lymphoma (118,152).

Differential Diagnosis. *Carcinoma and Melanoma.* Diffuse large cell lymphoma can be mistaken for carcinoma or melanoma. The lymphoma can appear deceptively cohesive (forming a sharp interface with the residual lymphoid tissue or forming trabeculae) (fig. 9-33). Histologic features that are helpful in making the distinction are discussed in chapter 21. Should there be any doubt, immunohistochemical studies must be performed to clarify the diagnosis.

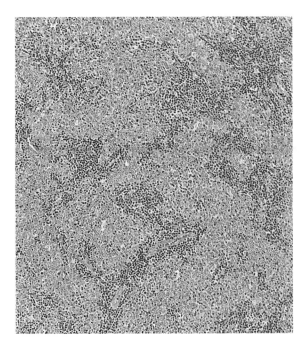

Figure 9-33
DIFFUSE LARGE B-CELL LYMPHOMA INVOLVING LYMPH NODE,
WITH CARCINOMA-LIKE GROWTH PATTERN
Left: This example shows a deceptively cohesive growth pattern.
Right: A trabecular growth pattern is seen in this case.

True Histiocytic Lymphoma. Diffuse large cell lymphoma of B- or T-cell lineage cannot be reliably distinguished from true histiocytic lymphoma without immunohistochemical or genotypic studies (see chapter 18), although the presence of an abundant eosinophilic cytoplasm may suggest the latter.

Hodgkin's Disease. Some cases of Hodgkin's disease (particularly the syncytial variant of nodular sclerosis type) can be difficult to distinguish from large cell lymphoma. This is especially true in the peripheral portion of a large cell lymphoma, where the large neoplastic cells are intermingled with the residual small lymphocytes (see fig. 9-12, right). In general, the neoplastic cells of Hodgkin's disease are larger and exhibit more prominent nucleoli, and there is almost always an inflammatory background in areas. Immunohistochemical studies are helpful in the distinction, because the Reed-Sternberg cells and variants of Hodgkin's disease are usually negative for CD45RB and T- and B-cell markers, and are usually positive for CD15 and CD30.

Small Noncleaved Cell Lymphoma. Large cell lymphoma composed of medium-sized cells overlaps morphologically with small noncleaved cell lymphoma, particularly the non-Burkitt's type. In fact, some non-Burkitt's lymphomas may be histogenetically related more to large cell lymphoma than Burkitt's lymphoma. A combination of the following features favors a diagnosis of small noncleaved cell lymphoma: nuclear moulding; "squaring off" of the cellular outline as the cells abut one another; very high mitotic count; coarse chromatin pattern; nucleoli centrally located rather than membrane bound; fairly monotonous population without multinucleated forms; low incidence of Leu-8, CD25, and CD35 expression; high incidence of CD10, CD24, and CD38 expression; and a high Ki-67 index (greater than 70 percent) (49). Some cases, however, defy proper classification.

Paraimmunoblastic Variant of Chronic Lymphocytic Leukemia. The paraimmunoblastic variant (tumor-forming subtype) of B-cell chronic lymphocytic leukemia or small lymphocytic lymphoma is characterized by a diffuse proliferation

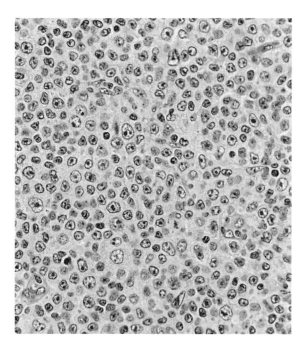

Figure 9-34
PARAIMMUNOBLASTIC VARIANT OF CHRONIC
LYMPHOCYTIC LEUKEMIA, MIMICKING
DIFFUSE LARGE CELL LYMPHOMA
Most of the large cells are only medium sized and lack
the basophilic cytoplasm characteristic of immunoblasts.
The intermingled prolymphocytes and the presence of pro-
liferation centers (not shown) indicate the correct diagnosis.

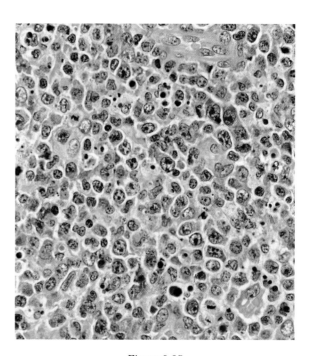

Figure 9-35
KIKUCHI'S NECROTIZING LYMPHADENITIS
The abundance of large lymphoid cells (some of which
have irregular nuclei) mimics lymphoma.

of medium-sized cells with round nuclei, a distinct central (often solitary) nucleolus, and a
moderate amount of light-staining cytoplasm
(77,117). In contrast to immunoblasts, paraimmunoblasts are smaller, the nucleoli are less
prominent, and the cytoplasm is much less basophilic (fig. 9-34). Furthermore, there are always
intermingled prolymphocytes. Although there
are no serious consequences of mistaking this
aggressive neoplasm for diffuse large cell lymphoma, it is important to segregate this entity
(which is related to small lymphocytic lymphoma
or chronic lymphocytic leukemia) from other
types of lymphoma so that its biologic behavior
can be better understood in future studies.

Plasmacytoma, Plasmablastic Type. Features
that distinguish large cell lymphoma from the
plasmablastic or anaplastic type of plasmacytoma
are discussed in chapter 16.

Diffuse Mixed Cell Lymphoma. Features that
distinguish diffuse large cell lymphoma from diffuse
mixed cell lymphoma are discussed in chapter 8.

Kikuchi's Necrotizing Lymphadenitis. This self-
limiting condition, most commonly involving the
cervical lymph nodes of young women, can mimic
large cell lymphoma because of the alarming
proliferation of activated lymphoid cells (mostly
T lineage), which can exhibit irregular foldings
of the nuclei (fig. 9-35) (18,20,38,41,115,146,
148). Histologic clues favoring this diagnosis
over lymphoma are: the pattern of involvement,
in the form of multiple well-delineated pale-
staining nodules (which may coalesce) scattered
in the parenchyma of the node (fig. 9-36); the
abundance of admixed karyorrhectic debris and
phagocytic histiocytes (with characteristic crescent-shaped nuclei and phagocytosed nuclear
debris or eosinophilic globules) (fig. 9-37); the
zonation phenomenon, with predominance of activated lymphoid cells in the peripheral portion
of the nodules and predominance of histiocytes
and karyorrhectic debris in the center; the presence of admixed plasmacytoid monocytes, which
are medium-sized cells with dispersed chromatin and an eccentric rim of amphophilic cytoplasm without a pale Golgi zone (fig. 9-38); and

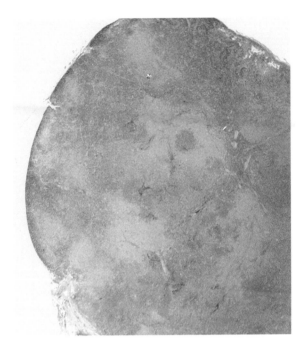

Figure 9-36
KIKUCHI'S NECROTIZING LYMPHADENITIS
The characteristic low-magnification appearance of this entity is seen. Multiple pale circumscribed foci are found in the node; note lack of extension of the process into the perinodal tissue.

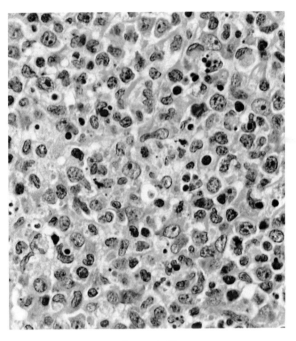

Figure 9-37
KIKUCHI'S NECROTIZING LYMPHADENITIS
Characteristically, the activated lymphoid cells are admixed with karyorrhectic debris and histiocytes. The histiocytes have crescentic nuclei and phagocytosed nuclear debris.

the confinement of the karyorrhectic process to the node, with little spillover into the perinodal tissue (fig. 9-39).

Infectious Mononucleosis and Reactive Immunoblastic Proliferations. Infectious mononucleosis or immunoblastic proliferations caused by viral infection, vaccination, or drug reaction (as with hydantoin) can produce a histologic picture (with large numbers of immunoblasts and even Reed-Sternberg–like cells) indistinguishable from that of diffuse large cell lymphoma, when taken out of context (23,39,61,123). A correct diagnosis requires a high index of suspicion. The possibility of infectious mononucleosis should be suspected when one or more of the following features are present: young age (a diagnosis of large cell lymphoma must be made with great caution in children and adolescents); incomplete effacement of architecture, at least in areas, such as patent sinuses and reactive lymphoid follicles (fig. 9-40); and foci of large cells in transition or admixed with small lymphocytes, plasma cells, and plasmablasts even though large cells (immunoblasts) may predominate. The proliferated immunoblasts usually (but not invariably) lack significant atypia such as marked irregular

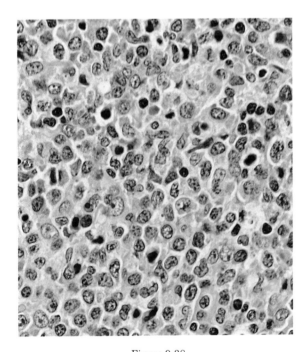

Figure 9-38
KIKUCHI'S NECROTIZING LYMPHADENITIS
Many plasmacytoid monocytes are seen. They are always found in variable numbers in Kikuchi's necrotizing lymphadenitis.

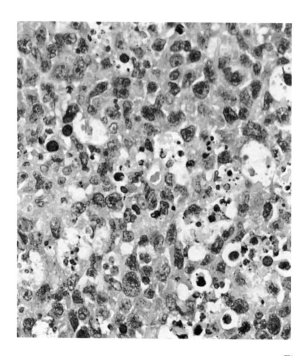 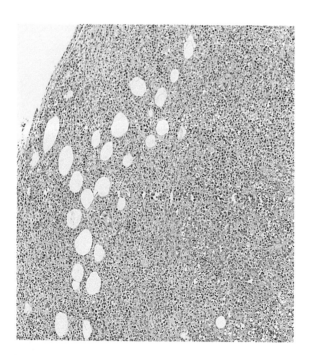

Figure 9-39
DIFFUSE LARGE CELL LYMPHOMA MIMICKING KIKUCHI'S NECROTIZING LYMPHADENITIS
Left: The abundance of karyorrhectic debris raises the possibility of Kikuchi's lymphadenitis. However, the nuclei are very atypical, plasmacytoid monocytes are not evident, and histiocytes with crescentic nuclei are lacking.
Right: The marked perinodal involvement renders the diagnosis of Kikuchi's lymphadenitis unlikely.

foldings of nuclei, granular clumping of chromatin, or clear cytoplasm (fig. 9-41).

Immunohistochemical studies may be helpful because the large cells represent a mixture of T cells and B cells or a predominance of T cells, and there is no light chain restriction (17,129). If all the large cells stain for B-lineage markers, lymphoma has to be strongly suspected (fig. 9-42). Difficult cases may necessitate genotypic studies to clarify the presence or absence of clonal populations.

Treatment. According to the Non-Hodgkin's Lymphoma Pathologic Classification Project study, the median survival for patients with diffuse large cell lymphoma is 1.3 to 1.5 years (105); the long-term survival is 25 percent (133). However, these figures were derived from patients treated in the early 1970s. The outcome has improved over the past two decades with the use of more aggressive treatment.

Localized stage I and II large cell lymphoma can sometimes be cured by radiation therapy or surgery, with 5-year relapse-free survival reported to be 25 to 50 percent (1). However, chemotherapy is used increasingly for treatment, either alone or in combination with radiation

therapy, and increases the 5-year relapse-free survival to 60 to 90 percent (1).

For more extensive disease (stage III, IV, or bulky stage II), systemic chemotherapy is the treatment of choice. The classic regime of cyclophosphamide, adriamycin, vincristine, and prednisone (CHOP) or a modified version produce complete remission rates of 50 to 60 percent, but 30 to 40 percent of the remissions are not durable (7). Overall, only one third of patients are cured (150). Some reports have shown that more aggressive chemotherapy regimes comprising more than five drugs (such as ProMACE-MOPP, MACOP-B, ProMACE-CytaBOM) result in a higher complete remission rate (75 to 85 percent) and hence survival rate, but lethal drug toxicity is more common (up to 10 percent in some studies) (44). The relapse rate in most series is 30 to 40 percent, and thus the overall predicted cure rate is about 60 percent (1,3,33,150). Some of the relapses can be delayed (over 30 months from beginning of therapy) (17). Unfortunately, the good results reported for these aggressive chemotherapy combinations have not always been reproducible in other studies, and most studies

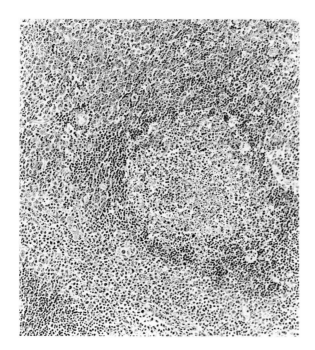

Figure 9-40
INFECTIOUS MONONUCLEOSIS
INVOLVING LYMPH NODE
There is partial preservation of architecture. The lymphoid follicle shows necrosis, as commonly observed in this condition.

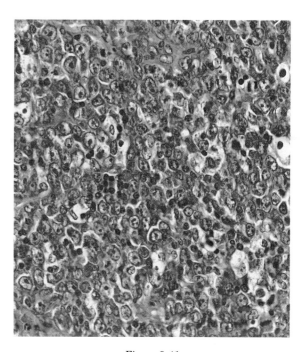

Figure 9-41
INFECTIOUS MONONUCLEOSIS
INVOLVING LYMPH NODE
There is striking proliferation of immunoblasts which lack significant atypia.

have not included a contemporary control group treated by CHOP for comparison of results (1,5,94,125). In fact, two recently published randomized cooperative group studies have shown the CHOP regimen to be comparable or superior to the more aggressive regimens (44,51).

For relapsed disease, salvage in at least a proportion of patients can be achieved by high-dose chemotherapy, with or without radiation therapy, followed by autologous or allogeneic bone marrow transplantation or peripheral blood stem cell reconstitution (83,150).

Prognosis. The following factors have been reported to have prognostic significance in diffuse large cell lymphoma. However, it should be noted that some prognostic variables may lose significance when more aggressive treatment protocols are used (1,3).

Age. Advanced age (over 60 or 65 years) is an adverse prognostic factor on complete remission rate and median survival (35,153).

Stage of Disease. High stage is a poor prognostic factor (43,69,78,133,135). According to the Non-Hodgkin's Lymphoma Pathologic Classification

Project study, the 10-year survival probabilities are 53 percent for stage I, 27 percent for stage II, and 15 percent for stages III and IV (133,135). The clinical implication of discordant bone marrow involvement has been discussed in a previous section.

Systemic Symptoms. Presence of systemic symptoms such as fever, sweats, and weight loss is associated with a worse prognosis (57,58,106,109).

Performance Status. The performance status of the patient, which reflects the ability to tolerate intensive therapy and response to the tumor, is of prognostic importance. Patients who are ambulatory (score 0-1) have a much better prognosis than those who are not (score 2-4) (116,131).

Primary versus Secondary Type of Diffuse Large Cell Lymphoma. Diffuse large cell lymphoma complicating low-grade lymphoma is generally associated with a worse prognosis (5,6,36,122,161).

Tumor Burden. The presence of bulky disease (any mass greater than 7 to 10 cm), involvement of two or more extranodal sites, and high titers of serum lactate dehydrogenase (which reflect a high tumor load) are poor prognostic factors on multivariate analysis (1,32,43,68,69,132).

173

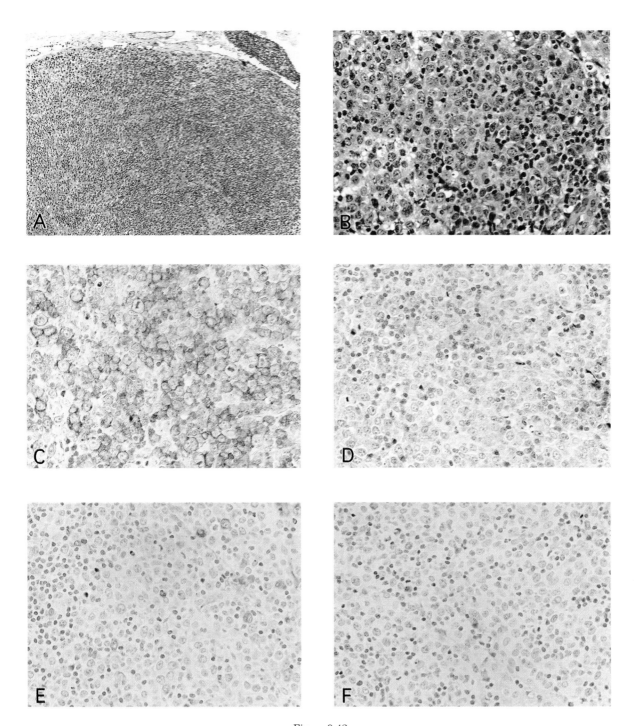

Figure 9-42
LYMPHOMA SIMULATING INFECTIOUS MONONUCLEOSIS IN LYMPH NODE

A: The lymph node is patchily infiltrated by large cells, with patent sinusoids.

B: The large lymphoid cells lack significant atypia. Therefore, the morphologic features do not allow a firm distinction between lymphoma and infectious mononucleosis.

C: Almost all the large cells are immunoreactive with CD20.

D: These cells are not immunoreactive with CD45RO; only the small lymphocytes are positive.

E: Immunostaining for immunoglobulin kappa light chain shows that many of the large cells exhibit Golgi or perinuclear staining.

F: These large cells fail to stain for lambda light chain, whereas some plasma cells in the background do. Thus, the monotonous B-cell proliferation with kappa light chain restriction supports a diagnosis of lymphoma in this case.

Histologic Type. Although some previous studies have shown histologic subdivision of diffuse large cell lymphoma to have prognostic implication (e.g., large noncleaved cell/centroblastic lymphoma showing a better prognosis than immunoblastic lymphoma) (14,82,145,155,160), recent studies have not confirmed these findings (16,40,45,76,99, 100,103,133). These studies are further plagued by lack of reproducible criteria for distinguishing the subtypes of diffuse large cell lymphoma.

Immunophenotype. T-cell versus B-cell Lineage. While some studies have shown that the lineage of a diffuse large cell lymphoma has no bearing on the prognosis (30,64,75,79,132), others have shown post-thymic T-cell lymphoma to be more aggressive and to relapse more frequently than diffuse large B-cell lymphoma (28,52,54,85, 130,135,142). The difference may be related to the treatment given, because study patients whose immunophenotypes lacked prognostic importance were treated by aggressive chemotherapy.

Aberrancy of the Immunophenotype. One study reported that lack of expression of CD20, CD22, or HLA-DR in a diffuse large B-cell lymphoma is correlated with a poorer survival (138). Another study suggested that absence of CD38 or presence of CD24 in high-grade B-cell lymphoma is correlated with better relapse-free survival (128).

Reactive Lymphoid Population. One study reported that a low percentage (less than 6 percent) of reactive CD8-positive T-cells in diffuse large B-cell lymphoma is correlated with a reduction in relapse-free survival (86).

Adhesion Molecule Expression. Some studies suggest that expression of CD44 (Hermes' antigen, the lymphocyte homing receptor), which apparently facilitates dissemination through promotion of adhesion to high endothelial venules, is associated with a less favorable prognosis (131).

Proliferative Fraction. In contrast to low-grade lymphomas, a high proliferative fraction (greater than 50 percent) has been found in several studies to be associated with a better survival in large cell lymphoma, probably attributable to greater susceptibility of the rapidly proliferating tumors to chemotherapy (15,50,56, 73,149). However, a retrospective study by the Southwest Oncology Group reports the opposite finding, with a Ki-67 index of greater than 60 percent predicting a worse prognosis in diffuse large cell lymphoma (55). This finding has recently been confirmed by a prospective study by the same group, who report 3-year survival rates of 29 percent and 59 percent in patients with a Ki-67 index of equal to or greater than 80 percent and a Ki-67 index of less than 80 percent, respectively (95). In fact, most patients with a Ki-67 index of over 80 percent die within 1 year (95). It has been suggested that the contrary results reported in earlier studies may be due to failure to balance all known prognostic or treatment factors (95). High-grade lymphomas with aneuploidy and a high percentage of S+G2 phase cells (more than 22 percent) have also been reported to have poorer survival (106).

Genetic Findings. The following cytogenetic abnormalities detected at diagnosis have been reported to confer a worse prognosis in diffuse large cell lymphoma: increased karyotypic complexity (more than four marker chromosomes), breaks at 1q21-23, trisomy 5, trisomy 6, trisomy 18, and abnormalities of chromosome 17 (80,81, 107,127,167). Those with breaks in the short arm of chromosome 2 or duplication of chromosome 3p have a longer survival than those without these changes (80,167). The t(14;18) or *bcl*-2 rearrangement identifies a patient population with a decreased remission duration and a trend for decreased overall survival (107,109,111,167). One study shows *bcl*-6 rearrangement to be an independent favorable prognostic factor, and another study has shown this feature to be associated with a slightly better overall survival, although not of statistic significance (103,110).

Treatment Variables. The use of less aggressive chemotherapy or suboptimal doses has been found to adversely affect response rate and survival (33,34,74,131,165). Patients who respond rapidly to treatment (complete remission with three or less cycles of therapy) have a more favorable outcome.

There is a trend towards the development of prognostic factor models incorporating variables that are of independent prognostic importance (such as the international index, which is calculated by the parameters of age, performance status, stage, number of extranodal sites of disease, and serum lactate dehydrogenase) to aid in selection of therapy (116). Patients in the high-risk group (low remission rate, high relapse rate, and low survival rate) are usually treated more aggressively, including newer therapies such as bone marrow transplantation, whereas those of low or

Table 9-5

UNUSUAL MORPHOLOGIC VARIANTS OF DIFFUSE LARGE CELL LYMPHOMA

Sinusoidal growth pattern

Interfollicular growth pattern

Myxoid stroma

Fibrillary "matrix"

Pseudorosettes

Multilobated nuclei

Spindly cells

Signet ring cells

Cytoplasmic granules

Microvillous large cell lymphoma (ultrastructural)

Intercellular junctions (ultrastructural)

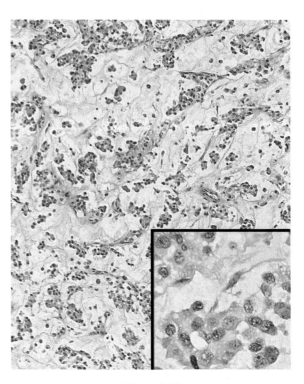

Figure 9-43

MYXOID LARGE B-CELL LYMPHOMA
OF SOFT TISSUES

Thick cords of tumor cells lie in an abundant myxoid matrix. Inset: The cytology of the tumor cells is compatible with that of lymphoma. Some nuclei show lobation.

standard risk are treated by standard therapy. Currently, most of the models only incorporate clinical or pathologic data, but biologic variables will probably be incorporated in the future (131).

UNUSUAL MORPHOLOGIC VARIANTS OF DIFFUSE LARGE CELL LYMPHOMA

The morphologic spectrum of diffuse large cell lymphoma is extremely broad. A number of unusual morphologic variants showing features traditionally considered to be more characteristic of nonlymphoid tumors have been recognized (Table 9-5). It is important not to mistake these variants for carcinoma or sarcoma, because they are potentially curable with chemotherapy, radiotherapy, or both. In case of doubt or in any unusual-looking malignant neoplasm, malignant lymphoma must be excluded by appropriate immunohistochemical studies. The variants are not mutually exclusive, for example, lymphomas with fibrillary matrix are almost always shown ultrastructurally to have features of microvillous lymphomas. Currently, there is no evidence that these morphologic variants, with the exception of those with cytoplasmic granules, are associated with distinctive clinical features or have prognostic significance.

Lymphoma with Myxoid Stroma. Rarely, lymphoma is accompanied by a prominent myxoid stroma, mimicking various sarcomas such as myxoid malignant fibrous histiocytoma

or myxoid chondrosarcoma. This pattern has been reported in large cell lymphoma of B lineage, anaplastic large cell lymphoma, and tumors of probable monocytic lineage (168–171). The large round, spindly, or stellate lymphoma cells form cords or are loosely suspended in a myxoid stroma which is Alcian blue positive and hyaluronidase sensitive (fig. 9-43). It appears that the myxoid matrix is produced by the stromal cells rather than by the lymphoma cells, and tissue edema may predispose to development of the myxoid stroma. The clue to the correct diagnosis is the cytology of the individual tumor cells and the presence of more typical foci of solid-growing lymphoma. The diagnosis can be readily confirmed by immunohistochemical studies.

Lymphoma with Spindly Cells. Lymphoma cells may assume a spindly configuration when they infiltrate fibrous tissue. This phenomenon is seen particularly in lymphomas of bone and soft tissues (173–175). However, lymphoma cells are also occasionally spindled in the absence

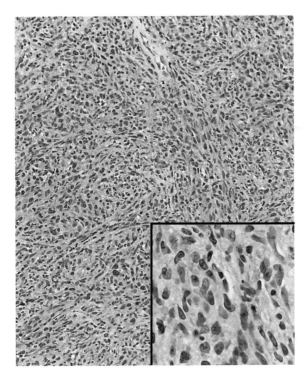

Figure 9-44
SPINDLY LARGE B-CELL LYMPHOMA
OF LYMPH NODE

Spindly cells arranged in short fascicles, producing a vague storiform pattern. Inset: The lymphoma cells possess elongated nuclei.

of stromal influence, presumably resulting from aberrations in the cytoskeleton (termed sarcomatoid lymphoma). Irregular fascicular growth of spindly lymphoma cells may result in patterns reminiscent of the storiform/pleomorphic type of malignant fibrous histiocytoma and other sarcomas (fig. 9-44) (172,176). However, areas more diagnostic of lymphoma are often found.

We have observed a remarkable example of chemotherapy-resistant large B-cell lymphoma transforming into a peculiar spindle cell tumor after treatment with high-dose cyclosporin A. The spindle cells, which possess serpentine nuclei, are oriented haphazardly or in fascicles, and are not readily recognizable as being lymphoid. The lymphomatous nature of the tumor is, however, confirmed by immunoreactivity for CD45RB and CD20 (fig. 9-45).

It should be noted that dendritic cell tumor, another hematolymphoid neoplasm, characteristically shows a spindle cell morphology (see chapter 18).

Lymphoma with Fibrillary Matrix and Pseudorosettes. Pseudorosette (rosette) formation, originally reported to be a rare morphologic manifestation of follicular lymphoma (177), can also occur in diffuse large cell lymphoma (178). The large lymphoma cells have an indistinct cellular outline, and are surrounded by a fibrillary eosinophilic "interstitial" material (fig. 9-46). Sometimes the lymphoma cells are oriented around a core of fibrillary material, forming pseudorosettes similar to those found in neuroblastoma and neuroepithelioma (fig. 9-47). Ultrastructurally, the fibrillary material is formed by entangled long cytoplasmic processes of the lymphoma cells, therefore also satisfying the diagnostic criteria of microvillous large cell lymphoma. Since the fibrillary material is composed mostly of cell membranes, it typically shows immunoreactivity for various cell surface antigens, including leukocyte common antigen (fig. 9-48). All the cases we have studied and those reported in the literature (178) are of B lineage, but there is no reason why this phenomenon cannot occur in T-cell lymphomas.

Microvillous Large Cell Lymphoma. The first example of microvillous large cell lymphoma was reported as an anemone cell tumor of uncertain histogenesis (189,190), because at that time it was not recognized that profuse long cytoplasmic projections could occur in lymphoid neoplasms (180). It is now well known that, besides mesothelioma, neoplasms of diverse histogenesis (such as lymphoma, Hodgkin's disease, adenocarcinoma, squamous cell carcinoma, Merkel's cell carcinoma) can exhibit myriads of villous cytoplasmic processes (179,184,188,189,191,193).

Microvillous lymphoma is also known as *anemone cell, filiform cell, villiform cell,* or *porcupine lymphoma* (180–183,185–187). Erlandson and Filippa (182) make a distinction between anemone cell and filiform large cell lymphoma, reserving the former designation for tumors in which the cells are completely surrounded by profuse, long, slender microvillus-like processes resembling those of mesothelial cells, and the latter designation for tumors with thicker filopodia which are not necessarily circumferential. Since there is no clear-cut dividing line between these two subtypes, we place both under the umbrella term microvillous large cell lymphoma.

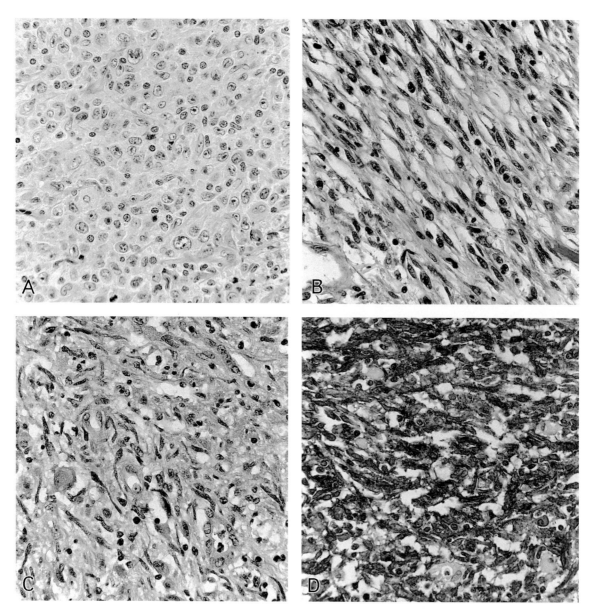

Figure 9-45
SPINDLE CELL TRANSFORMATION OF LARGE CELL LYMPHOMA AFTER CYCLOSPORIN A THERAPY
A: Before treatment with high-dose cyclosporin A, the large cell lymphoma has a conventional appearance.
B, C: After treatment, the tumor cells become strikingly spindly, and are disposed in fascicles or in a haphazard pattern. A diagnosis of lymphoma might not be suspected without such a history.
D: The lymphomatous nature of the spindly cells is confirmed by strong immunostaining with CD45RB.

Microvillous large cell lymphomas usually show no distinctive features at the light microscopic level, except for some that exhibit a sinusoidal growth pattern (181,186,187) and occasional cases that exhibit fibrillary interstitial material (192). Therefore, these lymphomas will not be recognized if ultrastructural studies are not

performed, although identification of this subtype is of no clinical importance. In fact, according to one study, abundant microvilli can be detected in approximately 10 percent of large cell lymphomas examined ultrastructurally (187). There are also no distinctive clinical features (181,186,187). Ultrastructurally, the neoplastic

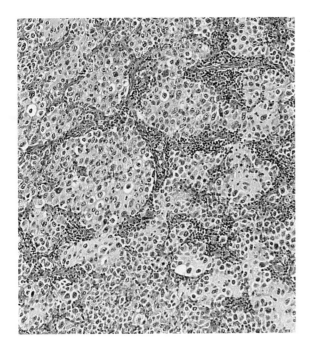
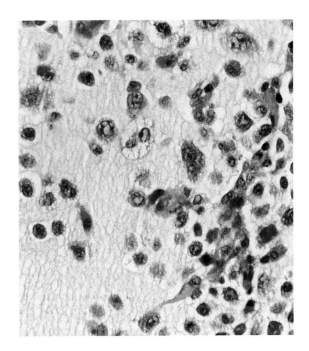

Figure 9-46
LARGE CELL LYMPHOMA WITH FIBRILLARY MATRIX
Left: Diffuse large cell lymphoma with abundant fibrillary matrix. This case simulates the architectural features of seminoma as a result of the delicate septa infiltrated by lymphocytes.
Right: Higher magnification shows large lymphoma cells (resembling ganglion-like cells) associated with abundant fibrillary matrix.

cells possess numerous long (but occasionally short) cytoplasmic processes which can be slender or broad, often disposed circumferentially but occasionally in one pole (fig. 9-49) (181,182,186, 187). The processes, particularly the thicker ones, may show interdigitations. In contrast to mesothelioma and adenocarcinoma, tight junctions and tonofilaments are lacking (182,191). The diagnosis can be readily confirmed by immunohistochemical studies. Microvillous large cell lymphomas are often of B lineage, and are usually CD30 negative (181,182,186,187,191).

Lymphoma with Intercellular Junctions. Although intercellular junctions are traditionally considered to negate a diagnosis of lymphoma at the ultrastructural level (195), they do occasionally occur in lymphoma (194,195,197,198,201). One study suggests that this phenomenon is not uncommon, since it was identified in 5 (9 percent) of 56 non-Hodgkin's lymphomas studied ultrastructurally (198). The cell junctions are usually few and primitive, composed of dense plaques on the closely apposed cytoplasmic membranes and

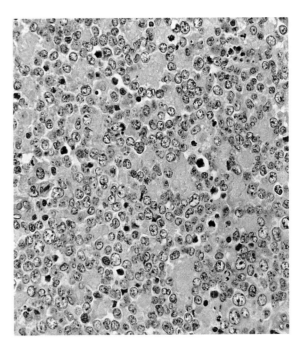

Figure 9-47
LARGE CELL LYMPHOMA WITH PSEUDOROSETTES
Pseudorosettes are formed by fibrillary cores surrounded by tumor cells.

179

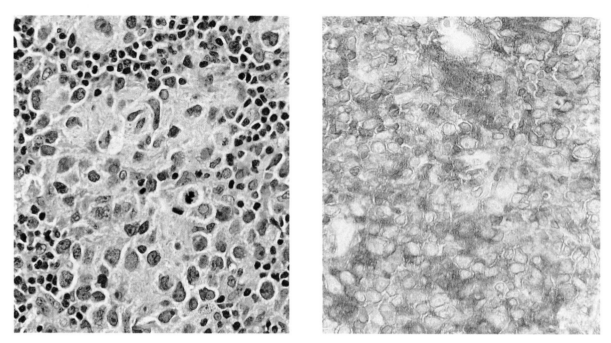

Figure 9-48
LARGE CELL LYMPHOMA WITH FIBRILLARY MATRIX
Left: The large lymphoma cells are associated with a moderate amount of fibrillary matrix.
Right: The tumor cells stain with CD45RB; the matrix is also positive.

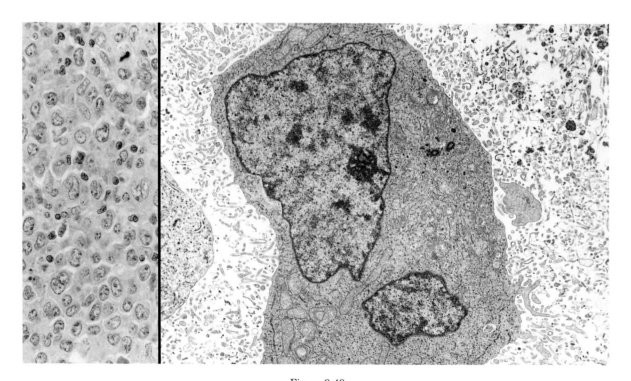

Figure 9-49
MICROVILLOUS LARGE CELL LYMPHOMA
Left: At the light microscopic level, this large cell lymphoma shows no distinctive features.
Right: Ultrastructurally, the lymphoma cells are shown to have numerous long microvilli.

unaltered intercellular gaps without a dense line (so-called paired subplasmalemmal densities) (198). Tonofilaments and true desmosomes are lacking. There may also be occasional tight junctions with focal fusion of cell membranes. This phenomenon can occur in both B- and T-cell lymphomas of large cell type (194,198). It is important to ascertain that the intercellular junctions indeed occur between the lymphoma cells and not between the entrapped follicular dendritic cells (196,199).

Thus, absence of cell junctions should not be considered an essential criterion for the ultrastructural diagnosis of lymphoma (198). Follicular dendritic cell tumors also characteristically exhibit intercellular junctions (see chapter 18) (200,202).

Signet Ring Large Cell Lymphoma. Signet ring cell morphology, a feature classically associated with adenocarcinoma, was first reported to occur as a rare phenomenon in follicular lymphoma (207). This feature can also rarely occur in large cell lymphomas of B-cell or T-cell lineage (203,204,206,211,215,216). The signet ring change may be a focal or prominent feature in an individual case.

Included under the designation signet ring cell lymphoma are two different cytologic types: clear vacuole type and eosinophilic globule (Russell body) type. Some authors reserve this term only for the former (209).

In the clear vacuole type, a solitary clear vacuole in the cytoplasm indents the nucleus or compresses it to a crescent-shaped structure (fig. 9-50). This appearance can occur in B- and T-cell lymphomas. The vacuole is mucin negative, but its rim may be stained by periodic acid–Schiff (PAS). For B-cell lymphomas, the rims of the vacuoles often stain for IgG (207,210,212,213). For T-cell lymphomas, the vacuoles show immunoreactivity for the surface antigens expressed by the tumor (206). Ultrastructurally, the electron-lucent vacuole is delimited by a cell membrane, but may contain multiple microspherules or irregular electron-dense clumps (205–207, 213,216). The vacuole is believed to be formed by endocytosis of the membrane and abnormal membrane recycling (206), or by fusion of multivesicular bodies (205).

In the eosinophilic globule (Russell body) type, a single cytoplasmic eosinophilic globule displaces and indents the nucleus of the lym-

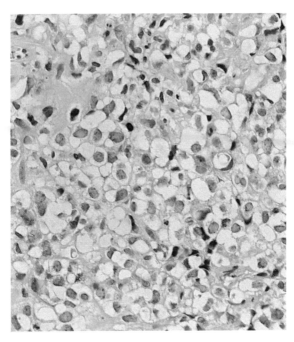

Figure 9-50
SIGNET RING LARGE CELL
LYMPHOMA OF B LINEAGE
This nasal tumor is composed of large cells whose nuclei are compressed by large clear cytoplasmic vacuoles. The diagnosis of lymphoma is confirmed by immunoreactivity with CD45RB and CD20. This lesion can potentially be mistaken for clear cell carcinoma or signet ring cell carcinoma.

phoma cell. This type has only been reported in B-cell lymphomas, probably resulting from failure of the secretory mechanism, leading to accumulation of immunoglobulin in the cytoplasm. Globules that are brightly eosinophilic are usually PAS positive and diastase resistant, and contain IgM; they are indistinguishable from Russell bodies (207). Ultrastructurally, the globule is composed of amorphous electron-dense material or, occasionally, crystals or fibrils within distended rough endoplasmic reticulum (204,207,208,214). A less common type of globule is weakly eosinophilic and PAS negative; it may contain IgA or IgG (fig. 9-51) (210,215). Ultrastructurally, the globules are usually composed of granular and fibrillar material without a limiting membrane. The major differential diagnosis is malignant rhabdoid tumor, which is usually cytokeratin positive and in which the cytoplasmic globule is formed by whorls of intermediate filaments.

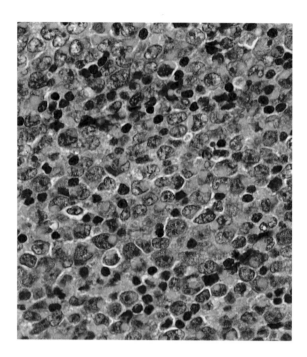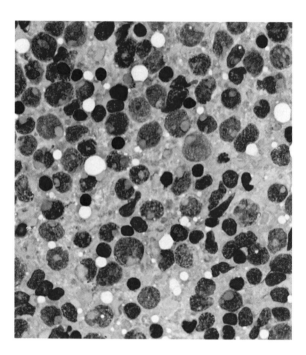

Figure 9-51
SIGNET RING LARGE CELL LYMPHOMA OF B LINEAGE
Left: The large lymphoma cells possess lightly eosinophilic cytoplasmic globules that displace and distort the nuclei.
Right: The cytoplasmic globules are more evident in this touch preparation stained with Giemsa. They appear as refractile light-staining globular inclusions.

Sinusoidal Large Cell Lymphoma. The nodal infiltrate of this lymphoma is confined entirely or predominantly to the sinuses, mimicking metastatic carcinoma or melanoma (fig. 9-52) (217,221). The correct diagnosis rests on recognition of the cytologic features of the neoplastic cells, which are often round to oval, noncohesive (although they may appear deceptively cohesive in areas), and pyroninophilic (fig. 9-52, inset). The diagnosis can be readily confirmed by immunohistochemical studies. A sinusoidal pattern is observed most characteristically in anaplastic large cell lymphoma and microvillous large cell lymphoma, but can occur in conventional large cell lymphoma of B- or T-cell lineage (217–222).

Interfollicular Large Cell Lymphoma. Large cell lymphoma can have an interfollicular distribution between hyperplastic lymphoid follicles (fig. 9-53). Although an interfollicular pattern is often considered to be a characteristic of T-cell lymphomas (227), it also occasionally occurs in large B-cell lymphomas, including T-cell–rich large B-cell lymphoma (223–226). Inter-

follicular large cell lymphoma can be mistaken for reactive paracortical hyperplasia; erosion of the follicular mantles by the infiltrate and presence of cytologic atypia strongly favor a diagnosis of lymphoma (fig. 9-53). If the majority of the large lymphoid cells in the interfollicular regions are B cells, this is strong evidence for a neoplastic process, particularly if supported by the demonstration of light chain restriction. For interfollicular T-cell proliferation, the demonstration of an aberrant immunophenotype strongly supports a diagnosis of neoplasia.

Multilobated Large Cell Lymphoma. Multilobated nuclei are characterized by three or more nuclear lobes connected to one another at a narrow point in the center, similar to the petals of a flower (fig. 9-54). Although previously thought to be a morphologic marker for post-thymic T-cell lymphoma (234,236), these nuclei are now known to occur more commonly in B-cell lymphomas (229, 231,237). It is not uncommon to find some multilobated nuclei in a large cell lymphoma (228–231,233,235,237), but the term multilobated lymphoma can be justifiably applied only when more

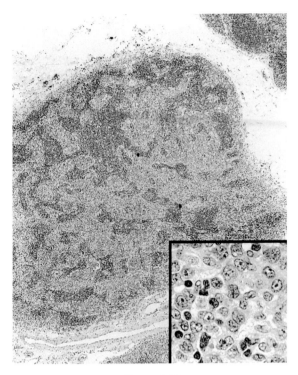

Figure 9-52
SINUSOIDAL LARGE CELL LYMPHOMA (T LINEAGE)

The sinuses of the lymph node are distended by lymphoma. Inset: Higher magnification shows the cytology of the lymphoma cells within the sinuses.

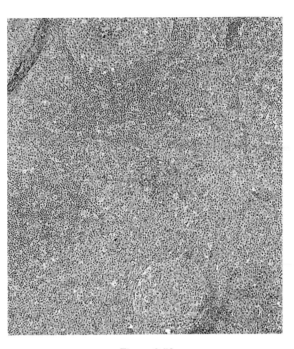

Figure 9-53
DIFFUSE LARGE B-CELL LYMPHOMA
WITH INTERFOLLICULAR GROWTH PATTERN

The interfollicular region is expanded by an abnormal lymphoid infiltrate, which has eroded the mantles of the reactive follicles.

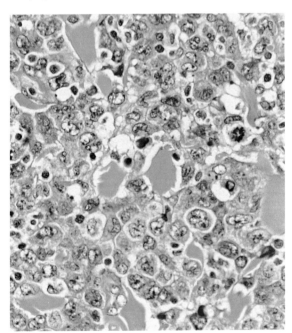

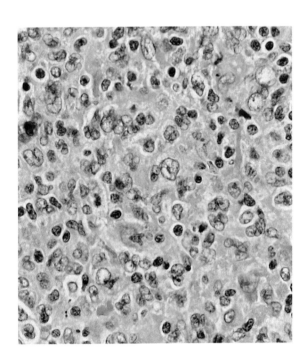

Figure 9-54
MULTILOBATED LARGE CELL LYMPHOMA

Left: This lymphoma, occurring in the skin, is of T lineage. The nuclei possess multiple lobes like the petals of a flower.
Right: This B-lineage lymphoma cannot be reliably distinguished from a T-lineage multilobated lymphoma on morphologic grounds.

than 50 percent of the lymphoma cells exhibit this feature (229), although the updated Kiel classification accepts a cut-off point of more than 10 to 20 percent for the multilobated subtype of centroblastic lymphoma (231).

Among B-cell lymphomas showing nuclear multilobation, most exhibit features of follicular center cell (centroblastic or centroblastic-centrocytic) lymphoma (229,231,232,235), such as follicle formation in some cases, intermingling with typical large noncleaved cells (centroblasts), and an occasional admixture with small cleaved cells (centrocytes). Similar multilobated cells can also be detected in small numbers in reactive germinal centers (229,235). However, in the absence of follicle formation, the lineage of a multilobated large cell lymphoma cannot be reliably predicted by morphologic assessment alone.

Malignant Lymphoma with Cytoplasmic Granules. Cytoplasmic granules can be demonstrated in rare cases of large cell lymphoma in Giemsa-stained cytologic preparations (a few to many fine or coarse azurophilic granules) or ultrastructurally (membrane-bound electron-dense granules) (fig. 9-55). The granules cannot be detected in conventional histologic sections. This phenomenon has been reported mostly in T-cell lymphomas that express natural killer cell markers and natural killer cell lymphomas (238, 240,242–244), and only rarely in B-cell lymphomas (241). There is some evidence that lymphomas expressing natural killer cell markers (almost invariably exhibiting cytoplasmic granules) are associated with an aggressive clinical course (239,242,244).

LARGE CELL LYMPHOMA VARIANTS WITH DISTINCTIVE CLINICOPATHOLOGIC FEATURES

Intravascular Lymphomatosis

Definition. Intravascular lymphomatosis is an uncommon and peculiar variant of large cell lymphoma that is characterized by multifocal, exclusive or predominant intravascular tumor growth (246,262,263,265,274,276). This term is preferred to the alternative designation, *angiotropic lymphoma* (269), which can be confused with the term angiocentric lymphoma. This entity was previously known as neoplastic angioendotheliomatosis, malignant angioendothelio-

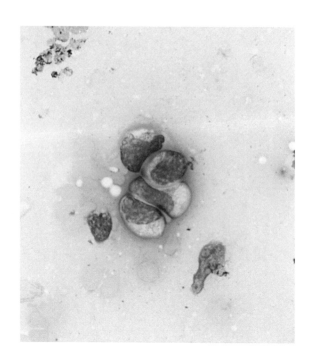

Figure 9-55
LARGE CELL LYMPHOMA
WITH AZUROPHILIC GRANULES
Touch preparation of a nasal CD56-positive T/NK cell lymphoma, showing azurophilic granules in the cytoplasm of the tumor cells.

matosis, proliferative angioendotheliomatosis, or angioendotheliomatosis proliferans systemisata, because it was thought to be a neoplasm of endothelial cells (250).

Clinical Features. Most patients are middle-aged or elderly, but a congenital case has also been reported (272). Patients usually present with symptoms attributable to involvement of the skin or central nervous system (CNS). Skin involvement usually manifests as erythematous or violaceous nodular subcutaneous masses or plaques which may ulcerate, often occurring in the trunk and extremities. CNS involvement usually manifests as confusing, bizarre, and nonspecific neurologic symptoms attributable to multiple infarcts due to vascular occlusion by lymphoma, and resulting in progressive dementia, nonlocalizing neurologic deficits, and focal neurologic signs. However, any organ or system, such as liver, kidney, adrenal gland, heart, lung, upper respiratory tract, breast, female genital tract, prostate, gastrointestinal tract, gall bladder, bone, and spleen, can be involved (247–249,252,258–260,262,267,277). There are usually

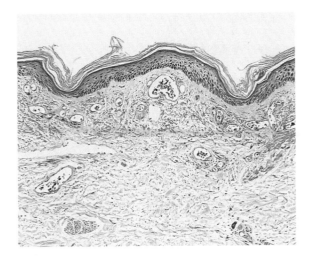

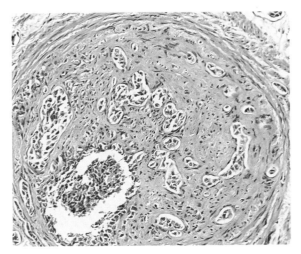

Figure 9-56
INTRAVASCULAR LYMPHOMATOSIS
INVOLVING SKIN
Top: The small blood vessels of the dermis are plugged with tumor cells.
Bottom: In the subcutaneous tissue, an involved large vessel, which is similarly filled with lymphoma cells, shows tortuous channels.

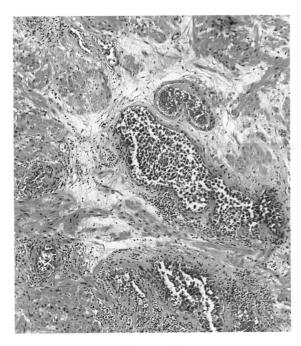

Figure 9-57
INTRAVASCULAR LYMPHOMATOSIS
INVOLVING PROSTATE
In this transurethral resection specimen, the medium-sized vessels are incidentally found to be filled with tumor cells (B lineage).

no circulating lymphoma cells and the bone marrow is rarely involved despite the extensive intravascular growth (253). Fever is common. Some patients show serologic evidence of disordered immune function, such as circulating antinuclear antibodies and rheumatoid factor (274). Rarely, renal involvement presents with clinicopathologic features of minimal change disease (251). One case of T-cell lineage was associated with human T-cell lymphotropic virus type I infection (270).

Microscopic Findings. The key feature of intravascular lymphomatosis, irrespective of site of involvement, is the filling of lumina of the small and intermediate-sized blood vessels by noncohesive, large, atypical mononuclear cells (figs. 9-56–9-59). These cells usually possess round nuclei, vesicular chromatin, multiple prominent nucleoli, and a moderate rim of amphophilic cytoplasm (fig. 9-59). Mitotic figures can often be seen. The tumor cells may be palisaded along the luminal side of the blood vessels, giving an impression that they represent endothelial lining (fig. 9-60), or they may proliferate in the subendothelial layer (256). There is a tendency for these intravascular tumor cells to be enmeshed in fibrin or platelet thrombi. The tumor can be associated with florid endothelial proliferation, resulting in glomeruloid structures. The blood vessels can also become tortuous or thrombosed, with or without recanalization (fig. 9-56). The resultant vascular occlusion can lead to multiple-site infarction of the involved organs (fig. 9-61). The

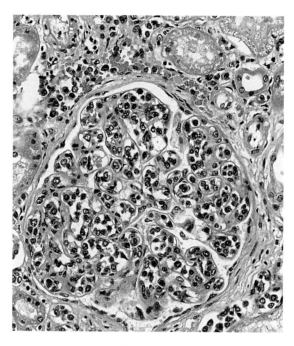

Figure 9-58
INTRAVASCULAR LYMPHOMATOSIS
INVOLVING KIDNEY
The glomerular capillaries are markedly expanded by lymphoma cells. The capillaries in the interstitium are similarly filled with lymphoma cells.

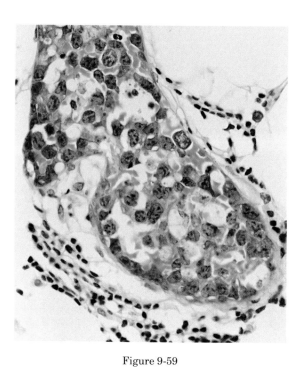

Figure 9-59
INTRAVASCULAR LYMPHOMATOSIS
The noncohesive intravascular tumor cells have nuclei with distinct nucleoli and the cells have amphophilic cytoplasm.

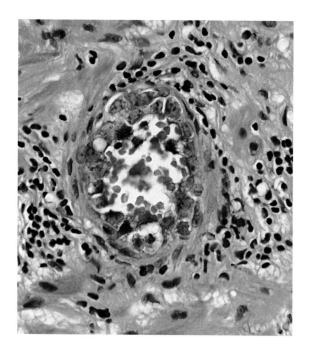

Figure 9-60
INTRAVASCULAR LYMPHOMATOSIS
The blood vessel is lined by tumor (lymphoma) cells, and erythrocytes are present in the lumen. This tumor can potentially be mistaken for a vascular (endothelial) neoplasm.

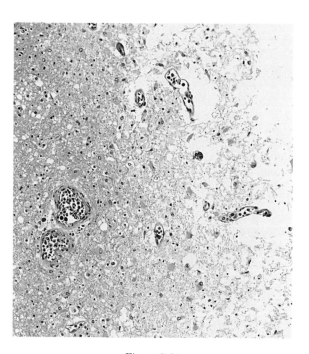

Figure 9-61
INTRAVASCULAR LYMPHOMATOSIS
INVOLVING BRAIN
The blood vessels are filled with lymphoma cells, and the adjacent brain tissue (right) shows rarefaction due to infarction.

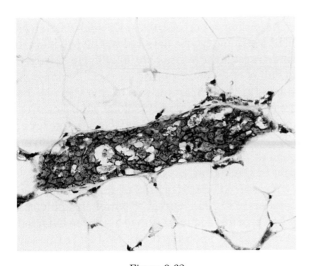

Figure 9-62
INTRAVASCULAR LYMPHOMATOSIS
The intravascular tumor cells show membrane staining with CD45RB.

presence of an extravascular component of lymphoma does not negate the diagnosis of intravascular lymphomatosis (255,271,273,274).

Immunologic and Genotypic Findings. The lymphoid nature of the lesion can be unequivocally confirmed by staining for CD45RB (leukocyte common antigen) and other lymphoid markers (fig. 9-62), and lack of staining for endothelial markers. Staining for factor VIII–related antigen has to be interpreted with care because entrapped endothelial cells or platelets can also stain. Almost all cases are of B-cell lineage, a finding further confirmed by immunoglobulin gene rearrangement studies (245,253); only a small percentage are of T-cell lineage (268-272). One case was reported to be of true histiocytic lineage (264), and a misleading designation, "intravascular histiocytosis," was proposed for this condition.

The homing receptor for high endothelial venules, as detected by the Hermes-3 antibody, is expressed by the lymphoma cells, and therefore this lymphocyte homing system appears to be intact (255,257). However, the lymphoma cells lack the leukocyte adhesion molecule CD11a/CD18, which may contribute to their inability to extravasate to extravascular spaces (257).

Differential Diagnosis. Disseminated carcinoma or melanoma may mimic intravascular lymphomatosis histologically. The lymphoid nature of the neoplastic cells of the latter can be suggested by the noncohesive growth pattern and the presence of amphophilic to basophilic cytoplasm. The clinical history is helpful in making the distinction, which can be further enhanced by staining with a panel of antibodies (CD45RB, cytokeratin, S-100 protein).

Intravascular lymphomatosis must be distinguished from reactive angioendotheliomatosis, a rare reactive vasoproliferative lesion associated with infective endocarditis, hypersensitivity reaction, or no obvious cause (261,266,275). Reactive angioendotheliomatosis is confined to the skin, the cellular proliferation is not obviously intravascular and composed of an admixture of plump spindled endothelial cells and pericytes, and nuclear atypia is lacking. The endothelial and pericytic nature of the cellular proliferation can be confirmed by immunostaining for factor VIII–related antigen and muscle-specific actin, respectively.

Treatment and Prognosis. Most cases are rapidly fatal; often the diagnosis is not made until autopsy (254). The poor prognosis might be related to delays in diagnosis and failure to receive appropriate treatment. In recent years, a correct diagnosis is more often made by biopsy (247,251). Complete remissions can sometimes be achieved with multiagent chemotherapy (264,269,271).

Anaplastic Large Cell Lymphoma

Definition. Anaplastic large cell lymphoma is characterized by a proliferation of large lymphoma cells with bizarre, anaplastic cytologic features (387a). Almost all cases show CD30 (Ki-1) immunoreactivity. This lymphoma is also commonly known in the literature as *Ki-1 lymphoma*, a term we and others do not endorse because it is unwise to classify a lymphoma based solely on the expression of a single marker (353).

In the past, anaplastic large cell lymphoma was often diagnosed as immunoblastic lymphoma, histiocytic malignancy, or metastatic carcinoma. It is now recognized as a distinct entity in the updated Kiel classification. In the Working Formulation, this lymphoma can be placed under the "large cell immunoblastic" category (382), but it is important to append the qualifying label "anaplastic large cell type" to draw attention to this clinicopathologically distinctive lymphoma type.

General Features. Most cases of anaplastic large cell lymphoma arise de novo (primary type); others arise in a setting of other lymphomas (secondary type) such as mycosis fungoides,

187

Lennert's lymphoma, T-zone lymphoma, angioimmunoblastic lymphadenopathy (AILD)-like T-cell lymphoma, and Hodgkin's disease, either at initial presentation or on follow-up (322,345). The secondary type occurs mostly in adults, and usually presents with high-stage disease; the prognosis is poor (387).

The CD30 antigen, recognized by the antibodies Ki-1, Ber-H2, and Hefi-1, was originally considered a specific marker for Reed-Sternberg cells and their variants in Hodgkin's disease (383). It is now recognized to be an activation marker, which is detectable on activated T cells, activated B cells, and even histiocytes (281, 387a). It has also been demonstrated in embryonal carcinoma and some mesenchymal tumors (351,361). CD30-positive cells are normally present as a minor lymphoid population located around lymphoid follicles, and are present in increased numbers in a variety of lymphoid hyperplasias, such as toxoplasmic lymphadenitis, infectious mononucleosis, Kikuchi's necrotizing lymphadenitis, and cutaneous reactive lymphoid proliferations (278,311,318,387a). CD30 expression can occur in non-Hodgkin's lymphomas in several settings: various types of conventional B-cell and T-cell lymphomas, in which there are scattered large neoplastic (activated) cells showing immunoreactivity with CD30; conventional large cell lymphoma, in which most of the neoplastic cells are CD30 positive; and anaplastic large cell lymphoma, in which most of the neoplastic cells are CD30 positive (313,345,352, 353,360,368,387a).

Occasional CD30-positive large cells are also frequently detected at the edges or within the neoplastic follicles in follicular lymphomas; they appear to be B cells but it is currently unclear whether they are neoplastic or reactive (352, 369). Therefore, use of the nondiscriminant term "Ki-1 lymphoma" is discouraged (360).

The CD30 molecule is a 120-kd transmembrane protein with an extracellular domain that is homologous to the tumor necrosis factor (TNF)/nerve growth factor (NGF) receptor superfamily. It is encoded by the CD30 gene localized at chromosome 1p36 (311a). The ligand that binds to CD30 belongs to a family of cytokines homologous to TNF, and the human gene encoding the CD30 ligand has been mapped to chromosome 9q33 (297,309,386).

According to some studies, Epstein-Barr virus (EBV) genome can be detected by the polymerase chain reaction or in situ hybridization in one third to half of cases of anaplastic large cell lymphoma, suggesting an important role of this virus in the genesis of this lymphoma (325,326,335). However, most recent studies have found a low frequency of EBV (0 to 12 percent) in anaplastic large cell lymphomas (292,328,349,376), except for those occurring in the setting of acquired immunodeficiency syndrome (AIDS) (frequency of approximately 80 percent) (290,295). Human T-lymphotropic virus type I proviral sequences have also been detected in rare cases, especially those involving skin, and this virus may be involved in the development of a small fraction of anaplastic large cell lymphomas (280,291,326,328,389).

Incidence. Anaplastic large cell lymphoma accounts for 2 to 7 percent of all non-Hodgkin's lymphomas (299,345,387). It has also been reported to occur in human immunodeficiency virus (HIV)-seropositive and iatrogenically immunosuppressed patients (282,345).

Natural History and Clinical Features. The following description applies to the primary type of anaplastic large cell lymphoma. There is a bimodal age distribution, with one peak in the second decade and the other in the fifth decade (306,345,356,362,375). The disease shows a male predominance, with a male to female ratio of 2 to 1 (279,299). The clinical presentation is variable. In addition to lymphadenopathy, presentation in extranodal sites (particularly the skin) is common. The cutaneous lesions are in the form of solitary or multiple nodules or papules; the larger nodules can ulcerate (306). A history of spontaneous regression or waxing and waning lesions may be obtained in some cases. The gastrointestinal tract, Waldeyer's ring, bone, and soft tissues are also common sites of extranodal presentation (279,284,286,298–301,306,336,339,345,363).

Half to two thirds of patients have stage I/II disease at presentation (322,342,345). Bone marrow involvement has been reported in 0 to 40 percent of cases (overall approximately 12 percent) (315a,397). Occasionally, the disease presents with generalized involvement of the lymphoreticular system, often accompanied by fever and reactive hemophagocytic syndrome, producing a picture of malignant histiocytosis (299,397). In fact, many cases previously diagnosed as malignant histio-cytosis have been reinterpreted as anaplastic large cell lymphoma.

Soluble CD30 antigen is frequently found in the sera of patients with anaplastic large cell lymphoma. Assay of this antigen can be used to monitor the activity of the disease and the response to treatment (311a,364).

Subsets of Primary T-Cell or Null-Cell Anaplastic Large Cell Lymphoma. It has been suggested that primary anaplastic large cell lymphomas of T-cell or null-cell type comprise two clinically and biologically distinctive subsets (286,303,320,344). The *primary cutaneous form* has solitary or multiple skin lesions with no evidence of extracutaneous disease at presentation; occurs predominantly in adults; commonly regresses spontaneously or pursues a regressing-relapsing course; and has an indolent behavior with a favorable prognosis (4-year survival of 92 percent). This form overlaps with lymphomatoid papulosis. In contrast to the primary systemic form, expression of cutaneous lymphocyte antigen (HECA-452) is common but expression of epithelial membrane antigen (EMA) is rare. The *primary systemic form* involves multiple sites which may include skin; has a bimodal age distribution; and is aggressive like other large cell lymphomas, but often shows a good response to chemotherapy (4-year survival of 65 percent). Cutaneous lymphocyte antigen is usually negative and EMA often positive.

Anaplastic large cell lymphoma of B-cell lineage does not show distinctive clinical or biologic features compared with usual forms of diffuse large B-cell lymphomas (353,357).

Microscopic Findings. The pattern of lymph node involvement can be complete, partial, or sinusoidal. The last pattern is a striking and characteristic feature in some cases (fig. 9-63). When the involvement is partial, the infiltrate tends to be paracortical and surrounds the residual lymphoid follicles or blood vessels (fig. 9-64). Fibrosis is common, taking the form of capsular thickening, fibrous bands, and delicate sclerotic strands enwrapping individual cells or packets of cells. The neoplastic proliferation can be relatively pure, or can be accompanied by variable numbers of reactive cells such as small lymphocytes, plasma cells, neutrophils, eosino-phils, and histiocytes (which can show erythro-phagocytosis) (fig. 9-65).

Cytologically, anaplastic large cell lymphoma is characterized by very large round, oval, or polygonal cells with bizarre pleomorphic nuclei (figs. 9-66–9-69). Sometimes the neoplastic cells grow in a cohesive pattern mimicking carcinoma (fig. 9-68), but they can also be individually dispersed within the residual lymphoid parenchyma and sinuses. The latter pattern of involvement can be so subtle that it may be missed on casual examination (fig. 9-64).

The nuclei of the lymphoma cells are round, oval, or irregularly shaped. The irregular nuclei often have an embryo-like appearance, with a smooth convex surface and a concave surface with multiple indentations (fig. 9-69). There can be binucleated cells resembling diagnostic Reed-Sternberg cells (fig. 9-67) or multinucleated forms with the individual nuclei disposed in a wreath-like pattern (fig. 9-67). The chromatin is usually coarsely clumped with areas of clearing, and multiple large round or comma-shaped nucleoli are present (299,301). The voluminous cytoplasm can be deeply basophilic, amphophilic, eosinophilic, pale, or clear. Cells with deeply basophilic cytoplasm often have a prominent pale-staining paranuclear hof (figs. 9-67, 9-69); cells with pale or clear cytoplasm often have a polygonal outline and a well-delineated pink-staining cell membrane, imparting a squamoid appearance (fig. 9-68) (299). In most cases, the tumor cells show considerable variation in size, although they can sometimes appear monomorphic (301). Erythro-phagocytosis is uncommon (279). Mitotic figures are typically abundant, and necrosis is common.

An unusual sarcomatoid variant, which may be mistaken for various types of sarcoma, has been recognized (298,310). It is characterized by spindly or stellate neoplastic cells suspended in a myxoid matrix (fig. 9-70, left), or spindly cells arranged in a storiform pattern (fig. 9-70, right). Attention to cytologic details, identification of areas with a more conventional growth pattern, and immunohistochemical studies should lead to a correct diagnosis.

In the secondary type of anaplastic large cell lymphoma, remnants of preexisting lymphoma can be seen as a separate component or intermingled with the anaplastic lymphoma cells.

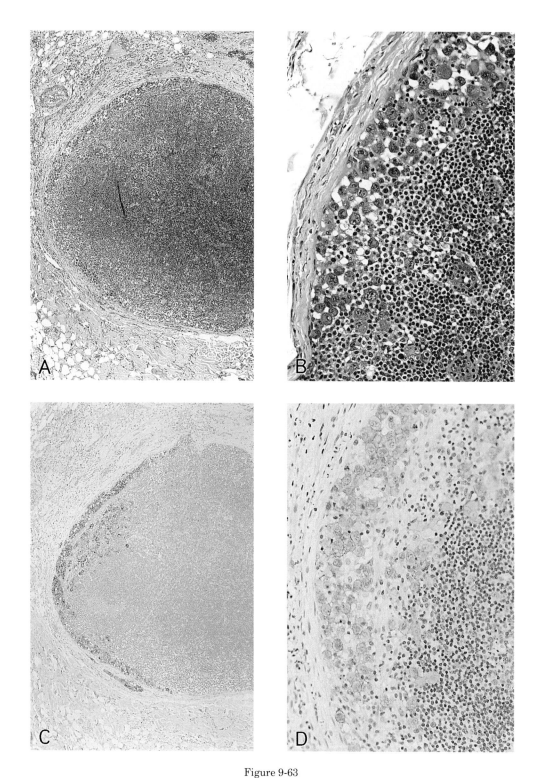

Figure 9-63
ANAPLASTIC LARGE CELL LYMPHOMA WITH SINUSOIDAL GROWTH PATTERN

A: The lymph node shows a predominantly sinusoidal infiltration by tumor.

B: Higher magnification shows the anaplastic appearance of the tumor cells in the subcapsular sinus.

C: Immunostaining for epithelial membrane antigen highlights the distribution of the tumor cells (predominantly in the subcapsular sinuses).

D: The tumor cells show cell membrane and Golgi immunostaining with CD30. This case is of non-T non-B lineage.

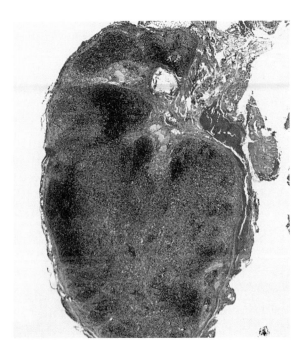
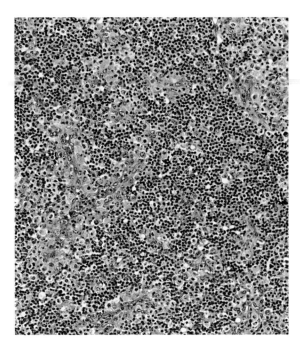

Figure 9-64
ANAPLASTIC LARGE CELL LYMPHOMA OF T LINEAGE
Left: Effacement of the nodal architecture is incomplete.
Right: The large neoplastic cells are individually dispersed in the paracortex, with a tendency to localize around the blood vessels.

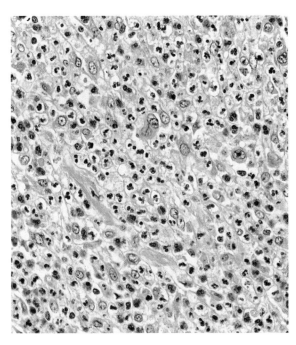

Figure 9-65
ANAPLASTIC LARGE CELL LYMPHOMA
OF T LINEAGE

In this case, the large lymphoma cells are mixed with (and masked by) a prominent infiltrate of neutrophils and eosinophils.

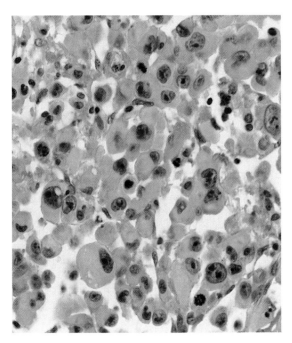

Figure 9-66
ANAPLASTIC
LARGE CELL LYMPHOMA

In this example, the large cells have abundant eosinophilic hyaline cytoplasm.

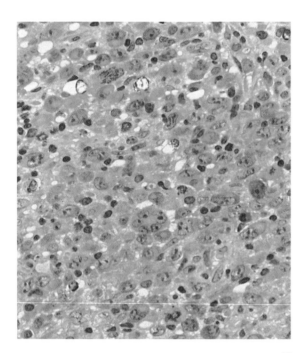
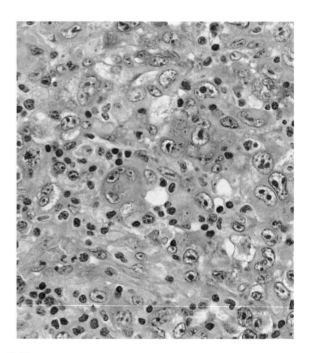

Figure 9-67
ANAPLASTIC LARGE CELL LYMPHOMA OF T LINEAGE

The large cells possess irregularly folded nuclei, vesicular chromatin, and prominent nucleoli. The cytoplasm is basophilic, and pale paranuclear Golgi zones are seen.

Left: A multinucleated cell with wreath-like nuclei is seen in the center field.

Right: Some binucleated and multinucleated forms are seen.

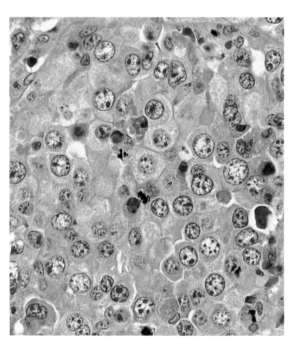

Figure 9-68
ANAPLASTIC LARGE CELL LYMPHOMA
(B LINEAGE)

In this case, large polygonal cells possess distinct cell membranes and pale cytoplasm, giving a squamoid appearance. The nuclei are mostly round.

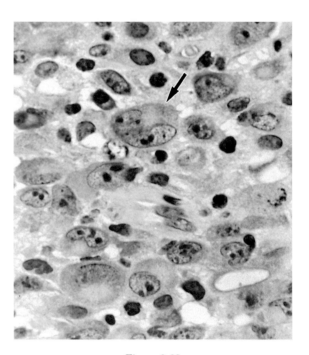

Figure 9-69
ANAPLASTIC LARGE CELL LYMPHOMA
OF T LINEAGE

The nuclei have an embryo-like appearance (arrow). Note the characteristic Golgi zone in the cytoplasm.

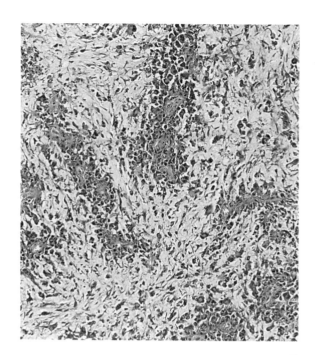 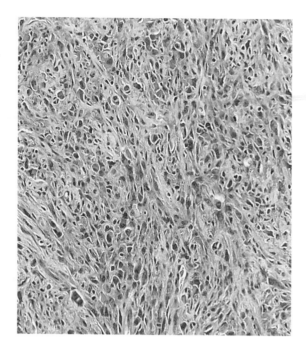

Figure 9-70
SARCOMATOID ANAPLASTIC LARGE CELL LYMPHOMA (T LINEAGE)
Left: Spindly, stellate, and ovoid large tumor cells are suspended in abundant myxoid stroma.
Right: Spindly tumor cells form short fascicles, resulting in a vague storiform pattern.

When anaplastic large cell lymphoma involves skin, the dermis, subcutaneous tissue, or both, are infiltrated. The overlying epidermis may show hyperplasia or ulceration (fig. 9-71); epidermotropism is variable. In the bone marrow, the infiltrate can be subtle or massive (397); the isolated lymphoma cells can be highlighted by immunostaining for CD30 (299). A significantly lower survival is seen in patients with marrow involvement (including subtle involvement) compared to those without marrow involvement (315a).

Immunologic Findings. Immunohistochemical studies show that approximately 60 percent of anaplastic large cell lymphomas are of T-cell lineage; 10 to 20 percent are of B-cell lineage; and 20 to 30 percent express no lineage-specific marker, express markers of both B-cell and T-cell lineage, or rarely, express histiocytic markers (283, 285,293,299,301,330,341,346,356,363,378,390, 393). Loss of multiple T-lineage markers is common in lymphomas of T-cell lineage (301,341,345).

Almost all cases stain for CD30. The antibodies Ki-1 and Hefi-1 work only on fresh or frozen tissues, while Ber-H2 can work on paraffin sections.

The reaction product should be localized to the cell membrane, Golgi zone, or both (figs. 9-63D, 9-72); diffuse cytoplasmic staining should not be regarded as true positive staining (384).

Over 50 percent of cases are immunoreactive for epithelial membrane antigen, in a cell membrane or Golgi pattern (fig. 9-63) (294,299,301, 306,317,321,342,346,356,368,374). This finding, coupled with the lack of CD45RB (leukocyte common antigen) expression in some cases (up to 40 percent), may give an erroneous impression of carcinoma (283,312,321,383). Rare cases have even been reported to stain with anticytokeratin antibodies (316,321,387). The lymphoma cells often stain for activation markers such as HLA-DR, transferrin receptor (CD71), and interleukin-2 receptor (CD25) (306,339,346,347,356, 365). Studies have reported variable frequencies of CD15 staining, from zero up to 100 percent of cases; most, however, report infrequent staining (279,283,294,306,322,368,377). Immunoreactive p53 protein is demonstrated in most cases (308). Staining for the putative intermediate filament–associated protein, restin, is common; restin is also expressed in the Reed-Sternberg cells of

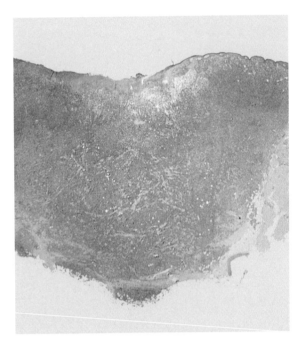
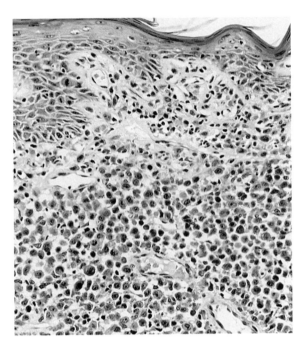

Figure 9-71
ANAPLASTIC LARGE CELL CD30-POSITIVE LYMPHOMA OF THE SKIN (T LINEAGE),
SO-CALLED REGRESSING ATYPICAL HISTIOCYTOSIS
Left: The skin shows ulceration and full-thickness infiltration by lymphoma.
Right: The neoplastic cells have an anaplastic appearance and amphophilic cytoplasm.

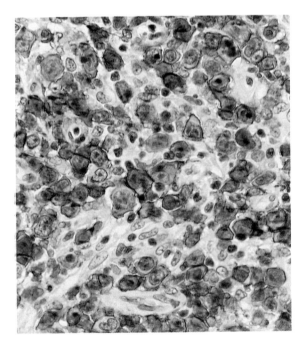

Figure 9-72
ANAPLASTIC LARGE CELL CD30-POSITIVE
LYMPHOMA OF T-CELL LINEAGE
Practically all the large neoplastic cells show membrane and/or Golgi staining for CD30.

Hodgkin's disease (305). Recently a paraffin section-reactive antibody has been produced against the chimeric protein (a protein kinase, p80) associated with t(2;5) (384a).

Molecular and Cytogenetic Findings. Although T-cell tumors often show rearrangements of the T-cell receptor genes and B-cell tumors rearrangements of the immunoglobulin genes, some anaplastic large cell lymphomas lack rearrangements of either gene type, show rearrangements of both, or show a discrepancy between the immunophenotype and genotype (327,356,358,393).

A characteristic chromosomal abnormality detected in some cases of anaplastic large cell lymphoma is translocation involving 5q35, usually in the form of t(2;5) (289,314,319,320,350, 359,373,392). This translocation appears to be largely specific for CD30-positive lymphomas (including those with anaplastic large cell and nonanaplastic large cell morphology). Previously reported examples of "malignant histiocytosis" exhibiting this translocation have been reinterpreted as CD30-positive large cell lymphomas (288,337,350). However, t(2;5) has also been occasionally reported in CD30-negative large cell lymphomas, including those of B-cell and null-cell lineage (381,392). The t(2;5) translocation results in the juxtaposition of the nucleophosmin gene (*NPM,* a nucleolar phosphoprotein gene) on chromosome 5q35 with anaplastic lymphoma kinase gene (*ALK,* a tyrosine kinase gene) on chromosome 2p23. The *ALK* gene is normally not transcribed in lymphoid cells, but the t(2;5) translocation results in a chimeric *NPM-ALK* gene and therefore aberrant production of the *ALK* fusion product (354). The breakpoints of the t(2;5) translocation appear to consistently involve the same introns of the *NPM* and *ALK* genes, leading to identical junctions in the chimeric mRNAs. Successful cloning of the translocated genes now permits the chromosomal translocation to be detected by Southern blot analysis or an RNA-based polymerase chain reaction. The t(2;5) translocation occurs in only a proportion of cases of anaplastic large cell lymphoma, predominantly those of T-cell or null-cell type (304). The frequency as determined by molecular analysis is approximately 12 percent in adult-predominant series (292a,348), and about 50 percent in child-predominant series (394a).

Other cytogenetic abnormalities have also been reported in anaplastic large cell lymphoma, such as 6q abnormalities, complex hyperdiploid karyotypes, and breakpoints at 14q32 or 2p12 (304,343,362,387).

Although immunoreactive p53 protein is detectable in 80 percent of anaplastic large cell lymphomas, structural alterations of the p53 gene are rare (6 percent) (296,308). C-*myc* gene abnormalities (mutation, translocation, or amplification) are detected in 32 percent of cases, and the positive cases are often of B lineage (328). On the other hand, bcl-2, K-*ras*, N-*ras,* and H-*ras* genes are not structurally altered (328).

Differential Diagnosis. Anaplastic large cell lymphoma must be distinguished from carcinoma or melanoma, for obvious reasons. This diagnosis should certainly be suspected or considered for any "undifferentiated carcinoma" of unknown primary or in young patients. A histologic clue to the diagnosis is the basophilia (plasmacytoid appearance) of the cytoplasm. Immunohistochemical studies are most helpful. However, the possibility of anaplastic large cell lymphoma cannot be dismissed by a negative leukocyte common antigen (CD45RB) reaction; application of further antibodies such as CD30, T-cell markers, and B-cell markers is advisable (299,313).

The borderline between conventional large cell lymphoma (particularly immunoblastic type) and anaplastic large cell lymphoma is not sharp, but the following features favor a diagnosis of the latter: large to giant size of all the neoplastic cells; nuclear pleomorphism, with significant variation in the shape of the nuclei; multiple medium-sized to large nucleoli; and abundant cytoplasm. A distinction should be made, since anaplastic large cell lymphoma has a supposed better prognosis (301,356). The exception is cutaneous lymphoma, because collaborative studies from Europe have shown that all cutaneous CD30-positive large cell lymphomas, irrespective of anaplastic or nonanaplastic morphology, have a similar favorable prognosis (versus CD30-negative ones) (287,362,395).

Distinction between anaplastic large cell lymphoma and Hodgkin's disease (especially the syncytial variant of the nodular sclerosis and lymphocyte depletion types) can be difficult. In fact, these two entities may lie on a continuous spectrum, with overlapping and borderline cases (340). The presence of a pure sinusoidal pattern favors a diagnosis of anaplastic large cell lymphoma, as does a more "sheet-like" growth of large neoplastic cells, at least focally; sparse or absent diagnostic Reed-Sternberg cells; and a more prominent pale Golgi zone. Immunohistochemical studies can be helpful (Table 9-6), although the immunophenotype can be indeterminate and therefore inconclusive.

Although anaplastic large cell lymphoma was often diagnosed in the past as malignant histiocytosis, the latter diagnosis is rarely made today. Bona fide malignant histiocytosis can be diagnosed with certainty only when fully supported by immunohistochemical and genotypic analyses (see chapter 18).

Although regressing atypical histiocytosis was originally considered to be a benign condition characterized by self-regressing large nodulo-ulcerative skin lesions (315,324), this entity is now widely believed to be a T-lineage anaplastic large cell lymphoma involving skin (fig. 9-71) (332,339,355). This is supported by subsequent recurrence and dissemination of the disease in most cases and the demonstration of clonal T-cell populations

Table 9-6

**IMMUNOPHENOTYPIC DIFFERENCES BETWEEN ANAPLASTIC
LARGE CELL LYMPHOMA AND CLASSIC HODGKIN'S DISEASE**

	Anaplastic Large Cell Lymphoma	Classic Hodgkin's Disease
Leukocyte common antigen (CD45RB)	Usually positive	Usually negative
CD15	Usually negative	Usually positive
CD30	Usually positive	Usually positive
Epithelial membrane antigen	Usually positive	Usually negative
T-cell markers	Often positive (~60 percent of cases)	Usually negative
B-cell markers	Positive in ~20 percent of cases	Occasional cells may be positive in some cases, particularly CD20
BNH.9*	Usually positive	Usually negative

* BNH.9 is a monoclonal antibody recognizing the blood group H and Y determinants (307).

(323,329). The tendency to regress spontaneously in the initial course of disease is also in keeping with the known natural history of cutaneous anaplastic large cell lymphoma (299).

The relationship between lymphomatoid papulosis and anaplastic large cell lymphoma is more controversial. Lymphomatoid papulosis is a recurrent self-healing cutaneous eruption (usually in the form of multiple papules of less than 2 cm) which is histologically malignant but clinically benign (391,396). Disseminated lymphoma has been documented to supervene in some cases (332,380). There are two histologic subtypes, one composed of anaplastic large lymphoid cells or even Reed-Sternberg–like cells mixed with inflammatory cells (type A), and the other composed mostly of lymphoid cells with cerebriform nuclei similar to those seen in the large cell variant of mycosis fungoides (type B) (396). The infiltrate in the dermis is usually dense and wedge shaped, and often invades the overlying epidermis (398). The histologic features of type A cases can be indistinguishable from anaplastic large cell lymphoma involving skin, although the clinical history and the small size of the lesions favor a diagnosis of lymphomatoid papulosis. The lymphoid infiltrate of lymphomatoid papulosis comprises mostly T cells, with frequent expression of CD30 (331,332,338,370,371). Genotypic studies have demonstrated clonal T-cell populations in most cases (334,394). Thus, at least some cases

of lymphomatoid papulosis may be viewed as a cutaneous anaplastic large cell lymphoma with a striking tendency to undergo regression and relapse (299,339). Some authors, however, consider lymphomatoid papulosis a non-neoplastic lesion related to pityriasis lichenoides (398).

Treatment and Prognosis. Despite the anaplastic cytology, anaplastic large cell lymphoma is not necessarily aggressive. In fact, several studies have shown this lymphoma to have a better outcome than other aggressive lymphomas, with overall survival of 50 to 60 percent (286,342,345, 353,356,359,365,381,385), although one study showed no difference in survival (368). Long-term survivals of 14 to 25 years have been reported despite the development of multiple recurrences in some patients (356,379).

Cutaneous involvement alone at presentation is associated with a highly favorable prognosis, and spontaneous regression is not uncommonly observed (299,342,345,395). Children appear to respond to treatment particularly well: the reported 5-year survival rate is greater than 80 percent, even including those with advanced stage disease (320,345,356,372,381). Complete remission is more common and the median survival is significantly longer in primary anaplastic large cell lymphoma compared with the secondary type (345) and high-stage disease is correlated with a lower probability of survival and a shorter remission duration (301,320,342,385).

Some studies suggest that cytologic subtyping of anaplastic large cell lymphoma may have prognostic relevance, a finding that requires confirmation by larger studies (299,301). Type I or group B, the more aggressive subtype, is characterized by a monomorphic population of cells with oval nuclei, relatively pale cytoplasm, infrequent paranuclear hof, and infrequent multinucleated forms (fig. 9-69). Type II or group A, the more favorable subtype, is characterized by pleomorphic cells with embryo-like nuclei, a prominent pale Golgi zone, deeply basophilic cytoplasm, and frequent multinucleated forms (figs. 9-67, 9-70).

Despite good initial response, radiotherapy alone fails to result in lasting remission (387). Therefore, aggressive chemotherapy is preferred (365). Since cutaneous disease may regress spontaneously and is associated with a good prognosis, a conservative approach may be adopted if there is no extracutaneous involvement and there is a history of regression. If the skin lesion is a new occurrence in a patient, it may be observed for several weeks for possible spontaneous regression before deciding whether or not to treat. However, for patients with extracutaneous involvement or noncutaneous presentation, prompt treatment by aggressive chemotherapy is indicated (299,342). Bone marrow transplant has been found to be an effective salvage therapy; 13-cis-retinoic acid, which has been reported to result in remission of chemotherapy-resistant cases, may also be considered as salvage therapy (302). In vitro studies suggest that retinoic acid causes upregulation of the retinoic acid receptor gene followed by activation of transforming growth factor β1, which in turn leads to apoptosis (333,388).

Variants of Anaplastic Large Cell Lymphoma

Lymphohistiocytic T-Cell Lymphoma. This uncommon type of lymphoma, considered by Pileri et al. (366) to be a variant of anaplastic large cell lymphoma with a high content of reactive nonepithelioid histiocytes, is more appropriately viewed as a peculiar form of post-thymic T-cell lymphoma. The large neoplastic cells (CD30 positive) do not have an anaplastic appearance and are intermingled with small and medium-sized neoplastic cells in addition to large numbers of reactive histiocytes (345). This

type of lymphoma occurs predominantly in young patients, who present with systemic symptoms and superficial lymphadenopathy. The disease responds well to aggressive chemotherapy. Recently, this tumor was also reported to occur in older patients (367). Since B-cell and null-cell variants are recognized, the term "lymphohistiocytic T-cell lymphoma" is inappropriate. Pileri et al. suggest the alternative designation, "anaplastic large cell lymphoma, lymphohistiocytic type" (367).

Small Cell Variant of CD30-Positive T-Cell Lymphoma. This variant shows many clinical and biologic similarities to anaplastic large cell lymphoma (340): it occurs predominantly in children and young adults; cutaneous involvement is frequently part of disseminated disease; the t(2;5) translocation is present; and some cases eventually evolve to a typical CD30-positive anaplastic large cell lymphoma.

However, since the CD30-positive cells are in the minority and do not have an anaplastic appearance, this lymphoma can also be viewed merely as a form of pleomorphic T-cell lymphoma. The reported actuarial 2-year disease-free survival is 14 percent and overall survival is 51 percent. Histologically, the lymph node shows partial or complete effacement of architecture, with predominance of small lymphoid cells with irregular ("cerebriform") nuclear membranes and dense chromatin. Scattered throughout are isolated small clusters of nonanaplastic large cells with more open chromatin and clear to weakly basophilic cytoplasm (fig. 9-73). The large cells are often accentuated around the venules. Both the small and large lymphoid cells show reactivity for T-cell markers (frequently with an "aberrant immunophenotype"), but only the large cells show CD30 positivity.

Anaplastic Large Cell Lymphoma, Hodgkin's-Like. This lymphoma is histologically characterized by overlapping features of nodular sclerosis Hodgkin's disease (nodule formation and fibrous bands) and the usual form of anaplastic large cell lymphoma (large anaplastic cells, cohesive of groups of tumor cells, and sinusoidal infiltration) (365,387). It is currently unclear as to whether it is biologically more related to the former or the latter, but the immunophenotype more closely resembles that of anaplastic large cell lymphoma. Some examples of the syncytial variant or

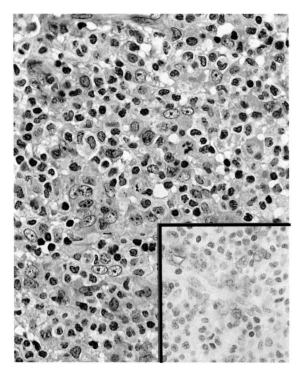

Figure 9-73
SMALL CELL PREDOMINANT
CD30-POSITIVE T-CELL LYMPHOMA
Among the small lymphoid cells with irregularly folded nuclei, there are small numbers of nonanaplastic large nuclei with distinct nucleoli. Inset: The large cell population is best shown by immunostaining for CD30. There is accentuation of large cells around the blood vessels.

the British National Lymphoma Investigation (BNLI) grade 2 nodular sclerosis Hodgkin's disease may also represent this entity.

Clinically, mediastinal involvement is common, often with bulky disease. There is preliminary evidence that the disease responds to treatment protocols used for aggressive non-Hodgkin's lymphoma but not to Hodgkin's disease protocols (365,387).

T-Cell–Rich Large B-Cell Lymphoma

Definition. T-cell–rich large B-cell lymphoma (TCRBL) is a neoplastic proliferation of large B cells associated with a prominent component of reactive T lymphocytes (constituting greater than 50 percent of the cellular population) (405,413, 418,420). These features have to be present throughout the entire lesion, to exclude examples of partial involvement of lymph node by a usual large B-cell lymphoma (405). One study requires

more than 90 percent T lymphocytes for inclusion under this category (417).

Some cases reported as TCRBL are small cell rather than large cell lymphomas (409,417). It is unclear whether "histiocyte-rich B-cell lymphoma" is a variant of TCRBL or is a paragranuloma type of lymphocyte predominance Hodgkin's disease (401).

Some authors suggest categorizing TCRBL under "diffuse mixed cell lymphoma" in the Working Formulation because this is a purely morphologic scheme (402,405), but we and others prefer placing it under the "diffuse large cell" category because only the large cell component is neoplastic (415,416).

Although it is currently unclear whether TCRBL is biologically different from conventional large B-cell lymphoma, it merits consideration in a separate section because of the diagnostic problems it poses.

Incidence. The exact incidence of TCRBL is unknown, in part due to lack of agreed definition. In one study, it comprises approximately 1 percent of all lymphomas (399); in another, it accounts for 8.4 percent of all B-cell lymphomas (413).

Clinical Features. TCRBL occurs predominantly in older adults (mean age 56 years), although younger patients can also be affected (399,400,405,408,409,413,416,417). There is a slight male predominance. The patients present with lymphadenopathy, but extranodal presentation also occurs. The disease is usually at high stage at presentation: more than 60 percent of patients present with stage III or IV disease. Spleen and bone marrow involvement are common (400,413,418,419).

Microscopic Findings. The infiltrate is usually diffuse, but a focal follicular or interfollicular growth pattern can be observed. The infiltrate comprises a mixture of lymphoid cells, and the large cell population can be inconspicuous (figs. 9-74–9-76). The small lymphoid cells (usually of T lineage) have dark round, irregular, or convoluted nuclei (figs. 9-75, 9-76). There can even be medium-sized cells with round or folded nuclei (mostly of T lineage) (fig. 9-76). Interspersed throughout are isolated or small clusters of large lymphoid cells with a broad range of appearances (figs. 9-74–9-78). In some cases, they are indistinguishable from large noncleaved cells (centroblasts) or immunoblasts; in other cases, they

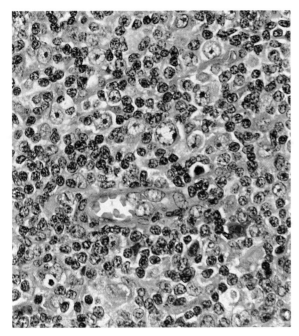

Figure 9-74
T-CELL–RICH LARGE B-CELL LYMPHOMA
The diffuse infiltrate comprises atypical large lymphoid cells dispersed in a background of small lymphocytes. (Figures 9-74, 9-79, and 9-80 are from the same case.)

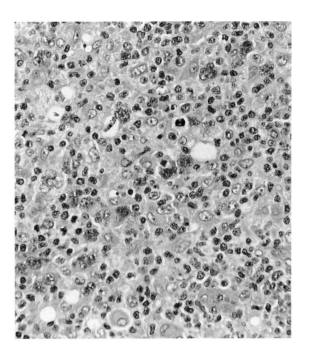

Figure 9-75
T-CELL–RICH LARGE B-CELL LYMPHOMA
In this example, the neoplastic large cells (B lineage) have irregularly folded nuclei and coarse chromatin.

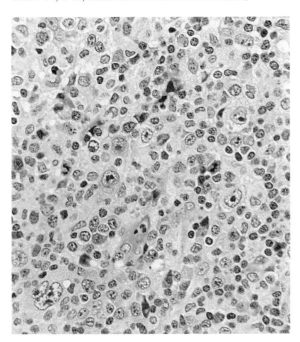

Figure 9-76
T-CELL–RICH LARGE B-CELL LYMPHOMA
There is a diffuse mixed cell infiltrate comprising small lymphoid cells and atypical large cells. Many of the background small lymphoid cells have an activated appearance (nuclei slightly larger and more irregular than those of small lymphocytes), and occasional medium-sized cells are seen. Morphologic distinction from a post-thymic T-cell lymphoma cannot be made.

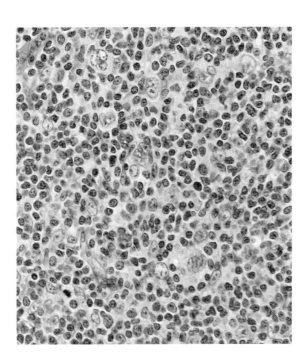

Figure 9-77
T-CELL–RICH LARGE B-CELL LYMPHOMA
The large cells show atypia in the form of irregular nuclear foldings and lobation; they resemble L&H cells of nodular lymphocyte predominance Hodgkin's disease.

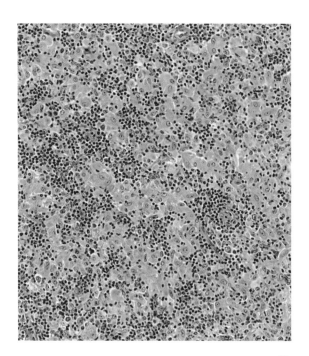
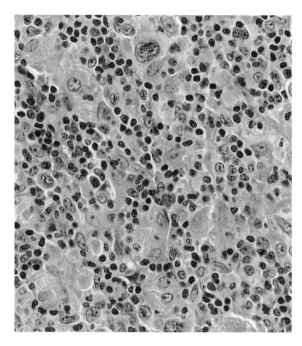

Figure 9-78
T-CELL–RICH LARGE B-CELL LYMPHOMA MIMICKING LENNERT'S LYMPHOMA
Left: This example is associated with numerous small aggregates of epithelioid histiocytes, mimicking the pattern of Lennert's lymphoma.
Right: Between the epithelioid histiocytes, isolated atypical large lymphoid cells (shown to be of B-cell lineage) are dispersed among small lymphocytes (mostly T-cell lineage).

possess irregularly folded or multilobated nuclei, vesicular or coarse chromatin, prominent nucleoli, and moderate to abundant amphophilic cytoplasm. There can be multinucleated forms resembling Reed-Sternberg cells.

High endothelial venules may or may not be prominent, but can be so striking as to mimic angioimmunoblastic lymphadenopathy–like T-cell lymphoma. Variable numbers of histiocytes, which may have an epithelioid appearance, are often intermingled, and a pattern mimicking lymphoepithelioid (Lennert's) lymphoma can occur. Plasma cells and eosinophils are prominent in some cases.

Immunologic Findings. Immunohistochemical studies reveal large numbers of T cells (more than 50 percent by definition, and often more than 70 percent) and scattered B cells (405,418). Suboptimal cytologic preservation in cryostat sections makes interpretation of the immunohistochemical staining difficult. In general, the T-cell antibodies stain the smaller cells, whereas the B-cell antibodies stain the larger ones. The

T cells are immunophenotypically normal, with CD4-positive cells usually predominating over CD8-positive cells. Correlation of cytology with the results of immunostaining is better achieved by applying the leukocyte antibodies on paraffin sections (417,420). Practically all the large atypical cells stain with the B markers, such as L26 (CD20), 4KB5 (CD45RA), mb-1 (CD79a), MB1 (CD45RA), MB2, LN1 (CDw75), or LN2 (CD74) (399,400,405,413). The background small lymphocytes are immunoreactive with T-cell markers such as MT1/Leu-22/L60 (CD43), UCHL1 (CD45RO), and CD3 (fig. 9-79). In many cases, monotypic surface or cytoplasmic immunoglobulin can be demonstrated on frozen and paraffin sections, respectively, thus confirming the neoplastic nature of the lymphoid proliferation (fig. 9-80) (409,413). Problems in interpretation of immunoglobulin immunohistochemistry related to the passive uptake of interstitial immunoglobulin can often be circumvented by in situ hybridization for immunoglobulin mRNA. The large cells are usually CD30 negative (400,405,408,413).

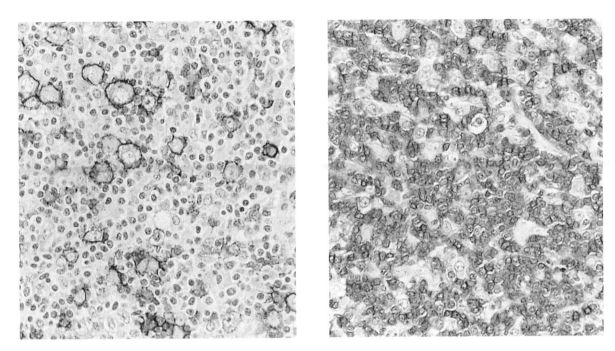

Figure 9-79

T-CELL–RICH LARGE B-CELL LYMPHOMA

Left: Only the scattered large cells stain with L26 (CD20).
Right: Most of the small lymphoid cells stain with UCHL1 (CD45RO), but the large cells are negative.

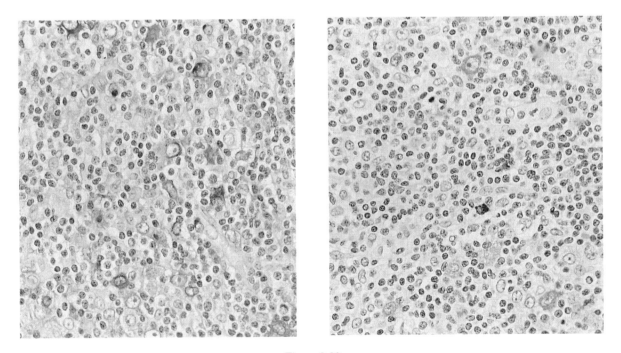

Figure 9-80

T-CELL–RICH LARGE B-CELL LYMPHOMA

Left: Most of the large cells show Golgi (dot) or perinuclear staining for kappa light chain.
Right: Some plasma cells stain for lambda light chain, whereas the large cells lack Golgi or perinuclear staining. Occasional large lymphoid cells show weak, diffuse cytoplasmic staining for lambda light chain, a phenomenon which can be due to absorption of immunoglobulin from the interstitium. This case should be interpreted as showing kappa light chain restriction.

Staining for epithelial membrane antigen is reported to be common in one study (400), but not in others (405,409,414).

Genotypic Findings. Genotypic analysis by the Southern blot technique or polymerase chain reaction has demonstrated rearrangements of the heavy and light chain immunoglobulin genes, but not the T-cell receptor genes (408,414,416). The rearranged immunoglobulin gene band on Southern blot analysis is usually faint compared with the germline band, because the neoplastic cells constitute only a minor population (409). Occasionally, rearrangements of immunoglobulin genes may not be detectable because of the low concentrations of neoplastic cells in the samples (409,416,417). There may be decreased intensity of the germline band of the T-cell receptor gene, indicating polyclonal T-cell proliferation.

In some cases, the *bcl*-2 gene is rearranged, suggesting that these cases may be related to follicular lymphoma (405,409,416). Epstein-Barr virus DNA has been detected in the neoplastic cells in a small proportion of cases (400,408).

Differential Diagnosis. It is most important to distinguish TCRBL from reactive immunoblastic proliferations such as infectious mononucleosis and viral infection. A distinction may be impossible, and immunohistochemical or genotypic studies are mandatory in such cases. Consistent staining of most or all of the large cells for B markers strongly favors a diagnosis of TCRBL over infectious mononucleosis (in which the blasts are predominantly T cells or a mixture of T and B cells), particularly when further supported by the demonstration of light chain restriction. In other cases, a diagnosis of lymphoma is more readily made on morphologic grounds because of definite atypia, such as multilobation and marked irregular nuclear contours, in a significant proportion of the large cells.

Distinguishing TCRBL from post-thymic T-cell lymphoma is often difficult, if not impossible, on morphologic grounds (412). In fact, many reported cases of TCRBL are identified from retrospective analysis of lymphomas diagnosed initially as post-thymic T-cell lymphomas (408–410, 417). It is important to distinguish the two because some studies suggest that post-thymic T-cell lymphomas are more aggressive (409). Lymphoid cells showing a continuous range of size and nuclear irregularity, features considered to be characteristic of post-

thymic T-cell lymphoma, can also be observed in TCRBL. Therefore, immunohistochemical or genotypic studies are required for distinction. The demonstration of an aberrant T-cell immunophenotype on frozen section immunohistochemistry favors a diagnosis of post-thymic T-cell lymphoma. One potential pitfall of immunohistochemical studies is that the B-cell proliferation that accompanies some post-thymic T-cell lymphomas may lead to an erroneous interpretation of TCRBL; the isolated immunoblasts in such cases do not exhibit nuclear atypia, have a more patchy distribution (particularly in the vicinity of reactive lymphoid follicles), and show polytypic staining for immunoglobulin.

TCRBL can be difficult to distinguish from classic Hodgkin's disease. In general, the nucleoli of the large cells of TCRBL are not as big as those in Reed-Sternberg cells and variants, and diagnostic Reed-Sternberg cells are rarely found. The background small lymphocytes in Hodgkin's disease rarely show the nuclear irregularities and activation commonly seen in TCRBL. Immunohistochemical studies are most helpful in the differential diagnosis (Table 9-7).

Distinction of TCRBL from diffuse lymphocyte predominance Hodgkin's disease is difficult, if not impossible, when the large cells are lobated, resembling lymphocytic and histiocytic (L&H) cells. The large cells in both entities are of B lineage, and the background is often rich in T cells, even for diffuse lymphocyte predominance Hodgkin's disease (in contrast to the nodular subtype). The presence of large numbers of Leu-7 (CD57)-positive cells rosetting around the large cells is a feature favoring a diagnosis of lymphocyte predominance Hodgkin's disease (404).

Treatment and Prognosis. Although some studies have shown that large numbers of reactive T lymphocytes are associated with a better prognosis in B-cell lymphomas (411), the issue has not been fully addressed for the diffuse large B-cell lymphomas. In one study, the percentage of T lymphocytes (CD2-positive) did not correlate with relapse-free survival (407). Current evidence suggests that TCRBL behaves and responds to therapy like conventional diffuse large B-cell lymphomas (418). Patients treated with single or triple agent chemotherapy usually relapse despite initial remission (409). Those given chemotherapy consisting of four or more drugs often achieve complete remission, although

Table 9-7

IMMUNOPHENOTYPIC DIFFERENCES BETWEEN T-CELL–RICH LARGE B-CELL LYMPHOMA AND CLASSIC HODGKIN'S DISEASE*

	Large Cells in T-Cell–Rich Large B-Cell Lymphoma	Reed-Sternberg Cells and Variants in Classic Hodgkin's Disease
Leukocyte common antigen (CD45RB)	Usually positive	Usually negative
B-cell markers	Positive	In some cases, a variable (usually small) proportion of Reed-Sternberg cells may be positive, especially for CD20
Cytoplasmic immunoglobulin	Monotypic immunoglobulin is demonstrable in many cases	Same cell staining for both kappa and lambda light chains (due to uptake of immunoglobulin from surroundings)
CD30	Usually negative	Usually positive
CD15	Usually negative	Usually positive
Epithelial membrane antigen	Sometimes positive	Usually negative

* The background is rich in T lymphocytes in both conditions.

some eventually relapse. According to one study, the overall actuarial survival at 10 years is 73 percent, and the disease-free survival is 37.5 percent (409). Patients with TCRBL should therefore be treated as for aggressive non-Hodgkin's lymphoma (405,418). One study suggests that TCRBL responds poorly to therapy conventionally given for Hodgkin's disease (400).

Is TCRBL a Distinct Entity? It is currently unclear whether TCRBL is a distinct entity or simply an unusual morphologic manifestation of conventional large B-cell lymphoma. Although some authors favor the former hypothesis (399), most believe that TCRBL is a heterogeneous entity encompassing follicular center cell lymphoma and nonfollicular center large B-cell lymphoma (405,409,413,415,416). The relationship with follicular lymphoma in some cases is supported by the occasional occurrence of a follicular pattern (403,405,415), relapse as follicular small cleaved cell lymphoma (366), and demonstration of *bcl*-2 gene rearrangements (405,409).

The florid T-cell reaction can often be demonstrated in the different sites of involvement (405, 413,418). However, the tumor can evolve into a conventional diffuse large cell lymphoma with loss of the T-cell reaction (402,409,416,418,419). Occasionally, a conventional diffuse large B-cell lymphoma relapses as TCRBL (420).

Alternative hypotheses have been proposed for the prominent T-cell infiltrate in addition to a host reaction. The T cells can conceivably be attracted to the vicinity by cytokines secreted by the neoplastic B cells (413). Lennert and Feller (406) propose that the T cells may be neoplastic and that the T-cell neoplasm may induce a monotypic proliferation of blast cells of B-cell type; this suggestion, however, is not supported by the genotypic findings. The relationship and overlap of TCRBL with the diffuse paragranuloma type of lymphocyte predominance Hodgkin's disease remain to be clarified (419).

Mediastinal Large B-Cell Lymphoma

Definition. This is a diffuse large cell non-Hodgkin's lymphoma of B lineage, presenting primarily with anterior mediastinal involvement. An origin in the thymus gland can be demonstrated in at least some cases (423). This entity is also commonly known as *mediastinal large cell lymphoma with sclerosis,* with the latter qualification emphasizing the frequent prominence of stromal sclerosis (437,438,443). Although mediastinal large B-cell lymphomas may be cytologically indistinguishable from large cell lymphomas of other sites, they merit separate consideration because of their distinctive clinicopathologic and immunohistochemical features.

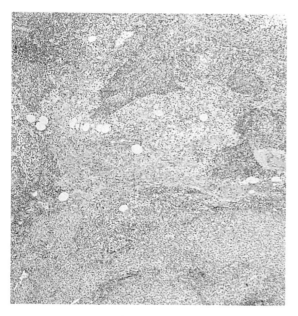

Figure 9-81
MEDIASTINAL LARGE B-CELL LYMPHOMA
The thymus (top) is involved by lymphoma (bottom).

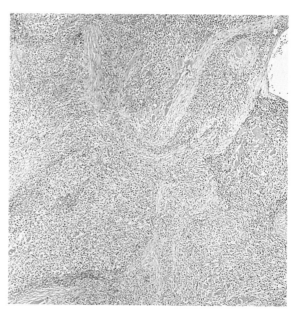

Figure 9-82
MEDIASTINAL LARGE B-CELL LYMPHOMA
Sclerotic bands traverse the tumor to produce nodules of variable sizes. An epithelium-lined cyst is seen on the top; this is a common finding in thymic lymphoma.

Incidence. Primary mediastinal large cell lymphoma is uncommon, accounting for 0.9 to 3.7 percent of all non-Hodgkin's lymphomas (429,430,440), and 2.4 to 6.5 percent of all large cell lymphomas (426,432,440,444).

Clinical Features. This lymphoma characteristically occurs in young adults (mean age, 32 years), although older adults are also affected. There is a female predominance, with a male to female ratio of approximately 1 to 2 (421–423, 427,428,430,432,435,437,439,441,443,444,446). The patients usually present with symptoms of superior vena cava obstruction or symptoms related to the mediastinal mass, such as cough, dyspnea, chest pain, and chest discomfort (421, 432,437). Pleural and pericardial effusions are also common. A small proportion of patients may have systemic symptoms (422,435). In others, the mediastinal mass is discovered incidentally. The tumor is usually large, and often invades the surrounding structures such as the pericardium, pleura, lung, trachea, sternum, and chest wall.

Microscopic Findings. Mediastinal large B-cell lymphoma exhibits diffuse infiltrative growth, permeating the fibrofatty tissue of the anterior mediastinum (fig. 9-81). In rare cases,

the tumor is confined predominantly to the medulla of the thymus (423). Sclerosis is often prominent, taking the form of hyaline twigs that compartmentalize the tumor cells into alveolar packets and cords, delicate interstitial fibrils intimately interspersed among tumor cells, and broad sclerotic bands (figs. 9-82, 9-83) (433,437).

The neoplastic cells possess medium-sized to large nuclei which can be round, oval, irregularly folded, elongated, multilobated, or multinucleated (435). The chromatin is vesicular or granular, and single or multiple distinct nucleoli are often observed. The cells may appear uniform or show significant pleomorphism (fig. 9-84). Frequently, there is a voluminous or moderate amount of pale to clear cytoplasm (fig. 9-84B), which has led some authors to adopt the nomenclature of *mediastinal clear cell lymphoma* (433). However, the cytoplasmic clearing appears to be an artifact of formalin fixation, because it is usually not evident in tissues fixed in B5 or Zenker's fixative (437). In other cases, the cytoplasm is amphophilic and less abundant, and the cells are cytologically indistinguishable from

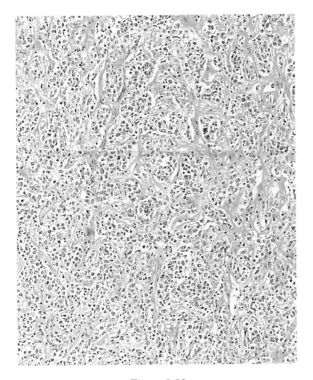

Figure 9-83
MEDIASTINAL LARGE B-CELL LYMPHOMA
Narrow sclerotic bands divide the tumor into packets.

large noncleaved cells (centroblasts). The neoplastic cells can be intermingled with variable numbers of small lymphocytes (which can be aggregated around the capillaries) and reactive histiocytes (437). Rare cases show prominent tropism for the reactive germinal centers (442).

Necrosis is common, and can be extensive. The subintima and walls of the large blood vessels are often permeated by lymphoma cells. There may be islands of residual thymic epithelium interspersed throughout the tumor or scattered at the periphery (figs. 9-81, 9-85). The thymic epithelium may undergo hyperplasia, forming irregular anastomosing strands or epithelium-lined cystic spaces (figs. 9-82; 9-85, left) (423, 437). It can also be infiltrated by the lymphoma cells (fig. 9-85, right).

Immunologic Findings. Most mediastinal large cell lymphomas are B-cell neoplasms; well-documented examples of T lineage tumors are rare (445,446). The mediastinal B-cell lymphomas are postulated to arise from the thymic B cells normally residing in the medulla, which are CD19+, CD20+, CD21-, CD22+, IgM+, and IgD+, and apparently unrelated to follicular center cells and mantle cells (424,425).

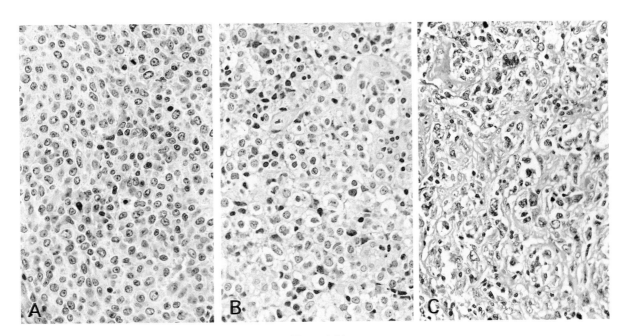

Figure 9-84
MEDIASTINAL LARGE B-CELL LYMPHOMA
A: In this example, the lymphoma cells are medium sized and appear monomorphous.
B: In this example, most of the cells have clear cytoplasm.
C: This case has a polymorphic appearance, with significant variation in the size of the tumor cells. Note the stromal sclerosis.

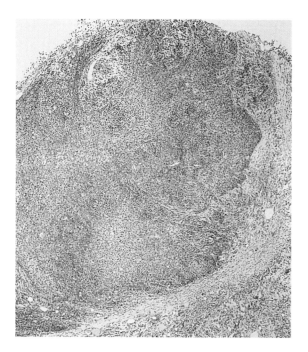 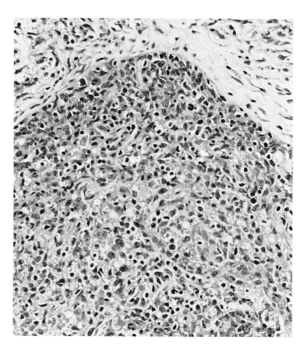

Figure 9-85
MEDIASTINAL LARGE B-CELL LYMPHOMA
Left: The islands of thymic epithelium can show remarkable proliferation around the neoplasm.
Right: In this case, the proliferated thymic epithelium is infiltrated by lymphoma cells.

Mediastinal large B-cell lymphomas stain with the various B-cell markers such as CD19, CD20, CD22, and CD37 (422,439,441,446). They are CD5-, CD21-, and CD10-, and often fail to express surface and cytoplasmic immunoglobulin (422,427,431,434,435,439). Surface immunoglobulin, if present, is usually of IgG or IgA type (427,430). The immunophenotypic profile therefore does not correspond to that of follicular center cells or immunoblasts, but closely resembles thymic B cells except for frequent lack of immunoglobulin expression. Most cases are CD25- and CD30- (422,435), and some are CD11c+ (434).

Lamarre et al. (427) postulated that mediastinal large B-cell lymphoma includes two distinct disease entities: immunoglobulin-negative tumors, which occur almost exclusively in young women and may originate from thymic B cells; and immunoglobulin-positive tumors, which occur in older men, and merely represent conventional large B-cell lymphomas that happen to involve predominantly mediastinal lymph nodes.

Moller et al. (434,435) postulated that these neoplastic cells correspond to a terminal step of B-cell differentiation in view of the expression of the plasma cell–associated marker PC-1, and suggested a relationship with marginal zone cell lymphoma.

Immunostaining for cytokeratin can reveal a surprisingly large number of positive cells in the form of irregular networks, which represent residual or hyperplastic thymic epithelium (437). These positive cells may lead to an erroneous interpretation of thymoma or thymic carcinoma, but careful attention to the cytology of the cytokeratin-positive cells reveals that they are not neoplastic.

Genotypic Findings. The B-cell nature of mediastinal large B-cell lymphoma is confirmed by the demonstration of rearrangements of the heavy and light chain immunoglobulin genes (427,438,439). In a study of six cases from Italy, c-*myc* gene alteration in the form of mutations or rearrangements was detected in three cases (439). Lack of rearrangement of the *bcl*-2 gene does not support a relationship with follicular lymphoma, although the number of cases studied is small (439). Epstein-Barr virus DNA sequences have not been detected by Southern blot hybridization technique (436,439).

Differential Diagnosis. It is important not to mistake the potentially curable mediastinal large cell lymphoma for thymic carcinoma. These tumors were commonly confused before the advent of immunohistochemical studies. Histologic features favoring a diagnosis of lymphoma over thymic carcinoma are lack of cohesive growth pattern, significant nuclear irregularities, and mural involvement of blood vessels. In case of doubt, immunohistochemical studies can readily clarify the diagnosis.

Some cases of Hodgkin's disease may be difficult to distinguish from mediastinal large B-cell lymphoma. This is particularly true with the syncytial variant of nodular sclerosis Hodgkin's disease, in which there are monotonous sheets of lacunar cells. In Hodgkin's disease, the neoplastic cells are generally larger; the nucleoli are more prominent; there is intermingling with eosinophils and neutrophils, at least in areas; and the immunophenotype is CD45-, CD15+, CD30+, and CD20± (Table 9-7).

Anaplastic large cell lymphoma, which can occur in the mediastinum, is distinguished from mediastinal large B-cell lymphoma by the larger size of the tumor cells, more bizarre nuclear features, and frequent CD30 expression.

Mediastinal large B-cell lymphoma can simulate seminoma by virtue of the packeting growth and cytoplasmic clearing. Irregular foldings of the nuclear membrane and lack of demonstrable glycogen strongly favor the former diagnosis, which can be confirmed by immunohistochemical studies.

Natural History, Treatment, and Prognosis. The extensive local infiltrative growth may involve vital structures in the thoracic cavity and mediastinum (such as heart, great vessels, lung, trachea, and esophagus) contributing to the morbidity and mortality of mediastinal large B-cell lymphoma. There is a tendency for the tumor to metastasize to unusual sites such as kidney, adrenal, and liver, while often sparing the bone marrow and peripheral lymph nodes (421,428, 431,432,437,443). Poor prognostic factors are large tumor size (greater than 10 cm), failure to achieve complete remission, and recurrence of tumor (426,437); age below 25 years and presence of tumor outside the thoracic cavity at presentation have been identifiied in one study to be associated with a worse prognosis (437), but not in another study (426).

According to some series, mediastinal large B-cell lymphoma is a highly aggressive lymphoma with a bad prognosis, because the tumor is often resistant to chemotherapy or radiotherapy, and the remission achieved is usually incomplete and short-lived (428,430,432,435,444). However, recent studies suggest that combined aggressive chemotherapy and involved-field radiation (dose approximately 40 Gy) can result in cure in a significant proportion of patients (422, 426,439,443). The complete remission rate ranges from 60 to 87 percent (422,426,442), and the actuarial 5-year survival is reported to be 57 percent (427). Patients who fail to achieve remission usually die within 2 years.

REFERENCES

Diffuse Large Cell Lymphoma

1. Aisenberg AC. Malignant lymphoma: biology, natural history, and treatment. Philadelphia: Lea & Febiger, 1991:111–310.
2. _____, Wilkes BM, Jacobson JO. The bcl-2 gene is rearranged in many diffuse B-cell lymphomas. Blood 1988;71:969–72.
3. _____, Wilkes BM, Jacobson JO, Harris NL. Immunoglobulin gene rearrangements in adult non-Hodgkin's lymphoma. Am J Med 1987;82:738–44.
4. Armitage JO. Treatment of non-Hodgkin's lymphoma. N Engl J Med 1993;328:1023–30.
5. _____, Cheson BD. Interpretation of clinical trials in diffuse large cell lymphoma. J Clin Oncol 1988;6: 1335–47.
6. _____, Dick FR, Corder MP. Diffuse histiocytic lymphoma after histologic conversion: a poor prognostic variant. Cancer Treat Rep 1981;65:413–8.
7. _____, Fyfe MA, Lewis J. Long-term remission durability and functional status of patients treated for diffuse histiocytic lymphoma with the CHOP regimen. J Clin Oncol 1984;2:898–902.
8. Arnold A, Cossman J, Bakhshi A, Jaffe ES, Waldmann TA, Korsmeyer SJ. Immunoglobulin gene rearrangements as unique clonal markers in human lymphoid neoplasms. N Engl J Med 1983;309:1593–9.
9. Bain B, Matutes E, Robinson D, et al. Leukaemia as a manifestation of large cell lymphoma. Br J Haematol 1991;77:301–10.

10. Baron BW, Nuciforma G, McCabe N, Espinosa R III, Le Beau MM, McKeithan TW. Identification of the gene associated with the recurring chromosomal translocations t(3;14)(q27;q32) and t(3;22)(q27;q11) in B-cell lymphomas. Proc Natl Acad Sci 1993;90:5262–6.

11. Bastard C, Deweindt C, Kerchaert JP, et al. LAZ3 rearrangement in non-Hodgkin's lymphoma: correlation with histology, immunophenotype, karyotype and clinical outcome in 217 patients. Blood 1994;83:2423–7.

12. Bertness V, Kirsch I, Hollis G, Johnson B, Bunn PA Jr. T-cell receptor gene rearrangements as clonal markers of human T-cell lymphomas. N Engl J Med 1985;313:534–8.

13. Borowitz MJ, Bousvaros A, Brynes RK, et al. Monoclonal antibody phenotyping of B-cell non-Hodgkin's lymphomas. The Southeastern Cancer Study Group experience. Am J Pathol 1985;121:514–21.

14. Brittinger G, Bartels H, Common H, et al. Clinical and prognostic relevance of the Kiel classification of non-Hodgkin's lymphomas, results of a prospective multicenter study by the Kiel Lymphoma Study Group. Hematol Oncol 1984;2:269–306.

15. Brown DC, Gatter KC. Monoclonal antibody Ki-67: its use in histopathology. Histopathology 1990;17:489–503.

16. Burke JS. The histopathologic classification of non-Hodgkin's lymphomas: ambiguities in the working formulation and two newly reported categories. Semin Oncol 1990;17:3–10.

17. Cabanillas F, Velasquez WS, Hagemeister FB, McLaughlin P, Redman JR. Clinical, biologic, and histologic features of late relapses in diffuse large cell lymphoma. Blood 1992;79:1024–8.

18. Chamulak GA, Brynes RK, Nathwani BN. Kikuchi-Fujimoto disease mimicking malignant lymphoma. Am J Surg Pathol 1990;14:514–23.

19. Chan JK, Ng CS, Isaacson PG. Relationship between high-grade lymphoma and low-grade B-cell mucosa-associated lymphoid tissue lymphoma (MALToma) of the stomach. Am J Pathol 1990;136:1153–64.

20. _____, Saw D. Histiocytic necrotizing lymphadenitis (Kikuchi's disease), a clinicopathologic study of 9 cases. Pathology 1986;18:22–8.

21. _____, Tsang WY, Ng CS, Wong CS, Lo ES. A study of the association of Epstein-Barr virus with Burkitt's lymphoma occurring in an Oriental population. Histopathology 1995;26:239–45..

22. _____, Yip TT, Tsang WY, et al. Detection of Epstein-Barr viral RNA in malignant lymphomas of the upper aerodigestive tract. Am J Surg Pathol 1994; 18:938–46.

23. Childs CC, Parham DM, Berard CW. Infectious mononucleosis. The spectrum of morphologic changes simulating lymphoma in lymph nodes and tonsils. Am J Surg Pathol 1987;11:122–32.

24. Cleary KR, Osborne BM, Butler JJ. Lymph node infarction foreshadowing malignant lymphoma. Am J Surg Pathol 1982;6:435-42.

25. Cleary ML, Chao J, Warnke R, Sklar J. Immunoglobulin gene rearrangement as a diagnostic criterion of B-cell lymphoma. Proc Natl Acad Sci USA 1984;81:593–7.

26. _____, Trela MJ, Weiss LM, Warnke R, Sklar J. Most null large cell lymphomas are B lineage neoplasms. Lab Invest 1985;53:521–5.

27. Cohen JI. Epstein-Barr virus gene expression in lymphoproliferative diseases. Leuk Lymphoma 1991;3:235–40.

28. Coiffier B, Brousse N, Peuchmaur M, et al. Peripheral T-cell lymphomas have a worse prognosis than B-cell lymphomas: a prospective study of 361 immunophenotyped patients treated with the LNH-84 regimen. Ann Oncol 1990;1:45–50.

29. Conlan MG, Bast M, Armitage JO, Weisenburger DD. Bone marrow involvement by non-Hodgkin's lymphoma: the clinical significance of morphologic discordance between the lymph node and bone marrow. Nebraska Lymphoma Study Group. J Clin Oncol 1990;8:1163–72.

30. Cossman J, Jaffe ES, Fisher RI. Immunologic phenotypes of diffuse, aggressive, non-Hodgkin's lymphomas, correlation with clinical features. Cancer 1984;54:1310–7.

31. Dalla-Favera R, Ye RH, Lo Coco F, et al. Identification of genetic lesions associated with diffuse large-cell lymphoma. Ann Oncol 1994;5:S55–60.

32. Danieu L, Wong G, Koziner B, Clarkson B. Predictive model for prognosis in advanced diffuse histiocytic lymphoma. Cancer Res 1986;46:5372–9.

33. DeVita VT Jr, Hubbard SM, Longo DL. The chemotherapy of lymphomas: looking back, moving forward—the Richard and Hinda Rosenthal Foundation Award lecture. Cancer Res 1987;47:5810–24.

34. _____, Hubbard SM, Young RC, Longo DL. The role of chemotherapy in diffuse aggressive lymphomas. Semin Hematol 1988;25(2 Suppl 2):2–10.

35. Dixon DO, Neilan B, Jones SE, et al. Effect of age on therapeutic outcome in advanced diffuse histiocytic lymphoma: the Southwest Oncology Group experience. J Clin Oncol 1986;4:295–305.

36. Dmitrovsky E, Matthews MJ, Bunn PA, et al. Cytologic transformation of cutaneous T-cell lymphoma: a clinicopathologic entity associated with poor prognosis. J Clin Oncol 1987;5:208–15.

37. Doggett RS, Wood GS, Horning S, et al. The immunologic characterization of 95 nodal and extranodal diffuse large cell lymphomas in 89 patients. Am J Pathol 1984;115:245–52.

38. Dorfman RF, Berry GJ. Kikuchi's histiocytic necrotizing lymphadenitis: an analysis of 108 cases with emphasis on differential diagnosis. Semin Diagn Pathol 1988;5:329–45.

39. _____, Warnke R. Lymphadenopathy simulating the malignant lymphomas. Hum Pathol 1974;5:519–50.

40. Ersboll J, Schultz HB, Hougaard P, Nissen NI, Hou-Jensen K. Comparison of the Working Formulation of non-Hodgkin's lymphoma with the Rappaport, Kiel and Lukes & Collins classifications. Translational value and prognostic significance based on review of 658 patients treated at a single institution. Cancer 1985;55:2442–58.

41. Feller AC, Lennert K, Stein H, Bruhn HD, Wuthe HH. Immunohistology and aetiology of histiocytic necrotizing lymphadenitis. Report of three instructive cases. Histopathology 1983;7:825–39.

42. Fisher DE, Jacobson JO, Ault KA, Harris NL. Diffuse large cell lymphoma with discordant bone marrow histology, clinical features and biological implications. Cancer 1989;64:1879–87.

43. Fisher RI, DeVita VT Jr, Johnson BL, Simon R, Young RC. Prognostic factors for advanced diffuse histiocytic lymphoma treated with combination chemotherapy. Am J Med 1977;63:177–82.

44. _____, Gaynor ER, Dahlberg S, et al. Comparison of a standard regimen (CHOP) with three intensive chemotherapy regimens for advanced non-Hodgkin's lymphoma. N Engl J Med 1993;329:580–1.

45. _____, Hubbard SM, DeVita VT Jr, et al. Factors predicting long-term survival in diffuse mixed, histiocytic, or undifferentiated lymphoma. Blood 1981;58:45–51.

46. Flug F, Pelicci PG, Bonetti F, Knowles DM II, Dalla-Favera R. T-cell receptor gene rearrangements as markers of lineage and clonality in human T-cell neoplasms. Proc Natl Acad Sci USA 1985;82:3460–4.

47. Freeman C, Berg JW, Cutler SJ. Occurrence and prognosis of extranodal lymphomas. Cancer 1972;29:252–60.

48. Gaidano G, Dalla-Favera R. Protooncogenes and tumor suppressor genes. In: Knowles DM, ed. Neoplastic hematopathology. Baltimore: Williams & Wilkins, 1992:245–61.

49. Garcia CF, Weiss LM, Warnke RA. Small noncleaved cell lymphoma: an immunophenotypic study of 18 cases and comparison with large cell lymphoma. Hum Pathol 1986;17:454–61.

50. Gerdes J, Stein H, Pileri S, et al. Prognostic relevance of tumor-cell growth fraction in malignant non-Hodgkin's lymphomas [Letter]. Lancet 1987;2:448–9.

51. Gordon LI, Harrington D, Andersen J, et al. Comparison of a second-generation combination chemotherapeutic reigmen (m-BACOD) with a standard regimen (CHOP) for advanced diffuse non-Hodgkin's lymphoma. N Engl J Med 1992;327:1342–9.

52. Greer JP, York JC, Cousar JB. Peripheral T-cell lymphoma: a clinicopathologic study of 42 cases. J Clin Oncol 1984;2:788–98.

53. Griesser H, Tkachuk D, Reis MD, Mak TW. Gene rearrangements and translocations in lymphoproliferative diseases. Blood 1989;73:1402–15.

54. Grogan TM, Fielder K, Rangel C, et al. Peripheral T-cell lymphoma: aggressive disease with heterogenous immunotypes. Am J Clin Pathol 1985;83:279–88.

55. _____, Lippman SM, Spier CM, et al. Independent prognostic significance of a nuclear proliferation antigen in diffuse large cell lymphomas as determined by the monoclonal antibody Ki-67. Blood 1988;71:1157–60.

56. Hall PA, Richards MA, Gregory WM, d'Ardenne AJ, Lister TA, Stansfeld AG. The prognostic value of Ki67 immunostaining in non-Hodgkin's lymphoma. J Pathol 1988;154:223–35.

57. Hamilton-Dutoit SJ, Pallesen G. A survey of Epstein-Barr virus gene expression in sporadic non-Hodgkin's lymphomas. Detection of Epstein-Barr virus in a subset of peripheral T-cell lymphomas. Am J Pathol 1992;140:1315–25.

58. Harousseau JL, Flandrin G, Tricot G, Brouet JC, Seligmann M, Bernard J. Malignant lymphoma supervening in chronic lymphocytic leukemia and related disorders. Richter's syndrome: a study of 25 cases. Cancer 1981;48:1302–8.

59. Harrington DS, Ye Y, Weisenburger DD, et al. Malignant lymphoma in Nebraska and Guangzhou, China: a comparative study. Hum Pathol 1987;18:924–8.

60. Harris NL, Jaffe ES, Stein H, et al. A revised European-American classification of lymphoid neoplasms: a proposal from the International Lymphoma Study Group. Blood 1994;84:1361–92.

61. Hartsock RJ. Postvaccinial lymphadenitis. Hyperplasia of lymphoid tissue that simulates malignant lymphomas. Cancer 1968;21:632–49.

62. Head DR, Avakian J, Kjeldsberg CR, Cerezo L. Relapse of intermediate or high-grade (unfavorable) non-Hodgkin's lymphoma as a low-grade (favorable) non-Hodgkin's lymphoma. Report of four cases. Am J Clin Pathology 1988;89:106–8.

63. Hodges GF, Lenhardt TM, Cotelingam JD. Bone marrow involvement in large-cell lymphoma. Prognostic implications of discordant disease. Am J Clin Pathol 1994;101:305–11.

64. Horning SJ, Weiss LM, Crabtree GS, Warnke RA. Clinical and phenotypic diversity of T-cell lymphomas. Blood 1986;67:1578–82.

65. Horwich A, Peckham M. "Bad risk" non-Hodgkin lymphomas. Semin Hematol 1983;20:35–56.

66. Hui PK, Feller AC, Lennert K. High grade non-Hodgkin's lymphoma of B-cell type. I. Histopathology. Histopathology 1988;12:127–43.

67. Jaffe ES, Strauchen JA, Berard CW. Predictability of immunologic phenotype by morphologic criteria in diffuse aggressive non-Hodgkin's lymphomas. Am J Clin Pathol 1982;77:46–9.

68. Jagannath S, Velasquez WS, Tucker SL, et al. Tumor burden assessment and its implication for a prognostic model in advanced diffuse large cell lymphoma. J Clin Oncol 1986;4:859–65.

69. Kaminski MS, Coleman CN, Colby TV, Cox RS, Rosenberg SA. Factors predicting survival in adults with stage I and II large-cell lymphoma treated with primary radiation therapy. Ann Intern Med 1986;104:747–56.

70. Kerckaert JP, Deweindt C, Tilly H, Quief S, Lecocq G, Bastard C. LAZ3, a novel zinc-finger encoding gene, is disrupted by recurring chromosomal 3q27 translocations in human lymphomas. Nature Genet 1993;5:66–70.

71. Kluin PM. Bcl-6 in lymphoma—sorting out a waste basket? [Editorial] N Engl J Med 1994;331:116–8.

72. _____, van Krieken JH, Kleiverda K, Kluin-Nelemans HC. Discordant morphologic characteristics of B-cell lymphomas in bone marrow and lymph node biopsies. Am J Clin Pathol 1990;94:59–66.

73. Kossakowska AE, Huchcroft S, Boras V, Urbanski SJ. Prognostic significance of proliferative activity of diffuse large cell lymphomas. Hematol Pathol 1991;5:101–7.

74. Kwak LW, Halpern J, Olshen RA, Horning SJ. Prognostic significance of actual dose intensity in diffuse large-cell lymphoma: results of a tree-structured survival analysis. J Clin Oncol 1990;8:963–77.

75. _____, Wilson M, Weiss LM, et al. Similar outcome of treatment of B-cell and T-cell diffuse large cell lymphomas: the Stanford experience. J Clin Oncol 1991;9:1426–31.

76. _____, Wilson M, Weiss LM, Horning SJ, Warnke RA, Dorfman RF. Clinical significance of morphologic subdivision in diffuse large cell lymphoma. Cancer 1991;68:1988–93.

77. Lennert K, Feller AC. Histopathology of non-Hodgkin's lymphomas (based on the updated Kiel classification). 2nd ed. Berlin: Springer-Verlag, 1992.

78. Levine AM, Goldstein M, Meyer PR, et al. Heterogeneity of response and survival in diffuse histiocytic lymphoma after BACOP therapy (bleomycin, doxorubicin, cyclophosphamide, vincristine, prednisone). Hematol Oncol 1985;3:87–98.

79. _____, Taylor CR, Schneider DR, et al. Immunoblastic sarcoma of T-cell versus B-cell origin: I. Clinical features. Blood 1981;58:52–61.

80. Levine EG, Arthur DC, Frizzera G, Peterson BA, Hurd DD, Bloomfield CD. Cytogenetic abnormalities predict clinical outcome in non-Hodgkin lymphoma. Ann Intern Med 1988;108:14–20.

81. _____, Bloomfield CD. Cytogenetics of non-Hodgkin's lymphoma. Monogr Natl Cancer Inst 1990;10:7–12.

82. Lieberman PH, Filippa DA, Straus DJ, Thaler HT, Cirrincione C, Clarkson BD. Evaluation of malignant lymphomas using three classifications and the Working Formulation. 482 cases with median follow-up of 11.9 years. Am J Med 1986;81:365–80.

83. Linch DC. Management of histologically aggressive non-Hodgkin's lymphomas. Br J Hematol 1994;86:691–4.

84. Lipford E, Wright JJ, Urba W, et al. Refinement of lymphoma cytogenetics by the chromosome 18q21 major breakpoint region. Blood 1987;70:1816–23.

85. Lippman SM, Miller TP, Spier CM, Slymen DJ, Grogan TM. The prognostic significance of the immunotype in diffuse large-cell lymphoma: a comparative study of the T-cell and B-cell phenotype. Blood 1988;72:436–41.

86. _____, Spier CM, Miller TP, Slymen DJ, Rybski JA, Grogan TM. Tumor-infiltrating T-lymphocytes in B-cell diffuse large cell lymphoma related to disease course. Mod Pathol 1990;3:361–7.

87. Lo Coco F, Ye BH, Lista F, et al. Rearrangements of the BCL6 gene in diffuse large cell non-Hodgkin's lymphoma. Blood 1994;83:1757–9.

88. Marazuela M, Yebra M, Giron JA, et al. Late relapse with nodular lymphoma after treatment for diffuse non-Hodgkin's lymphoma. Cancer 1991;67:1950–3.

89. Maurer R, Schmid U, Davies JD, Mahy NJ, Stansfeld AG, Lukes RT. Lymph node infarction and malignant lymphoma: a multicenter survey of European, English and American cases. Histopathology 1986;10:571-88.

90. _____, Taylor CR, Parker JW, Cramer A, Lukes RJ. Immunoblastic sarcoma: morphologic criteria and the distinction of B and T cell types. Oncology 1982;39:42–50.

91. Medeiros LJ, Bagg A, Cossman J. Application of molecular genetics to the diagnosis of hematopoietic neoplasms. In: Knowles DM, ed. Neoplastic hematopathology. Baltimore: Williams & Wilkins, 1992:263–98.

92. Michie SA, Garcia CF, Strickler JG, Dailey MO, Rouse RV, Warnke RA. Expression of the Leu-8 antigen by B-cell lymphomas. Am J Clin Pathol 1987;88:486–90.

92a. Migliazza A, Ye BH, Martinotti S, et al. Mutation of the 5' non-coding region of bcl-6 in non-Hodgkin lymphoma [Abstract]. Blood 1994;84(Suppl 1):41a.

93. Miki T, Kawamata N, Hirosawa S, Aoki N. Gene involved in the 3q27 translocation associated with B-cell lymphoma, BCL5, encodes a Kruppel-like zinc-finger protein. Blood 1994;83:26–32.

94. Miller TP, Dana BW, Weick JK, et al. Southwest Oncology Group clinical trials for intermediate- and high-grade non-Hodgkin's lymphomas. Semin Hematol 1988;25(2 Suppl 2):17–22.

95. _____, Grogan TM, Dahlberg S, et al. Prognostic significance of the Ki-67 associated proliferative antigen in aggressive non-Hodgkin's lymphomas: a prospective Southwest Oncology Group trial. N Engl J Med 1994;83:1460–6.

96. Morgello S. Epstein-Barr and human immunodeficiency viruses in AIDS-related primary central nervous system lymphoma. Am J Pathol 1992;141:441–50.

97. Nakamine H, Masih AS, Strobach RS, et al. Immunoblastic lymphoma with abundant clear cytoplasm, a comparative study of B- and T-cell types. Am J Clin Pathol 1991;96:177–83.

98. Nathwani BN. Classifying non-Hodgkin's lymphomas. In: Berard CW, Dorfman RF, Kaufman N, eds. Malignant lymphoma. International Academy of Pathology Monograph. No. 29. Baltimore: Williams & Wilkins, 1987:18–80.

99. _____, Dixon DO, Jones SE, et al. The clinical significance of the morphological subdivision of diffuse "histiocytic" lymphoma: a study of 162 patients treated by the Southwest Oncology Group. Blood 1982;60:1068–74.

100. _____, Griffith RC, Kelly DR, et al. A morphologic study of childhood lymphoma of the diffuse "histiocytic" type. The Pediatric Oncology Group experience. Cancer 1987;59:1138–42.

101. _____, Winberg CD. Non-Hodgkin's lymphomas: an appraisal of the "Working Formulation" of non-Hodgkin's lymphomas for clinical usage. In: Sommers SC, Rosen PP, eds. Malignant lymphomas, a pathology annual monograph. Norwalk: Appleton-Century Crofts, 1983:1–63.

102. Neiman RS. Immunoblastic sarcoma. Am J Surg Pathol 1982;6:755–60.

103. _____, Cain K, Ben Arieh Y, Harrington D, Mann RB, Wolf BC. A comparison between the Rappaport classification and Working Formulation in Cooperative Group Trials: the ECOG experience: the ECOB experience. Hematol Pathol 1992;6:61–70.

104. Ng CS, Chan JK, Lo ST, Poon YF. Immunophenotypic analysis of non-Hodgkin's lymphomas in Chinese. A study of 75 cases in Hong Kong. Pathology 1986;18:419–25.

105. Non-Hodgkin's Lymphoma Pathologic Classification Project. National Cancer Institute sponsored study of classifications of non-Hodgkin's lymphomas: summary and description of a working formulation for clinical usage. Cancer 1982;49:2112–35.

106. O'Brien CJ, Holgate C, Quirke P, et al. Correlation of morphology, immunophenotype, and flow cytometry with remission induction and survival in high grade non-Hodgkin's lymphoma. J Pathol 1989;158:31–9.

107. Offit K. Chromosome analysis in the management of patients with non-Hodgkin's lymphoma. Leuk Lymphoma 1992;7:275–82.

108. _____, Jhanwar S, Ebrahim SA, Filippa D, Clarkson BD, Chaganti RS. t(3;22)(q27;q11): a novel translocation associated with diffuse non-Hodgkin's lymphoma. Blood 1989;74:1876–9.

109. _____, Koduru PR, Hollis R, et al. 18q21 rearrangement in diffuse large cell lymphoma: incidence and clinical significance. Br J Haematol 1989;72:178–83.

110. _____, Lo Coco F, Louie DC, et al. Rearrangement of the bcl-6 gene as a prognostic marker in diffuse large-cell lymphoma. N Engl J Med 1994;331:74–80.

111. _____, Wong G, Filippa DA, Tao Y, Changati RS. Cytogenetic analysis of 434 consecutively ascertained specimens of non-Hodgkin's lymphoma: clinical correlations. Blood 1991;77:1508–15.

112. Ott MM, Ott G, Kuse R, et al. The anaplastic variant of centrocytic lymphoma is marked by frequent rearrangements of the bcl-1 gene and high proliferation indices. Histopathology 1994;24:329–34.

113. Pellicci PG, Knowles DM, Dalla-Favera R. Lymphoid tumors displaying rearrangements of both immunoglobulin and T-cell receptor genes. J Exp Med 1985;162:1015–24.

114. Picker LJ, Weiss LM, Medeiros LJ, Wood GS, Warnke RA. Immunophenotypic criteria for the diagnosis of non-Hodgkin's lymphoma. Am J Pathol 1987;128:181–201.

115. Pileri S, Kikuchi M, Helbron D, Lennert K. Histiocytic necrotizing lymphadenitis without granulocytic infiltration. Virchows Arch [A] 1982;395:257–71.

116. Predictive model for aggressive non-Hodgkin's lymphoma. The International Non-Hodgkin's Lymphoma Prognostic Factors Project. N Engl J Med 1993;329:987–94.

117. Pugh WC, Manning JT, Butler JJ. Paraimmunoblastic variant of small lymphocytic lymphoma/leukemia. Am J Surg Pathol 1988;12:907–17.

118. Raghoebier S, Kramer MH, Van Krieken JH, et al. Essential differences in oncogene involvement between primary nodal and extranodal large cell lymphoma. Blood 1991;78:2680–5.

119. Ree HJ, Leone LA, Crowley JP. Sclerosis in diffuse histiocytic lymphoma: a clinicopathologic study of 25 cases. Cancer 1982;49:1636–48.

120. Robertson LE, Redman JR, Butler JJ, et al. Discordant bone marrow involvement in diffuse large-cell lymphoma: a distinct clinical-pathologic entity associated with a continuous risk of relapse. J Clin Oncol 1991;9:236–42.

121. Rowe M. Epstein-Barr virus and lymphoid malignancy. In: Hoffbrand AV, Brenner MK, eds. Recent advances in haematology. No. 6. Edinburgh: Churchill Livingstone, 1992:209–26.

122. Salhany KE, Cousar JB, Greer JP, Casey TT, Fields JP, Collins RD. Transformation of cutaneous T-cell lymphoma to large cell lymphoma. A clinicopathologic and immunologic study. Am J Pathol 1988;132:265–77.

123. Saltzstein SL, Ackerman LV. Lymphadenopathy induced by anticonvulsant drugs and mimicking clinically and pathologically malignant lymphomas. Cancer 1959;12:164–82.

124. Sandlund JT, Pui CH, Santana VM, et al. Clinical features and treatment outcome for children with CD30+ large-cell non-Hogkin's lymphoma. J Clin Oncol 1994;12:895–8.

125. Schneider AM, Straus DJ, Schluger AE, et al. Treatment results with an aggressive chemotherapeutic regimen (MACOP-B) for intermediate- and some high-grade non-Hodgkin's lymphomas. J Clin Oncol 1990;8:94–102.

126. Schneider DR, Taylor CR, Parker JW, Cramer AC, Meyer PR, Lukes RJ. Immunoblastic sarcoma of T- and B-cell types: morphologic description and comparison. Hum Pathol 1985;16:885–900.

127. Schouten HC, Sanger WG, Weisenburger DD, Anderson J, Armitage JO. Chromosomal abnormalities in untreated patients with non-Hodgkin's lymphoma: associations with histology, clinical characteristics, and treatment outcome. The Nebraska Lymphoma Study Group. Blood 1990;75:1841–7.

128. Schuurman HJ, Huppes W, Verdonck LF, van Baarlen J, Van Unnik JA. Immunophenotyping of non-Hodgkin's lymphoma. Correlation with relapse-free survival. Am J Pathol 1988;131:102–11.

129. Segal GH, Kjeldsberg CR, Smith GP, Perkins SL. CD30 antigen expression in florid immunoblastic proliferations, a clinicopathologic study of 14 cases. Am J Clin Pathol 1994;102:292–8.

130. Shimoyama M, Oyama A, Tajima K, et al. Differences in clinicopathological characteristics and major prognostic factors between B-lymphoma and peripheral T-lymphoma excluding adult T-cell leukemia/lymphoma. Leuk Lymphoma 1993;10:335–42.

131. Shipp MA. Prognostic factors in aggressive non-Hodgkin's lymphoma: who has high risk disease? Blood 1994;83:1165–73.

132. _____, Harrington DP, Klatt MM, et al. Identification of major prognostic subgroups of patients with diffuse large cell lymphoma treated with m-BACOD or M-BACOD. Ann Intern Med 1986;104:757–65.

133. Simon R, Durrelman S, Hoppe RT, et al. The Non-Hodgkin Lymphoma Pathologic Classification Project. Long-term follow-up of 1153 patients with non-Hodgkin lymphomas. Ann Intern Med 1988;109:939–45.

134. Slater DM, Krajewski AS, Cunningham S. Activation and differentiation antigen expression in B-cell non-Hodgkin's lymphoma. J Pathol 1988;154:209–22.

135. Slymen DJ, Miller TP, Lippman SM, et al. Immunobiologic factors predictive of clinical outcome in diffuse large-cell lymphoma. J Clin Oncol 1990;8:986–93.

136. Smith JL, Jones DB, Bell AJ, Wright DH. Correlation between histology and immunophenotype in a series of 322 cases of non-Hodgkin's lymphoma. Hematol Oncol 1989;7:37–48.

137. Soini Y, Paakko P, Alavaikko M, Vahakangas K. p53 expression in lymphatic malignancies. J Clin Pathol 1992;45:1011–4.

138. Spier CM, Grogan TM, Lippman SM, Slymen DJ, Rybski JA, Miller TP. The aberrancy of immunophenotype and immunoglobulin status as indicators of prognosis in B cell diffuse large cell lymphoma. Am J Pathol 1988;133:118–26.

139. Stansfeld AG. High-grade malignant lymphomas. In: Stansfeld AG, d'Ardenne AJ, eds. Lymph node biopsy interpretation. 2nd ed. Edinburgh: Churchill Livingstone, 1992:333–66.

140. _____. Peripheral T-cell lymphomas. In: Stansfeld AG, d'Ardenne AJ, eds. Lymph node biopsy interpretation. 2nd ed. Edinburgh: Churchill Livingstone, 1992:285–331.

141. Stein H, Dallenbach F. Diffuse large cell lymphoma of B and T cell type. In: Knowles DM, ed. Neoplastic hematopathology. Baltimore: Williams & Wilkins, 1992: 675–714.

142. Stein RS, Greer JP, Flexner JM, et al. Large-cell lymphomas: clinical and prognostic features. J Clin Oncol 1990;8:1370–9.

143. _____, Magee MJ, Lenox RK, et al. Malignant lymphomas of follicular center cell origin in man. VI. Large cleaved cell lymphoma. Cancer 1987;60:2704–11.

144. Stewart ML, Felman IE, Nichols PW, Pagnini-Hill A, Lukes RJ, Levine AM. Large noncleaved follicular center cell lymphoma. Clinical features in 53 patients. Cancer 1986;57:288–97.

145. Strauchen JA, Young JC, DeVita VT Jr, Anderson T, Fantone TC, Berard CW. Clinical relevance of the histopathological subclassification of diffuse "histiocytic" lymphoma. N Engl J Med 1978;299:1382–7.

145a. Tsang WY, Chan JK. Spectrum of morphologic changes in lymph nodes attributable to fine needle aspiration. Hum Pathol 1992;23:562–5.

146. _____, Chan JK, Ng CS. Kikuchi's lymphadenitis: a morphologic analysis of 75 cases with special reference to unusual features. Am J Surg Pathol 1994;18:219–31.

147. Tubbs RR, Fishleder A, Weiss RA, Savage RA, Sebek BA, Weick JK. Immunohistologic cellular phenotypes of lymphoproliferative disorders. Comprehensive evaluation of 564 cases including 257 non-Hodgkin's lymphomas classified by the International Working Formulation. Am J Pathol 1983;113:207–21.

148. Turner RR, Martin J, Dorfman RF. Necrotizing lymphadenitis, a study of 30 cases. Am J Surg Pathol 1983;7:115–23.

149. Tusenius KJ, Bakker PJ, Van Oers MH. Measurement of proliferation indices in non-Hodgkin's lymphoma—is it useful? Leuk Lymphoma 1992;7:181–7.

150. Urba WJ, Duffey PL, Longo DL. Treatment of patients with aggressive lymphomas: an overview. Monogr Natl Cancer Inst 1990;10:29–37.

151. Van Krieken JH, Medeiros J, Pals ST, Raffeld M, Kluin PM. Diffuse aggressive B-cell lymphomas of the gastrointestinal tract. An immunophenotypic and gene rearrangement analysis of 22 cases. Am J Clin Pathol 1992;97:170–8.

152. _____, Raffeld M, Raghoebier S, Jaffe ES, van Ommen GJ, Kluin PH. Molecular genetics of gastrointestinal non-Hodgkin's lymphomas: unusual prevalence and pattern of c-myc rearrangements in aggressive lymphomas. Blood 1990;76:797–800.

153. Vose JM, Armitage JO, Weisenburger DD, et al. The importance of age in survival of patients treated with chemotherapy for aggressive non-Hodgkin's lymphoma. J Clin Oncol 1988;6:1838–44.

154. Waldmann TA, Davis MM, Bongiovanni KF, Korsmeyer SJ. Rearrangements of genes for the antigen receptor on T cells as markers of lineage and clonality in human lymphoid neoplasms. N Engl J Med 1985;313:776–83.

155. Warnke RA, Strauchen JA, Burke JS, Hoppe HT, Campbell BA, Dorfman RF. Morphologic types of diffuse large-cell lymphoma. Cancer 1982;50:690–5.

156. _____, Weiss LM. B-cell malignant lymphomas, an immunologic perspective. In: Berard CW, Dorfman RF, Kaufman N, eds. Malignant lymphoma. Baltimore: Williams & Wilkins, 1987:88–103. (International Academy of Pathology monograph. No. 29.)

157. Weiss LM, Michie SA, Medeiros LJ, Strickler JG, Garcia CF, Warnke RA. Expression of Tac antigen by non-Hodgkin's lymphomas. Am J Clin Pathol 1987;88:483–5.

158. _____, Movahed LA. In situ demonstration of Epstein-Barr viral genome in viral-associated B-cell lymphoproliferation. Am J Pathol 1989;134:651–9.

159. _____, Warnke RA, Sklar J, Cleary ML. Molecular analysis of the t(14;18) chromosomal translocation in malignant lymphomas. N Engl J Med 1987;317:1185–9.

160. Whitcomb CC, Cousar JB, Flint A, et al. Subcategories of histiocytic lymphoma: associations with survival and reproducibility of classification. The Southeastern Cancer Study Group experience. Cancer 1981;48:2464–74.

161. Williams ME, Innes DJ, Borowitz MJ, et al. Immunoglobulin and T-cell receptor gene rearrangements in human lymphoma and leukemia. Blood 1987;69:79–86.

162. Wong KF, Chan JK, Ng CS, Chu YC, Li LP, Chan CH. Large cell lymphoma with initial presentation in the bone marrow. Hematol Oncol 1993;10:261–71.

163. Ye BH, Lista F, Lo Coco F, et al. Alterations of a zinc finger-encoding gene, BCL-6, in diffuse large-cell lymphoma. Science 1993;262:747–50.

164. _____, Rao PH, Chaganti RSK, Dalla-Favera R. Cloning of bcl-6, the locus involved in chromosomal translocations affecting band 3q27 in B-cell lymphoma. Cancer Res 1993;43:2732–5.

165. Yi PI, Coleman M, Saltz L, et al. Chemotherapy for large cell lymphoma: a status update. Semin Oncol 1990;17:60–73.

166. York JC, Glick AD, Cousar JB, Collins RD. Changes in the appearance of hematopoietic and lymphoid neoplasms: clinical, pathologic, and biologic implications. Hum Pathol 1984;15:11–38.

167. Yunis JJ, Mayer MG, Arnesen MA, Aeppli DP, Oken MM, Frizzera G. bcl-2 and other genomic alterations in the prognosis of large cell lymphoma. N Engl J Med 1989;320:1047–54.

Lymphoma with Myxoid Stroma

168. Chan JK, Buchanan R, Fletcher CD. Sarcomatoid variant of anaplastic large cell Ki-1 lymphoma. Am J Surg Pathol 1990;14:983–8.

169. Fung DT, Chan JK, Tse CC, Sze WM. Myxoid change in malignant lymphoma. Pathogenetic considerations. Arch Pathol Lab Med 1992;116:103–5.

170. Strauchen JA. Sarcomatoid neoplasm of monocytic lineage [Letter]. Am J Surg Pathol 1991;15:1206–7.

171. Tse CC, Chan JK, Yuen RW, Ng CS. Malignant lymphoma with myxoid stroma: a new pattern in need of recognition. Histopathology 1991;18:31–5.

Lymphoma with Spindly Cells

172. Chan JK, Buchanan R, Fletcher CD. Sarcomatoid variant of anaplastic large cell Ki-1 lymphoma. Am J Surg Pathol 1990;14:983–8.

173. Dahlin DC, Unni KK. Bone tumors, general aspects and data on 8542 cases. 4th ed. Springfield: Charles C Thomas, 1986:208–26.

174. Kluin PM, Slootweg PJ, Schuurman JH, et al. Primary B-cell malignant lymphoma of the maxilla with a sarcomatous pattern and multilobated nuclei. Cancer 1984;54:1598–605.

175. Perrone T, Frizzera G, Rosai J. Mediastinal diffuse large-cell lymphoma with sclerosis. A clinicopathologic study of 60 cases. Am J Surg Pathol 1986;10:176–91.

176. Weiss LM, Berry GJ, Dorfman RJ, et al. Spindle cell neoplasms of lymph nodes of probable reticulum cell lineage: true reticulum cell sarcoma? Am J Surg Pathol 1990;14:405–14.

Lymphoma with Fibrillary Matrix

177. Frizzera G, Gajl-Peczalska K, Sibley RK, Rosai J, Cherwitz D, Hurd DD. Rosette formation in malignant lymphoma. Am J Pathol 1985;119:351–6.

178. Tsang WY, Chan JK, Tang SK, Tse CC, Cheung MM. Large cell lymphoma with fibrillary matrix. Histopathology 1992;20:80–2.

Microvillous Lymphoma

179. Battifora H. Comments by the panel, re: anemone cell tumor. Ultrastruct Pathol 1985;8:369–73.

180. _____, Kaiserling E, Lennert K, Kim H, Mackay B. Comments by the panel, re: anemone cell tumor. Ultrastruct Pathol 1980;1:450–3.

181. Bernier V, Azar HA. Filiform large-cell lymphomas: an ultrastructural and immunohistochemical study. Am J Surg Pathol 1987;11:387–96.

182. Erlandson RA, Filippa DA. Unusual non-Hodgkin's lymphomas and true histiocytic lymphomas. Ultrastruct Pathol 1989;13:249–73.

183. Font RL, Shields J. Large cell lymphoma of the orbit with microvillous projections ("porcupine lymphoma"). Arch Ophthalmol 1985;103:1715–9.

184. Huntrakoon M, Bhatia P. Anemone cell tumor. Ultrastruct Pathol 1985;8:369–73.

185. Ishihara T, Takahashi M, Uchino F, Matsumoto N. A filiform large cell lymphoma in the spleen: a case report with immunohistochemical and electron microscopic study. Ultrastruct Pathol 1990;14:193–9.

186. Kinney MC, Glick AD, Stein H, Collins RD. Comparison of anaplastic large cell Ki-1 lymphomas and microvillous lymphomas in their immunologic and ultrastructural features. Am J Surg Pathol 1990;14:1047–60.

187. Osborne BM, Mackay B, Butler JJ, Ordonez NG. Large cell lymphoma with microvillus-like projections: an ultrastructural study. Am J Clin Pathol 1983;79:443–50.

188. Schwarz R, Marquet E, Sobel HJ. Another look at the "anemone cell." Ultrastruct Pathol 1982:3:209–11.

189. Sibley R, Rosai J. Reply from the authors, re: another look at the "anemone cell." Ultrastruct Pathol 1982;3:212–4.

190. _____, Rosai J, Froehlich W. A case for the panel: anemone cell tumor. Ultrastruct Pathol 1980;1:449–53.

191. Taxy JB, Almanaseer IY. "Anemone" cell (villiform) tumors: electron microscopy and immunohistochemistry of five cases. Ultrastruct Pathol 1984;7:143–50.

192. Tsang WY, Chan JK, Tang SK, Tse CC, Cheung MM. Large cell lymphoma with fibrillary matrix. Histopathology 1992;20:80–2.

193. Wills EJ. Anemone cell tumor with neuroendocrine differentiation (presumed Merkel cell carcinoma). Ultrastruct Pathol 1990;14:161–71.

Lymphoma with Intercellular Junctions

194. Eyden BP, Harris M. An immunohistochemically defined non-Hodgkin's lymphoma showing intercellular junctions. A case report. Virchows Arch [A] 1989;415:297–300.

195. Huntrakoon M, Bhatia P. Anemone cell tumor. Ultrastruct Pathol 1985;8:369–73.

196. Kaiserling E. Ultrastructure of non-Hodgkin's lymphomas. In: Lennert K, ed. Malignant lymphomas other than Hodgkin's disease, histology, cytology, ultrastructure, immunology. Berlin: Springer-Verlag, 1978:471–528.

197. Kojima M, Imai Y, Mori N. A concept of follicular lymphoma, a proposal for the existence of a neoplasm originating from the germinal center. GANN Monogr Cancer Res 1973;15:195–207.

198. Lamoureux D, Daya D, Simon GT. Cell junctions in lymphomas: study of a primary ovarian T-cell lymphoma and review of fifty-six other cases of lymphoma. Ultrastruct Pathol 1990;14:247–52.

199. Levine GD, Dorfman RF. Nodular lymphoma, an ultrastructural study of its relationship to germinal centers and a correlation of light and electron microscopic findings. Cancer 1975;35:148–64.

200. Monda L, Warnke R, Rosai J. A primary lymph node malignancy with features suggestive of dendritic reticulum cell differentiation. Am J Pathol 1986;122:562–72.

201. Perrone T, Frizzera G, Rosai J. Mediastinal diffuse large cell lymphoma with sclerosis. A clinicopathologic study of 60 cases. Am J Surg Pathol 1986;10:176–91.

202. Weiss LM, Berry GJ, Dorfman RF, et al. Spindle cell neoplasms of lymph nodes of probable reticulum cell lineage. True reticulum cell sarcoma? Am J Surg Pathol 1990;14:405–14.

Signet Ring Cell Lymphoma

203. Cross PA, Eyden BP, Harris M. Signet ring cell lymphoma of T cell type. J Clin Pathol 1989;42:239–45.

204. Dardick I, Srinivasan R, Al-Jabi M. Signet ring cell variant of large cell lymphoma. Ultrastruct Pathol 1983;5:195–200.

205. Eyden BP, Cross PA, Harris M. The ultrastructure of signet-ring cell non-Hodgkin's lymphoma. Virchows Arch [A] 1990;417:395–404.

206. Grogan TM, Payne CM, Richter LC, Rangel CS. Signet ring cell lymphoma of T-cell origin. Am J Surg Pathol 1985;9:684–92.

207. Kim H, Dorfman RF, Rappaport H. Signet ring cell lymphoma. A rare morphologic and functional expression of nodular (follicular) lymphoma. Am J Surg Pathol 1978;2:119–32.

208. Kurotaki H, Suga M, Kaimori M, Kumagai H, Yoshioka H, Nagai K. Fibril formation in the rough endoplasmic reticulum of lymphoma cells, a case report with histopathologic, immunohistochemical, electron and immunoelectron microscopic studies. Pathol Res Pract 1994;190:84–96.

209. Lennert K, Feller AC. Histopathology of the non-Hodgkin's lymphomas (based on the updated Kiel classification). 2nd ed. Berlin: Springer-Verlag, 1992:93.

210. Navas-Palacios JJ, Valdes MD, Lahuerta-Palacios JJ. Signet ring cell lymphoma. Ultrastructural and immunohistochemical features of these varieties. Cancer 1983;52:1613–23.

211. Perrone T, Frizzera G, Rosai J. Mediastinal diffuse large-cell lymphoma with sclerosis. A clinicopathologic study of 60 cases. Am J Surg Pathol 1986;10:176–91.

212. Silberman S, Fresco R, Steinecker PH. Signet ring cell lymphoma. A report of the case and review of the literature. Am J Clin Pathol 1984;81:358–63.

213. Spagnolo DV, Papadimitriou JM, Matz LR, Walters MN. Nodular lymphomas with intracellular immunoglobulin inclusions: report of three cases and a review. Pathology 1982;14:415–27.

214. Uccini S, Pescarmona E, Ruco LP, Baroni CD, Monarca B, Modesti A. Immunohistochemical characterization of B-cell signet ring cell lymphoma. Report of a case. Pathol Res Pract 1988;183:497–504.

215. Van den Tweel JG, Taylor CR, Parker JW, Lukes RJ. Immunoglobulin inclusions in non-Hodgkin's lymphomas. Am J Clin Pathol 1978;69:306–13.

216. Weiss LM, Wood GS, Dorfman RF. T-cell signet ring lymphoma. A histologic, ultrastructural, and immunohistochemical study of two cases. Am J Surg Pathol 1985;9:273–80.

Sinusoidal Large Cell Lymphoma

217. Chan JK, Ng CS, Chu YC, Wong KF. S-100 protein-positive sinusoidal large cell lymphoma. Hum Pathol 1987;18:756–9.

218. _____, Ng CS, Hui PK, Leung TW, Lo ES, Lau WH, McGuire LJ. Anaplastic large cell Ki-1 lymphoma. Delineation of two morphological types. Histopathology 1989;15:11–34.

219. Jaffe ES. Malignant histiocytosis and true histiocytic lymphomas. In: Jaffe ES, ed. Surgical pathology of the lymph nodes and related organs. Major problems in pathology series. Philadelphia: WB Saunders, 1985:381.

220. Kinney MC, Glick AD, Stein H, Collins RD. Comparison of anaplastic large cell Ki-1 lymphomas and microvillous lymphomas in their immunologic and ultrastructural features. Am J Surg Pathol 1990;14:1047–60.

221. Osborne BM, Butler JJ, MacKay B. Sinusoidal large cell (histiocytic) lymphoma. Cancer 1980;46:2484–91.

222. Stein H, Mason DY, Gerdes J, et al. The expression of the Hodgkin's disease associated antigen Ki-1 in reactive and neoplastic lymphoid tissue: evidence that Reed-Sternberg cells and histiocytic malignancies are derived from activated lymphoid cells. Blood 1985;66:848–58.

Interfollicular Large Cell Lymphoma

223. Macon WR, Williams ME, Greer JP, Stein RS, Collins RD, Cousar JB. T-cell-rich B-cell lymphomas, a clinicopathologic study of 19 cases. Am J Surg Pathol 1992;16:351–63.

224. Ng CS, Chan JKC, Hui PK. Heterogeneity of interfollicular lymphomas [Abstract]. Surg Pathol 1991;4:372.

225. _____, Chan JK, Hui PK, Lau WH. Large B-cell lymphomas with a high content of reactive T cells. Hum Pathol 1989;20:1145–54.

226. Osborne BM, Butler JJ, Pugh WC. The value of immunophenotyping on paraffin sections in the identification of T-cell rich B-cell large-cell lymphomas: lineage confirmed by JH rearrangement. Am J Surg Pathol 1990;14:933–8.

227. Stansfeld AG. Peripheral T-cell lymphomas. In: Stansfeld AG, d'Ardenne AJ, eds. Lymph node biopsy interpretation. 2nd ed. Edinburgh: Churchill Livingstone, 1992:285–331.

Multilobated Large Cell Lymphoma

228. Cerezo L. B-cell multilobated lymphoma. Cancer 1983;52:2277–80.

229. Chan JK, Ng CS, Tung S. Multilobated B-cell lymphoma, a variant of centroblastic lymphoma. Report of four cases. Histopathology 1986;10:601–12.

230. Hui PK, Feller AC, Lennert K. High-grade non-Hodgkin's lymphoma of B-cell type. I. Histopathology. Histopathology 1988;12:127–43.

231. Lennert K, Feller AC. Histopathology of non-Hodgkin's lymphomas (based on the updated Kiel classification). 2nd ed. Berlin: Springer-Verlag, 1992:115–20, 252.

232. O'Hara CJ, Said JW, Pinkus GS. Non-Hodgkin's lymphoma, multilobated B-cell type: report of nine cases with immunohistochemical and immunoultrastructural evidence for a follicular center cell derivation. Hum Pathol 1986;17:593–9.

233. Pileri S, Brandi G, Rivano MT, Govoni E, Martinelli G. Report of a case of non-Hodgkin's lymphoma of large multilobated cell type with B-cell origin. Tumori 1982;68:543–8.

234. Pinkus GS, Said JW, Hargreaves H. Malignant lymphoma, T-cell type. A distinct morphologic variant with large multilobated nuclei, with a report of four cases. Am J Clin Pathol 1979;72:540–50.

235. van der Putte SC, Schuurman HJ, Rademakers LH, Kluin P, van Unnik JA. Malignant lymphoma of follicle center cells with marked nuclear lobation. Virchows Arch [B] 1984;46:93–107.

236. _____, Toonstra J, de Weger RA, van Unnik JA. Cutaneous T-cell lymphoma, multilobated type. Histopathology 1982;6:35–54.

237. Weiss RL, Kjeldsberg CR, Colby TV, Marty J. Multilobated B-cell lymphomas. A study of 7 cases. Hematol Oncol 1985;3:79–86.

Lymphoma with Cytoplasmic Granules

238. Kanavaros P, Lavergne A, Galian A, et al. A primary immunoblastic T malignant lymphoma of the small bowel, with azurophilic intracytoplasmic granules: a histologic, immunologic, and electron microscopic study. Am J Surg Pathol 1988;12:641–7.

239. Kern WF, Spier CM, Hanneman EH, Miller TP, Matzner M, Grogan TM. Neural cell adhesion molecule-positive peripheral T-cell lymphoma: a rare variant with a propensity for unusual sites of involvement. Blood 1992;79:2432–7.

240. Longacre TA, Listrom MB, Spigel JH, William CL, Dressler L, Clark D. Aggressive jejunal lymphoma of large granular lymphocytes, immunohistochemical, ultrastructural, molecular and DNA content analysis. Am J Clin Pathol 1990;93:124–32.

241. Pileri S, Martinelli G, Rivano MT, Biagini G, Govoni E. Neurosecretory-like granules in non-Hodgkin's malignant lymphomas. Hum Pathol 1984;15:588–9.

242. Sun T, Schulman P, Kolitz J, et al. A study of lymphoma of large granular lymphocytes with modern modalities, report of two cases and review of the literature. Am J Hematol 1992;40:135–45.

243. Wong KF, Chan JK, Ng CS. CD56 (NCAM)-positive malignant lymphoma. Leuk Lymphoma 1994;14:29–36.

244. _____, Chan JK, Ng CS, Lee KC, Tsang WY, Cheung MMC. CD56 (NKH1)-positive hematolymphoid malignancies: an aggressive neoplasm featuring frequent cutaneous/mucosal involvement, cytoplasmic azurophilic granules, and angiocentricity. Hum Pathol 1992;23:798–804.

Intravascular Lymphomatosis

245. Abe S, Kumanishi T, Yoshida Y, Higuchi M, Hirono S. Neoplastic angioendotheliosis: demonstration of immunoglobulin gene rearrangements by the Southern blot hybridization technique. Virchows Arch [A] 1990;58:241–4.

246. Ansell J, Bhawan J, Cohen S, Sullivan J, Sherman D. Histiocytic lymphoma and malignant angioendotheliomatosis: one disease or two? Cancer 1982;50:1506–12.

247. Axelsen RA, Laird PP, Horn M. Intravascular large cell lymphoma: diagnosis on renal biopsy. Pathology 1991;23:241–3.

248. Banerjee SS, Harris M. Angiotropic lymphoma presenting in the prostate. Histopathology 1988;12:667–70.

249. Ben-Ezra J, Sheibani K, Kendrick FE, Winberg CD, Rappaport H. Angiotropic large cell lymphoma of the prostate: an immunohistochemical study. Hum Pathol 1986;17:964–7.

250. Bhawan J. Angioendotheliomatosis proliferans systemisata, an angiotropic neoplasm of lymphoid origin. Semin Diagn Pathol 1987;4:18–27.

251. D'agati V, Sablay LB, Knowles DM, Walter L. Angiotropic large cell lymphoma (intravascular malignant lymphomatosis) of the kidney: presentation as minimal change disease. Hum Pathol 1989;20:263–8.

252. Davey DD, Muun R, Smith LW, Cibull ML. Angiotropic lymphoma: presentation in uterine vessels with cytogenetic studies. Arch Pathol Lab Med 1990;114:879–82.

253. Demirer T, Dail DH, Aboulafia DM. Four varied cases of intravascular lymphomatosis and a literature review. Cancer 1994;73:1738–45.

254. Domizio P, Hall PA, Cotter F, et al. Angiotropic large cell lymphoma (ALCL): morphological, immunohistochemical and genotypic studies with analysis of previous reports. Hematol Oncol 1989;7:195–206.

255. Ferry JA, Harris NL, Picker LJ, et al. Intravascular lymphomatosis (malignant angioendotheliomatosis). A B-cell neoplasm expressing surface homing receptors. Mod Pathol 1988;1:444–52.

256. Fulling KH, Gersell DJ. Neoplastic angioendotheliomatosis: histologic, immunohistochemical and ultrastructural findings in two cases. Cancer 1983;51:1107–18.

257. Jalkanen S, Aho R, Kallajoki M, et al. Lymphocyte homing receptors and adhesion molecules in intravascular malignant lymphomatosis. Int J Cancer 1989;44:777–82.

258. Kamesaki H, Matsui Y, Ohno Y et al. Angiocentric lymphoma with histologic features of neoplastic angioendotheliomatosis presenting with predominant respiratory and hematologic manifestations. Report of a case and review of the literature. Am J Clin Pathol 1990;94:768–72.

259. Kayano H, Katayama I. Primary hepatic lymphoma presenting as intravascular lymphomatosis. Arch Pathol Lab Med 1990;114:580–4.

260. Laurino L, Melato M. Malignant angioendotheliomatosis (angiotropic lymphoma) of the gall bladder. Virchows Arch [A] 1990;417:243–6.

261. Martin S, Pitcher D, Tschen J, Wolf JE Jr. Reactive angioendotheliomatosis. J Am Acad Dermatol 1980;2:117–23.

262. Molina A, Lombard C, Donlon T, Bangs CD, Dorfman RF. Immunohistochemical and cytogenetic studies indicate that malignant angioendotheliomatosis is a primary intravascular (angiotropic) lymphoma. Cancer 1990;66:474–9.

263. Mori S, Itoyama S, Mohri N, et al. Cellular characteristics of neoplastic angioendotheliomatosis, an immunohistological marker study of six cases. Virchows Arch [A] 1985;407:167–75.

264. O'Grady JT, Shadidullah H, Doherty VR, Al-Nafussi A. Intravascular histiocytosis. Histopathology 1994;24: 265–8.

265. Otrakji CL, Voigt W, Amador A, Nadji M, Gregorios JB. Malignant angioendotheliomatosis—a true lymphoma: a case of intravascular lymphomatosis studied by southern blot hybridization analysis. Hum Pathol 1988;19:475–8.

266. Pasyk K, Depowski M. Proliferating systematized angioendotheliomatosis of 5-month-old infant. Arch Dermatol 1978;114:1512–5.

267. Prayson RA, Segal GH, Stoler MH, Licata AA, Tubbs RR. Angiotropic large cell lymphoma in a patient with adrenal insufficiency. Arch Pathol Lab Med 1991;115:1039–41.

268. Sepp N, Schuler G, Romani N, et al. Intravascular lymphomatosis (angioendotheliomatosis): evidence for a T cell origin in two cases. Hum Pathol 1990;21:1051–8.

269. Sheibani K, Battifora H, Winberg CD, et al. Further evidence that malignant angioendotheliomatosis is an angiotropic large cell lymphoma. N Engl J Med 1986;314:943–8.

270. Shimokawa I, Higami Y, Sakai H, Moriuchi Y, Murase K, Ikeda T. Intravascular malignant lymphoma: a case of T-cell lymphoma probably associated with human T-cell lymphotropic virus. Hum Pathol 1991;22:200–2.

271. Stroup RM, Sheibani K, Moncada A, Purdy LJ, Battifora H. Angiotropic (intravascular) large cell lymphoma. A clinicopathologic study of seven cases with unique clinical presentations. Cancer 1990;66:1781–8.

272. Tateyama H, Eimoto T, Tada T, Kamiya M, Fujiyoshi Y, Kajiura S. Congenital angiotropic lymphoma (intravascular lymphomatosis) of the T-cell type. Cancer 1991;67:2131–6.

273. Theaker JM, Gatter KC, Esiri MM, Easterbrook P. Neoplastic angioendotheliomatosis—further evidence supporting a lymphoid origin. Histopathology 1986;10:1261–70.

274. Wick MR, Mills SE, Scheithauer BW, Cooper PH, Davitz MA, Parkinson K. Reassessment of malignant angioendotheliomatosis: evidence in favor of its reclassification as intravascular lymphomatosis. Am J Surg Pathol 1986;10:112–23.

275. _____, Rocamora A. Reactive and malignant angioendotheliomatosis: a discriminant clinicopathologic study. J Cutan Pathol 1988;15:260–71.

276. Wrotnowski U, Mills SE, Cooper PH. Malignant angioendotheliomatosis: an angiotropic lymphoma? Am J Clin Pathol 1985;83:244–8.

277. Yousem SA, Colby TV. Intravascular lymphomatosis presenting in the lung. Cancer 1990;65:349–53.

Anaplastic Large Cell Lymphoma

278. Abbondanzo SL, Sato N, Straus SE, Jaffe ES. Acute infectious mononucleosis. CD30 (Ki-1) antigen expression and histologic correlations. Am J Clin Pathol 1990;93:698–702.

279. Agnarsson BA, Kadin ME. Ki-1 positive large cell lymphoma. A morphologic and immunologic study of 19 cases. Am J Surg Pathol 1988;12:264–74.

280. Anagnostopoulos I, Hummel M, Kaudewitz P, Herbst H, Braun-Falco O, Stein H. Detection of HTLV-I proviral sequences in CD30-positive large cell cutaneous T-cell lymphomas. Am J Pathol 1990;137:1317–22.

281. Andreesen R, Brugger W, Lohr GW, Bross KJ. Human macrophages can express the Hodgkin's cell-associated antigen Ki-1 (CD30). Am J Pathol 1989;134:187–92.

282. Audouin J, Le Tourneau A, Diebold J, Reynes M, Tabbah I, Bernadou A. Primary intestinal lymphoma of Ki-1 large cell anaplastic type with mesenteric lymph node and spleen involvement in a renal transplant recipient. Hematol Oncol 1989;7:441–9.

283. Bacchi MM, Bacchi CE, Gown AM, Kidd PG. Diversity of morphologic, immunocytochemical, and molecular biological findings in Ki-1 (CD30-positive) large cell lymphomas [Abstract]. Mod Pathol 1991;4:67A.

284. Banerjee SS, Heald J, Harris M. Twelve cases of Ki-1 positive anaplastic large cell lymphoma of skin. J Clin Pathol 1991;44:119–25.

285. Banks PM, Metter J, Allred DC, et al. Anaplastic large cell (Ki-1) lymphoma with histiocytic phenotype simulating carcinoma. Am J Clin Pathol 1990;94:445–52.

286. Beljaards RC, Meijer CJ, Scheffer E, et al. Prognostic significance of CD30 (Ki-1/Ber-H2) expression in primary cutaneous large-cell lymphomas of T-cell origin. A clinicopathologic and immunohistochemical study of 20 patients. Am J Pathol 1989;135:1169–78.

287. _____, Meijer CJ, Scheffer E, et al. Primary cutaneous CD30+ large cell lymphoma: definition of a new type of cutaneous lymphoma with a favorable prognosis. Cancer 1993;71:2097–104.

288. Benz-Lemoine E, Brizard A, Huret JL, et al. Malignant histiocytosis: a specific t(2;5)(p23;q35) translocation? Review of the literature. Blood 1988;72:1045–7.

289. Bitter MA, Franklin WA, Larson RA, et al. Morphology in Ki-1 (CD30)-positive non-Hodgkin's lymphoma is correlated with clinical features and the presence of a unique chromosomal abnormality, t(2;5)(p23;q35). Am J Surg Pathol 1990;14:305–16.

290. Boiocchi M, De Re V, Gloghini A, et al. High incidence of monoclonal EBV episomes in Hodgkin's disease and anaplastic large-cell Ki-1-positive lymphoma in HIV-1-positive patients. Int J Cancer 1993;54:53–9.

291. Borisch B, Boni J, Burki K, Laissue JA. Recurrent cutaneous anaplastic large cell (CD30+) lymphoma associated with Epstein-Barr virus, a case report with 9-year follow-up. Am J Surg Pathol 1992;16:796–801.

292. Brousset P, Rochaix P, Chittal S, Rubie H, Robert A, Delsol G. High incidence of Epstein-Barr virus detection in Hodgkin's disease and absence of detection in anaplastic large-cell lymphoma in children. Histopathology 1993;23:189–91.

292a. Bullrich F, Morris SW, Hummel M, Pileri S, Stein H, Croce CM. Nucleophosmin (NPM) gene rearrangements in Ki-1-positive lymphomas. Cancer Res 1994;54:2873–7.

293. Carbone A, Gloghini A, De Re V, Tamaro P, Boiocchi M, Volpe R. Histopathologic, immunophenotypic, and genotypic analysis of Ki-1 anaplastic large cell lymphomas that express histiocyte-associated antigens. Cancer 1990;66:2547–56.

294. _____, Gloghini A, Volpe R. Paraffin section immunohistochemistry in the diagnosis of Hodgkin's disease and anaplastic large cell (CD30+) lymphoma. Virchows Arch [A] 1992;420:527–32.

295. _____, Gloghini A, Zanette I, Canal B, Volpe R. Demonstration of Epstein-Barr viral genomes by in situ hybridization in acquired innumodeficiency syndrome-related high grade and anaplastic large cell lymphomas (CD30+ lymphoma). Am J Clin Pathol 1993;99:289–97.

296. Cesarman E, Inghirami G, Chadburn A, Knowles DM. High levels of p53 protein expression do not correlate with p53 gene mutations in anaplastic large cell lymphoma. Am J Pathol 1993;143:845–56.

297. Chan JK. CD30+ (Ki-1) lymphoma: t(2;5) translocation, the implicated genes, and more. Adv Anat Pathol 1995 (in press).

298. _____, Buchanan R, Fletcher CD. Sarcomatoid variant of anaplastic large cell Ki-1 lymphoma. Report of a case. Am J Surg Pathol 1990;14:983–8.

299. _____, Ng CS, Hui PK, et al. Anaplastic large cell Ki-1 lymphoma, delineation of two morphological types. Histopathology 1989;15:11–34.

300. _____, Ng CS, Hui PK, et al. Anaplastic large cell Ki-1 lymphoma of bone. Cancer 1991;68:2186–91.

301. Chott A, Kaserer K, Augustin I, et al. Ki-1-positive large cell lymphoma. A clinicopathologic study of 41 cases. Am J Surg Pathol 1990;14:439–48.

302. Chow JM, Cheng AL, Su IJ, Wang CH. 13-cis-retinoic acid induces cellular differentiation and durable remission in refractory cutaneous Ki-1 lymphoma. Cancer 1991;67:2490–4.

303. de Bruin PC, Belijaards RC, van Heerde P, et al. Differences in clinical behaviour and immunophenotype between primary cutaneous and primary nodal anaplastic large cell lymphoma of T-cell and null cell phenotype. Histopathology 1993;23:127–35.

304. Dekmezian R, Goodacre A, Cabanillas F. The 2;5 translocation: is it specific for anaplastic (Ki-1) large cell lymphomas? [Abstract] Mod Pathol 1990;3:25A.

305. Delabie J, Shipman R, Bruggen J, et al. Expression of the novel intermediate filament-associated protein restin in Hodgkin's disease and anaplastic large-cell lymphoma. Blood 1992;80:2891–6.

306. Delsol G, Al Saati T, Gatter KC, et al. Coexpression of epithelial membrane antigen (EMA), Ki-1, and interleukin-2 receptor by anaplastic large cell lymphomas. Diagnostic value in so-called malignant histiocytosis. Am J Pathol 1988;130:59–70.

307. _____, Blancher A, Al Saati T, et al. Antibody BNH9 detects red blood cell-related antigens on anaplastic large cell (CD30+) lymphomas. Br J Cancer 1991;64:321–6.

308. Doglioni C, Pelosio P, Mombello A, Scarpa A, Chilosi M. Immunohistochemical evidence of abnormal expression of the antioncogene-encoded p53 phosphoprotein in Hodgkin's disease and CD30+ anaplastic lymphomas. Hematol Pathol 1991;5:67–73.

309. Durkop H, Latza U, Hummel M, Eitelbach F, Seed B, Stein H. Molecular cloning and expression of a new member of the nerve growth factor receptor family that is characteristic for Hodgkin's disease. Cell 1992;68:421–7.

310. Dusenbery D, Jones DB, Sapp KW, Lemons FM. Cytologic findings in the sarcomatoid variant of large cell anaplastic (Ki-1) lymphoma, a case report. Acta Cytol 1993;37:508–14.

311. Eckert F, Schmid U, Kaudewitz P, Burg G, Braun-Flaco O. Follicular lymphoid hyperplasia of the skin with high content of Ki-1 positive lymphocytes. Am J Dermatopathol 1989;11:345–52.

311a. Falini B, Pileri S, Pizzolo G, et al. CD30 (Ki-1) molecule: a new cytokine receptor of the tumor necrosis factor receptor superfamily as a tool for diagnosis and immunotherapy. Blood 1995;85:1–14.

312. _____, Pileri S, Stein H, et al. Variable expression of leukocyte common (CD45) antigen in CD30 (Ki-1)-positive anaplastic large cell lymphoma: implications for the differential diagnosis between lymphoid and nonlymphoid malignancies. Hum Pathol 1990;21:624–9.

216

313. Feller AC, Sterry W. Large cell anaplastic lymphoma of the skin. Br J Dermatol 1989;121:593–602.

314. Fischer P, Nacheva E, Mason DY, et al. A Ki-1 (CD30)-positive human cell line (Karpas 299) established from a high-grade non-Hodgkin's lymphoma, showing a 2;5 translocation and rearrangement of the T-cell receptor ß-chain gene. Blood 1988;72:234–40.

315. Flynn KJ, Dehner LP, Gajl-Peczalska KH, Dahl MV, Ramsay N, Wang N. Regressing atypical histiocytosis: a cutaneous proliferation of atypical neoplastic histiocytes with unexpectedly indolent biologic behavior. Cancer 1982;49:959–70.

315a. Fraga M, Brousset P, Schlaifer D, et al. Bone marrow involvement in anaplastic large cell lymphoma. Immunohistochemical detection of minimal disease and its prognostic significance. Am J Clin Pathol 1995;103:82–9.

316. Frierson HF Jr, Bellafiore FJ, Gaffey MJ, McCary WS, Innes DJ Jr, Williams ME. Cytokeratin in anaplastic large cell lymphoma. Mod Pathol 1994;7:317–21.

317. Fujimoto J, Hata J, Ishii E, et al. Ki-1 lymphomas in childhood: immunohistochemical analysis and the significance of epithelial membrane antigen (EMA) as a new marker. Virchows Arch [A] 1988;412:307–14.

318. Gerdes J, Schwarting R, Stein H. High proliferative activity of Reed Sternberg associated antigen Ki-1 positive cells in normal lymphoid tissue. J Clin Pathol 1986;39:993–7.

319. Gordon BG, Weisenburger DD, Warkentin PI, et al. Peripheral T-cell lymphoma in childhood and adolescents. A clinicopathologic study of 22 patients. Cancer 1993;71:257–63.

320. Greer JP, Kinney MC, Collins RD, et al. Clinical features of 31 patients with Ki-1 anaplastic large-cell lymphoma. J Clin Oncol 1991;9:539–47.

321. Gustmann C, Altmannsberger M, Osborn M, Griesser H, Feller AC. Cytokeratin expression and vimentin content in large cell anaplastic lymphomas and other non-Hodgkin's lymphomas. Am J Pathol 1991;138:1413–22.

322. Hansmann ML, Fellbaum C, Bohm A. Large cell anaplastic lymphoma: evaluation of immunophenotype on paraffin and frozen sections in comparison with ultrastructural features. Virchows Arch [A] 1991;418:427–33.

323. Headington JT, Roth MS, Ginsburg D, Lichter AS, Hyder D, Schnitzer B. T-cell receptor gene rearrangement in regressing atypical histiocytosis. Arch Dermatol 1987;123:1183–7.

324. _____, Roth MS, Schnitzer B. Regressing atypical histiocytosis: a review and critical appraisal. Semin Diagn Pathol 1987;4:28–37.

325. Herbst H, Dallenbach F, Hummel M, et al. Epstein-Barr virus DNA and latent gene products in Ki-1 (CD30)-positive anaplastic large cell lymphomas. Blood 1991;78:1–10.

326. _____, Stein H. Tumor virus in CD30+ anaplastic large cell lymphomas. Leuk Lymphoma 1993;9:321–8.

327. _____, Tippelmann G, Anagnostopoulos I, et al. Immunoglobulin and T-cell receptor gene rearrangements in Hodgkin's disease and Ki-1-positive anaplastic large cell lymphoma: dissociation between phenotype and genotype. Leuk Res 1989;13:103–16.

328. Inghirami G, Macri L, Cesarman E, Chadburn A, Zhong J, Knowles DM. Molecular characterization of CD30+ anaplastic large-cell lymphoma: high frequency of c-myc proto-oncogene activation. Blood 1994;83:3581–90.

329. Jaworsky C, Cirillo-Hyland V, Petrozzi JW, Lessin SR, Murphy GF. Regressing atypical histiocytosis. Aberrant prothymocyte differentiation, T-cell receptor gene rearrangements, and nodal involvement. Arch Dermatol 1990;126:1609–16.

330. Jones DB, Gerdes J, Stein H, Wright DH. An investigation of Ki-1 positive large cell lymphoma with antibodies reactive with tissue macrophages. Hematol Oncol 1986;4:315–22.

332. Kadin ME. Characteristic immunologic profile of large atypical cells in lymphomatoid papulosis. Possible implications for histogenesis and relationship to other diseases [Editorial]. Arch Dermatol 1986;122:1388–90.

333. _____. Ki-1/CD30+ (anaplastic) large cell lymphoma: maturation to a clinicopathologic entity with prospects of effective therapy [Editorial]. J Clin Oncol 1994;12:884–7.

331. _____, Sako D, Berliner N, et al. Childhood Ki-1 lymphoma presenting with skin lesions and peripheral lymphadenopathy. Blood 1986;68:1042–9.

334. _____, Vonderheid EC, Sako D, Clayton LK, Olbrict S. Clonal composition of T cells in lymphomatoid papulosis. Am J Pathol 1987;126:13–7.

335. Kanavaros P, Jiwa NM, De Bruin PC, et al. High incidence of EBV genome in CD30-positive non-Hodgkin's lymphomas. J Pathol 1992;168:307–15.

336. _____, Lavergne A, Galian A, Houdart R, Bernard JF. Primary gastric peripheral T-cell malignant lymphoma with helper/inducer phenotype. First case report with a complete histological, ultrastructural and immunochemical study. Cancer 1988;61:1602–10.

337. Kaneko Y, Frizzera G, Edamura S, et al. A novel translocation, t(2;5)(p23;q35), in childhood phagocytic large T-cell lymphoma mimicking malignant histiocytosis. Blood 1989;73:806–13.

338. Kaudewitz P, Stein H, Burg G, Mason DY, Braun-Falco O. Atypical cells in lymphomatoid papulosis express the Hodgkin cell-associated antigen Ki-1. J Invest Dermatol 1986;86:350–4.

339. _____, Stein H, Dallenbach F, et al. Primary and secondary cutaneous Ki-1+ (CD30+) anaplastic large cell lymphomas: morphologic, immunohistologic, and clinical characteristics. Am J Pathol 1989;135:359–67.

340. Kinney MC, Collins RD, Greer JP, et al. A small cell variant of Ki-1 (CD30+) T-cell lymphoma. Am J Surg Pathol 1993;17:859–68.

341. _____, Glick AD, Stein H, Collins RD. Comparison of anaplastic large cell Ki-1 lymphomas and microvillous lymphomas in their immunologic and ultrastructural features. Am J Surg Pathol 1990;14:1047–60.

342. _____, Greer JP, Glick AD, Salhany KE, Collins RD. Anaplastic large-cell Ki-1 malignant lymphomas: recognition, biological and clinical implications. Pathol Annu 1991;26(Pt 1):1–24.

343. Knuutila S, Lakkala T, Teerenhovi L, Peltomaki P, Kovanen R, Franssila K. t(2;5)(p23;q35)—a specific chromosome abnormality in large cell anaplastic (Ki-1) lymphoma. Leuk Lymphoma 1990;3:53–9.

344. Krishnan J, Tomaszewski MM, Kao GF. Primary cutaneous CD30+ anaplastic large cell lymphoma. Report of 27 cases. J Cutan Pathol 1993;20:193–202.

345. Lennert K, Feller AC. Histopathology of non-Hodgkin's lymphomas (based on the updated Kiel classification). Berlin: Springer-Verlag, 1992:152–3; 229–44; 256–8.

346. Leoncini L, Del Vecchio MT, Kraft R, et al. Hodgkin's disease and CD30-positive anaplastic large cell lymphomas—a continuous spectrum of malignant disorders. A quantitative morphometric and immunohistologic study. Am J Pathol 1990;137:1047–57.

347. Le Tourneau A, Audouin J, Diebold J. Ultrastructural study of 4 cases of Ki-1 positive large anaplastic cell malignant lymphoma. Virchows Arch [A] 1988;413:215–22.

349. Lopategui JR, Sun LH, Chan JK, et al. Low frequency association of the t(2;5)(p23;q35) chromosomal translocations with CD30+ lymphomas from American and Asian patients. A reverse transcriptase-polymerase chain reaction study. Am J Pathol 1995;146:323–8.

349a. _____, Gaffey MJ, Chan JK, et al. Infrequent association of Epstein Barr virus with CD3-positive anaplastic large cell lymphoma from American and Asian patients. Am J Surg Pathol 1995;19:42–9.

350. Mason DY, Bastard C, Rimokh R, et al. CD30-positive large cell lymphomas ("Ki-1 lymphoma") are associated with a chromosomal translocation involving 5q35. Br J Haematol 1990;74:161–8.

351. Mechtersheimer G, Moller P. Expression of Ki-1 antigen (CD30) in mesenchymal tumors. Cancer 1990;66:1732–7.

352. Miettinen M. CD30-distribution: immunohistochemical study on formalin-fixed, paraffin-embedded Hodgkin's and non-Hodgkin's lymphomas. Arch Pathol Lab Med 1992;116:1197–201.

353. Miyake K, Yoshino T, Sarken AB, Teramot N, Akagi T. CD30 antigen in non-Hodgkin's lymphoma. Pathol Int 1994;44:428–34.

354. Morris SW, Kirstein MN, Valentine MB, et al. Fusion of a kinase gene, ALK, to a nucleolar protein gene, NPM, in non-Hodgkin's lymphoma. Science 1994;263:1281–4.

355. Motley RJ, Jasani B, Ford AM, Poynton CH, Calonje-Daly JE, Holt PJ. Regressing atypical histiocytosis, a regressing cutaneous phase of Ki-1 positive anaplastic large cell lymphoma. Cancer 1992;70:476–83.

356. Nakamura S, Takagi N, Kojima M, et al. Clinicopathologic study of large cell anaplastic lymphoma (Ki-1-positive large cell lymphoma) among the Japanese. Cancer 1991;68:118–29.

357. Noorduyn LA, de Bruin PC, van Heerde P, van de Sandt MM, Ossenkoppele GJ, Meijer CJ. Relation of CD30 expression to survival and morphology in large cell B cell lymphomas. J Clin Pathol 1994;47:33–7.

358. O'Connor NT, Stein H, Gatter KC, et al. Genotypic analysis of large cell lymphomas which express the Ki-1 antigen. Histopathology 1987;11:733–40.

359. Offit K, Ladanyi M, Gangi MD, Ebrahim SA, Filippa D, Changati RS. Ki-1 antigen expression defines a favorable clinical subset of non-B cell non-Hodgkin's lymphoma. Leukemia 1990;4:625–30.

360. Pallesen G. The diagnostic significance of the CD30 (Ki-1) antigen [Commentary]. Histopathology 1990; 16:409–13.

361. _____, Hamilton-Dutoit SJ. Ki-1 (CD30) antigen is regularly expressed by tumor cells of embryonal carcinoma. Am J Pathol 1988;133:446–50.

362. Paulli M, Berti E, Rosso R. CD30/Ki-1+ lymphoproliferative disorders of the skin: clinicopathologic correlation and statistical analysis of 86 cases [Abstract]. Mod Pathol 1994;7:118A.

363. Penny RJ, Blaustein JC, Longtine JA, Pinkus GS. Ki-1-positive large cell lymphomas, a heterogeneous group of neoplasms. Morphologic, immunophenotypic, genotypic and clinical features of 24 cases. Cancer 1991;68:362–73.

364. Pfreundschuh M, Pohl C, Berenbeck C, et al. Detection of a soluble form of the CD30 antigen in sera of patients with lymphoma, adult T-cell leukemia and infectious mononucleosis. Int J Cancer 1990;45:869–74.

365. Pileri S, Bocchia M, Baroni CD, et al. Anaplastic large cell lymphoma (CD30+/Ki-1+), results of a prospective clinicopathological study of 69 cases. Br J Hematol 1994;86:513–23.

366. _____, Falini B, Delsol G, et al. Lymphohistiocytic T-cell lymphoma (anaplastic large cell lymphoma CD30+/Ki-1+ with a high content of reactive histiocytes). Histopathology 1990;16:383–91.

367. _____, Sabattini E, Poggi S, Amini M, Falini B, Stein H. Lymphohistiocytic T-cell lymphoma [Letter]. Histopathology 1994;25:191–3.

368. Piris M, Brown DC, Gatter KC, Mason DY. CD30 expression in non-Hodgkin's lymphoma. Histopathology 1990;17:211–8.

369. _____, Gatter KC, Mason DY. CD30 expression in follicular lymphoma. Histopathology 1991;18:25–9.

370. Ralfkiaer E, Bosq J, Gatter KC, et al. Expression of a Hodgkin and Reed-Sternberg cell associated antigen (Ki-1) in cutaneous lymphoid infiltrates. Arch Dermatol Res 1987;279:285–92.

371. _____, Stein H, Wantzin GL, Thomsen K, Ralfkiaer N, Mason DY. Lymphomatoid papulosis. Characterization of skin infiltrates by monoclonal antibodies. Am J Clin Pathol 1985;84:587–93.

372. Reiter A, Schrappe M, Tiemana M, et al. Successful treatment strategy for Ki-1 anaplastic large-cell lymphoma of childhood: a prospective analysis of 62 patients enrolled in three consecutive Berlin-Frankfurt-Munster group studies. J Clin Oncol 1994;12:899–908.

373. Rimokh R, Magaud JP, Berger F, et al. A translocation involving a specific breakpoint (q35) on chromosome 5 is characteristic of anaplastic large cell lymphoma ("Ki-1 lymphoma"). Br J Haematol 1989;71:31–6.

374. Rivas C, Piris MA, Gamallo C, et al. Ultrastructure of 26 cases of Ki-1 lymphomas: morphoimmunologic correlation. Ultrastruct Pathol 1990;14:381–97.

375. Rodriguez J, Pugh W, Romaguera J, Cabanillas F. Anaplastic Ki-1+ large-cell lymphoma. Cancer Invest 1993;11:554–8.

376. Ross CW, Schlegelmilch JA, Grogan TM, Weiss LM, Schnitzer B, Hanson CA. Detection of Epstein-Barr virus genome in Ki-1 (CD30)-positive large cell anaplastic lymphomas using the polymerase chain reaction. Am J Pathol 1992;141:457–65.

377. Rosso R, Paulli M, Magrini U, et al. Anaplastic large cell lymphoma, CD30/Ki-1 positive, expressing the CD15/Leu-M1 antigen, immunohistochemical and morphological relationships to Hodgkin's disease. Virchows Arch [A] 1990;416:229–35.

378. Sakurai S, Nakajima T, Oyama T, Sano T, Hosomura Y. Anaplastic large cell lymphoma with histiocytic phenotypes. Acta Pathol Jpn 1993;43:142–5.

379. Salhany KE, Collins RD, Greer JP, Kinney MC. Long-term survival in Ki-1 lymphoma. Cancer 1991;67:516–22.

380. Sanchez NP, Pittelkow MR, Muller SA, Banks PM, Winkelmann RK. The clinicopathologic spectrum of lymphomatoid papulosis: study of 31 cases. J Am Acad Dermatol 1983;8:81–94.

381. Sandlund JT, Pui CH. Santana VM, et al. Clinical features and treatment outcome for children with CD30+ large-cell non-Hodgkin's lymphoma. J Clin Oncol 1994;12:895–8.

382. Schnitzer B, Roth MS, Hyder DM, Ginsburg D. Ki-1 lymphomas in children. Cancer 1988;61:1213–21.

383. Schwab U, Stein H, Gerdes J, et al. Production of a monoclonal antibody specific for Hodgkin and Sternberg-Reed cells of Hodgkin's disease and a subset of normal lymphoid cells. Nature 1982;299:65–7.

384. Schwarting R, Gerdes J, Durkop H, Falini B, Pileri S, Stein H. Ber-H2: a new anti-Ki-1 (CD30) monoclonal antibody directed at a formol-resistant epitope. Blood 1989;74:1678–89

384a. Shiota M, Fujimoto J, Takenaga M, et al. Diagnosis of t(2;5)(p23;q35)-associated Ki-1 lymphoma with immunohistochemistry. Blood 1994;84:3648–52..

385. Shulman LN, Frisard B, Antin JH, et al. Primary Ki-1 anaplastic large cell lymphoma in adults: clinical characteristics and therapeutic outcome. J Clin Oncol 1993;11:937–42.

386. Smith CA, Gruss HJ, Davis T, et al. CD30 antigen, a marker for Hodgkin's lymphoma, is a receptor whose ligand defines an emerging family of cytokines with homology to TNF. Cell 1993;73:1349–60.

387. Stein H, Dallenbach F. Diffuse large cell lymphomas of B and T cell type. In: Knowles DM, ed. Neoplastic Hematopathology. Baltimore: Williams & Wilkins. 1992;675–714.

387a. _____, Mason DY, Gerdes J, et al. The expression of the Hodgkin's disease associated antigen Ki-1 in reactive and neoplastic lymphoid tissue: evidence that Reed-Sternberg cells and histiocytic malignancies are derived from activated lymphoid cells. Blood 1985;66:848–58.

388. Su IJ, Cheng AL, Kadin M. Retionic acid-induced differentiation and regression of cutaneous Ki-1 anaplastic large cell lymphoma: in vivo and in vitro observations [Abstract]. Mod Pathol 1994;7:144A.

389. Takimoto Y, Tanaka H, Tanabe O, Kuramoto A, Sasaki N, Nanba K. A patient with anaplastic large cell lymphoma (Ki-1 lymphoma) showing clonal integration of HTLV-1 proviral DNA. Leukemia 1994;8:507–9.

390. Tashiro K, Kikuchi M, Takeshita M, Yoshida T, Ohshima K. Clinicopathological study of Ki-1-positive lymphomas. Pathol Res Pract 1989;185:461–7.

391. Valentino LA, Helwig EB. Lymphomatoid papulosis. Arch Pathol 1973;96:409–16.

392. Weisenburger DD, Vose JM, Gordon BG, et al. Is the 2;5 chromosomal translocation specific for CD30+ anaplastic large cell lymphoma [Abstract]? Mod Pathol 1993;6:103A.

393. Weiss LM, Picker LJ, Copenhaver CM, Warnke RA, Sklar J. Large-cell hematolymphoid neoplasms of uncertain lineage. Hum Pathol 1988;19:967–73.

394. _____, Wood GS, Trela M, Warnke RA, Sklar J. Clonal T-cell populations in lymphomatoid papulosis: evidence of a lymphoproliferative origin for a clinically benign disease. N Engl J Med 1986;315:475–9.

394a. Wellmann A, Clark HM, Otsuki T, Jaffe ES, Raffeld M. Detection of the t(2;5)(p23;q35) in classical anaplastic large cell lymphoma by reverse transcriptase-polymerase chain reaction [Abstract]. Mod Pathol 1995;8:123A.

395. Willemze R, Beljaards RC, Meijer CJ. Classification of primary cutaneous T-cell lymphomas. Histopathology 1994;24:405–15.

396. _____, Meyer CJ, Van Vloten WA, Scheffer E. The clinical and histological spectrum of lymphomatoid papulosis. Br J Dermatol 1982;107:131–44.

397. Wong KF, Chan JK, Ng CS, Chu YC, Lam PW, Yuen HL. Anaplastic large cell Ki-1 lymphoma involving bone marrow. Marrow findings and association with reactive hemophagocytosis. Am J Hematol 1991;37:112–9.

398. Wood GS. Benign and malignant cutaneous lymphoproliferative disorders including mycosis fungoides. In: Knowles DM, ed. Neoplastic hematopathology. Baltimore: Williams & Wilkins, 1992:917–52.

T-Cell–Rich Large B-Cell Lymphoma

399. Baddoura FK, Chan WC. T-cell rich B-cell lymphoma: a clinicopathologic study [Abstract]. Mod Pathol 1991;4:68A.

400. Chittal SM, Brousset P, Voigt JJ, Delsol G. Large B-cell lymphoma rich in T-cells and simulating Hodgkin's disease. Histopathology 1991;19:211–20.

401. Delabie J, Vandenberghe E, Kennes C, et al. Histiocyte-rich B-cell lymphoma. A distinct clinicopathologic entity possibly related to lymphocyte predominant Hodgkin's disease, paragranuloma subtype. Am J Surg Pathol 1992;16:37–48.

402. Jaffe ES, Gonzalez CL, Medeiros LJ, Raffeld M. T-cell-rich B-cell lymphomas [Letter]. Am J Surg Pathol 1991;15:491–2.

403. _____, Longo DL, Cossman J, Hsu S, Arnold A, korsmeyer SJ. Diffuse B cell lymphomas with T cell predominance in patients with follicular lymphoma or "pseudo T cell lymphoma" [Abstract]. Lab Invest 1984;50:27A–8A.

404. Kamel OW, Gelb AB, Shibuya RB, Warnke RA. Leu 7 (CD57) reactivity distinguishes nodular-lymphocyte predominance Hodgkin's disease from nodular sclerosing Hodgkin's disease, T-cell-rich B-cell lymphoma and follicular lymphoma. Am J Pathol 1993;142:541–6.

405. Krishnan J, Wallberg K, Frizzera G. T-cell-rich large B-cell lymphoma. A study of 30 cases, supporting its histologic heterogeneity and lack of clinical distinctiveness. Am J Surg Pathol 1994;18:455–65.

406. Lennert K, Feller AC. Histopathology of non-Hodgkin's lymphomas (based on the updated Kiel classification). 2nd ed. Berlin: Springer-Verlag, 1992:162–3.

407. Lippman SM, Spier CM, Miller TP, Slymen DJ, Rybski JA, Grogan TM. Tumor-infiltrating T-lymphocytes in B-cell diffuse large cell lymphoma related to disease course. Mod Pathol 1990;3:361–7.

408. Loke SL, Ho F, Srivastava G, Fu KH, Leung B, Liang R. Clonal Epstein-Barr virus genome in T-cell-rich lymphomas of B or probable B lineage. Am J Pathol 1992;140:981–9.

409. Macon WR, Williams ME, Greer JP, Stein RS, Collins RD, Cousar JB. T-cell-rich B-cell lymphomas, a clinicopathologic study of 19 cases. Am J Surg Pathol 1992;16:351–63.

410. Medeiros LJ, Lardelli P, Stetler-Stevenson M, Longo DL, Jaffe ES. Genotypic analysis of diffuse, mixed cell lymphomas: comparison with morphologic and immunophenotypic findings. Am J Clin Pathol 1991;95:547–55.

411. Mikata A, Suzuki H, Ohkawa H. Immunohistochemical studies on B cell lymphomas with special reference to T cell infiltration and its significance as a prognostic factor. Acta Pathol Jpn 1988;38:47–58.

412. Mirchandani I, Palutke M, Tabaczka P, Goldfarb S, Eisenberg L, Pak MS. B-cell lymphoma morphologically resembling T-cell lymphomas. Cancer 1985;56:1578–83.

413. Ng CS, Chan JK, Hui PK, Lau WH. Large B-cell lymphomas with a high content of reactive T cells. Hum Pathol 1989;20:1145–54.
414. Ohshima K, Masuda Y, Kikuchi M, et al. Monoclonal B cells and restricted oligoclonal T cells in T-cell rich B-cell lymphoma. Pathol Res Pract 1994;190:15–24.
415. Osborne BM, Butler JJ, Pugh WC. T-cell-rich B-cell lymphomas: the authors' response [Letter]. Am J Surg Pathol 1991;15:492.
416. _____, Butler JJ, Pugh WC. The value of immunophenotyping on paraffin sections in the identification of T-cell rich B-cell large-cell lymphomas: lineage confirmed by JH rearrangement. Am J Surg Pathol 1990;14:933–8.

417. Ramsay AD, Smith WJ, Isaacson PG. T-cell-rich B-cell lymphoma. Am J Surg Pathol 1988;12:433–43.
418. Rodriguez J, Pugh WC, Cabanillas F. T-cell rich B-cell lymphomas. Blood 1993;82:1586–9.
419. Stansfeld AG. Low grade B-cell lymphomas. In: Stansfeld AG, d'Ardenne AJ, eds. Lymph node biopsy interpretation. 2nd ed. Edinburgh, Churchill Livingstone, 1992:229–83.
420. Winberg CD, Sheibani K, Burke JS, Wu A, Rappaport H. T-cell-rich lymphoproliferative disorders: morphologic and immunologic differential diagnoses. Cancer 1988;62:1539–55.

Mediastinal Large B-Cell Lymphoma

421. Addis BJ, Isaacson PG. Large cell lymphoma of the mediastinum: a B-cell tumor of probable thymic origin. Histopathology 1986;10:379–90.
422. Al-Sharabati M, Chittal S, Duga-Neulat I, et al. Primary anterior mediastinal B-cell lymphoma. A clinicopathologic and immunohistochemical study of 16 cases. Cancer 1991;67:2579–87.
423. Davis RE, Dorfman RF, Warnke RA. Primary large cell lymphoma of the thymus: a diffuse B-cell neoplasm presenting as primary mediastinal lymphoma. Hum Pathol 1990;21:1262–8.
424. Hofmann WJ, Momburg F, Moller P. Thymic medullary cells expressing B lymphocyte antigens. Hum Pathol 1988;19:1280–7.
425. Isaacson PG, Norton AJ, Addis BJ. The human thymus contains a novel population of B lymphocytes. Lancet 1987;2:1488–91.
426. Jacobson JO, Aisenberg AC, Lamarre L, et al. Mediastinal large cell lymphoma: an uncommon subset of adult lymphoma curable with combined modality therapy. Cancer 1988;62:1893–8.
427. Lamarre L, Jacobson JO, Aisenberg AC, Harris NL. Primary large cell lymphoma of the mediastinum: a histologic and immunophenotypic study of 29 cases. Am J Surg Pathol 1989;13:730–9.
428. Lavabre-Bertrand T, Donadio D, Fegueux N, et al. A study of 15 cases of primary mediastinal lymphoma of B-cell type. Cancer 1992;69:2561–6.
429. Levitt LJ, Aisenberg AC, Harris NL, Linggood RM, Poppema S. Primary non-Hodgkin's lymphoma of the mediastinum. Cancer 1982;50:2486–92.
430. Lichtenstein AK, Levine A, Taylor CR, et al. Primary mediastinal lymphoma in adults. Am J Med 1980;68:509–14.
431. Menestrina F, Chilosi M, Bonetti F, et al. Mediastinal large-cell lymphoma of B-type, with sclerosis: histopathological and immunohistochemical study of eight cases. Histopathology 1986;10:589–600.
432. Miller JB, Variakojis D, Bitran JD, et al. Diffuse histiocytic lymphoma with sclerosis: a clinicopathologic entity frequently causing superior vena caval obstruction. Cancer 1981;47:748–56.
433. Moller P, Lammler B, Eberlein-Gonska M, et al. Primary mediastinal clear cell lymphoma of B-cell type. Virchows Arch [A] 1986;409:79–92.

434. _____, Matthaei-Mauer DU, Hofmann WJ, Dorken B, Moldenhauer G. Immunophenotypic similarities of mediastinal clear-cell lymphoma and sinusoidal (monocytoid) B cells. Int J Cancer 1989;43:10–6.
435. _____, Moldenhauer G, Momburg F, et al. Mediastinal lymphoma of clear cell type is a tumor corresponding to terminal steps of B-cell differentiation. Blood 1987;69:1087–95.
436. Nakagawa A, Nakamura S, Kohsikawa T, et al. Clinicopathologic study of primary mediastinal non-lymphoblastic non-Hodgkin's lymphomas among the Japanese. Acta Pathol Jpn 1993;43:44–54.
437. Perrone T, Frizzera G, Rosai J. Mediastinal diffuse large-cell lymphoma with sclerosis: a clinicopathologic study of 60 cases. Am J Surg Pathol 1986;10:176–91.
438. Scarpa A, Bonetti F, Menestrina F, et al. Mediastinal large-cell lymphoma with sclerosis: genotypic analysis establishes its B-nature. Virchows Arch [A] 1987;412:17–21.
439. _____, Borgato L, Chilosi M, et al. Evidence of c-myc gene abnormalities in mediastinal large B-cell lymphoma of young adult age. Blood 1991;78:780–8.
440. Stein H, Dallenbach F. Diffuse large cell lymphomas of B and T cell type. In: Knowles DM, ed. Neoplastic hematopathology. Baltimore: Williams & Wilkins, 1992:675–714.
441. Strickler JG, Kurtin PJ. Mediastinal lymphoma. Semin Diagn Pathol 1991;8:2–13.
442. Suster S. Large cell lymphoma of the mediastinum with marked tropism for germinal center. Cancer 1992;69:2910–6.
443. Todeschini G, Ambrosetti A, Meneghini UV, et al. Mediastinal large B-cell lymphoma with sclerosis: a clinical study of 21 patients. J Clin Oncol 1990;8:804–8.
444. Trump DL, Mann RB. Diffuse large cell and undifferentiated lymphomas with prominent mediastinal involvement. A poor prognostic subset of patients with non-Hodgkin's lymphoma. Cancer 1982;50:277–82.
445. Waldron JA Jr, Dohring EJ, Farber LR. Primary large cell lymphomas of the mediastinum: an analysis of 20 cases. Semin Diagn Pathol 1985;2:281–95.
446. Yousem SA, Weiss LM, Warnke RA. Primary mediastinal non-Hodgkin's lymphomas: a morphological and immunologic study of 19 cases. Am J Clin Pathol 1985;83:676–80.

10

MALIGNANT LYMPHOMA, SMALL NONCLEAVED CELL

Definition. Small noncleaved cell lymphoma (SNCL) is a highly proliferative lymphoma composed of a relatively monomorphic population of cells with blastic-appearing nuclei and a moderate rim of basophilic cytoplasm. SNCL encompasses Burkitt's lymphoma (BL) and lymphomas that were designated as *undifferentiated non-Burkitt's type* in the Rappaport classification (45) and *non-Burkitt's type* in the Working Formulation (38). In the updated Kiel classification (47), Burkitt's lymphoma has been removed from the B-lymphoblastic category and assigned separate status. However, SNCL is biologically similar to some cases of L3 acute lymphoblastic leukemia.

Incidence. Endemic BL is the most common malignancy of childhood in equatorial Africa, 10 times more frequent than the next most common tumor, Wilms' tumor. BL is also endemic in Papua, New Guinea (5,50). North Africa and South America are regions of intermediate incidence. Incidence peaks at 4 to 7 years, with an overall male to female ratio of 2 to 1. In children with jaw tumors, the male to female ratio is 3.2 to 1. There is a distinctive geographic distribution of BL in Africa, correlating with climatic factors such as rainfall and altitude and mirroring that of many viral diseases; this initially suggested dissemination by an arthropod-borne vector (7–9,12). This geographic distribution also corresponds closely to that of holoendemic malaria. Approximately 95 percent of cases of endemic BL are associated with the Epstein-Barr virus (EBV) (25). Since there is evidence of defective T-cell regulation of EBV-infected B cells in patients with malaria, it has been theorized that T-cell suppression and B-cell stimulation may play a role in the pathogenesis of BL.

Sporadic BL in the United States was first reported in 1965 (15,40). However, confirmed cases clearly occurred earlier (figs. 10-1, 10-2) (6,46). In the United States and western Europe, SNCL accounts for approximately 2 percent of lymphomas, with a median age of 30 years (38). There is a high frequency of occurrence in children, accounting for 30 to 50 percent of childhood lymphomas, but SNCL is rare below the age of 2

years (30–32). BL occurs in a younger age group than the non-Burkitt's type (20,26,37), probably accounting for the bimodal age distribution found for SNCL in the Working Formulation study (38). The male to female ratio is about 2.5 to 1 (38).

The Burkitt Lymphoma Registry (27) compared the incidence and epidemiology of BL in the United States and Africa: in the United States fewer cases are EBV-associated (less than 30 percent have the viral genome); the lymphoma occurs in somewhat older patients (70 percent are more than 12 years old); and there is a more diffuse geographic disease distribution. Similarities include time-space clustering (reported in California, Virginia, and Pennsylvania); a male

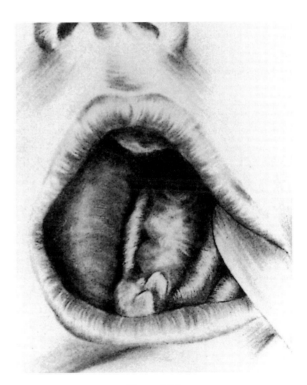

Figure 10-1
BURKITT'S LYMPHOMA: JAW
AND GINGIVAL INVOLVEMENT

First case of Burkitt's lymphoma in the United States, recorded in 1928 (unrecognized by the authors at that time) and confirmed as BL in 1964 (15). The patient was a 16-year-old girl from St. Louis, Missouri. This illustration demonstrates tumors presenting in the mouth, displacing teeth. (Fig. 1 from Brown JB, O'Keefe CD. Sarcoma of the ovary with unusual oral metastases. Ann Surg 1928;87:467-71.)

221

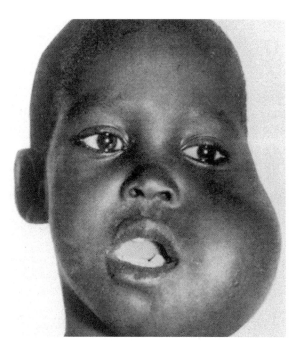

Figure 10-2
BURKITT'S LYMPHOMA: MANDIBLE
A large tumor of the mandible in a 5-year-old African boy. (Fig. 2.9 from Burkitt DP, Wright DH. Burkitt's lymphoma. Edinburgh and London: E & S Livingston, 1970:11.)

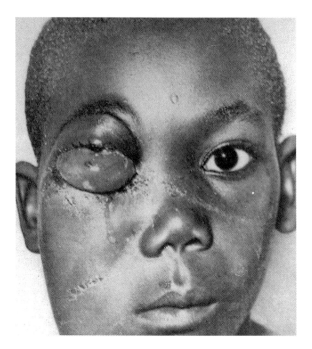

Figure 10-3
BURKITT'S LYMPHOMA: MANDIBLE, MAXILLA, AND ORBIT
Involvement of the right mandible, maxilla, and orbit producing proptosis in an African boy. (Fig. 5 from Burkitt DP, O'Conor GT. Lymphoma in African children. I. A clinical syndrome. Cancer 1961;14:258–69.)

preponderance in children below age 13 years; and an excellent response to chemotherapy.

There is an increased incidence of SNCL in patients with immunodeficiency disorders and it is the most common form of lymphoma in patients with acquired immunodeficiency syndrome (AIDS) (55).

Natural History and Clinical Features. SNCL is classified as a high-grade tumor in both the Working Formulation (38) and the Kiel classification (47). The neoplasms rapidly proliferate, with very high growth fractions and potential doubling times. Measured doubling times of BL are reported to vary from 12 hours to several days (31).

In Africa, endemic BL shows a predilection for bones of the jaw and face (figs. 10-2, 10-3), including the orbital bones, and may involve all four quadrants of the jaw with loosening of deciduous teeth (11,12). Other frequent sites of involvement include ovary (fig. 10-4) (a presenting feature in some young African girls), testis, thyroid, salivary gland, kidney (fig. 10-5), breast in pregnant women, and central nervous system. Paraspinal tumors may manifest with paraplegia. Bone marrow involvement is found in only 8 percent of cases.

In most cases of SNCL in the United States and Europe, abdominal involvement is the most frequent manifestation (fig. 10-6). The small intestine is most often affected, but the stomach, large intestine, peritoneum, and retroperitoneal tissues may be involved. The central nervous system, ovary, facial bones, testis, and lymph nodes are less frequently involved. Bone marrow involvement at presentation occurs in about 10 to 30 percent of patients. The mediastinum, liver, and spleen are not usually involved (2).

It is a matter of controversy whether BL has a different pattern of presentation than the non-Burkitt's type, partly due to the difficulty in histologically distinguishing the two entities and partly because the non-Burkitt's type presents in an older population, thus confounding the analysis with age differences. SNCL of non-Burkitt's type, particularly in adults, may show a higher incidence of peripheral lymphadenopathy and nasopharyngeal involvement and a lower incidence of gastrointestinal involvement (2,26,

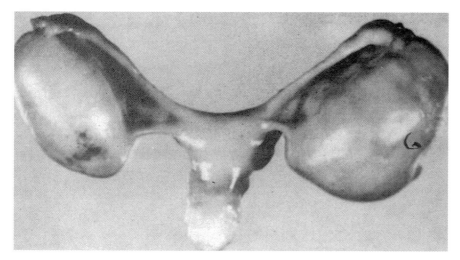

Figure 10-4
BURKITT'S LYMPHOMA:
OVARIES
Bilateral ovarian tumors in
a 4-year-old girl from St. Louis,
Missouri with Burkitt's lymphoma.

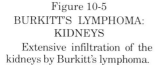

Figure 10-5
BURKITT'S LYMPHOMA:
KIDNEYS
Extensive infiltration of the
kidneys by Burkitt's lymphoma.

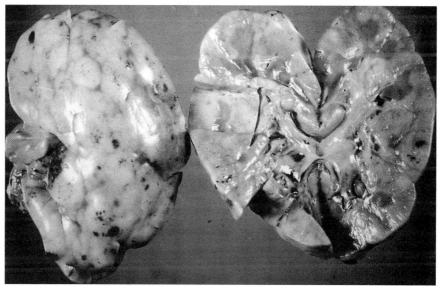

37,43). In one study, a higher incidence of bone marrow involvement was seen in non-Burkitt's as opposed to Burkitt's SNCL (4.5 versus 37.5 percent) (26); however, another study showed a higher incidence of bone marrow involvement in the Burkitt's type (33 versus 15 percent) (37). In two large pediatric series, no differences in extent of disease or primary site of involvement were found between the two types (23,24).

There is an overlap between SNCL involving the bone marrow (fig. 10-7) and the L3 subtype of acute lymphoblastic leukemia, also known as Burkitt's cell leukemia (fig. 10-8) (31,32). The latter may represent the initial clinical presentation without solid lymphomatous masses, apart from lymphadenopathy and hepatosplenomegaly.

Microscopic Findings. SNCLs almost always have a diffuse growth pattern, often infiltrating soft tissues like the retroperitoneum, and sparing lymph nodes (fig. 10-9). On rare occasions, BL, or less commonly non-Burkitt's type, may selectively involve the germinal centers of lymph nodes (fig. 10-10) or lymphoid tissues of the intestinal tract (35). A true follicular pattern similar to that seen in follicular center cell lymphoma is rare.

In formalin-fixed histologic sections, BL is characterized by cellular monotony. The neoplastic cells are of uniform size and shape and their round to oval nuclei, which may possess slight indentations, are comparable in size to those of reactive histiocytes or endothelial cells (fig. 10-11). Since the nuclei of small noncleaved cells are

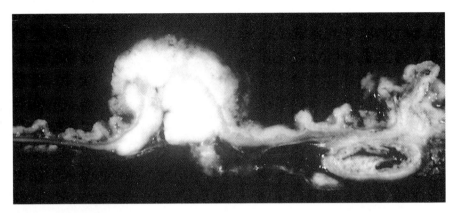

Figure 10-6
BURKITT'S LYMPHOMA:
INTESTINE
Cross section of small intestine involved by Burkitt's lymphoma.

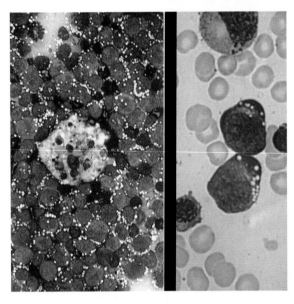

Figure 10-7
BURKITT'S LYMPHOMA
Left: *Touch Imprint of Lymph Node*. Small noncleaved cells possess a thin rim of basophilic cytoplasm containing numerous vacuoles. Macrophage in center contains abundant cellular debris.
Right: *Bone Marrow Aspirate*. Two small noncleaved cells with eccentric nuclei and a thin rim of basophilic cytoplasm contain vacuoles aggregated at one pole of the cell.

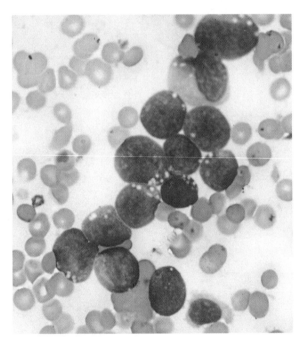

Figure 10-8
BURKITT'S LYMPHOMA: BONE MARROW
The cytologic features of Burkitt's lymphoma cells are similar to those of lymphoblasts in the L3 type of acute lymphoblastic leukemia.

larger than those of small lymphocytes, it must be recognized that the term "small noncleaved" is relative to the size of the large noncleaved cells (centroblasts). Nuclear chromatin is coarsely reticulated, with relatively clear parachromatin. Two to five basophilic nucleoli are usually evident. When fixation has been delayed, nuclei may become vesicular and nucleoli more prominent, a phenomenon that is also evident after B5 fixation (3). The neoplastic cells possess a thin rim of amphophilic and intensely pyroninophilic cytoplasm which characteristically squares off as one cell abuts another, imparting a jigsaw puzzle–like appearance particularly evident in formalin-fixed tissue (fig. 10-11). Multinucleated forms are almost never seen except in the non-Burkitt's type (fig. 10-12). Mitoses are numerous. Karyorrhexis may be a prominent feature and a starry sky appearance, imparted by cell debris-laden histiocytes scattered evenly among the neoplastic cells, is characteristic but not pathognomonic of BL (figs. 10-9–10-11).

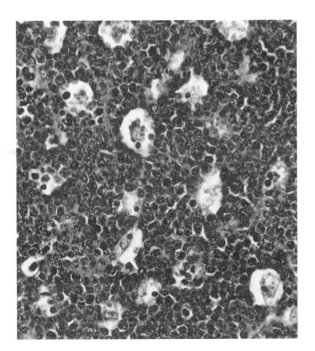

Figure 10-9
BURKITT'S LYMPHOMA: OVARY
H&E stained section of an ovarian tumor in the 16-year-old girl from St. Louis, Missouri seen in figure 10-1, showing the characteristic architectural features of Burkitt's lymphoma.

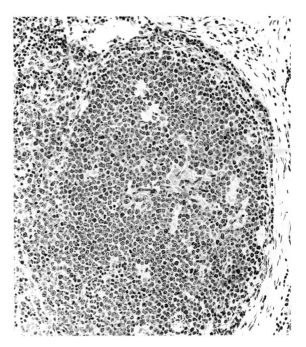

Figure 10-10
BURKITT'S LYMPHOMA: LYMPH NODE
Selective involvement of a germinal center by Burkitt's lymphoma.

In Wright-Giemsa–stained imprint preparations or fine needle aspirations the nuclei may be round, oval, or clefted, with stippled chromatin and two to five relatively inconspicuous nucleoli (fig. 10-7). There is a well-defined narrow rim of deeply basophilic cytoplasm. Varying numbers of cytoplasmic vacuoles are always evident, usually at one pole of the cytoplasm. These correspond to lipid granules, demonstrable in frozen sections with neutral fat stains (fig. 10-13), in addition to dilated mitochondria. Large histiocytes laden with pyknotic cells or cell debris are often present.

Electron microscopic studies of BL show the nuclei to be round or oval, but deep evaginations of the nuclear membranes may be present (fig. 10-14) (16). Nuclear chromatin is relatively fine, but is often densely clumped at the nuclear membrane and around nucleoli. The latter are large, multiple, and usually attached to the nuclear membrane. Nuclear blebs, sometimes containing cytoplasmic organelles, may be prominent (fig. 10-15). The cytoplasm contains numerous free ribosomes and polysomes, in addition to vacuoles,

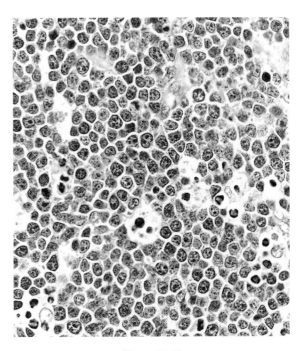

Figure 10-11
BURKITT'S LYMPHOMA: INTESTINE
Uniform round to oval nuclei possess coarsely reticulated chromatin with relatively clear parachromatin and two or more nucleoli. A thin rim of cytoplasm squares off as one cell abuts another ("jigsaw-puzzle" effect). A starry sky pattern is evident.

225

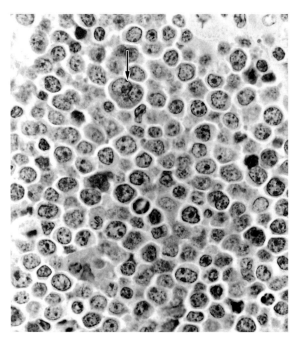

Figure 10-12
SMALL NONCLEAVED, NON-
BURKITT'S TYPE LYMPH NODE
Neoplastic cells are more variable in size and shape (note multinucleated cell, arrow) and nuclei possess more prominent nucleoli. The "jigsaw puzzle" effect is still evident.

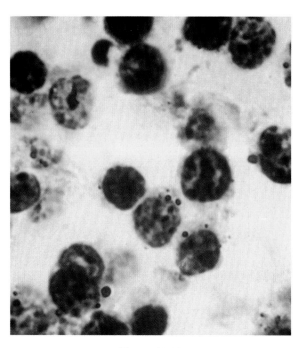

Figure 10-13
BURKITT'S LYMPHOMA:
LYMPH NODE TOUCH PREPARATION
Oil red O stain demonstrates lipid droplets within the cytoplasm of small noncleaved cells.

lipid droplets, and large swollen mitochondria aggregated at one pole of the cell (fig. 10-14).

SNCL of the non-Burkitt's type shows a much greater degree of cellular pleomorphism and cytologic heterogeneity compared with the Burkitt's type (fig. 10-12). Nuclear membranes are delicate and the chromatin is finely dispersed around one or more nucleoli, which may be inconspicuous in some nuclei but prominent in others. The cytoplasm is variable in character and amount: it may be amphophilic and moderate in amount, and the cells may be cohesive; more frequently it is pale and scant. A starry sky pattern may or may not be present. However, the diagnostic reproducibility of these differences is not high (51).

Immunologic Findings. Following the application of monoclonal antibodies against lymphocyte differentiation antigens it is clear that virtually all SNCLs are of B lineage; however, rare SNCLs of T-cell phenotype have been described (42). The B-lineage cases all express surface immunoglobulins, predominantly IgM, often with IgD and rarely IgG. This is invariably

associated with either kappa or lambda light chain restriction. Based on reports in the literature and the results of our own studies (19), a number of B-cell–specific antigens (CD19, CD20, CD22) and B-cell–associated antigens (non-lineage specific) such as CD24 and HLA-DR, are present on the cell surface of SNCLs. Moreover, CD10, the common acute lymphocytic leukemia (ALL) antigen (CALLA) present on the surface of precursor B cells and some mature germinal center cells, is also detectable in vivo on most SNCLs. The observation that this antigen is frequently lost during cultivation of BL cell lines in vitro, particularly those containing the EBV genome, has exposed differences in phenotype between sporadic and endemic BL. CD21, which represents the receptor for both the C3d component of human complement and EBV, is more commonly expressed on the cell surface of endemic BL than on sporadic BL, consistent with the observation that the endemic form usually contains the EBV genome and possesses receptors for C3d, whereas the sporadic cases are usually negative

226

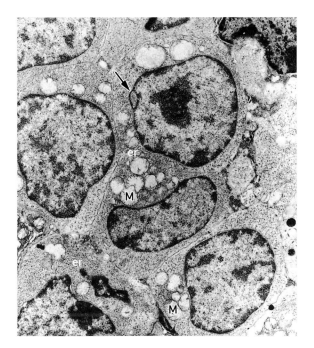

Figure 10-14
BURKITT'S LYMPHOMA: OMENTUM
Electron micrograph shows small noncleaved cells with rounded or oval nuclei and narrow cytoplasm packed with free ribosomes. Endoplasmic reticulum (er) is scanty. Swollen, altered mitochondria (M) are aggregated at one pole. A nuclear projection enclosing cytoplasmic material is present in one cell (arrow). A degenerating nucleus is seen in the upper right corner. (Fig. 5 from Dorfman RF. The fine structure of a malignant lymphoma in a child from St. Louis, MO. JNCI 1967;38:491-504.)

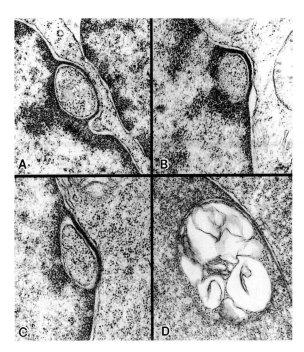

Figure 10-15
BURKITT'S LYMPHOMA: OMENTUM
Composite electron micrographs showing nuclear projections. In A, B, and C the projections bulge into the cytoplasm. Extensions of perinuclear space are bounded by membranes continuous with the outer membrane of the nucleus. Between these membranes is a dense, compressed zone of chromatin continuous with that of the adjacent nucleoplasm. B shows two distinct membranes on either side of this dense zone, representing reduplication of the inner and outer membranes. Projections enclose cytoplasmic material containing free ribosomes similar to those in the surrounding cytoplasm. D shows a cytoplasmic inclusion, containing a myelin figure surrounded by free ribosomes. A compressed zone of nucleoplasm bounded on both sides by extensions of the perinuclear space overlays this, but there is no bulging of the nuclear envelope toward the cytoplasm.

for both (31,32). Sporadic SNCL may secrete IgM, which can be detected in the serum by immunoelectrophoresis. IgM secretion has not been described in patients with endemic BL.

In vivo studies of endemic and sporadic SNCL have shown that both types express B-cell markers, including surface IgM and CD10, but not activation markers such as CD25 and CD30. The absence of the latter suggests that the tumor cells may represent the neoplastic counterpart of a resting B cell. The observation that a significantly higher proportion of SNCLs have mμ and delta heavy chains and fewer gamma and alpha chains, suggests that SNCL may represent a neoplasm of B lymphocytes arrested at an immature stage of development since mμ and delta heavy chains are present on B lymphocytes prior to the development of gamma heavy chains. Magrath (30–32) maintains that there are no

reported phenotypic differences at the level of cell surface markers between large cell lymphomas of B-cell type and SNCL. Our studies (19) have delineated significant differences between these lymphomas when studied with a large panel of monoclonal antibodies applied to frozen sections. For example, a significant number of large cell lymphomas express CD25, CD44, and Leu-8, markers that are rarely expressed by BL.

All SNCLs have a very high Ki-67 index, a marker of growth rate. In contrast to lymphoblastic lymphomas (of pre-B- and T-cell types), SNCLs do not possess the enzyme terminal deoxyribonucleotidyl transferase (TdT). It should be noted, however, that some cases of Burkitt's leukemia (L3 of the FAB classification) that have the t(8;14) translocation may express TdT.

Molecular and Cytogenetic Findings. Characterization of the chromosomal translocations of SNCL has played an important role in understanding the genetic mechanisms underlying the pathogenesis of malignant lymphomas in general. More than 80 percent of the Burkitt's subtype of SNCL carry the t(8;14) (q23;q21) translocation, the first recurring translocation reported to be associated with a lymphoproliferative disease (36,54). Two other, less frequent variant translocations, t(8;22) and t(2;8), occur in approximately 16 percent and 8 percent of BLs, respectively (21,22). All three translocations have in common the involvement of chromosome 8 band q23, now known to be the site of the *myc* gene. The breakpoints on chromosomes 14, 2, and 22 involve the site of immunoglobulin (Ig) heavy chain, and kappa and lambda light chain genes, respectively (31,32). There is a correlation between variant translocations and the type of light chain expressed: BL cells with t(8;22) have lambda light chains and those with the t(2;8) variant express kappa chains.

Molecular studies indicate that a consistent feature of BL translocations is the juxtaposition of the *myc* gene with one of the Ig heavy or light chain genes (13,32). This reconfiguration results in deregulated *myc* gene expression, presumably by loss or mutation of its own controlling elements and the overriding effects of adjacent regulatory elements from Ig loci. The *myc* gene product is a nuclear protein with properties of a transcription factor whose intracellular concentration appears to affect B-cell growth and differentiation, presumably by its regulation of specific target genes (24).

Molecular epidemiologic studies have shown that breakpoints within the *myc* and Ig genes have different distributions in endemic versus sporadic BL (44), perhaps reflecting their origin from Ig gene rearrangement mistakes during different stages of B-lymphocyte development or maturation. Both immunophenotypic data and molecular evidence suggest that endemic BL arises in a pre-B cell, actively rearranging its Ig genes. In contrast, the translocation in sporadic BL probably occurs at a later stage of B-cell differentiation. *Myc* translocations are not an invariant feature of BL and are observed in a

lower percentage of sporadic compared to endemic BLs (22). *Myc* gene rearrangements are observed by Southern blot analyses in many BLs, although some variant breakpoints and t(8;14) breakpoints in endemic BL, which tend to occur more distant from the *myc* gene, may escape detection with this technique. In a study of 10 cases of non-Burkitt's SNCL, *myc* gene rearrangements were not seen; in contrast, *bcl-2* gene rearrangements were found in 3 cases (53). This suggests that the majority of cases of the non-Burkitt's subtype may represent a heterogeneous group of lymphomas distinct from the Burkitt's subtype. *Bcl-2* gene rearrangements were found in patients who presented with nodal disease only; none of the patients who presented with extranodal disease had evidence of *bcl-2* involvement. This suggests that the non-Burkitt's subtype may actually represent at least two entities, one arising from a lymph node germinal center and the other arising in extranodal lymphoid tissue (53).

A significant percentage of BLs harbor latent EBV genomes; indeed, the virus was originally discovered in primary explants of BL. The EBV genome is present in a higher proportion of endemic BLs than sporadic BLs (95 versus less than 20 percent), and has also been identified in occasional cases of non-Burkitt's SNCL. The viral genome is clonally homogeneous within the tumor cell population, indicating it was present in lymphoma cell precursors prior to their clonal expansion, consistent with a role for EBV in the pathogenesis of some BLs. The specific contribution of EBV and its interrelationship with deregulated *myc* expression and altered T-cell immunity remain controversial and unresolved. EBV-infected B lymphocytes are normally subject to T-cell regulation in immune competent hosts; however, in equatorial Africa, where malaria is endemic, defective T-cell regulation is frequent and may contribute to unregulated B-cell proliferation. Subsequent genetic errors, i.e., chromosomal translocations resulting in "activation" of the *myc* proto-oncogene, may represent a critical, but perhaps insufficient event in the development of BL. A similar course of events is likely in acquired immunodeficiency syndrome (AIDS) patients who develop SNCL, where HIV infection results in altered T-cell regulation of EBV-infected or polyclonally activated B cells.

Molecular genetic studies of high-grade lymphomas in patients with AIDS have indicated that they resemble sporadic BL at the molecular level (48).

Although the t(8;14) translocation and its variants are commonly observed in SNCL, they are not specific for this subtype: up to 15 percent of diffuse large cell lymphomas have this translocation (41). A subset of acute lymphoblastic leukemia (ALL) of the B-cell type has cytogenetic and molecular features indistinguishable from BL, providing additional evidence that ALL of the L3 subtype represents the bone marrow/peripheral blood counterpart of SNCL (31,32).

Studies of transgenic animal models suggest that genetic changes, in addition to *myc* activation, are necessary for the development of full malignant potential (1), underscoring the multistep nature of lymphomagenesis. Indeed, up to 70 percent of BLs contain cytogenetic abnormalities in addition to one of the three characteristic primary abnormalities (22). The frequent presence of EBV, particularly in endemic BL, suggests an accessory but not essential role for viral gene products such as EBNA-1. A significant percentage of SNCLs contain mutant p53 tumor suppressor genes in addition to activated myc genes (18).

Progression from follicular lymphoma to SNCL possessing the t(8;14) or variant translocation and the t(14;18) translocation has been described.

Differential Diagnosis. Before its clinical description by Burkitt in 1958 (11) and its definition as a malignant lymphoma by O'Conor in 1960 (39), a number of different tumors of the jaw and orbit affecting African children were considered in the differential diagnosis of BL. Jaw tumors included embryonal rhabdomyosarcoma, Ewing's sarcoma, and from a clinical point of view, fibrous dysplasia (ossifying fibroma) and adamantinoma (ameloblastoma); orbital tumors included retinoblastoma, neuroblastoma, embryonal rhabdomyosarcoma, and so-called chloroma (granulocytic sarcoma), recognized as having a predilection for orbital bones in African children. The majority of these tumors can clearly be differentiated on morphologic grounds, assisted by the application of appropriate histochemical and immunohistochemical studies. In regions of the world where BL is sporadic, the principal differential diagnosis includes lymphoblastic lymphoma, large cell lymphoma (large noncleaved/centro blastic and immunoblastic) and other round cell tumors of childhood.

Lymphoblastic Lymphoma (LBL) (see chapter 11). In contrast to the tendency of BL to involve abdominal organs including the intestinal tract, kidney, and ovary, the initial manifestation of LBL is nearly always supradiaphragmatic, especially mediastinal. Adolescent boys are particularly affected.

The nuclei of the lymphoblasts possess a finely dispersed chromatin, inconspicuous nucleoli, and often convoluted nuclear membranes. The cytoplasm is scanty and lacks the intense pyroninophilia of BL; however, like the latter tumor, numerous mitoses are evident and macrophages scattered among the lymphoblasts may impart a starry sky pattern. Further distinctions between LBL (mostly T lineage) and BL can be made with appropriate immunophenotypic, cytogenetic, and molecular genetic analyses as indicated above.

Large Cell Lymphoma (see chapter 9). Inadequate fixation and technically poor sections may result in an artifactual size increase of the nuclei of BL cells; these may appear more vesicular, with lack of chromatin clumping, thus being confused with large noncleaved cell (centroblastic) lymphoma. Large noncleaved cells usually possess a narrow rim of cytoplasm which may be amphophilic or basophilic and pyroninophilic. Their oval vesicular nuclei generally contain fewer but more prominent basophilic nucleoli that are typically apposed to the nuclear membrane on the short axis of the oval nucleus. In addition, large cell lymphomas are usually more heterogeneous from one neoplastic cell to another and generally have more admixed non-neoplastic cells.

Large cell immunoblastic lymphoma of the plasmacytoid type is characterized by neoplastic cells that are larger than those of SNCL. The immunoblasts usually have uniformly round to oval vesicular nuclei containing a prominent, centrally placed nucleolus which may be basophilic or eosinophilic. The plasmacytoid variant possesses an eccentrically placed nucleus with abundant amphophilic or basophilic and intensely pyroninophilic cytoplasm, greater in amount than that of SNCL.

Although a morphologic distinction between large cell lymphoma and SNCL can be made in most instances, some cases appear to be transitional between large cell lymphoma and SNCL of non-Burkitt's type. This observation is consistent with the molecular data suggesting a biologic overlap between some cases of SNCL of non-Burkitt's type and large cell lymphoma (53).

Granulocytic Sarcoma (so-called Chloroma) (see chapter 19). In African children, extra-medullary granulocytic sarcoma has a predilection for the orbital bones and may also involve the ovary. The leukemic cells often possess eosinophilic cytoplasm which may be granular, differing from the basophilic cytoplasm of BL. The distinction between granulocytic sarcoma and non-Hodgkin's lymphomas can be facilitated by the demonstration of nonspecific cytoplasmic esterase activity in immature myeloid cells, by the naphthol-ASD-chloroacetate method (the Leder stain), or by the demonstration of myeloperoxidase or other myeloid-related antigens with immunohistochemical studies.

Immediate and proper fixation of tissue and the preparation of technically good sections are essential for the accurate distinction of BL, SNCL of the non-Burkitt's type, other non-Hodgkin's lymphomas, and small round cell tumors of childhood.

Treatment and Prognosis. Prompt staging and early treatment are essential because of the short doubling time of the tumor. Staging systems have been devised by the National Cancer Institute and St. Jude National Children's Hospital (Table 10-1) (33). Recognizing the importance of tumor volume in the management of SNCL, these systems separate patients with limited stage disease from those with extensive intrathoracic or intra-abdominal disease. Although in Africa, bone marrow involvement is less frequent in endemic BL and cure rate for patients with central nervous system disease is high (50 percent), it is recognized that these two sites of involvement presage a poorer prognosis in patients from the United States. Surgical resection and debulking of abdominal tumors are important in the therapy of SNCL (30–32,34).

The prognostic significance of BL versus non-Burkitt's SNCL has been widely debated in the literature. Some groups have observed a shorter median survival for patients with BL (51), others have reported a shorter median survival for patients with non-Burkitt's SNCL, (27) while oth-

Table 10-1

STAGING FOR SMALL NONCLEAVED CELL LYMPHOMA*

Stage A	A single extra-abdominal tumor site
Stage AR	Completely resected intra-abdominal tumor (tumor volume reduced by more than 90 percent)
Stage B	Multiple extra-abdominal sites
Stage C	Intra-abdominal tumor without involvement at other sites
Stage D	Intra- and extra-abdominal sites

*From reference 33.

ers have found no significant differences in survival between the two subtypes (4,23,24,26,37).

Endemic BL is remarkably sensitive to various chemotherapeutic agents, initially given in doses now considered inadequate (10,12). The response of SNCL to a wide range of chemotherapeutic agents very likely reflects its high growth fraction. The response to treatment is related to stage of the disease, to the type of drugs used, and to the patients biologic defense mechanisms: spontaneous remissions of biopsy-proven BL in Africa were recorded by Burkitt and other clinicians (12).

Currently available combination chemotherapeutic regimens result in reported cure rates of up to 90 percent in patients with low-stage disease and 70 to 80 percent in patients with advanced disease (4,33). Patients with adverse prognostic features such as large unresected tumors greater than 10 cm, a high pretreatment serum lactate dehydrogenase level, or involvement of the central nervous system or bone marrow still have a poor survival (4), and may be candidates for consolidative bone marrow transplantation.

It has been noted that relapses in SNCL usually occur within 1 year and, in the United States, there is a lower frequency of late relapse. After 2 years without evidence of relapse, BL appears to be cured. Long-term survival with non-Burkitt's SNCL may be less frequent (37).

REFERENCES

1. Adams JM, Harris AW, Pinkert CA, et al. The c-myc oncogene driven by immunoglobulin enhancers induces lymphoid malignancy in transgenic mice. Nature 1985;318:533–8.

2. Aine R. Small non-cleaved follicular center cell lymphoma: clinicopathologic comparison of Burkitt and non-Burkitt variants in Finnish material. Eur J Cancer Clin Oncol 1985;21:1179–85.

3. Berard C, O'Conor GT, Thomas LB, et al. Histopathological definition of Burkitt's tumor. No. 40. Geneva: World Health Organization, 1969.

4. Bernstein JI, Coleman CN, Strickler JG, Dorfman RF, Rosenberg SA. Combined modality therapy for adults with small non-cleaved cell lymphoma (Burkitt's and non-Burkitt's types). J Clin Oncol 1986;4:847–58.

5. Booth K, Burkitt DP, Bassett DJ, Cooke RA, Biddulph J. Burkitt lymphoma in Papua, New Guinea. Br J Cancer 1967;21:657–64.

6. Brown JB, O'Keefe CD. Sarcoma of the ovary with unusual oral metastases. Ann Surg 1928;87:467–71.

7. Burkitt DP. Determining the climatic limitations of a children's cancer common in Africa. Br Med J 1962; 2:1019–23.

8. _____. Etiology of Burkitt's lymphoma—an alternative hypothesis to a vectored virus. JNCI 1969;42:19–28.

9. _____. A lymphoma syndrome dependent on environment. I. Clinical aspects. In: Roulet FC, ed. The lymphoreticular tumors in Africa. Basel: S Karger, 1964:83.

10. _____, O'Conor GT. Malignant lymphoma in African children. I. A clinical syndrome. Cancer 1961;14:258–69.

11. _____. A sarcoma involving the jaws in African children. Brit J Surg 1958;197:218–223.

12. _____, Wright DH. Burkitt's lymphoma. Edinburgh: Livingstone, 1970.

13. Dalla-Favera R. Chromosomal translocations involving the c-myc oncogene and their role in the pathogenesis of B cell neoplasia. In: Brugge J, Curran T, Harlow E, McCormick F, eds. Origin of human cancer. Cold Spring Harbor: Cold Spring Harbor Laboratory Press, 1991.

14. _____, Bregni M, Erikson J, Patterson D, Gallo RC, Croce CM. Human c-myc oncogene is located on the region of chromosome 8 that is translocated in Burkitt lymphoma cells. Proc Natl Acad Sci USA 1982;79:7824–7.

15. Dorfman RF. Childhood lymphosarcoma in St. Louis, Missouri, clinically and histologically resembling Burkitt's tumor. Cancer 1965;18:418–30.

16. _____. The fine structure of a malignant lymphoma in a child from St. Louis, Missouri. JNCI 1967;38:491–504.

17. Epstein MA, Achong BG, Barr YM. Virus particles in cultured lymphoblasts from Burkitt's lymphoma. Lancet 1964;1:702–3.

18. Gaidano G, Ballerini P, Gong JZ, et al. p53 mutations in human lymphoid malignancies: association with Burkitt lymphoma and chronic lymphocytic leukemia. Proc Natl Acad Sci USA 1991;88:5413–7.

19. Garcia CF, Weiss LM, Warnke RA. Small non-cleaved cell lymphoma: an immunophenotypic study of 18 cases and comparison with large cell lymphoma. Hum Pathol 1986;17:454–61.

20. Grogan TM, Warnke RA, Kaplan HS. A comparative study of Burkitt's and non-Burkitt's "undifferentiated" malignant lymphoma: immunologic, cytochemical, ultrastructural, cytologic, histopathologic, clinical and cell culture features. Cancer 1982;49:1817–28.

21. Haluska FG, Tsujimoto Y, Croce CM. The molecular genetics of non-Hodgkin's lymphomas. In: Magrath I, ed. The non-Hodgkin's lymphomas. Baltimore: Williams & Wilkins, 1990;96–108.

22. Heim S, Mitelman F. Cancer cytogenetics. New York: Liss, 1987:203–6.

23. Hutchison RE, Murphy SB, Fairclough DL, et al. Diffuse small noncleaved cell lymphoma in children, Burkitt's versus non-Burkitt's types. Results from the Pediatric Oncology Group and St. Jude Children's Research Hospital. Cancer 1989;64:23–8.

24. Kelly DR, Nathwani BN, Griffith RC, et al. A morphologic study of childhood lymphoma of the undifferentiated type. The Pediatric Oncology Group experience. Cancer 1987;59:1132–7.

25. Lenoir G, O'Conor GT, Olweny CL, eds. Burkitt's lymphoma. A human cancer model. International Agency for Research on Cancer. IARC scientific publication, No. 60. New York: Oxford University Press, 1985.

26. Levine AM, Pavlova Z, Pockros AW, et al. Small noncleaved follicular center cell (FCC) lymphoma: Burkitt and non-Burkitt variants in the United States. I. Clinical features. Cancer 1983;52:1073–9.

27. Levine PH, Karamaju LS, Connelly RR et al. The American Burkitt Lymphoma Registry: eight years of experience. Cancer 1982;49:1016–22.

28. Longo DL, Wilson W. Follicular lymphomas. In: Magrath IT, ed. The non-Hodgkin's lymphomas. Baltimore: Williams & Wilkins, 1990:96–108.

29. Luscher B, Eisenman RN. New light on myc and myb. Part I. Myc Genes Dev 1990;4:2025–35.

30. Magrath IT. The pathogenesis of Burkitt's lymphoma. In: Van de Woude GF, Klein G, eds. Advances of cancer research. San Diego: Academic Press, 1990:133–270.

31. _____. Small non-cleaved cell lymphomas. In: Magrath IT, ed. The non-Hodgkin's lymphomas. Baltimore: Williams & Wilkins, 1990:256–78.

32. _____, Jain V, Jaffe ES. Small noncleaved cell lymphoma. In: Knowles DM, ed. Neoplastic hematopathology. Baltimore, Williams & Wilkins, 1992:749–72.

33. _____, Janus C, Edwards BK, et al. An effective therapy for both undifferentiated (including Burkitt's) lymphomas and lymphoblastic lymphomas in children and young adults. Blood 1984;63:1102-11.

34. _____, Lwanga S, Carswell W, et al. Surgical reduction of tumor bulk in the management of abdominal Burkitt's lymphoma. Br Med J 1974;2:308–12.

35. Mann RB, Jaffe ES, Braylan RC, et al. Non-endemic Burkitt's lymphoma: a B-cell tumor related to germinal centers. N Engl J Med 1976;295:685–91.

36. Manolov G, Manolova Y. Marker band in one chromosome 14 from Burkitt lymphomas. Nature 1972;237:33–4.

37. Miliauskas JR, Berard CW, Young RC, Garvin AJ, Edwards BK, DeVita VT Jr. Undifferentiated non-Hodgkin's lymphomas (Burkitt's and non-Burkitt's types). The relevance of making this histologic distinction. Cancer 1982;50:2115–21.

38. The Non-Hodgkin's Lymphoma Pathologic Classification Project. National Cancer Institute sponsored study of classifications of non-Hodgkin's lymphomas: summary and description of a working formulation for clinical usage. Cancer 1982;49:2112–35.

39. O'Conor GT, Rappaport H, Smith EB. Childhood lymphoma in African children. II. A pathological entity. Cancer 1961;14:270–83.

40. _____, Rappaport H, Smith EB. Childhood lymphoma resembling "Burkitt tumor" in the United States. Cancer 1965;18:411–7.

41. Offit K, Chaganti SK. Chromosomal aberrations in non-Hodgkin's lymphoma: biologic and clinical correlations. Hematol Oncol Clin North Am 1991;5:853–69.

42. Oliver JD, Grogan TM, Payne CM, Spier C, Richter LC, Rangel CS. Burkitt's-like lymphoma of T-cell type. Mod Pathol 1988;1:15–22.

43. Pavlova Z, Parker JW, Taylor CR, Levine AM, Feinstein DI, Lukes RJ. Small noncleaved follicular center cell lymphoma: Burkitt's and non-Burkitt's variants in the US. II. Pathologic and immunologic features. Cancer 1987;59:1892–902.

44. Pelicci PG, Knowles DM, Magrath I, Dalla-Favera R. Chromosomal breakpoints and structural alterations of the c-myc locus differ in endemic and sporadic forms of Burkitt lymphoma. Proc Natl Acad Sci USA 1986;83:2984–8.

45. Rappaport H. Braylan R. Changing concepts in the classification of malignant neoplasms of the hematopoietic system. In: Rebuck J, Berard CW, Abell MR, eds. The reticuloendothelial system. Baltimore: Williams & Wilkins, 1975:1–19, (International Academy of Pathology, Vol. 16.)

46. Recant L, Lacy P, eds. Lymphosarcoma in a St. Louis girl, clinically and histologically resembling Burkitt's African lymphoma (clinicopathologic conference, Washington University School of Medicine. Am J Med 1965;38:96–104.

47. Stansfeld AG, Diebold J, Noel H, et al. Updated Kiel classification for lymphomas [Letter]. Lancet 1988;1:292–3.

48. Subar M, Neri A, Inghirami G, Knowles DM, Dalla-Favera R. Frequent c-myc oncogene activation and infrequent presence of Epstein-Barr virus genome in AIDS-associated lymphoma. Blood 1988;72:667–71.

49. Taub R, Kirsch I, Morton C, et al. Translocation of the c-myc gene into the immunoglobulin heavy chain locus in human Burkitt lymphoma and murine plasmacytoma cells. Proc Natl Acad Sci USA 1982;79:7837–41.

50. ten Seldam RE, Cooke R, Atkinson L. Childhood lymphoma in the territories of Papua and New Guinea. Cancer 1966;19:437–46.

51. Wilson JF, Kjeldsberg CR, Sposto R, et al. The pathology of non-Hodgkin's lymphoma of childhood: II. Reproducibility and relevance of the histologic classification of "undifferentiated" lymphomas (Burkitt's versus non-Burkitt's). Hum Pathol 1987;18:1008–14.

52. Wright DH. Burkitt's tumour in England: a comparison with childhood lymphosarcoma. Int J Cancer 1966;1:503–514.

53. Yano T, van Krieken JH, Magrath IT, Longo DL, Jaffe ES, Raffeld M. Histogenetic correlations between subcategories of small noncleaved cell lymphomas. Blood 1992;79:1282–90.

54. Zech L, Hagland U, Nilsson K, Klein G. Characteristic chromosomal abnormalities in biopsies and lymphoid-cell lines from patients with Burkitt and non-Burkitt lymphomas. Int J Cancer 1976;17:47–56.

55. Ziegler JL, Beckstead JA, Volberding PA, et al. Non-Hodgkin's lymphoma in 90 homosexual men. Relation to generalized lymphadenopathy and the acquired immunodeficiency syndrome. N Engl J Med 1984;311:565–70.

✧✧✧

11

MALIGNANT LYMPHOMA, LYMPHOBLASTIC

Definition. Malignant lymphoma, lymphoblastic type, is a neoplasm composed of lymphoid cells with the morphologic appearance of immature lymphocytes (thymocytes) of the thymic cortex, and a primary site of presentation other than peripheral blood or bone marrow. The cells are cytologically identical to the lymphoblasts of acute lymphoblastic leukemia. In the original Kiel classification, Burkitt's lymphoma was included among these lymphomas (29); it is considered a separate entity in the updated Kiel classification (30).

Incidence. Although lymphoblastic lymphoma may present at any age, it is typically seen in older children and young adolescents, with a median age of incidence of about 17 years (39). The incidence is roughly twice as high in males (38). Lymphoblastic lymphoma accounted for 4 percent of all lymphomas in the Working Formulation study (39). In children, this neoplasm represents approximately one third of non-Hodgkin's lymphomas (36).

Natural History and Clinical Features. About half of patients present with a generally large mediastinal mass (37,38). The critical location and rapid growth of the tumor occasionally cause acute respiratory compromise due to tracheal compression and superior vena cava syndrome; this neoplasm is the most common of the non-Hodgkin's lymphomas to present as a medical emergency. The mediastinal involvement is often associated with pleural and pericardial effusions, and occasionally with pericardial tamponade. Fever or weight loss occur in half the cases. A wide variety of other sites may be involved, including peripheral lymph nodes (usually supradiaphragmatic), Waldeyer's ring, breast, skin, bone, central nervous system, gonads, liver, spleen, and, particularly, bone marrow. Lymphoblastic lymphoma of B-cell lineage shows a propensity to present as multiple cutaneous nodules (6,31,47).

Prominent bone marrow involvement raises the possibility of acute lymphoblastic leukemia. Acute lymphoblastic leukemia and lymphoblastic lymphoma represent two ends of one biologic spectrum, to which arbitrary criteria are applied for separation into two clinical diseases. These criteria vary: the Pediatric Oncology Group uses a cutoff of 25 percent or less bone marrow blasts for a diagnosis of lymphoblastic lymphoma (36); in adults the cutoff is less than 10 percent circulating blasts in the peripheral blood and absence of pancytopenia (15). Even with these distinctions, patients frequently present with stage IV disease, generally due to some degree of bone marrow involvement.

Rare cases of lymphoblastic lymphoma may be associated with peripheral eosinophilia, as well as myeloid hyperplasia with eosinophilia in the marrow (1). These patients may be at high risk for subsequent myeloid neoplasia.

Lymphoblastic lymphoma is considered a high-grade lymphoma in the Working Formulation and Kiel classifications (30,39). Without aggressive treatment, wide dissemination usually occurs very rapidly, particularly to the bone marrow, central nervous system, and gonads (38). In one study, the incidence of leukemia during the course of the disease was 82 percent (37). Once leukemic conversion occurs, wide dissemination of disease often follows. About half of autopsied patients have central nervous system involvement and one third have gonadal involvement. When appropriate treatment is given, a rapid response to therapy is often seen.

Microscopic Findings. Lymphoblastic lymphoma typically effaces nodal architecture in a diffuse fashion, usually with capsular involvement and extension into the perinodal soft tissues (fig. 11-1) (38). Within the lymph node, the neoplastic infiltrate may be rimmed by fibrous trabeculae, creating a lobular or pseudonodular pattern; however, true follicle formation is not seen (fig. 11-2) (25). When only partial lymph node involvement is present, the neoplastic infiltrate is generally paracortical, leaving islands of residual lymphoid tissue, including germinal centers, intact (38). A starry sky appearance may be prominent focally (fig. 11-3), but is not usually present uniformly throughout the tumor. The mitotic rate may be variable, but is generally

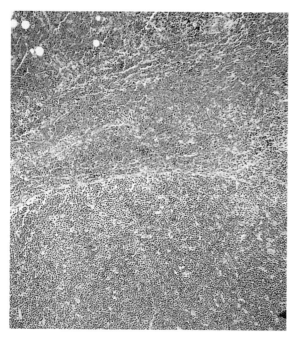

Figure 11-1
LYMPHOBLASTIC LYMPHOMA
Note the massive extension of the neoplasm outside the
lymph node capsule and into the pericapsular adipose tissue.

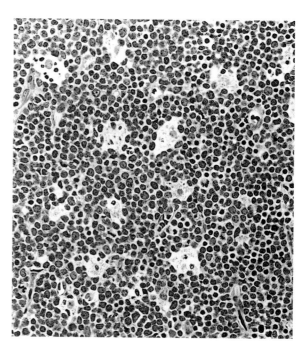

Figure 11-3
LYMPHOBLASTIC LYMPHOMA
A starry sky pattern is seen in this case.

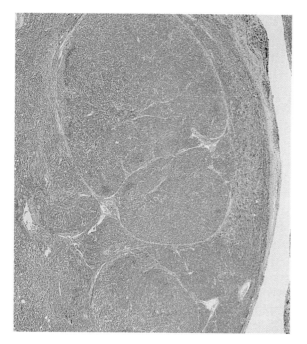

Figure 11-2
LYMPHOBLASTIC LYMPHOMA
A follicular appearance is simulated by expanded lobules of
neoplasm. True neoplastic follicles are not present in this tumor.

high, averaging between 5 and 15 per high-power field. A higher mitotic rate is seen in patients younger than 30 years of age (38). In less optimal preparations, a characteristic crush artifact may be found, particularly in the pericapsular areas, but also within the lymph node parenchyma (fig. 11-4). When soft tissues are involved, single file infiltration between individual collagen bundles is often present, a distinctive feature that this neoplasm shares with granulocytic sarcoma (fig. 11-5). The tumor cells may infiltrate around blood vessels, expanding the fibrous tissues in a concentric fashion (fig. 11-6).

The neoplastic cells of lymphoblastic lymphoma are small to medium in size, averaging 12 to 14 µm in diameter (fig. 11-7) (37). The nuclear-cytoplasmic ratio is high, and cytoplasm can be discerned in only the best histologic preparations. The nuclei are round to ovoid in shape, and the nuclear membranes are thin, but distinct. In most cases, the nuclear membranes have deep subdivisions, imparting a multilobed appearance to the nuclei; this is the *convoluted variant* (fig. 11-8). The nuclei in this histologic subtype may show a small degree of variation from cell to cell. In the *nonconvoluted subtype*, either very fine

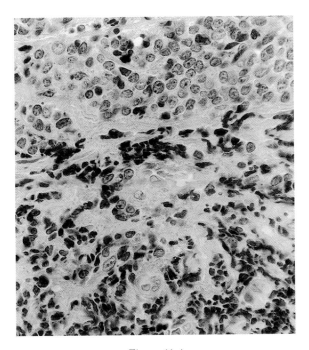

Figure 11-4
LYMPHOBLASTIC LYMPHOMA
A characteristic crush artifact is seen in this photomicrograph.

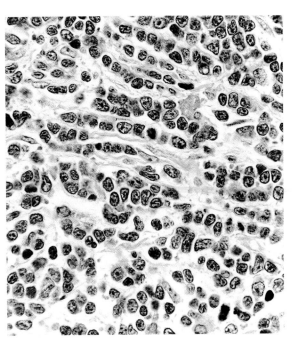

Figure 11-5
LYMPHOBLASTIC LYMPHOMA
Single file infiltration is seen.

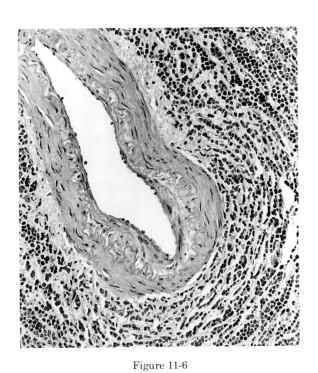

Figure 11-6
LYMPHOBLASTIC LYMPHOMA
A characteristic "targetoid" pattern of infiltration around
the adventitia of vessels is seen.

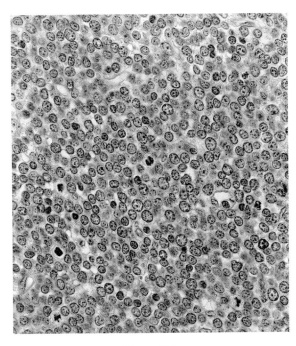

Figure 11-7
LYMPHOBLASTIC LYMPHOMA
A homogeneous population of medium-sized cells is pres-
ent with only rare host cells discernable.

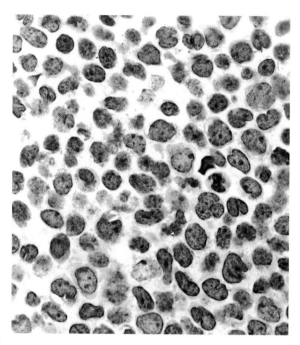

Figure 11-8
LYMPHOBLASTIC LYMPHOMA
This case represents the convoluted variant.

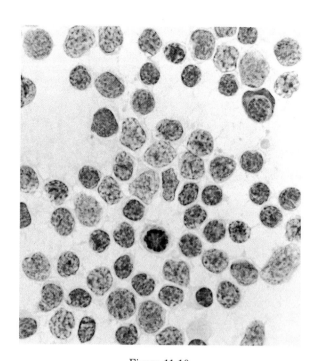

Figure 11-10
LYMPHOBLASTIC LYMPHOMA
Note the blastic character of the chromatin and the mitotic figure in this cytologic preparation.

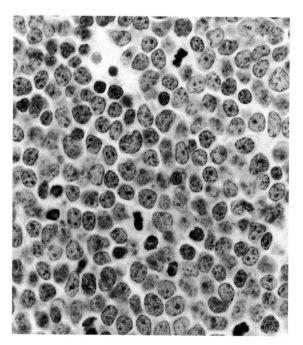

Figure 11-9
LYMPHOBLASTIC LYMPHOMA
This case represents the nonconvoluted variant.

linear subdivisions are present or no irregularities are discerned (fig. 11-9). In this subtype, the nuclei from cell to cell are uniform. In both groups, the nucleoli are either very small and single or not discernable, and the chromatin is extremely fine. The character of the chromatin is probably the most distinctive feature of this neoplasm. A few cells have a slightly coarser chromatin pattern, intermediate in character between the other lymphoblasts and small, mature lymphocytes. Multinucleated tumor cells are not seen. Generally, other cells are not present in the infiltrate, with the exception of macrophages in areas with the starry sky appearance, and plasma cells or eosinophils in occasional cases (56).

Imprints may be useful in the diagnosis of lymphoblastic lymphoma (fig. 11-10) (27). The character of the chromatin and the presence of convolutions are often better appreciated in these preparations. The neoplastic cells are morphologically indistinguishable from blasts of the L2 or, less commonly, L1 subtype of acute lymphoblastic leukemia (French-American-British [FAB] classification). The lymphoblastic cytoplasm can be

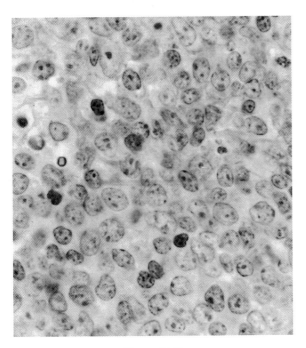

Figure 11-11
LYMPHOBLASTIC LYMPHOMA: ATYPICAL VARIANT
Although a fine chromatin pattern is still present, the nuclei are larger and have more prominent nucleoli than those seen in most cases of lymphoblastic lymphoma.

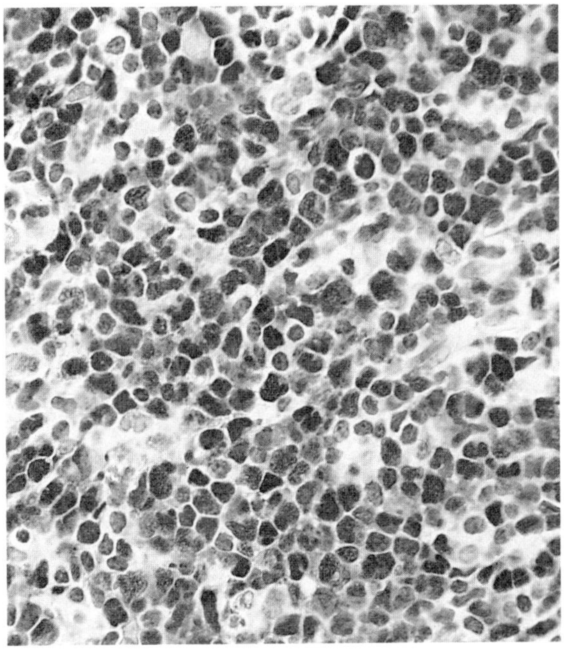

Figure 11-12
LYMPHOBLASTIC LYMPHOMA
This case is TdT positive in paraffin sections.

appreciated in these preparations, and often contains coarsely clumped periodic acid-Schiff (PAS)–positive material. Small cytoplasmic vacuoles may be seen, but not in large numbers.

Variants. As mentioned above, lymphoblastic lymphoma can be divided into convoluted and nonconvoluted subtypes, based on the contours of the nuclear membranes of the neoplastic cells. In the National Cancer Institute–sponsored study of lymphoma classification, as well as other studies, the presence or absence of convolutions did not influence the clinical parameters or survival (39). Also, a division between these two types is often arbitrary, since cases have variable numbers of convoluted cells which may be related to factors such as the fixation of the tissues and the technical preparation of the sections. Therefore, at the current time, there is little practical value in distinguishing these variants.

An *atypical* or *large cell variant* of lymphoblastic lymphoma has also been described, comprising about 10 percent of cases (21). The neoplastic cells are slightly larger than in the usual cases, with larger nuclei that may contain one or

two evident nucleoli (fig. 11-11). Although this variant is associated more with a B- rather than T-cell phenotype, there are no other histologic or clinical differences.

Immunologic Findings. Virtually all lymphoblastic neoplasms express terminal deoxynucleotidyl transferase (TdT) (9). Fortunately, this antigen can now be demonstrated in either frozen or paraffin sections, including acid-decalcified, paraffin-embedded bone marrow biopsies (fig. 11-12) (40,46). In contrast, other non-Hodgkin's lymphomas, including small noncleaved cell lymphoma, are TdT negative.

Approximately 80 to 85 percent of lymphoblastic lymphomas are T-cell neoplasms (16,55). The phenotypes of T-cell lymphoblastic lymphoma and T-cell acute lymphoblastic leukemia have been correlated to stages of intrathymic T-cell differentiation (5,43). In stage I of thymic differentiation, the cells express pan-T-cell markers but lack the subset markers CD4 and CD8, as well as CD1. In stage II, the cells express CD1 and either lack expression of both CD4 and CD8 or coexpress these subset markers (fig. 11-13). In stage III, a mature

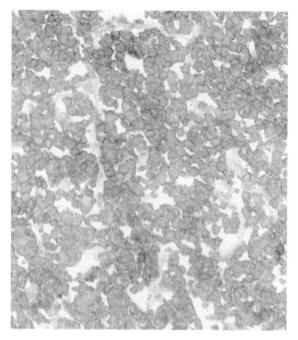

Figure 11-13
LYMPHOBLASTIC LYMPHOMA
Staining for CD1 is seen in this frozen section.

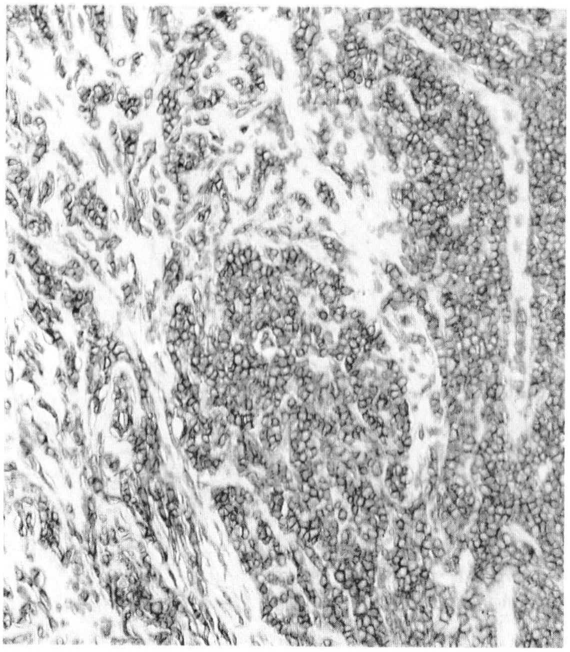

Figure 11-14
LYMPHOBLASTIC LYMPHOMA
Staining for CD43 is seen in this paraffin section.

T-cell phenotype is noted, with either a CD4+, CD8- helper phenotype or a CD4-, CD8+ cytotoxic/suppressor phenotype. CD1 is no longer expressed in this stage. While most cases of acute lymphoblastic leukemia show a phenotype that most closely resembles stage I or, less commonly, stage II differentiation, most T-cell lymphoblastic lymphomas demonstrate a phenotype consistent with either stage II or, less commonly, stage III differentiation. However, there is a great deal of overlap, the immunophenotype may not conform to the defined stages, and the phenotype cannot be used to predict the clinical outcome.

In about 90 percent of cases, the neoplastic cells of T-lymphoblastic lymphoma express each of the pan-T antigens: CD1, CD2, CD7, cytoplasmic CD3, and CD43 (48,55). The latter two markers work well in paraffin sections, and may be useful in combination with other markers in differentiating T-lymphoblastic lymphoma from small, noncleaved or other B-lineage lymphomas (fig. 11-14). CD45RB (leukocyte common antigen), another marker useful in paraffin sections, is expressed in about 80 percent of cases (54); but since this is one of the lower rates of positivity among the non-Hodgkin's lymphomas, lymphoblastic lymphoma should be considered in the evaluation of a neoplasm that appears to be hematolymphoid, but lacks expression of this antigen.

Virtually all cases of T-lymphoblastic lymphoma express the transferrin receptor antigen CD71, about half express the T-activation antigen CD38, one third express CD10 (CALLA), 20 percent express HLA-DR, and 20 percent show strong reactivity for CD16 and CD57, markers for natural killer cells (48,55). The tumor cells do not express the B-cell lineage markers CD19, CD20, CD21, and CD24. Rare tumors may show evidence of both T-cell lineage and myeloid differentiation (13), however, the presence of myeloid markers is more indicative of acute nonlymphocytic leukemia.

Approximately 15 to 20 percent of cases of lymphoblastic lymphoma lack T-lineage markers, but express the B-lineage markers CD19, CD20, CD21, and CD24 and the CALLA antigen CD10 (16,48,55). Most of these cases do not express surface immunoglobulin, and therefore can be classified as having either a pre-pre-B-cell (if cytoplasmic immunoglobulin is absent) or a pre-B-cell phenotype (if only cytoplasmic immunoglobulin is present). These phenotypes are similar to most cases of acute lymphoblastic leukemia. A few cases possess surface immunoglobulin, despite having histologic features diagnostic of lymphoblastic lymphoma (51,55). These rare cases may be the only type of lymphoblastic lymphoma that is TdT negative and must be distinguished from the blastic variant of mantle cell lymphoma: lack of CD5 expression would favor lymphoblastic lymphoma.

Neoplasms that express a T-cell phenotype are frequently associated with a mediastinal mass and tend to occur in males (48); those that possess natural killer antigens in addition to T-cell antigens, according to one study, have a female predominance and a more aggressive clinical course (49). Cases with a pre-pre-B- or pre-B-cell phenotype may have a propensity for skin or osteolytic bone involvement and only rarely present as mediastinal masses (6,16,46a). The number of reported cases is small but these patients may have a less aggressive clinical course than patients with T-lymphoblastic lymphoma. The number of reported cases of immunoglobulin-expressing B-cell lymphoblastic lymphoma is currently too small to suggest clinicopathologic correlations.

Molecular and Cytogenetic Findings. The cytogenetic and molecular features of T-lineage lymphoblastic lymphoma significantly overlap those of T-lineage acute lymphoblastic leukemia and they are considered here as a common group. Gene rearrangement analyses have shown that lymphoblastic neoplasms generally contain rearrangements of the T-cell receptor β-chain gene, as expected, given the T-lineage derivation of most lymphoblastic lymphomas and the fact that T-cell receptor rearrangement is an early event in T-cell differentiation (34,35,52). However, these rearrangements, as well as those of other T-cell receptor (TCR) genes (α, γ, δ), cannot serve as lineage-specific markers since they are also observed in up to 25 percent of B-cell precursor acute lymphoblastic leukemias and a smaller percentage of other non-Hodgkin's lymphomas. T-cell receptor gene configurations are, however, useful tumor-specific clonal markers. In fact, since the antigen-specific properties of individual T-cell receptor proteins derive in part from random nucleotide insertions at the junctions of rearranged T-cell receptor gene segments, the junctional sequences in any given T-lymphoblastic neoplasm constitute clonotypic markers

unique to each patient's malignancy. Various polymerase chain reaction–based strategies have been devised for amplification, characterization, and detection of δ and γ TCR junctional segments and these have been employed as clonotypic molecular markers for longitudinal assessment of disease status in patients with T-lymphoblastic neoplasms (17,22).

Most lymphoblastic lymphomas contain cytogenetic abnormalities of which chromosomal translocations are particularly common and best characterized at the molecular level. Unlike B-lineage lymphomas such as follicular small cleaved cell lymphoma and small noncleaved cell lymphoma, there is no single recurrent translocation or chromosomal abnormality that is observed in most lymphoblastic lymphomas (24, 42). Up to 30 percent, however, contain one of several possible translocations involving chromosome band 14q11 or 7q35, which are now known to be the sites of the T-cell receptor α/δ and β gene complexes, respectively (42). A variety of different chromosomal loci have been reported to exchange with chromosome bands 14q11 and 7q35 in T-lymphoblastic neoplasms (Table 11-1). These translocations result from apparent errors in the T-cell receptor rearrangement process that relocates cellular proto-oncogenes into a T-cell receptor locus analogous to the translocation of *myc* into immunoglobulin genes, as seen in Burkitt's lymphoma. In a small subset of lymphoblastic lymphomas, the *myc* gene is translocated to the T-cell receptor α/δ locus at 14q11 (20). Similar to *myc*, most of the novel genes translocated in T-lymphoblastic lymphoma (Table 11-1) code for proteins that likely function as transcription factors since they share homology with known transcriptional proteins (for review, see reference 14). These data suggest that a number of different cellular genes may serve as oncogenes following deregulated expression in early lineage T cells.

The most consistently involved gene in T-lymphoblastic lymphoma reported to date is *TAL* (also called *SCL*), which may be structurally altered in up to one third of T-lymphoblastic lymphomas (10). *TAL/SCL* was originally discovered following its translocation into a T-cell receptor α/δ locus as a result of a t(1;14) chromosomal translocation, which occurs in approximately 5 percent of T-lymphoblastic lymphomas. However,

Table 11-1

GENES INVOLVED BY CHROMOSOMAL TRANSLOCATIONS IN T-LINEAGE LYMPHOBLASTIC LYMPHOMA/LEUKEMIA

Gene	Chromosome Location	Frequency	Protein Features	References
LYL1	19p13.1	Rare	HLH protein	33
TAL1/SCL*	1p32-34	5%	HLH protein	4,12
TAL2	9q32	Rare	HLH protein	57
TTG1/Rhomobotin	11p15	Rare	LIM protein	7,8,32
TTG2/Rhom2	11p13	10%	LIM protein	7,45
HOX11	10q24	7%	Homeodomain protein	23
TAN	9q34.3	Rare	Membrane protein	18
LCK	1p34	Rare	Tyrosine kinase	53
MYC	8q24	5-10%	bHLH-ZIP protein	19

*TAL1/SCL rearrangements occur in up to 25 percent of T-lineage leukemias/lymphomas as a result of submicroscopic deletions in fusions with the gene called SIL (see text).

TAL/SCL was subsequently reported to be rearranged in at least 25 percent of T-lymphoblastic neoplasms following submicroscopic deletions of chromosome band 1p32 in the absence of observable translocations (2,10). These deletions are clustered and thus amenable to detection by the polymerase chain reaction, a potentially useful marker for longitudinal assessment of minimal residual disease status in a significant proportion of T-lymphoblastic neoplasms (26).

Differential Diagnosis. *Small Noncleaved Cell Lymphoma.* Small noncleaved cell lymphoma may be easily confused with lymphoblastic lymphoma, particularly in suboptimal histologic preparations. Both lymphomas show diffuse infiltration by a monomorphic neoplastic population. A starry sky appearance is generally more prominent, and the mitotic rate is higher, in small noncleaved cell lymphoma. The individual neoplastic cells are slightly larger than those of lymphoblastic lymphoma, and these cells possess more abundant cytoplasm which is intensely pyroninophilic and tends to square off when one cell abuts another. The nuclei are larger than those of lymphoblastic lymphoma, and have a more vesicular chromatin pattern

with multiple nucleoli rather than the single small nucleolus that is usually present in lymphoblastic lymphoma. In touch preparations, the cells of small noncleaved lymphoma often have basophilic cytoplasm containing large cytoplasmic vacuoles identical with those of the L3 subtype of acute lymphoblastic leukemia.

Small noncleaved cell lymphoma is invariably a B-lineage neoplasm, while the majority of lymphoblastic lymphomas are of T lineage. In paraffin sections, the B-lineage antibodies CD20, CD74, and CDw75 may help identify the former (11). TdT is positive in almost all cases of lymphoblastic lymphoma, but negative in small noncleaved cell lymphoma.

Diffuse Small Cleaved Cell Lymphoma. Prior to the delineation of lymphoblastic lymphoma as a distinct clinicopathologic entity, many cases were diagnosed as diffuse small cleaved cell lymphoma (diffuse poorly differentiated lymphocytic lymphoma). The nuclei of the neoplastic cells of the latter have a coarse chromatin pattern rather than the fine, delicate chromatin seen in lymphoblastic lymphoma; the mitotic rate is much lower; and a starry sky appearance is never found. In addition, small areas of follicular architecture

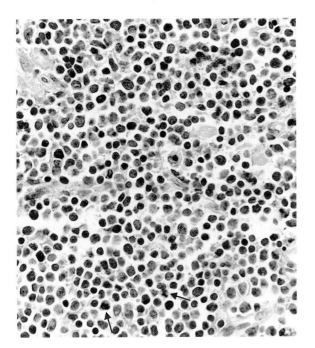

Figure 11-15
LYMPHOBLASTIC LYMPHOMA
This mediastinoscopic biopsy shows compression artifact and degenerative changes, obscuring the nuclear features. A diagnosis of small lymphocytic lymphoma could easily be made, unless special attention is given to the high mitotic rate (at arrows).

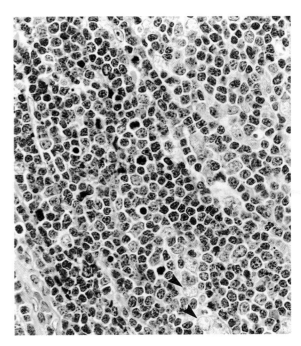

Figure 11-16
LYMPHOCYTE-RICH THYMOMA
The immature lymphoid cells closely mimic the neoplastic cells of lymphoblastic lymphoma. Note the pale epithelial cells diagnostic of thymoma, highlighted by the arrows.

identify diffuse small cleaved cell lymphoma as a follicular center lymphoma; true follicular architecture is never seen in lymphoblastic lymphoma.

Small Lymphocytic Lymphoma. The monotonous cellular infiltrate found in small lymphocytic lymphoma and variants can be easily confused with lymphoblastic lymphoma, particularly in suboptimal preparations (fig. 11-15). The chromatin pattern is coarser and the mitotic rate lower in small lymphocytic lymphoma. In addition, prolymphocytes, within or outside of pseudofollicular proliferation centers, are characteristic of small lymphocytic lymphoma, but are not seen in lymphoblastic lymphoma. A blastic variant of mantle cell lymphoma has been described which can closely resemble lymphoblastic lymphoma (28). The proliferating cells in this neoplasm possess scant, indistinct cytoplasm and nuclei with finely dispersed chromatin. Identification of a focal or widespread mantle zone pattern is helpful in identifying this variant. Scattered epithelioid histiocytes with granular eosinophilic cytoplasm are more common in the blastic variant of mantle cell

lymphoma. Demonstration of a typical mantle cell lymphoma in a previous or concurrent biopsy supports the diagnosis. Immunologically, most cases of lymphoblastic lymphoma can be distinguished from blastic mantle cell lymphoma by the T-cell phenotype and the presence of TdT. The rare cases of B-cell lymphoblastic lymphoma lack CD5 expression while the blastic variant of mantle cell lymphoma usually expresses this antigen, similar to the more common low-grade mantle cell lymphoma (28).

Thymoma. A lymphocytic component predominates in approximately one third of thymomas. In most cases of this type, the lymphocytes are mature looking and easily distinguished from lymphoblastic lymphoma, but in a small subset, the lymphocytes resemble immature thymic lymphocytes (fig. 11-16). The immunophenotype of these thymoma lymphocytes often corresponds to that of immature T cells (44), and these neoplasms can therefore be mistaken for lymphoblastic lymphoma, particularly if the diagnosis is based on flow cytometric analysis without proper morphologic correlation. Clinically, thymomas are uncommon in childhood and adolescence, a common age for lymphoblastic lymphoma. One histologic key to the recognition of thymoma is identification of the characteristic thick fibrous capsule continuous with wide fibrous strands. In addition, the neoplastic elements in thymoma, the epithelial cells, should be identified throughout the tumor, regardless of the number of lymphocytes. While lymphoblastic lymphoma may infiltrate the thymus, it does not uniformly enlarge it; rather, the epithelial elements are found in one portion, while most of the lymphoma is devoid of epithelial cells. Keratin stains may facilitate recognition of the epithelial cells.

Acute Leukemia. As discussed above, the distinction between lymphoblastic lymphoma and acute lymphoblastic leukemia is an arbitrary one, and without real biologic or clinical significance. Distinguishing lymphoblastic lymphoma and acute nonlymphocytic leukemia may also be difficult, and has major clinical implications. Acute nonlymphocytic leukemia presenting outside the peripheral blood and bone marrow (granulocytic sarcoma) may show a pattern of tissue infiltration identical to lymphoblastic lymphoma, with extensive involvement of fibrous tissue, single file infiltration between individual collagen bundles, and a preferential paracortical localization when lymph node involvement is partial. In addition, both neoplasms may have a high mitotic rate and be composed of intermediate-sized cells. In acute nonlymphocytic leukemia, there is usually more variation from cell to cell, often with some cells possessing more cytoplasm than generally seen in lymphoblastic lymphoma. Although some cases of lymphoblastic lymphoma may contain occasional eosinophils, acute nonlymphocytic leukemia usually has more eosinophils, and often contains neutrophils and myeloid precursors. When the diagnosis is in doubt, particularly when unusual sites such as breast, skin, or ovary are involved, the application of histochemical stains such as chloroacetate esterase, or immunologic markers such as CD15, CD68, myeloperoxidase, or neutrophil elastase, may resolve the diagnostic dilemma.

Nonhematopoietic Small Cell Neoplasms. Small cell undifferentiated (oat cell) carcinoma may simulate lymphoblastic lymphoma, particularly in small or suboptimal specimens (fig. 11-17).

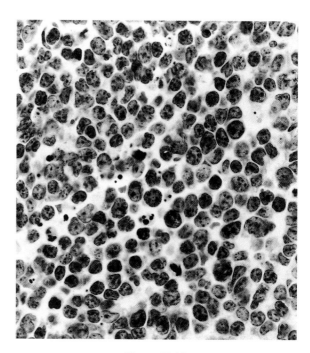

Figure 11-17
SMALL CELL UNDIFFERENTIATED
(OAT CELL) CARCINOMA
SIMULATING LYMPHOBLASTIC LYMPHOMA
Note occasional nuclear molding.

The cells of small cell undifferentiated carcinoma are usually larger than those of lymphoblastic lymphoma, and generally show a greater degree of single cell necrosis. Although the cells of small cell undifferentiated carcinoma usually show nuclear molding, this may be simulated in cases of lymphoblastic lymphoma with crush artifact. Occasionally, there is precipitation of DNA on the walls of blood vessels in cases of small cell undifferentiated carcinoma. In difficult cases, immunostains for keratin, CD45RB, and CD43 should be definitive in separating the two entities.

Small round cell tumors of childhood, including Ewing's sarcoma, neuroblastoma, and rhabdomyosarcoma may also be difficult to distinguish from lymphoblastic lymphoma. The differential diagnosis is further discussed in chapter 21.

Treatment. Treatment of lymphoblastic lymphoma with standard non-Hodgkin's lymphoma regimens proved unsuccessful, and led to the recognition of lymphoblastic lymphoma as a high-grade lymphoma. In the past decade, lymphoblastic lymphoma has been treated more successfully, using aggressive multi-agent chemotherapy in a manner analogous to that used in acute lymphoblastic leukemia (15,41,50). Local irradiation to sites of massive involvement is sometimes added (50). Since there is a high likelihood of relapse in the central nervous system, intrathecal chemotherapy or intracranial radiotherapy are often used. Bone marrow transplantation appears to be a promising therapy for the future (3).

Prognosis. In the Working Formulation classification, lymphoblastic lymphoma is regarded as a high-grade lymphoma, with a median survival of 2 years and a 5-year survival rate of 26 percent (39). The median time to relapse is 1 year,

the shortest of any of the non-Hodgkin's lymphomas. With modern treatment protocols, the survival rate has dramatically increased, with a 3-year actuarial freedom from relapse of 56 percent (15). The prognosis is not affected by any known histologic factors. High-risk disease has been defined as Ann Arbor stage IV disease with bone marrow or central nervous system involvement and a high initial serum lactate dehydrogenase level (15). Other clinical parameters, including B symptoms, Karnofsky status, sex, age, site of initial presentation, or presence of bulk disease have not been shown to predict outcome in multivariate analyses.

REFERENCES

1. Abruzzo LV, Jaffe ES, Cotelingam JD, Whang-Peng J, Del Duca V Jr, Medeiros LJ. T-cell lymphoblastic lymphoma with eosinophilia associated with subsequent myeloid malignancy. Am J Surg Pathol 1992;16:236–45.

2. Aplan PD, Lombardi DP, Ginsberg AM, Cossman J, Bertness VL, Kirsch IR. Disruption of the human SCL locus by "illegitimate" V-(D)-J recombinase activity. Science 1990;250:1426–9.

3. Appelbaum FR, Sullivan KM, Buckner CD, et al. Treatment of malignant lymphoma in 100 patients with chemotherapy, total body irradiation, and marrow transplantation. J Clin Oncol 1987;5:1340–7.

4. Begley CG, Aplan PD, Denning SM, Haynes BF, Waldmann TA, Kirsch IR. The gene SCL is expressed during early hematopoiesis and encodes a differentiation-related DNA-binding motif. Proc Natl Acad Sci USA 1989;86:10128–32.

5. Bernard A, Boumsell L, Reinherz EL, et al. Cell surface characterization of malignant T cells from lymphoblastic lymphoma using monoclonal antibodies: evidence for phenotypic differences between malignant T cells from patients with acute lymphoblastic leukemia and lymphoblastic lymphoma. Blood 1981;57:1105–10.

6. _____, Murphy SB, Melvin S, et al. Non-T, non-B lymphomas are rare in childhood and associated with cutaneous tumor. Blood 1982;59:549–54

7. Boehm T, Foroni L, Kaneko Y, Preutz MF, Rabbitts TH. The rhomobotin family of cystein-rich LIM-domain oncogenes: distinct members are involved in T-cell translocations to human chromosomes 11p15 and 11p13. Proc Natl Acad Sci USA 1991;88:4367–71.

8. _____, Greenberg JM, Buluwela L, Lavenir I, Forster A, Rabbitts TH. An unusual structure of a putative T-cell oncogene which allows production of a similar proteins from distinct mRNAs. EMBO J 1990;9:857–68.

9. Braziel RM, Keneklis T, Donlon JA, et al. Terminal deoxynucleotidyl transferase in non-Hodgkin's lymphoma. Am J Clin Pathol 1983;80:655–9.

10. Brown L, Cheng JT, Chen Q, et al. Site-specific recombination of the tal-1 gene is a common occurrence in human T-cell leukemia. EMBO J 1990;9:3343–51.

11. Brownell MD, Sheibani K, Battifora H, Winberg CD, Rappaport H. Distinction between undifferentiated (small noncleaved) and lymphoblastic lymphoma. An immunohistologic study on paraffin-embedded, fixed tissue sections. Am J Surg Pathol 1987;11:779–87.

12. Chen Q, Cheng JT, Tasi LH, et al. The tal gene undergoes chromosome translocation in T cell leukemia and potentially encodes a helix-loop-helix protein. EMBO J 1990;9:415–24.

13. Childs CC, Chrystal GS, Strauchen JA. Biphenotypic lymphoblastic lymphoma. An unusual tumor with lymphocytic and granulocytic differentiation. Cancer 1986;57:1019–23.

14. Cleary ML. Oncogenic conversion of transcription factors by chromosomal translocations. Cell 1991;66:619–22.

15. Coleman CN, Picozzi VJ Jr, Cox RS, et al. Treatment of lymphoblastic lymphoma in adults. J Clin Oncol 1986;4:1628–37.

16. Cossman J, Chused TM, Fisher RI, Magrath I, Bollum F, Jaffe ES. Diversity of immunological phenotypes of lymphoblastic lymphoma. Cancer Res 1983;43:4486–90.

17. d'Auriol L, Macintyre E, Galibert E, Sigaux F. In vitro amplification of T-cell gamma gene rearrangements: a new tool for the assessment of minimal residual disease in acute lymphoblastic leukemias. Leukemia 1989;3:155–8.

18. Ellisen LW, Bird J, West DC, et al. TAN-1, the human homolog of the Drosophila notch gene, is broken by chromosomal translocation in T lymphoblastic neoplasms. Cell 1991;66:649–61.

19. Erikson J, Finger L, Sun L, et al. Deregulation of c-myc by translocation of the alpha-locus of T-cell receptor in T-cell leukemias. Science 1986;232:884–6.

20. Finger LR, Harvey RC, Moore RC, Showe LC, Croce CM. A common mechanism of chromosomal translocation in T- and B-cell neoplasia. Science 1986;234:982–5.

21. Griffith RC, Kelly DR, Nathwani BN, et al. A morphologic study of childhood lymphoma of the lymphoblastic type. The Pediatric Oncology Group experience. Cancer 1987;59:1126–231.

22. Hansen-Hagge TE, Yokota S, Bartram CR. Detection of minimal residual disease in acute lymphoblastic leukemia by in vitro amplification of rearranged T-cell receptor delta chain sequences. Blood 1989;74:1762–7.

23. Hatano M, Roberts CW, Minden M, Crist WM, Korsmeyer SJ. Deregulation of a homeobox gene, HOX11, by the t(10;14) in T cell leukemia. Science 1991;253:79–82.

24. Heim S, Mitelman F. Cancer cytogenetics. New York: A.R.Liss Inc., 1987.

25. Ioachim HL, Finkbeiner JA. Pseudonodular pattern of T-cell lymphoma. Cancer 1980;145:1370–8.

26. Jonnson OG, Kitchens RL, Baer RJ, Buchanan GR, Smith RG. Rearrangements of the tal-1 locus as clonal markers for T cell acute lymphoblastic leukemia. J Clin Invest 1991;87:2029–35.

27. Koo CH, Rappaport H, Sheibani K, Pangalis GA, Nathwani BN, Winberg CD. Imprint cytology of non-Hodgkin's lymphomas. Based on a study of 212 immunologically characterized cases: correlation of touch imprints with tissue sections. Hum Pathol 1989;20(12 Suppl 1):1–137.

28. Lardelli P, Bookman MA, Sundeen J, Longo DL, Jaffe ES. Lymphocytic lymphoma of intermediate differentiation. Morphologic and immunophenotypic spectrum and clinical correlations. Am J Surg Pathol 1990;14:752–63.

29. Lennert K. Histopathology of non-Hodgkin's lymphoma (based on the Kiel classification). Berlin: Springer-Verlag, 1981.

30. _____, Feller AC. Histopathology of non-Hodgkin's lymphomas (based on the updated Kiel classification). 2nd ed. Berlin: Springer-Verlag, 1992.

31. Link MP, Roper M, Dorfman RF, Crist WM, Cooper MD, Levy R. Cutaneous lymphoblastic lymphoma with pre-B markers. Blood 1983;61:838–41.

32. McGuire EA, Hockett RD, Pollock KM, Bartholdi MF, O'Brien SJ, Korsmeyer SJ. The t(11;14)(p15;q11) in a T cell acute lymphoblastic leukemia cell line activates multiple transcripts, including Ttg-1, a gene encoding a potential zinc finger protein. Mol Cell Biol 1989;9:2124–32.

33. Mellentin JD, Smith SD, Cleary ML. Lyl-1, a novel gene altered by chromosomal translocation in T cell leukemia, codes for a protein with a helix-loop-helix DNA binding motif. Cell 1989;58:77–83.

34. Minden MD, Mak TW. The structure of the T cell antigen receptor genes in normal and malignant T cells. Blood 1986;327–39.

35. Mirro J, Kitchingman G, Behm FG, et al. T cell differentiation stages identified by molecular and immunologic analysis of the T cell receptor complex in childhood lymphoblastic leukemia. Blood 1987;69:908–12.

36. Murphy SB. Childhood non-Hodgkin's lymphoma. N Engl J Med 1978;299:1446–8.

37. Nathwani BN, Diamond LW, Winberg CD, et al. Lymphoblastic lymphoma: a clinicopathologic study of 95 patients. Cancer 1981;48:2347–57.

38. _____, Kim H, Rappaport H. Malignant lymphoma, lymphoblastic. Cancer 1976;38:964–83.

39. The Non-Hodgkin's Lymphoma Pathologic Classification Project. National Cancer Institute sponsored study of classifications of non-Hodgkin's lymphomas: summary and description of a working formulation for clinical usage. Cancer 1982;49:2112–35.

40. Orazi A, Caggoretti G, John K, Neiman RS. Terminal deoxynucleotidyl transferase staining of malignant lymphomas in paraffin sections. Mod Pathol 1994;7:582–6.

41. Picozzi VJ Jr, Coleman CN. Lymphoblastic lymphoma. Semin Oncol 1990;17:96–103.

42. Raimondi SC, Behm FG, Roberson PK, et al. Cytogenetics of childhood T-cell leukemia. Blood 1988;72:1560–6.

43. Roper M, Crist WM, Metzgar R, et al. Monoclonal antibody characterization of surface antigens in childhood T-cell lymphoid malignancies. Blood 1983;61:830–7.

44. Rouse RV, Weiss LM. Human thymomas: evidence of immunologically defined normal and abnormal microenvironmental differentiation. Cell Immunol 1988;111:94–106.

45. Royer-Pokora B, Loos U, Ludwig WD. TTG-2, a new gene encoding a cysteine-rich protein with the LIM motif, is overexpressed in acute T-cell leukaemia with the t(11;14)(p13;q11). Oncogene 1991;6:1887–93.

46. Said JW, Shintaku IP, Pinkus GS. Immunohistochemical staining for terminal deoxynucleotidyl transferase (TDT). An enhanced method in routinely processed formalin-fixed tissue sections. Am J Clin Pathol 1988;89:649–52.

46a. Sander CA, Jaffe ES, Gebhardt FC, Yano T, Medeiros LJ. Mediastinal lymphoblastic lymphoma with an immature B-cell immunophenotype. Am J Surg Pathol 1992;16:300–5.

47. _____, Medeiros LJ, Abruzzo LV, Horak ID, Jaffe ES. Lymphoblastic lymphoma in cutaneous sites: a clinicopathologic analysis of six cases. J Am Acad Dermatol 1991;25(6 Pt 1):1023–31.

48. Sheibani K, Nathwani BN, Winberg CD, et al. Antigenically defined subgroups of lymphoblastic lymphoma. Relationship to clinical presentation and biologic behavior. Cancer 1987;60:183–90.

49. _____, Winberg CD, Burke JS, et al. Lymphoblastic lymphoma expressing natural killer cell-associated antigens: a clinicopathologic study of six cases. Leuk Res 1987;11:371–7.

50. Slater DE, Mertelsmann R, Koziner B, et al. Lymphoblastic lymphoma in adults. J Clin Oncol 1986;4:57–67.

51. Stroup R, Sheibani K, Misset JL, Szekely AM, Tremblay G, Rappaport H. Surface immunoglobulin-positive lymphoblastic lymphoma. A report of three cases. Cancer 1990;65:2559–63.

52. Tawa A, Hozumi N, Minden M, Mak TW, Gelfard EW. Rearrangement of the T-cell receptor β-chain gene in non-T cell, non-B cell acute lymphoblastic leukemia of children. N Engl J Med 1985;313:1033–7.

53. Tycko B, Smith SD, Sklar J. Chromosomal translocations joining LCK and TCRB loci in human T cell leukemia. J Exp Med 1991;174:867–73.

54. Warnke RA, Gatter KC, Falini B, et al. Diagnosis of human lymphoma with monoclonal antileukocyte antibodies. N Engl J Med 1983;309:1275–81.

55. Weiss LM, Bindl JM, Picozzi VJ, Link MP, Warnke RA. Lymphoblastic lymphoma: an immunophenotype study of 26 cases with comparison to T cell acute lymphoblastic leukemia. Blood 1986;67:474–8.

56. Wilson JF, Jenkin RD, Anderson JR, et al. Studies on the pathology of non-Hodgkin's lymphoma of childhood. l. The role of routine histopathology as a prognostic factor. A report from the Children's Cancer Study Group. Cancer 1984;53:1695–704.

57. Xia Y, Brown L, Yang CY, et al. TAL2, a helix-loop-helix gene activated by the (7;9)(q34;q32) translocation in human T-cell leukemia. Proc Natl Acad Sci USA 1991;88:11416–20.

12

MYCOSIS FUNGOIDES

Definition. Mycosis fungoides is a neoplasm composed of T lymphocytes that have a cerebriform nuclear appearance and a marked propensity for infiltration of skin or, rarely, other epithelia.

Incidence. Patients with mycosis fungoides are typically adults, with a median age of about 55 years (21). However, there are rare reports of the disease occurring in children. The incidence is twice as high in men than women and twice as high in blacks than whites. It is a rare lymphoma, with only about 500 new cases (0.29 per 100,000) occurring annually (54).

There appear to be no strong predisposing occupational or environmental exposures for mycosis fungoides (61). Currently, there is intense study concerning the possibility of an associated retrovirus, but a definitive link has not been established (20). Patients may have an increased incidence of other hematolymphoid neoplasms, including Hodgkin's disease (10,46,47).

Natural History and Clinical Features. The disease has an extremely long natural history (21). In the premycotic stage, patients generally present with a long history of nonspecific skin lesions. The typical, slightly scaling macules present over a variety of sites and simulate many chronic skin disorders clinically and pathologically (8). The median duration from the onset of skin symptoms to the diagnosis of mycosis fungoides is nearly 6 years. A histologic diagnosis can sometimes be established in the next stage, the erythematous or patch stage, in which the macules coalesce to form flat erythematous patches, sometimes associated with atrophy. When infiltration with increasing numbers of cells occurs, the disease progresses to the plaque stage, where the individual lesions become indurated. The histologic diagnosis is usually easily established at this time. In time and without treatment, the tumor stage is reached with the formation of obvious raised tumors, often with secondary ulceration. This progression of disease is not invariable, and is not always as orderly as described. Not all patients with premycotic or patch stage mycosis fungoides progress to higher stages, and occasional patients present with

tumor masses, the tumor d'emblee form of mycosis fungoides.

Another presentation of mycosis fungoides is generalized erythroderma. This is particularly common in conjunction with generalized lymphadenopathy, splenomegaly, and circulating tumor cells in the peripheral blood, known as Sézary's syndrome. At times, mycosis fungoides can take on unusual skin presentations, such as verrucous/hyperkeratotic, pustular, bullous, folliculocentric, acanthosis nigricans–like, hypopigmented, and pigmented purpura-like lesions (28). Rarely, epithelia other than skin may be the presenting site, such as the oral cavity or pharynx.

Although skin involvement is usually the most obvious clinical manifestation, extracutaneous involvement also occurs (5,40). A summary of the TNBM classification for mycosis fungoides is given in Table 12-1 and the staging classification is outlined in Table 12-2 (6). Regional lymph node infiltration is particularly common, although it is often difficult to distinguish clinically from lymphadenopathy due to dermatopathic changes. At autopsy, visceral involvement can be found in over two thirds of patients (18,40). The lung, liver, and spleen are preferentially affected, although any organ may show infiltration in the late stages of the disease. Patients with mycosis fungoides often die of causes other than the neoplasm, which is not surprising given the indolent nature of the disease (21). Patients with advanced stage disease usually die from tumor infiltration or intercurrent infection as a direct result of the disease.

Microscopic Findings. The histologic appearance of mycosis fungoides in the skin depends upon the stage at which the lesion is biopsied. Lesions biopsied in the premycotic stage may show nonspecific findings. The earliest changes consist of a sparse, superficial perivascular lymphocytic infiltrate with slight or no epidermal hyperplasia and with rare lymphocytes in the lower epidermis (45). Later, the epidermis shows acanthosis with broad areas of slight hyperorthokeratosis that is compact or laminated, although atrophy may also be seen. Focal parakeratosis is common. A mild to moderate

Table 12-1

TNBM CLASSIFICATION OF MYCOSIS FUNGOIDES

Classification	Description
T: Skin	
T0	Clinically and/or histopathologically suspicious lesions
T1	Limited plaques, papules, or eczematous patches covering >10% of the skin surface
T2	Generalized plaques, papules, or erythematous patches covering ≥10% of the skin surface
T3	Tumors
T4	Generalized erythroderma
N: Lymph nodes	
N0	No clinically abnormal lymph nodes, pathology negative
N1	Clinically abnormal lymph nodes, pathology negative
N2	No clinically abnormal lymph nodes, pathology positive
N3	Clinically abnormal lymph nodes, pathology positive
B: Peripheral blood	
B0	<5% atypical circulating cells
B1	>5% atypical circulating cells
M: Visceral organs	
M0	No visceral organ involvement
M1	Visceral involvement

Table 12-2

STAGING CLASSIFICATION OF MYCOSIS FUNGOIDES

Stage	Classification		
	T	N	M
IA	1	0	0
IB	2	0	0
IIA	1-2	1	0
IIB	3	0,1	0
III	4	0,1	0
IVA	1-4	2,3	0
IVB	1-4	0-3	1

(epidermotropism) as single cells, small clusters of cells, large clusters of cells (Pautrier microabscesses), lined up along the basal layer, or as a diffuse infiltration of all levels of the epidermis (figs. 12-5, 12-6). Well-defined Pautrier microabscesses are found in only a few cases, but atypical lymphocytes can be identified in at least 50 percent of cases (36,45). Identical atypical lymphocytes are sometimes present in the peripheral blood (fig. 12-7). The epidermis sometimes shows rounded, hyperplastic rete ridges adjacent to flattened rete. It is usually nonspongiotic, but slight spongiosis may be found in one third of cases. Vacuolar alteration may also be present, but is usually only mild.

In biopsies from tumor lesions from skin, nodules of atypical lymphocytes are found within the dermis and subcutaneous tissue. Occasionally, transformation of the atypical lymphocytes to large lymphoid cells having nuclei with a vesicular chromatin pattern may occur (fig. 12-8) (14, 41,42). This transformation may closely resemble large cell lymphoma or even Hodgkin's disease. However, cerebriform atypical lymphocytes are usually still identifiable, and the typical epidermal infiltration remains in most of these lesions.

Lymph nodes draining sites of skin involvement may show reactive follicular hyperplasia or, more commonly, dermatopathic lymphadenopathy, or involvement by mycosis fungoides, with or without superimposed dermatopathic changes (11). Dermatopathic lymphadenopathy, compared to other reactive patterns, occurs more frequently in black patients and in patients with

mixed infiltrate consisting of lymphoid cells, histiocytes, eosinophils, and plasma cells is usually present in a dermal perivascular location, and occasional lymphocytes are found in the overlying epidermis (figs. 12-1, 12-2).

The diagnostic features of mycosis fungoides are usually present in the more advanced patch and plaque lesions (fig. 12-3). The dermis shows a moderate to marked mixed inflammatory infiltrate, often in a band-like distribution beneath the epidermis, which now includes significant numbers of atypical lymphocytes. These atypical lymphocytes have hyperchromatic nuclei with cerebriform contours, and range from the size of a normal lymphocyte nucleus (known as mycosis or small Sézary cells) to approximately twice that size (true mycosis or large Sézary cells) (fig. 12-4). These atypical lymphocytes are also typically identified in the overlying epidermis

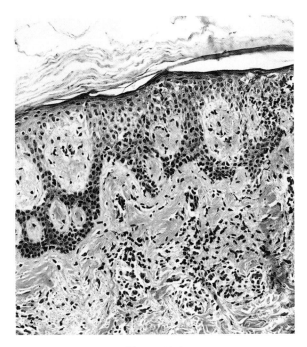

Figure 12-1
MYCOSIS FUNGOIDES, PATCH STAGE
A moderate dermal lymphoid infiltrate is present. (Figures 12-1 and 12-2 are from the same case.)

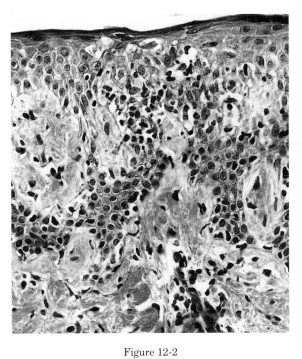

Figure 12-2
MYCOSIS FUNGOIDES, PATCH STAGE
Preferential infiltration of the epidermis is seen, without significant amounts of spongiosis.

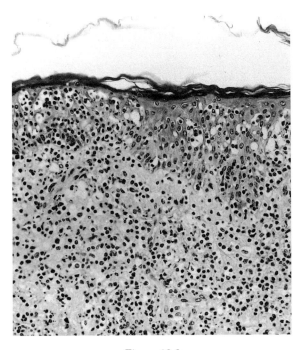

Figure 12-3
MYCOSIS FUNGOIDES, PLAQUE STAGE
A heavy dermal lymphoid infiltrate is present. The epidermis shows a significant degree of lymphocytic infiltration.

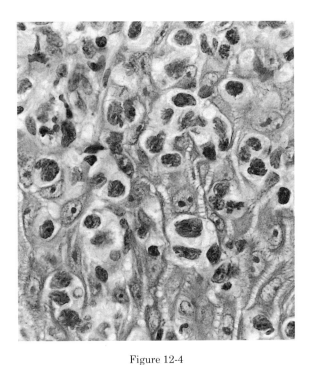

Figure 12-4
MYCOSIS FUNGOIDES
Atypical lymphocytes of various sizes are seen infiltrating the epidermis.

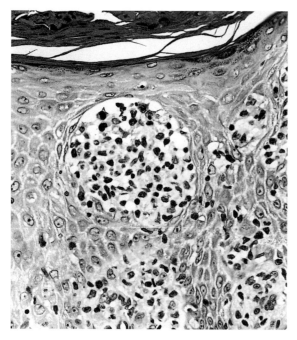

Figure 12-5
MYCOSIS FUNGOIDES
Multiple Pautrier microabscesses are present.

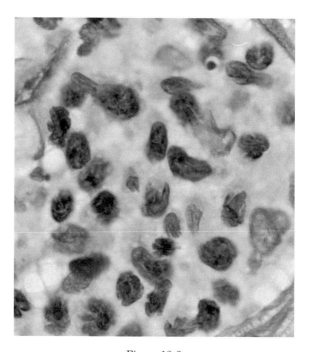

Figure 12-6
MYCOSIS FUNGOIDES
The atypical lymphocytes in this Pautrier's microabscess
show cerebriform contours. Langerhans cells are also present.

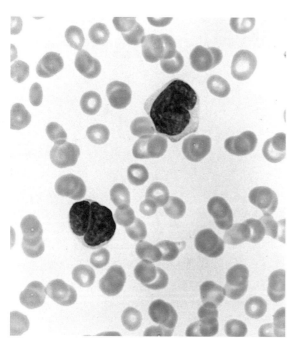

Figure 12-7
SÉZARY'S SYNDROME
Two circulating mycosis (or Sézary) cells are seen.

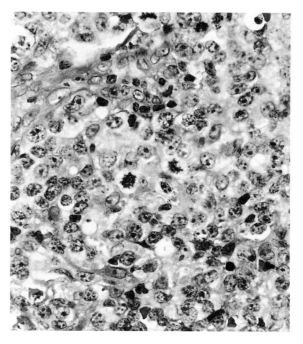

Figure 12-8
MYCOSIS FUNGOIDES, TUMOR STAGE
Transformation to large lymphoid cells has occurred.

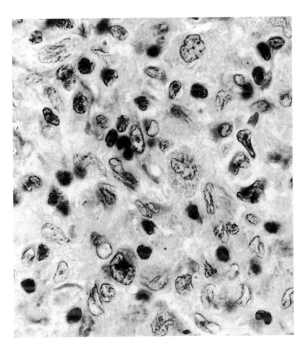

Figure 12-9
DERMATOPATHIC LYMPHADENOPATHY,
IN A PATIENT WITH MYCOSIS FUNGOIDES
Single atypical lymphoid cells are present (LN-1).

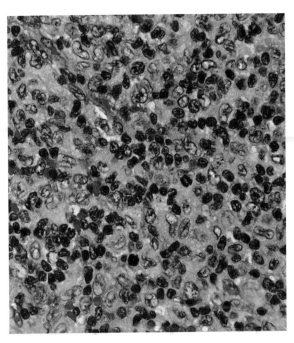

Figure 12-10
DERMATOPATHIC LYMPHADENOPATHY,
IN A PATIENT WITH MYCOSIS FUNGOIDES
Small clusters of atypical lymphocytes are present (LN-2).

more extensive skin involvement (52). The lymph node involvement ranges from histologically undetectable to complete obliteration of architecture by atypical lymphocytes. These histologic changes are graded: LN-0, in which reactive changes are present, but no atypical lymphocytes are evident; LN-1, in which only few atypical lymphocytes are noted in the paracortex; LN-2, in which atypical lymphocytes occur both singly or in small clusters, generally of fewer than three to six cells in the paracortex; LN-3, in which large clusters of atypical lymphocytes, generally in aggregates of 15 or more cells, are interspersed between and tend to separate the paracortical histiocytes, often accompanied by large immunoblastic cells; and LN-4, in which partial or complete obliteration of architecture by atypical lymphocytes occurs (figs. 12-9, 12-10) (43). Generally, all nodes showing changes of LN-3 or -4 and the majority of nodes showing changes of LN-2 show involvement by mycosis fungoides when assessed by other independent techniques (5,33). This classification of lymph node histopathology correlates with the extent of skin, blood, and visceral involvement, as well as

with survival (43). Another classification system for lymph node morphology is based more on cell size and the degree of nuclear convolution of the atypical lymphocytes. Lymph nodes containing numerous, large convoluted mononuclear cells (nuclei up to 11.5 µm) are considered positive for mycosis fungoides in this scheme (44).

Similar to the transformation that may occur in skin lesions, some lymph nodes show partial or complete replacement by large, and occasionally highly pleomorphic, lymphoid cells simulating large cell lymphoma or even Hodgkin's disease (fig. 12-11) (41,52).

The characteristic atypical lymphocytes are generally seen in mycosis fungoides involving visceral sites. Here, however, evidence of transformation to a large cell neoplasm is more common than in the skin or lymph nodes. The architecture of the involved organ is usually preserved; interestingly, a predilection of the atypical lymphocytes for epithelia is often seen (40).

On ultrastructural examination, the atypical lymphocyte of mycosis fungoides has a markedly irregular nuclear contour (fig. 12-12) (32). However, reactive lymphocytes may at times have

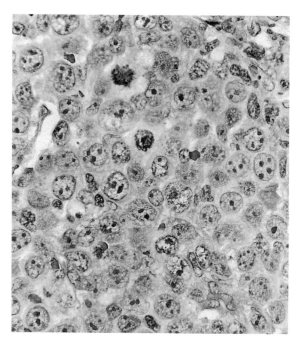

Figure 12-11
MYCOSIS FUNGOIDES
Complete lymph node effacement by large lymphoid cells is seen. Without a clinical history, this appearance may be indistinguishable from other large cell lymphomas.

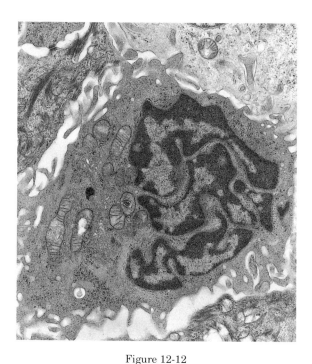

Figure 12-12
MYCOSIS FUNGOIDES
A cerebriform cell is seen. (Courtesy of Dr. Dominic V. Spagnolo, Perth, Western Australia.)

highly irregular nuclear membranes simulating those seen in mycosis fungoides. A diagnosis of mycosis fungoides is suggested when clusters or sheets of cells with highly irregular nuclear outlines are found. Because of these nuclear irregularities, morphometric analyses have been used as a diagnostic tool. If the nuclear contour index (NCI), defined as the nuclear perimeter per square root of nuclear area, is high in a large proportion of cells or very high in some cells, then a diagnosis of mycosis fungoides, rather than a reactive infiltrate, is supported (34).

Variants and Related Disorders. *Small Cell and Large Cell Variants.* Lutzner and colleagues (31) described large cell and small cell variants of mycosis fungoides, depending on the size of the atypical lymphocytes. However, since then it has become clear that individual cases of mycosis fungoides have differing proportions of atypical lymphocytes that are large, small, and intermediate-sized; thus, there is no clear separation between these morphologic variants.

Pagetoid Reticulosis (Woringer-Kolopp Disease). Pagetoid reticulosis is a clinical entity in

which patients present with single or multiple hyperkeratotic or verrucous plaques on the hands or feet (13). Skin biopsy shows clusters and nests of atypical lymphocytes within a markedly acanthotic epidermis, with only a mild inflammatory infiltrate within the underlying dermis (fig. 12-13). Progression to disseminated skin or systemic disease may occur, although the probability is not yet known given the rarity of the disease. Pagetoid reticulosis is best regarded as a distinct clinical variant of mycosis fungoides with a good prognosis.

Granulomatous Slack Skin Disease. Granulomatous slack skin disease affects patients younger than the typical patient with mycosis fungoides (29). Patients present with boggy plaques, frequently in the axilla and groin, which progress to pendulous folds of wrinkled erythematous skin. The epidermis and papillary dermis show histologic changes similar to those seen in conventional mycosis fungoides. However, the reticular dermis and subcutaneous tissue exhibit numerous granulomas containing giant cells with numerous nuclei (fig. 12-14). Atypical lymphoid cells and Langerhans cells can sometimes

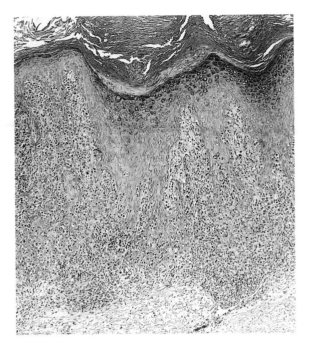

Figure 12-13
PAGETOID RETICULOSIS

A highly acanthotic epidermis containing numerous atypical lymphoid cells is seen. Other than a "hugging" lymphoid infiltrate in the dermis directly adjacent to the epidermis, the dermis is devoid of lymphoid cells. (Courtesy of Dr. Bruce R. Smoller, Stanford, CA.)

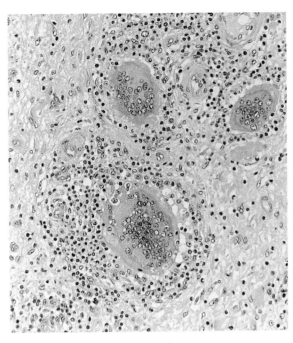

Figure 12-14
GRANULOMATOUS SLACK SKIN DISEASE

Multinucleated giant cells with numerous nuclei and containing engulfed small lymphoid cells and dendritic cells are present in a background of atypical lymphoid cells within the dermis.

be found in the cytoplasm of these multinucleated histiocytes. There is also marked destruction of the elastic fibers in the dermis.

Other Histologic Variants. At times, mycosis fungoides can have an unusual histologic appearance (28,45). Rarely, a significant epidermal component is lacking or an infiltrate can be centered around hair follicles. The epidermis may be pseudo-epitheliomatous, papillomatous, acanthosis nigricans–like, or depigmented. Spongiotic vesicles, pustules, or bullae may be the most prominent histologic feature. Presentation as a vasculitis or panniculitis may occur. Rarely, numerous granulomas dominate the histologic appearance. Another interesting change is mucin deposition, either within the dermis or presenting as follicular mucinosis (fig. 12-15).

Immunologic Findings. Invariably, the presumed neoplastic component of mycosis fungoides, the atypical lymphocytes with cerebriform nuclei, possess a T-cell phenotype. In paraffin sections, the cells express the leukocyte common antigen CD45RB and the T-lineage–associated antigens

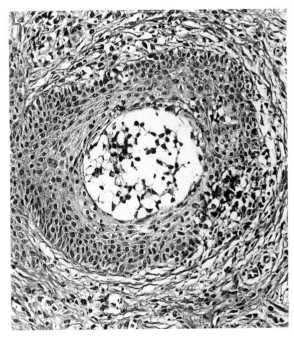

Figure 12-15
FOLLICULAR MUCINOSIS, IN A PATIENT
WITH MYCOSIS FUNGOIDES

Note the infiltration of the epithelium by lymphoid cells.

CD3, CD45RO, and CD43 (38,65). In frozen sections, the cells express a CD4+, CD8- helper T-lymphocyte phenotype in at least 95 percent of cases. A few cases express a CD4-, CD8+ suppressor T-cell phenotype, or, more rarely, a CD4+, CD8+ phenotype (2,41). In early skin lesions, retention of the pan-T antigens CD2, CD3, CD5, and the β-T-cell chain antigen, recognized by the monoclonal antibody βF1, is found in over 95 percent of cases. However, these may be absent in tumor lesions of skin and lesions with advanced lymph node involvement (37), particularly in cases with large cell transformation (41). CD15, CD30, and CD74 are often expressed in mycosis fungoides that has transformed to large cell lymphoma, a phenotype whose cells may be confused with the Reed-Sternberg cells of Hodgkin's disease (41,62). In both early and late lesions of mycosis fungoides, absence of the main T-cell antigens CD7 and Leu-8 is usually seen (37). In fact, absence of CD7 is an almost invariant feature of the leukemic type mycosis fungoides (Sézary's syndrome). However, since both CD7, and particularly Leu-8, may be deficient in benign inflammatory skin lesions, their absence as a diagnostic marker of mycosis fungoides skin lesions is limited.

Pan-T-cell antigen loss may be particularly common in cases of suppressor phenotype mycosis fungoides (2). Two subtypes of suppressor phenotype mycosis fungoides have been delineated based on the pattern of pan-T-cell antigen expression: a CD2+, CD7- phenotype associated with a chronic disease course and a CD2-, CD7+ phenotype associated with rapid progression. The neoplastic cells of mycosis fungoides often express the activation markers CD71, CD38, BE1, and BE2, and sometimes express CD25, but none of these antigens has diagnostic significance (4,24,35,65). The nonneoplastic infiltrate is usually a mixture of helper and suppressor T cells, histiocytes, Langerhans cells, and indeterminate cells, as well as B cells on occasion. (65).

Molecular and Cytogenetic Findings. Gene rearrangement studies to determine the status of the β-T-cell receptor gene have demonstrated that mycosis fungoides represents a clonal T-cell proliferation (55). Different sites of disease from the same patient generally show identical clonal bands, indicating that the disease is monoclonal and systemic in patients with multiple lesions. Clonal rearrangements of the β-T-cell receptor gene have also been found in pagetoid reticulosis and granulomatous slack skin disease, providing additional evidence that these entities represent variants of mycosis fungoides (29,64).

Gene rearrangement studies have been shown to have great utility in the diagnosis of subtle lymph node involvement by mycosis fungoides, and for the diagnosis of blood involvement (33,55,57). Clonal T-cell receptor gene rearrangements are more frequently detected in dermatopathic lymph nodes with clusters of atypical cells (LN-3) than with earlier histologic changes (LN-1 and -2), and are associated with a worse survival (33). Although there may be a role for these studies in the initial diagnosis of mycosis fungoides, and particularly Sézary's syndrome, through the analysis of peripheral blood lymphocytes, it must be kept in mind that clonal rearrangements of the β-T-cell receptor gene can occasionally be found in DNA derived from peripheral blood lymphocytes of patients without lymphoid neoplasms. For example, multiclonal gene rearrangements of the β-T-cell receptor gene have been reported in acute infectious mononucleosis, presumably representing a host reaction to the viral infection (48). Gene rearrangement studies may also be of use in the initial diagnosis of mycosis fungoides in skin, as almost all inflammatory dermatoses show a germline configuration for the β-T-cell receptor gene (56,66). However, clonal β-T-cell receptor gene rearrangements may be found in other T-cell lymphomas involving the skin as well as in lymphomatoid papulosis and pityriasis lichenoides et varioliformis acuta (Mucha-Habermann disease) (56,58). Conversely, clonal gene rearrangements are not always detectable in the earliest skin lesions of mycosis fungoides, presumably due to insufficient numbers of neoplastic cells for the 1- to 5-percent sensitivity of the Southern blot analysis (15,39,66). Analysis of gene rearrangements using the polymerase chain reaction may provide a more sensitive method of diagnosis in the future (3).

In most patients with mycosis fungoides, cytogenetic abnormalities are found in cells analyzed from biopsies in which involvement by neoplasm is suspected, even in sites where the involvement cannot be proven morphologically (5,17,19,60). In contrast to many of the other lymphomas, no consistent cytogenetic abnormality has been found in mycosis fungoides. Chromosome banding studies have shown extensive heteroploidy. In one study, numerical abnormalities of chromosomes 11, 21, and 22 were most common, while structural abnormalities were most common in chromosome 1 (60). Patients with more extensive chromosomal changes tend to have more advanced clinical disease. Clone formation is associated with a poor prognosis. DNA cytophotometric studies have also shown an aneuploid DNA population in involved tissues from mycosis fungoides patients (51).

Differential Diagnosis. *Skin: Inflammatory Dermatoses, including Large Plaque Parapsoriasis and Actinic Reticuloid.* Skin biopsies taken from patients with the earliest lesions of mycosis fungoides are easily mistaken for an inflammatory process, particularly a type of spongiotic, interface, or psoriasiform dermatitis. The distinction between mycosis fungoides and inflammatory dermatoses rests upon the definitive identification of atypical lymphocytes with cerebriform, hyperchromatic nuclei in the former. Their identification is easier when they are found in the epidermis, particularly as discrete collections unaccompanied by significant spongiosis (Pautrier microabscesses). Although some early lesions of mycosis fungoides may lack overtly atypical cells, it is best to defer the histologic diagnosis in their absence until additional or future lesions are biopsied; it is not uncommon for multiple biopsies to be required over time for the definitive diagnosis to be established. Large plaque parapsoriasis very closely simulates mycosis fungoides including exocytosis of lymphocytes, but lacks significant numbers of atypical lymphocytes (fig. 12-16). The pertinence of distinguishing this disorder from mycosis fungoides has come into question as long-term follow-up studies have shown a progression to overt mycosis fungoides in a percentage of patients (27).

Actinic reticuloid may be viewed as the most extreme variant of chronic photosensitivity dermatitis (49). Clinically, mycosis fungoides may be closely simulated, with the formation of papules, plaques, or even generalized erythroderma. Histologically, dense lymphoid infiltrates may be present and highly irregular lymphocytes may be found in skin, lymph nodes, and blood (fig. 12-17). Demonstration of photosensitivity to a broad spectrum of wavelengths, including ultra-

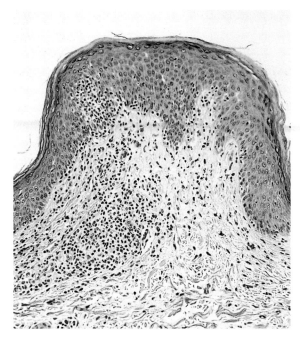

Figure 12-16
LARGE PLAQUE PARAPSORIASIS
This biopsy shows a moderate dermal lymphoid infiltrate with exocytosis of lymphocytes that could easily be mistaken for mycosis fungoides. (Figures 12-16 and 12-19 are from the same case.)

violet (UV)-A, UV-B, and part of the visible spectrum may help to establish the diagnosis.

Immunologic studies may be of some use in the differential diagnosis of mycosis fungoides versus actinic reticuloid: in actinic reticuloid, the dermal lymphoid infiltrate is composed primarily of CD4-, CD8+ cells as opposed to the usual CD4+, CD8- infiltrate in mycosis fungoides, and the peripheral blood often shows a reversed CD4+ to CD8+ ratio (49). Gene rearrangement analysis may help differentiate mycosis fungoides and inflammatory skin disorders, however, early lesions of mycosis fungoides may lack detectable clonal gene rearrangements. In addition, although most inflammatory skin disorders lack clonal T-cell gene rearrangements, there are exceptions, including pityriasis lichenoides et varioliformis acuta (PLEVA) in which clonal rearrangements of the β- and γ-T-cell receptor genes may be identified (56).

Skin: Lymphomatoid Papulosis. When atypical lymphocytes are clearly identified in the skin biopsy, the histologic differential diagnosis should include lymphomatoid papulosis and nonmycosis

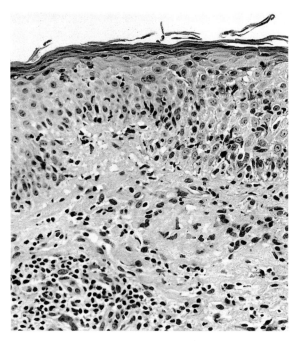

Figure 12-17
ACTINIC RETICULOID
This biopsy demonstrates a significant degree of exocytosis of lymphocytes into the epidermis. Clinical history and immunologic studies may be useful in distinguishing actinic reticuloid from mycosis fungoides. (Courtesy of Dr. Bruce R. Smoller, Stanford, CA.)

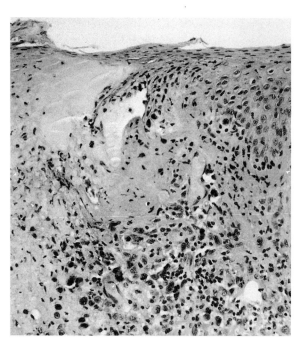

Figure 12-18
LYMPHOMATOID PAPULOSIS
The epidermis is ulcerated and an underlying, highly atypical lymphoid infiltrate is present in the dermis.

fungoides malignant lymphomas involving the skin. Lymphomatoid papulosis generally presents as multiple papules which appear and disappear spontaneously, often over a 3- to 4-week cycle (53). Any cutaneous site may be involved, although there is a predilection for the trunk and limbs. There is a wide age distribution, but adults between 20 and 40 years are most commonly affected. The individual lesions vary in appearance, depending on the age of the lesion biopsied. In fully developed lesions, the type of lesion that may be most confused with mycosis fungoides, a superficial and deep perivascular and diffuse mixed lymphoid infiltrate is present, often with exocytosis into the epidermis (fig. 12-18). This infiltrate is composed of small lymphocytes, histiocytes, granulocytes, and variable numbers of atypical lymphocytes (fig. 12-19). The atypical lymphocytes vary in size and shape from small and cerebriform, similar to the atypical lymphocytes seen in mycosis fungoides, to large and pleomorphic, similar to cells found in anaplastic large cell lymphoma. When the former cells pre-dominate, in the so-called type B lesion, the confusion with mycosis fungoides is greatest.

Immunologic studies may aid in the differential diagnosis of lymphomatoid papulosis versus mycosis fungoides, but are not diagnostic alone. The atypical cells of lymphomatoid papulosis are usually CD30+ and often express other activation-associated markers such as CD25 and HLA-DR (23). Although rare, cases of mycosis fungoides in transformation to large cell morphology may also express these markers. Gene rearrangement studies are not helpful in the differential diagnosis, since both of these disorders may have clonal rearrangements of the β-T-cell receptor gene.

Skin and Lymph Node: Malignant Lymphomas other than Mycosis Fungoides. Malignant lymphomas, particularly peripheral T-cell lymphomas other than mycosis fungoides, may involve the skin and simulate mycosis fungoides. These lymphomas generally form tumor nodules, either based in the dermis or based in the subcutaneous tissue, with secondary extension into the reticular dermis. Often, a prominent angiocentric component is seen (9), a histologic

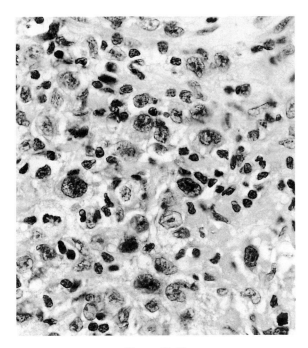

Figure 12-19
LYMPHOMATOID PAPULOSIS
Numerous pleomorphic lymphoid cells are present. The clinical history was critical in distinguishing this from mycosis fungoides and other post-thymic T-cell lymphomas.

appearance that was called lymphomatoid granulomatosis in the past. The most critical feature distinguishing these neoplasms from mycosis fungoides is the absence of epidermotropism in the neoplastic cells. In addition, the neoplastic cells in nonmycosis fungoides malignant lymphomas involving skin generally have more pleomorphic infiltrates that include lymphoid cells with large vesicular nuclei as opposed to the smaller cerebriform cells generally found in mycosis fungoides. As noted above, some advanced lesions from patients with mycosis fungoides have nodules of tumor in which the lymphoid cells are indistinguishable from large cell lymphoma. However, cerebriform lymphocytes, often with epidermotropism, are usually still present in these lesions. When these cells cannot be found, the only clues to the diagnosis of mycosis fungoides may be in the clinical history and review of previous biopsies.

The neoplastic infiltrate in adult T-cell leukemia/lymphoma (ATLL) is composed of hyperlobated cells which may closely simulate the cerebriform cells of mycosis fungoides, and may even show epidermotropism with the formation of Pautrier microabscesses (22). The clinical features, including the geographic origin of the patient, the calcium level (usually elevated in ATLL), and the presence of HTLV-1 infection, are essential in recognizing this neoplasm when it presents in skin.

In a lymph node biopsy it may be impossible to histologically distinguish transformation of mycosis fungoides to large cell lymphoma from other large cell lymphomas. Knowledge of the clinical history and review of previous or concurrent skin biopsies for features of mycosis fungoides are mandatory for correct diagnosis. Immunologic and genotypic studies may be helpful in distinguishing mycosis fungoides from a B-cell lymphoma or Hodgkin's disease, but are not generally useful in distinguishing mycosis fungoides from other post-thymic T-cell lymphomas.

Lymph Node: Dermatopathic Lymphadenopathy. As noted above, lymph nodes draining skin lesions of mycosis fungoides may show nonspecific reactive follicular hyperplasia, dermatopathic lymphadenopathy, or involvement with mycosis fungoides (11). Dermatopathic lymphadenopathy is a reactive change of the lymph node due to a disruption of the skin barrier, marked by a proliferation of histiocytes, interdigitating reticulum cells, and Langerhans cells in the paracortical region along with the deposition of melanin pigment (12). The abundant pale to eosinophilic cytoplasm present in these cell types imparts a mottled look to the interfollicular regions on low magnification examination. Variable numbers of small atypical lymphocytes and immunoblasts may also be present, both in the lymphadenopathy associated with mycosis fungoides as well as that associated with nonneoplastic skin lesions such as hypersensitivity reactions and nonspecific chronic dermatitis (7). Since even large numbers of atypical lymphocytes may be found in benign conditions, the histologic diagnosis of mycosis fungoides in a lymph node may only be made with certainty when there is partial or complete replacement of the nodal architecture by atypical lymphocytes or frankly neoplastic cells. Immunologic studies are of limited value in differentiating subtle cases of mycosis fungoides involving lymph nodes and dermatopathic lymphadenopathy (59). In contrast, gene rearrangement studies may be quite useful in this distinction, as clonal rearrangements of the β-T-cell receptor gene can be detected by Southern blot hybridization when as few as 1 to 5 percent of the cells in the lymph node are neoplastic (55).

Lymph Node: Hodgkin's Disease. Since Hodgkin's disease rarely presents in skin in the absence of widespread disease elsewhere, differentiating it from mycosis fungoides generally only arises within the context of a lymph node biopsy. Rarely, in cases of mycosis fungoides with transformation, the large cells can be highly pleomorphic and resemble Reed-Sternberg cells. The overlap with Hodgkin's disease is compounded if plasma cells, eosinophils, and fibrosis are present. Attention should be focused on the spectrum of atypical cells present in the background of mycosis fungoides. However, an increased incidence of Hodgkin's disease may be found in patients with longstanding mycosis fungoides, and coexisting Hodgkin's disease and mycosis fungoides in the same lymph node biopsy have also been described (10,47).

Treatment. There are four generally accepted treatment options available for patients with mycosis fungoides: photochemotherapy, topical chemotherapy, systemic chemotherapy, and radiation therapy (21). Biologic response modifiers, mainly the interferons, and monoclonal antibody therapy are still experimental (25,26). Administration of psoralin followed by exposure to high-intensity long-wave ultraviolet-A radiation (PUVA) is the most common form of photochemotherapy available (1). This treatment is usually effective, when given alone, in patients with early but not late stage disease. It may represent the treatment of choice for erythroderma. Extracorporeal PUVA therapy is a promising experimental approach to therapy; it may be most beneficial in patients with Sézary's syndrome (16). Nitrogen mustard is the most commonly used topical chemotherapeutic agent

(50). Similar to PUVA therapy, the treatment is effective in most patients with patches and plaques, but not tumors. Because it is convenient and has only limited side effects, it may represent the treatment of choice for patients with limited plaque disease. Total skin electron beam therapy is the most effective single agent for the treatment of mycosis fungoides, but the equipment is expensive and a high degree of technical expertise is required (30). It is most beneficial in the treatment of tumorous disease. The initial response rate approaches 100 percent. Although long-term disease-free survivals may be achieved, the disease recurs in most patients. Systemic chemotherapy is usually reserved for patients with extracutaneous disease. Numerous regimens have been tried, and none result in complete remission of long duration. Chlorambucil combined with prednisone is a common treatment for patients with Sézary's syndrome (63). A recent trend in the treatment of mycosis fungoides is toward combining several modalities of therapy.

Prognosis. Mycosis fungoides is generally an indolent disease. The prognosis is most closely related to the stage of the disease, but age, sex, race, and interval between onset of symptoms and diagnosis all affect survival (42). Patients with disease limited to the skin have a median survival of greater than 10 years. Patients with cutaneous tumors or erythroderma, peripheral blood involvement, or lymphadenopathy without histologic involvement of the lymph nodes have a median survival of about 5 years. Evidence of large cell transformation in the skin is associated with a significantly decreased survival period (41,42). The median survival time in patients with histologically documented lymph node involvement or visceral involvement is only 12 to 18 months, with very few long-term survivors. Transformation to large cell histology in the lymph nodes has an even worse prognosis than transformation occurring in cutaneous sites (41).

REFERENCES

1. Abel EA, Sendagorta E, Hoppe RT, Hu CH. PUVA treatment of erythrodermic and plaque-type mycosis fungoides: ten-year follow-up study. Arch Dermatol 1987;123:897–901.

2. Agnarsson BA, Vonderheid EC, Kadin ME. Cutaneous T cell lymphoma with suppressor/cytotoxic (CD8) phenotype: identification of rapidly progressive and chronic subtypes. J Am Acad Dermatol 1990;22:569–77.

3. Bahler DW, Berry G, Okesenberg J, Warnke RA, Levy R. Diversity of T-cell antigen receptor variable genes used by mycosis fungoides cells. Am J Pathol 1992;140:1–8.

4. Berger CL, Morrison S, Chu A, et al. Diagnosis of cutaneous T cell lymphoma by use of monoclonal antibodies reactive with tumor-associated antigens. J Clin Invest 1982;70:1205–15.

5. Bunn PA Jr, Huberman MS, Whang-Peng J, et al. Prospective staging evaluation of patients with cutaneous T-cell lymphomas. Demonstration of a high frequency of extracutaneous dissemination. Ann Intern Med 1980;93:223–30.

6. _____, Lamberg SI. Report of the Committee on Staging and Classification of Cutaneous T Cell Lymphomas. Cancer Treat Rep 1979;63:725–8.

7. Burke JS, Colby TV. Dermatopathic lymphadenopathy. Comparison of cases associated and unassociated with mycosis fungoides. Am J Surg Pathol 1981;5:343–52.

8. Carney DN, Bunn PA Jr. Manifestations of cutaneous T cell lymphoma. J Dermatol Surg Oncol 1980;6:369–77.

9. Chan JK, Ng CS, Ngan KC, Hui PK, Lo ST, Lau WH. Angiocentric T-cell lymphoma of the skin. An aggressive lymphoma distinct from mycosis fungoides. Am J Surg Pathol 1988;12:861–76.

10. Chan WC, Griem ML, Grozea PN, Freel RJ, Variakojis D. Mycosis fungoides and Hodgkin's disease occurring in the same patient. Report of three cases. Cancer 1979;44:1408–13.

11. Colby TV, Burke JS, Hoppe RT. Lymph node biopsy in mycosis fungoides. Cancer 1981;47:351–9.

12. Cooper RA, Dawson PJ, Rambo ON. Dermatopathic lymphadenopathy. A clinicopathologic analysis of lymph node biopsy over a fifteen-year period. Calif Med 1967;106:170–5.

13. Degreef H, Holvoet C, Van Vloten WA, De Wolf-Peeters C, Desmet V. Woringer-Kolopp disease: an epidermotropic variant of mycosis fungoides. Cancer 1976;38:2154–65.

14. Dmitrovsky E, Matthews MJ, Bunn PA, et al. Cytologic transformation in cutaneous T cell lymphoma: a clinicopathologic entity associated with poor prognosis. J Clin Oncol 1987;5:208–15.

15. Dosaka N, Tanaka T, Fujita M, Miyachi Y, Horio T, Imamura S. Southern blot analysis of clonal rearrangements of T-cell receptor gene in plaque lesions of mycosis fungoides. J Invest Dermatol, 1989;93:626–9.

16. Edelson R, Berger C, Gasparro F, et al. Treatment of cutaneous T-cell lymphoma by extracorporeal photochemotherapy. Preliminary results. N Engl J Med 1987;316:297–303.

17. _____, Berger C, Raafat J, Warburton D. Karyotype studies of cutaneous T cell lymphoma: evidence for clonal origin. J Invest Dermatol 1979;73:548–50.

18. Epstein EH, Devin DL, Croft JD, Lutzner MA. Mycosis fungoides. Survival, prognostic features, response to therapy, and autopsy findings. Medicine 1972;51:61–72.

19. Erkman-Balis B, Rappaport H. Cytogenetic studies in mycosis fungoides. Cancer 1974;34:626–33.

20. Hall WW, Liu CR, Schneewind O, et al. Deleted HTLV-I provirus in blood and cutaneous lesions of patients with mycosis fungoides. Science 1991;253:317–20.

21. Hoppe RT, Wood GS, Abel EA. Mycosis fungoides and the Sézary syndrome: pathology, staging, and treatment. Curr Probl Cancer 1990;14:293–371.

22. Jaffe ES, Blattner WA, Blayney DW, et al. The pathologic spectrum of adult T-cell leukemia/lymphoma in the United States. Human T-cell leukemia/lymphoma virus-associated lymphoid malignances. Am J Surg Pathol 1984;8:263–75.

23. Kaudewitz P, Burg G. Lymphomatoid papulosis and Ki-1 (CD30)-positive cutaneous large cell lymphomas. Semin Diagn Pathol 1991;8:117–24.

24. _____, Soldner R, Burg G, et al. Reactivity of monoclonal antibody BE2 in different stages of mycosis fungoides and in benign dermal infiltrates. Arch Dermatol Res 1986;279:83–8.

25. Knox SJ, Levy R, Hodgkinson S, et al. Observations on the effect chimeric anti-CD4 monoclonal antibody in patients with mycosis fungoides. Blood 1991;77:20–30.

26. Kohn EC, Steis RG, Sausville EA, et al. Phase II trial of intermittent high-dose recombinant interferon alfa-2a in mycosis fungoides and the Sézary syndrome. J Clin Oncol 1990;8:155–60.

27. Lambert WC, Everett MA. The nosology of parapsoriasis. J Am Acad Dermatol 1981;5:373–95.

28. LeBoit PE. Variants of mycosis fungoides and related cutaneous T-cell lymphomas. Semin Diagn Pathol 1991;8:73–81.

29. _____, Beckstead JH, Bond B, Epstein WL, Frieden IJ, Parslow TG. Granulomatous slack skin: clonal rearrangement of the T-cell receptor beta gene is evidence for the lymphoproliferative nature of a cutaneous elastolytic disorder. J Invest Dermatol 1987;89:183–6.

30. Lo TC, Salzman FA, Moschella SL, Tolman EL, Wright KA. Whole body surface electron irradiation in the treatment of mycosis fungoides. An evaluation of 200 patients. Radiology 1979;130:453–7.

31. Lutzner MA, Emerit I, Durepaire R, Grupper C, Prunieras M. Cytogenetic, cytophotometric, and ultrastructural study of large cerebriform cells of the Sézary syndrome and description of a small cell variant. J Natl Cancer Inst 1973;50:1145–62.

32. _____, Hobbs, JW, Horvath P. Ultrastructure of abnormal cells in Sezary syndrome, mycosis fungoides and parapsoriasis en plaque. Arch Dermatol 1971;103:375–86.

33. Lynch JW Jr, Linoilla I, Sausville EA, et al. Prognostic implications of evaluation for lymph node involvement by T-cell antigen receptor gene rearrangement in mycosis fungoides. Blood 1992;79:3293–9.

34. Meijer CJ, van der Loo EM, van Vloten WA, van der Velde EA, Scheffer E, Cornelisse CJ. Early diagnosis of mycosis fungoides and Sézary's syndrome by morphometric analysis of lymphoid cell in the skin. Cancer 1980;45:2864–71.

35. Michie SA, Abel EA, Hoppe RT, Warnke RA, Wood GS. Expression of T-cell receptor antigens in mycosis fungoides and inflammatory skin lesions. J Invest Dermatol 1989;93:116–20.

36. Nickoloff BJ. Light-microscopic assessment of 100 patients with patch/plaque-stage mycosis fungoides. Am J Dermatopathol 1988;10:469–77.

37. Picker LJ, Weiss LM, Medeiros LJ, Wood GS, Warnke RA. Immunophenotypic criteria for the diagnosis of non-Hodgkin's lymphoma. Am J Pathol 1987;128:181–201.

38. Ralfkiaer E. Immunohistological markers for the diagnosis of cutaneous lymphomas. Semin Diagn Pathol 1991;8:62–72.

39. _____, O'Connor NT, Crick J, Wantzin GL, Mason DY. Genotypic analysis of cutaneous T-cell lymphomas. J Invest Dermatol 1987;88:762–5.

40. Rappaport H, Thomas LB: Mycosis fungoides: the pathology of extracutaneous involvement. Cancer 1974;34:1198–229.

41. Salhany KE, Cousar JB, Greer JP, Casey TT, Fields JP, Collins RD. Transformation of cutaneous T-cell lymphoma to large cell lymphoma: a clinicopathologic and immunologic study. Am J Pathol 1988;132:265–77.

42. Sausville EA, Eddy JL, Makuch RW, et al. Histopathologic staging at initial diagnosis of mycosis fungoides and the Szary syndrome: definition of three distinctive prognostic groups. Ann Intern Med 1988;109:372–82.

43. _____, Worsham GF, Matthews MJ, et al. Histologic assessment of lymph nodes in mycosis fungoides/Sézary syndrome (cutaneous T-cell lymphoma): clinical correlations and prognostic import of a new classification system. Hum Pathol 1985;16:1098–109.

44. Scheffer E, Meijer C, Van Vloten WA. Dermatopathic lymphadenopathy and lymph node involvement in mycosis fungoides. Cancer 1980;45:137–48.

45. Shapiro PE, Pinto FJ. The histologic spectrum of mycosis fungoides/Sezary syndrome (cutaneous T-cell lymphoma). A review of 222 biopsies, including newly described patterns and the earliest pathologic changes. Am J Surg Pathol 1994;18:645–67.

46. Sheen SR III, Banks PM, Winkelmann RK. Morphologic heterogeneity of malignant lymphomas developing in mycosis fungoides. Mayo Clin Proc 1984;59:95–106.

47. Simrell CR, Boccia RV, Longo DL, Jaffe ES. Coexisting Hodgkin's disease and mycosis fungoides. Immunohistochemical proof of existence. Arch Pathol Lab Med 1986;110:1029–34.

48. Strickler JG, Movahed LA, Gajl-Peczalska KJ, Horwitz CA, Brunning RD, Weiss LM. Oligoclonal T cell receptor gene rearrangements in blood lymphocytes of patients with acute Epstein-Barr virus-induced infectious mononucleosis. J Clin Invest 1990;86:1358–63.

49. Toonstra J. Actinic reticuloid. Semin Diagn Pathol 1991;8:109–16.

50. Van Scott EJ, Kalmanson JD. Complete remissions of mycosis fungoides lymphoma induced by topical nitrogen mustard (HN2). Control of delayed hypersensitivity to HN2 by desensitization and by induction of specific immunologic tolerance. Cancer 1973;32:18–30.

51. Van Vloten WA, Scheffer E, Meijer CJ. DNA-cytophotometry of lymph node imprints from patients with mycosis fungoides. J Invest Dermatol 1979;73:275–7.

52. Vonderheid EC, Diamond LW, Lai SM, Au F, Dellavecchia MA. Lymph node histopathologic findings in cutaneous T-cell lymphoma. A prognostic classification system based on morphologic assessment. Am J Clin Pathol 1992;97:121–9.

53. Weinman VF, Ackerman AB. Lymphomatoid papulosis. A critical review and new findings. Am J Dermatopathol 1981;3:129–63.

54. Weinstock MA, Horm JW. Mycosis fungoides in the United States. Increasing incidence and descriptive epidemiology. JAMA 1988;260:42–6.

55. Weiss LM, Hu E, Wood GS, et al. Clonal rearrangements of the T-cell receptor gene in mycosis fungoides and dermatopathic lymphadenopathy. N Engl J Med 1985;313:539–44.

56. _____, Wood GS, Ellisen LW, Reynolds TC, Sklar J. Clonal T-cell populations in pityriasis lichenoides et varioliformis acuta (Mucha-Habermann disease). Am J Pathol 1987; 126:417–21.

57. _____, Wood GS, Hu E, Abel EA, Hoppe RT, Sklar J. Detection of clonal T-cell receptor gene rearrangements in the peripheral blood of patients with mycosis fungoides/Sezary syndrome. J Invest Dermatol 1989;92:601–4.

58. _____, Wood GS, Trela M, Warnke RA, Sklar J. Clonal T-cell populations in lymphomatoid papulosis. Evidence for a lymphoproliferative origin for a clinically benign disease. N Engl J Med 1986;315:475–9.

59. _____, Wood GS, Warnke RA. Immunophenotypic differences between dermatopathic lymphadenopathy and lymph node involvement in mycosis fungoides. Am J Pathol 1985;120:179–85.

60. Whang-Peng J, Bunn PA, Knutsen T, Matthews MJ, Schechter G, Minna JD. Clinical implications of cytogenetic studies in cutaneous T-cell lymphoma (CTCL). Cancer 1982;50:1539–53.

61. Whittemore AS, Holly EA, Lee IM, et al. Mycosis fungoides in relation to environmental exposures and immune response: a case control study. JNCI 1989; 81:1560–7.

62. Wieczorek R, Suhrland M, Ramsay D, Reed ML, Knowles DM II. Leu-M1 antigen expression in advanced (tumor) stage mycosis fungoides. Am J Clin Pathol 1986;86:25–32.

63. Winkelmann RK, Diaz-Perez JL, Buechner SA. The treatment of Sézary syndrome. J Am Acad Dermatol 1984;10:1000–4.

64. Wood GS, Weiss LM, Hu C-H, et al. T-cell antigen deficiencies and clonal rearrangements of T-cell receptor genes in pagetoid reticulosis (Woringer-Kolopp disease). N Engl J Med 1988;318:164–7.

65. _____, Weiss LM, Warnke RA, Sklar J. The immunopathology of cutaneous lymphomas: immunophenotypic and immunogenotypic characteristics. Semin Dermatol 1986;5:334–45.

66. Zelickson BD, Peters MS, Muller SA, et al. T-cell receptor gene rearrangement analysis: cutaneous T cell lymphoma, peripheral T cell lymphoma, and premalignant and benign cutaneous lymphoproliferative disorders. J Am Acad Dermatol 1991;25:787–96.

13
POST-THYMIC T-CELL LYMPHOMA

Definition. Post-thymic T-cell lymphoma is a malignant lymphoma of T lymphocytes whose morphologic appearance and phenotype are consistent with mature T lymphocytes, in contrast to the immature morphologic appearance and phenotype of T-cell lymphoblastic lymphoma. A synonym is *peripheral T-cell lymphoma*. In the updated Kiel classification, T-cell chronic lymphocytic leukemia, T-prolymphocytic leukemia, and mycosis fungoides are considered part of post-thymic T-cell lymphomas (seen in table 5-3). In this chapter, post-thymic T-cell lymphomas other than mycosis fungoides are discussed (see chapter 12 for a discussion of mycosis fungoides and the Fascicle on Tumors of the Bone Marrow (12) for a discussion of the chronic T-cell leukemias; T-lineage anaplastic large cell lymphoma is discussed in chapter 9).

Incidence. Post-thymic T-cell lymphoma is usually a disease of the elderly, although it can affect a wide age range, including children (30,35,75,100). The median age is 60 years. The male to female ratio is about 3 to 2. About 25 percent of patients have a history of a previous lymphoproliferative or immune disease: both B-cell lymphoma and Hodgkin's disease (30,100), as well as immune disorders such as celiac sprue, rheumatoid arthritis, a sarcoidosis-like syndrome, Sjögren's syndrome, Hashimoto's thyroiditis, and immune thrombocytopenia have preceded post-thymic T-cell lymphoma (30,35,100). Occasionally, the presenting site of the lymphoma is at the previous site of immune disease; this is reported most frequently in cases of celiac sprue (36).

Post-thymic T-cell lymphoma accounts for 10 to 20 percent of diffuse non-Hodgkin lymphomas in Western countries (103). The incidence is higher in areas where human T-cell lymphotropic virus type 1 (HTLV-1) infection is endemic (97). HTLV-1 is a complex retrovirus endemic to the southernmost islands of Japan, areas of the Caribbean, the southeastern United States (affecting mainly blacks), equatorial Africa, and possibly southern Italy (6,7,9,13). The virus travels via sexual transmission from male to female, by blood transfusion, by intravenous drug abuse,

or from mother to child, probably during breast feeding (6). It remains latent for many years, but a few patients develop adult T-cell leukemia/lymphoma, a leukemia/lymphoma with distinct clinical and pathologic characteristics (see below). It is estimated that 1 of every 900 male carriers and 1 of every 2000 female carriers older than 40 years develop adult T-cell leukemia/lymphoma each year (93).

Some T-cell lymphomas may be associated with Epstein-Barr virus (EBV). This virus has been identified within the tumor cells in a high percentage of angiocentric lymphomas, particularly those occurring in the upper respiratory tract (5,33,60,90,104). In addition, T-cell lymphomas have occurred in patients with a chronic mononucleosis-like syndrome in which EBV was found (42). EBV genomes have been identified in many cases of angioimmunoblastic lymphadenopathy and angioimmunoblastic lymphadenopathy–like T-cell lymphoma. In situ hybridization studies have localized the virus to scattered B and T lymphocytes in most cases (106), although one study identified EBV in a minority of the neoplastic cells in some instances (2). Increased amounts of EBV in these two disorders may be a result of impairment of the immune system of affected patients.

Natural History and Clinical Features. Patients with post-thymic T-cell lymphoma usually present with generalized lymphadenopathy, with frequent retroperitoneal disease but relative sparing of the mediastinum (30,35,75,100). Mediastinal involvement may occur, however, particularly in younger patients (8,31,75). Skin manifestations are common, either as the presenting symptom or associated with lymphadenopathy. The skin lesions are highly variable in appearance and include maculopapular lesions, plaques, nodules, and ulcers (16,35,100). Often, there is a long history of waxing and waning skin lesions, sometimes responsive to topical steroids, and usually interpreted pathologically as showing benign or atypical lymphocytic infiltration (35). B symptoms, i.e., weight loss, fever, and night sweats, are present in about half of patients, usually those with more advanced disease

(30,35,75,100). Visceral involvement is common at presentation, particularly of liver, spleen, and lung as well as bone marrow. Hepatic and splenic involvement are most often seen in malignant lymphomas with a high content of epithelioid histiocytes. However, virtually any site, including gastrointestinal tract (particularly the small intestine), sinonasal tract and nasopharynx (especially in Asians) (14), heart, bone, testis, central nervous system, skeletal muscle, and adrenal gland may be involved. Overall, approximately two thirds of patients present with stage III or stage IV disease.

Anemia is present in approximately one third of patients, and is occasionally Coombs positive (30,100). Peripheral blood involvement is uncommon, and usually correlates with extensive skin or bone marrow involvement. In addition to containing circulating lymphoma cells, the peripheral blood may exhibit eosinophilia; this sometimes correlates with the presence of a hyperplastic bone marrow with myelodysplastic features (30,35, 100). Rarely, the eosinophilia may be quite striking. Other laboratory abnormalities that may occur include a polyclonal hypergammaglobulinemia and a Coombs-positive hemolytic anemia. Hypercalcemia is often found in those patients with adult T-cell leukemia/lymphoma associated with HTLV-1, but may also be found occasionally in other patients (9,75).

The clinical course for patients with post-thymic T-cell lymphoma is quite variable. In rare patients, spontaneous regression may occur; in others, death due to disease occurs rapidly. The disease may wax and wane for many years. During the course of disease, a high percentage of patients develop extranodal disease (75). Rebiopsy of lymph nodes of patients in relapse occasionally shows transformation to a lymphoma with a greater component of large cells. At autopsy, a high incidence of extranodal involvement is found.

Microscopic Findings. Post-thymic T-cell neoplasia exhibits a wide degree of morphologic heterogeneity, and cannot be easily characterized (49,91,99,103). However, there are several features common to most of these lymphomas. First, they invariably have a diffuse or sinusoidal architecture; a truly follicular pattern is never seen. Typically, they first involve the paracortical region of the lymph node (so-called T-zone lymphoma) and only secondarily replace the cortical region

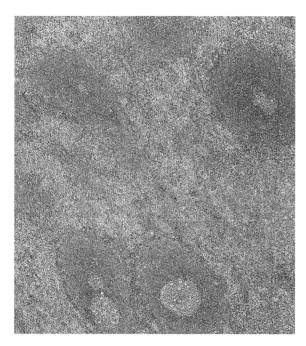

Figure 13-1
POST-THYMIC T-CELL LYMPHOMA
Preferential involvement of the paracortical region is seen.

(fig. 13-1). The neoplastic population varies widely from case to case, but generally shows a spectrum of atypical cells (fig. 13-2). Some are the size of small cleaved cells (fig. 13-3), many are intermediate in size (fig. 13-4), while others can be large and pleomorphic, simulating Hodgkin cells (T-immunoblastic lymphoma or pleomorphic T-cell lymphoma) (fig. 13-5). Occasionally, multinucleated tumor giant cells can be seen. The nuclei of both the small and large cells often exhibit marked irregularities, and may vary from round with vesicular chromatin, to hyperlobated with marked chromatin condensation (fig. 13-6) (76). The cytoplasm is generally moderate to abundant in amount, and may be clear, pale, eosinophilic, or basophilic (fig. 13-7). Uncommonly, the lymphoid infiltrate is monomorphous (monomorphous medium-sized T-cell lymphoma). Rarely, the neoplastic cells are signet ring shaped or plasmacytoid (fig. 13-8) (32,103,109).

In addition to the neoplastic elements, other cells are often admixed: eosinophils, plasma cells, small lymphocytes, and histiocytes (often epithelioid histiocytes) in varying proportions (fig. 13-9). Generally, there is increased vascularity and the venules often have plump endothelial cells

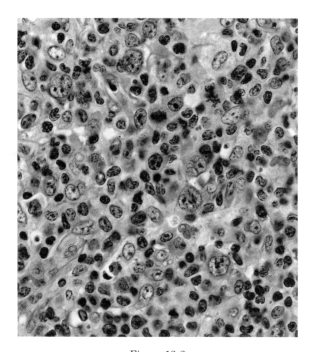

Figure 13-2
POST-THYMIC T-CELL LYMPHOMA
A diffuse obliteration of lymph node architecture by a mixed population of atypical cells is present.

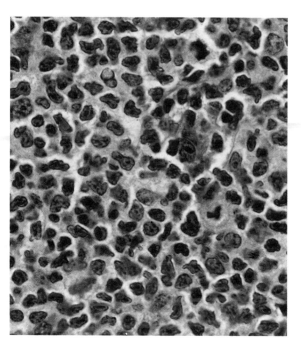

Figure 13-3
POST-THYMIC T-CELL LYMPHOMA
There is a relatively homogeneous population of small cells with irregularly shaped nuclei. This case might be classified as diffuse, predominantly small cleaved cell lymphoma in the Working Formulation.

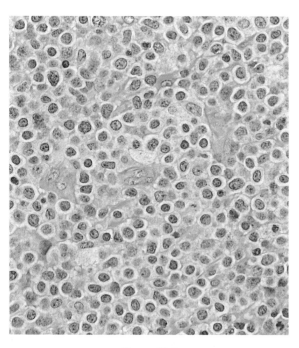

Figure 13-4
POST-THYMIC T-CELL LYMPHOMA
A relatively homogeneous population of medium-sized neoplastic cells is present (so-called monomorphous medium-sized post-thymic T-cell lymphoma).

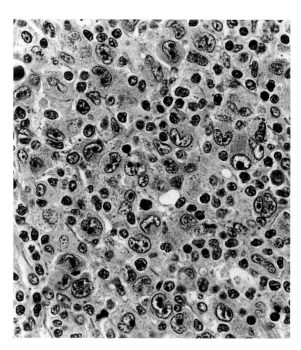

Figure 13-5
POST-THYMIC T-CELL LYMPHOMA
Pleomorphic lymphoid cells are seen, including cells that could be mistaken for Hodgkin cells.

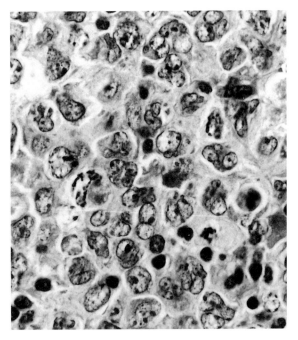

Figure 13-6
POST-THYMIC T-CELL LYMPHOMA
Hyperlobated cells are present in this case.

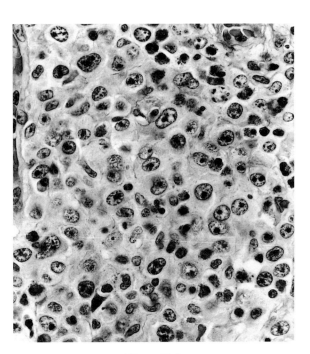

Figure 13-7
POST-THYMIC T-CELL LYMPHOMA
There is a predominance of cells with pale cytoplasm.

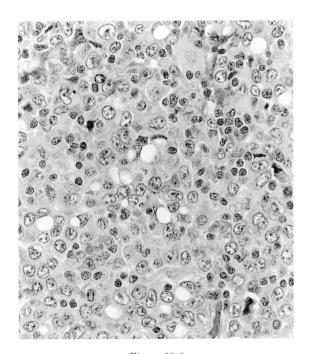

Figure 13-8
POST-THYMIC T-CELL LYMPHOMA
WITH SIGNET RING CELLS
Note occasional cells with clear vacuoles compressing the nucleus to the side of the cell.

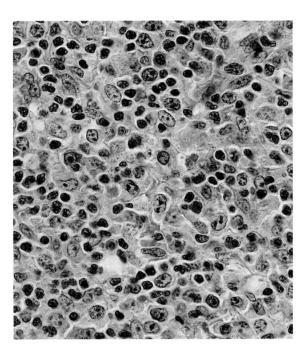

Figure 13-9
POST-THYMIC T-CELL LYMPHOMA
In addition to the neoplastic T cells, scattered plasma cells, eosinophils, and histiocytes are present.

(high endothelial venules). Fibrosis is generally not marked, although exceptions may occur, particularly in the mediastinum. Occasionally, small groups of cells are compartmentalized by a delicate reticulin framework. Necrosis, which may involve both the infiltrated tissue and normal tissue, is particularly common in angiocentric lymphomas.

Given the wide variability in both the neoplastic and reactive components of these neoplasms, it is not surprising that diagnosis and classification of these tumors has been difficult. One common practice is to try to fit the cases into the closest equivalent in the International Working Formulation (103). Using this classification, most post-thymic T-cell lymphomas would be classified into the categories of diffuse mixed small and large cell, diffuse large cell, and large cell immunoblastic lymphomas, with occasional cases representing small lymphocytic and diffuse small cleaved cell neoplasms. A criticism of this practice is that the descriptive categories were created with B-cell lymphomas in mind. For example, one cannot truly consider T-cell lymphomas to be composed primarily or even partially of cleaved cells, since cleaved cells are usually equated with follicular B lymphocytes. Nonetheless, the International Working Formulation study was a histologic and not an immunologic study (96). Advantages to using the Working Formulation include practicality, as well as the absence of data demonstrating the superiority of other proposed classifications created specifically for T-cell lymphomas.

The classification system for peripheral T-cell lymphomas proposed by a group of Chinese, European, and Japanese pathologists and used as the basis for the updated Kiel classification is shown in Table 5-3 (85,91). Unfortunately, this classification is difficult to apply in practice and poorly reproducible, even among experienced hematopathologists (34). The classification is based on cytologic criteria, and divides post-thymic T-cell lymphomas into a low-grade and higher grade categories. In general, the low-grade lymphomas contain significant numbers of non-neoplastic cells or are composed of a relatively homogeneous population of small to intermediate, but atypical cells, while high-grade lymphomas are usually composed of a more homogeneous population of intermediate to large atypical cells. Unique to the Kiel classification is the subtype of T-zone lymphoma, which is recognized by the distribution of small to intermediate and occasional large atypical cells in a distinct interfollicular pattern.

In the spleen, post-thymic T-cell lymphomas usually form microscopic nodules, which may be present in the white pulp, the red pulp, localized to the peripheral portion of the marginal zones, or in the main T-cell zone of the spleen, the periarteriolar sheath (89). Rarely, diffuse infiltration of the red pulp may be seen, resembling what was formerly described in malignant histiocytosis. The cytologic composition of the splenic neoplasm is identical to its appearance in the lymph nodes.

Variants. *Adult T-Cell Leukemia/Lymphoma.* Adult T-cell leukemia/lymphoma is a distinct clinicopathologic entity associated with HTLV-1 infection (see above) (9,39). The patients are usually adults, but about 10 years younger than patients with other T-cell lymphomas. They are invariably stage IV at presentation, with generalized lymphadenopathy and skin, liver, spleen, and bone involvement (often with lytic lesions). Hypercalcemia is present in most patients, and the peripheral blood contains highly pleomorphic hyperlobated neoplastic cells (fig. 13-10). The latter finding is highly characteristic of this disease and if not seen at presentation, almost always occurs at some time during the clinical course. Unfortunately, these cells cannot always be distinguished from the circulating cells of Sézary's syndrome. The lymph node findings are variable: the histologic appearance ranges from a predominance of small or medium-sized cells, to a mixture of small and large cells, to a predominance of large cells. The neoplastic cells are usually highly pleomorphic, with markedly irregular and polylobated nuclear contours (fig. 13-11). The small and medium-sized cells tend to have condensed nuclear chromatin, while the large cells often have a more vesicular appearance with multiple nuclei. Giant cells, including Reed-Sternberg–like cells, may be found. The lymph node findings are not pathognomonic for this entity. Post-thymic T-cell lymphomas not associated with HTLV-1 infection may have lymph node findings identical to those described above.

Angioimmunoblastic Lymphadenopathy with Dysproteinemia (AILD)/AILD-like T-Cell Lymphoma. AILD is a rare lymphoid disorder first recognized in the 1970s (28,29,58). Patients usually present with generalized lymphadenopathy,

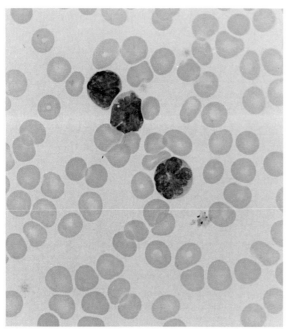

Figure 13-10
HUMAN T-CELL LEUKEMIA/LYMPHOMA
The peripheral blood contains lymphoid cells with hyperlobated nuclei.

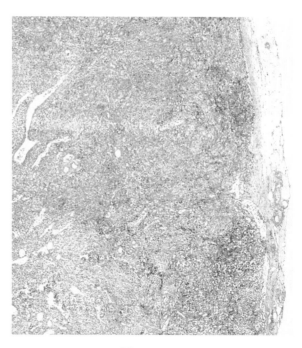

Figure 13-12
ANGIOIMMUNOBLASTIC LYMPHADENOPATHY
The submarginal and medullary sinuses are patent. The lymph node appears lymphocyte depleted.

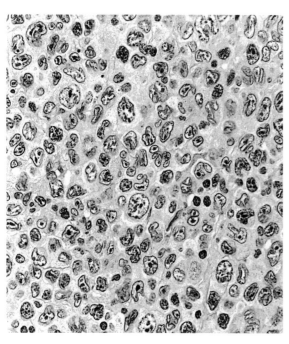

Figure 13-11
HUMAN T-CELL LEUKEMIA/LYMPHOMA
This case shows highly pleomorphic neoplastic cells.

and often have hepatosplenomegaly, fever, and a rash. Laboratory studies typically reveal anemia, often Coombs positive, and polyclonal hypergammaglobulinemia. Involved lymph nodes show diffuse effacement of architecture, although the sinuses may remain patent (fig. 13-12). Germinal centers are either absent or "burnt-out," and there is a conspicuous increase in the number and prominence of high endothelial venules, with an overall lymphocyte-depleted appearance (fig. 13-13). A mixture of small lymphocytes, immunoblasts, epithelioid histiocytes, plasma cells, and eosinophils is present (fig. 13-14) . Occasionally, there is a high content of epithelioid histiocytes (69). Fibrosis is absent, but intercellular deposits of a periodic acid–Schiff (PAS)-positive amorphous substance are seen, both in cortical and paracortical areas of involved nodes. Large irregular networks of dendritic reticulum cells (better highlighted by immunostaining) are often present (51).

AILD-like T-cell lymphoma is histologically similar to AILD (63,81). However, the cellularity is increased rather than decreased. More importantly, there are usually clusters and islands of

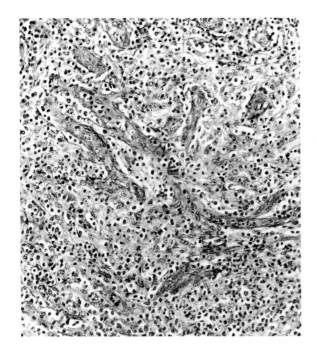

Figure 13-13
ANGIOIMMUNOBLASTIC LYMPHADENOPATHY
A cell-depleted mixed infiltrate is present, with prominent postcapillary venules.

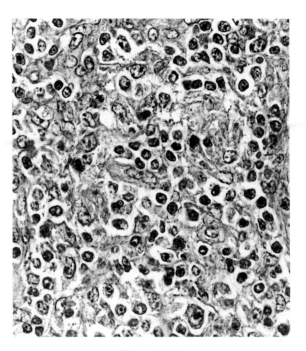

Figure 13-14
ANGIOIMMUNOBLASTIC LYMPHADENOPATHY
There is a mixed infiltrate, including small lymphocytes, immunoblasts, eosinophils, plasma cells, and histiocytes.

large atypical cells, often with clear cytoplasm (fig. 13-15). The atypical cells are particularly prominent around blood vessels. Phenotypic, cytogenetic, and genotypic studies (see below) of cases previously regarded as AILD have revealed frequent abnormal findings, such as aneuploid clonal populations with aberrant phenotypes, suggesting that the histologic distinction between AILD and AILD-like lymphoma may be difficult to define. While some hematopathologists now regard all cases previously designated AILD as representing T-cell lymphoma, we prefer to retain the term AILD for those cases with the characteristic histologic findings described above for AILD, and without evident clonal populations found on special studies.

A small proportion of cases of both AILD and AILD-like lymphomas terminate in a diffuse, large cell lymphoma, often of immunoblastic subtype (69). These lymphomas may be of B- or T-cell phenotype. The B-immunoblastic lymphomas sometimes contain Epstein-Barr virus, and possibly arise as a result of the depression of cellular immunity seen in AILD and AILD-like lymphoma (1).

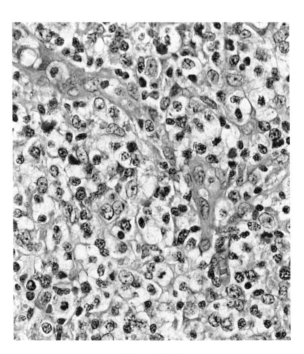

Figure 13-15
ANGIOIMMUNOBLASTIC LYMPHADENOPATHY–
LIKE POST-THYMIC T-CELL LYMPHOMA
In addition to features reminiscent of angioimmunoblastic lymphadenopathy, atypical lymphoid cells with clear cytoplasm are present in this field.

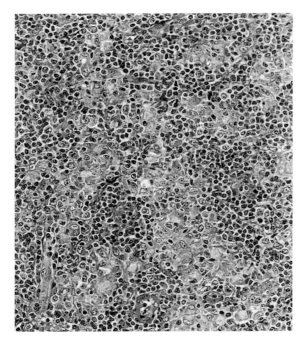

Figure 13-16
POST-THYMIC T-CELL LYMPHOMA WITH
HIGH CONTENT OF EPITHELIOID HISTIOCYTES
(SO-CALLED LENNERT'S LYMPHOMA)
Numerous clusters of epithelioid histiocytes are present throughout the section.

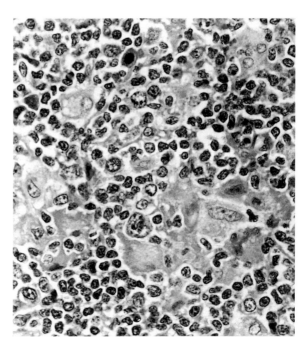

Figure 13-17
POST-THYMIC T-CELL LYMPHOMA WITH HIGH
CONTENT OF EPITHELIOID HISTIOCYTES
(SO-CALLED LENNERT'S LYMPHOMA)
Scattered atypical lymphoid cells are found among the epithelioid histiocytes.

T-Cell Lymphoma with High Content of Epithelioid Histiocytes (Lymphoepithelioid or so-called Lennert's Lymphoma). In this lymphoma, the lymph node architecture is effaced by a proliferation of epithelioid histiocytes and a polymorphic population of lymphoid cells (10,47,71). The epithelioid histiocytes dominate the histologic picture, generally occurring as single cells and in small, ill-defined clusters (fig. 13-16). They may occasionally form large aggregates, but well-formed epithelioid granulomas resembling those seen in sarcoidosis are not present. Multinucleated Langhans-type giant cells are only present in a few cases. Although the epithelioid histiocytes are the most prominent histologic finding, careful observation reveals atypical small and medium to large lymphoid cells in these cases (fig. 13-17). The smaller cells are often located between the clusters of epithelioid cells, while the medium to large cells are usually adjacent to the epithelioid histiocytes, generally as single cells. While the small lymphocytes often have condensed chromatin, the larger cells have nuclei with vesicular chromatin and prominent nucleoli, and may occasionally simulate Reed-Sternberg cells. Scattered plasma cells and eosinophils may also be present. Residual germinal centers, significant fibrosis, and extensive necrosis are generally absent. With progression, the component of epithelioid histiocytes often decreases.

Angiocentric Lymphoma and Other Angiocentric Immunoproliferative Lesions. Angiocentric immunoproliferative lesions encompass a spectrum of T-cell lymphoproliferative disorders with a marked predilection for the walls of blood vessels, including many cases of lymphomatoid granulomatosis, benign lymphocytic angiitis and granulomatosis, polymorphic reticulosis, and midline malignant reticulosis (16,22,44,45,55,56,79). Distinct from angiotropic lymphoma (intravascular lymphomatosis), in which the neoplastic cells are predominantly found within the blood vessel lumen, the cells in angiocentric immunoproliferative lesions infiltrate the muscular walls and surrounding adventitial tissues of small arteries and veins (fig. 13-18). Despite a marked degree of

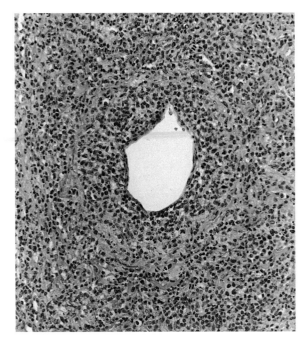

Figure 13-18
ANGIOCENTRIC T-CELL LYMPHOMA
In this post-thymic T-cell lymphoma involving the lung,
there is extensive invasion of the walls of blood vessels.

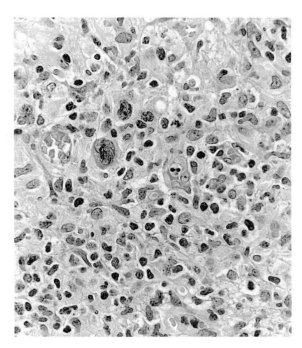

Figure 13-19
ANGIOCENTRIC T-CELL LYMPHOMA
Grade II cytologic features are present in this case.

infiltrate, the vessel wall itself is rarely necrotic. These lesions have a predilection for the upper respiratory tract (previously designated polymorphic reticulosis or lethal midline granuloma) the skin, and the lungs (previously designated lymphomatoid granulomatosis). However, recent reassessment of pulmonary lymphomatoid granulomatosis has indicated that many cases represent EBV-associated B-cell lymphoproliferations rather than T-cell lymphoma (32a).

An attempt has been made to grade these lesions (56). Grade I lesions consist of an angiocentric and angiodestructive lymphoid proliferation composed of a polymorphous infiltrate of lymphocytes, plasma cells, and histiocytes, with or without eosinophils, and with infrequent or absent large lymphoid cells. Cytologic atypia is minimal and necrosis is generally not present. It is not clear that this lesion represents lymphoma; it is probably identical to what has been described in the literature as benign angiitis and granulomatosis. The cellular composition of grade II lesions is similar to that seen in grade I lesions; however, some cytologic atypia in small lymphoid cells is evident. This histologic appearance is

equivalent to diffuse small cleaved cell or diffuse mixed small and large cell lymphoma (fig. 13-19). Necrosis, due to vascular compromise, may be seen. It is believed that although the lesions are polymorphic they represent a subtle form of T-cell lymphoma. Grade III lesions, also termed angiocentric lymphomas, are more monomorphic with greater numbers of large lymphoid cells, and cytologic atypia is present in both the small and large lymphoid cells. Necrosis is usually a prominent feature. These lesions are easily recognized histologically as lymphoma and, in the Working Formulation, can be classified as diffuse mixed small and large cell, diffuse large cell, and large cell immunoblastic lymphomas.

Intestinal T-Cell Lymphoma. This subtype was previously called ulcerative jejunitis and malignant histiocytosis of the intestine (37). It commonly, but not exclusively, occurs in adults with a history of malabsorption, and often presents with abdominal pain, often as a result of perforation. It usually presents in the jejunum, but may occur in the colon. Multiple foci of disease are common at presentation (18). Grossly, ulcers with or without a mass are seen.

267

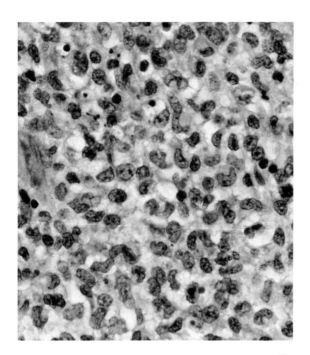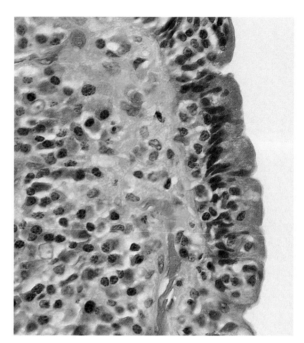

Figure 13-20
INTESTINAL T-CELL LYMPHOMA
Left: A population of atypical lymphoid cells is seen in the wall of the small intestine.
Right: Atypical lymphoid cells are penetrating the surface epithelium.

The lymphomas are most often composed of a mixture of small and large atypical cells (diffuse, mixed) or contain a predominance of large cells (diffuse, large cell or immunoblastic) (fig. 13-20, left). Characteristically, atypical lymphoid cells are seen penetrating the overlying epithelium or adjacent mucosa (fig. 13-20, right). The adjacent mucosa may show band-like lymphoma infiltrates spreading along the mucosa. Distant uninvolved mucosa may or may not show severe villous atrophy. The tumor cells express CD103, an antigen present on mucosa-associated T lymphocytes (84).

Post-Thymic T-Cell Lymphoma with Erythrophagocytosis. Occasional post-thymic T-cell lymphomas, especially but not necessarily angiocentric T-cell type, may be associated with erythrophagocytosis (23,38,40). Two clinical syndromes exist. In the first, patients with a history of lymphoma abruptly develop an acute illness characterized by hepatosplenomegaly, fever, and pancytopenia (38,40). Cytologically bland histiocytes containing numerous erythrocytes, as well as neutrophils and platelets, are found distending the sinuses of the bone marrow and lymph nodes, the red pulp of the spleen, and the sinus-

oids of the liver. This histiocytic proliferation is distinct from the sites of involvement by lymphoma. In the second presentation, patients with no prior lymphoma develop a hemophagocytic syndrome (23). Histologically, malignant lymphoma and benign hemophagocytizing histiocytes are seen in direct proximity to one another (fig. 13-21).

It has been postulated that the hemophagocytic syndrome is caused by cytokines released by the lymphoma, leading to the histiocytic proliferation (83). Alternatively, since angiocentric lymphomas have recently been recognized to contain Epstein-Barr virus in a high proportion of cases (60), it is possible that release of the virus stimulates other cells to produce cytokines, similar to Epstein-Barr virus–associated hemophagocytic syndrome.

Hepatosplenic T-Cell Lymphoma. This is a rare form of post-thymic T-cell lymphoma in which the liver and spleen are preferentially involved (24). In the spleen, there is preferential infiltration of the red pulp, while in the liver, the neoplastic cells are found in the sinusoids. The bone marrow is also involved, with a preference

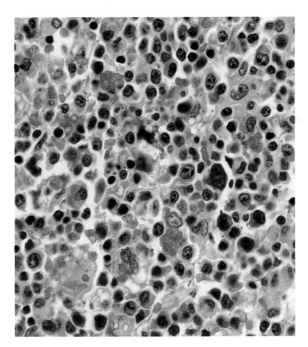

Figure 13-21
POST-THYMIC T-CELL LYMPHOMA
WITH BENIGN ERYTHROPHAGOCYTOSIS
Benign histiocytes with numerous engulfed erythrocytes in their cytoplasm are present in the midst of malignant lymphoid cells which phenotyped as T lineage.

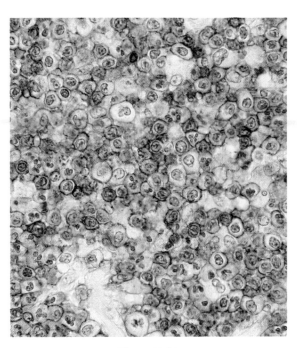

Figure 13-22
POST-THYMIC T-CELL LYMPHOMA
The neoplastic cells, including cells in mitosis, are positive for the T-cell–associated marker CD43.

for sinusoids. The neoplastic cells display a gamma/delta T-cell receptor rather than the usual alpha/beta receptor, and they lack CD5 and CD7 antigens (see below). This entity is further discussed in chapter 20.

Erythrophagocytic T-Gamma Lymphoma. In this rare neoplasm, patients typically present with fever and hepatosplenomegaly (43). Histologically, large tumor cells with abundant erythrophagocytosis are seen in the paracortical regions of lymph nodes, the sinusoids of the red pulp of the spleen, the sinusoids of the liver, and diffusely throughout the bone marrow. The tumor cells lack the prominent azurophilic granules usually found in most normal T-gamma cells. This entity is further discussed in chapter 20.

Anaplastic Large Cell Lymphoma (Ki-1 Lymphoma). Most cases of anaplastic large cell lymphoma phenotype as post-thymic T-cell lymphoma. This entity is described in greater detail in chapter 9.

Small Lymphocytic Lymphoma of T-Cell Type. This rare entity is discussed in chapter 7.

Immunologic Findings. By definition, post-thymic T-cell lymphomas should express the phenotype of mature T cells (49,99). In paraffin sections, the panleukocyte marker CD45RB is expressed in about 90 percent of cases (102). The T-lineage–associated markers CD45RO, CD43, and CD3 (the latter recognized by a polyclonal reagent) are expressed in approximately 80 to 85 percent of cases (fig. 13-22) (12,46,88,102). Expression of B-lineage markers in paraffin sections is generally not seen. CD15 expression may be seen in about 10 to 15 percent of cases (3), but is often granular and cytoplasmic, distinct from the paranuclear or membranous staining seen in Hodgkin's disease (77). However, some cases show a pattern of staining identical to that of Reed-Sternberg cells (111).

Many more antigens can be evaluated in frozen sections, and studies have revealed aberrant phenotypes in most cases (fig. 13-23) (8,31,103). Rather than being a source of confusion, these abnormal phenotypes can be utilized to establish an immunologic diagnosis of T-cell malignancy. Post-thymic T-cell lymphomas show aberrant absence of one or more of the pan-T-cell markers

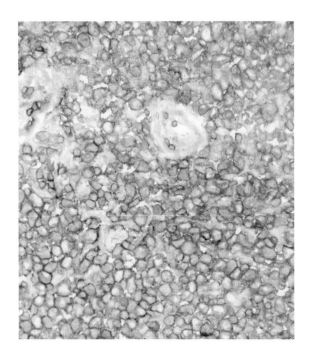 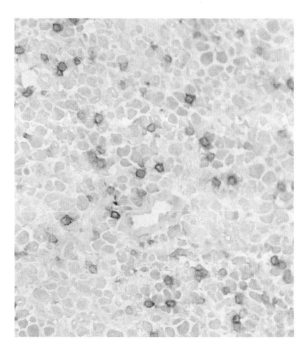

Figure 13-23
POST-THYMIC T-CELL LYMPHOMA
The neoplastic cells in this case expressed the T-lineage markers CD2 and CD3, and the helper subset marker CD4, but lacked expression of CD7. A CD3 stain is shown at left, while a CD7 stain is shown at right.

CD2, CD3, and CD5, and the major T-cell marker CD7, in three quarters of cases (74); absence of one marker is seen in one third of cases, absence of two markers in one quarter of cases, and absence of three markers in one fifth of cases. CD7 and CD5 are the antigens most likely to be absent, in 56 and 46 percent of cases, respectively, while CD3 and CD2 are more often conserved, with antigen absence found in 19 and 18 percent of cases, respectively. CD7 is reported to be invariably negative in human adult T-cell leukemia/lymphoma (52).

Most post-thymic T-cell lymphomas express the alpha/beta T-cell receptor. However, aberrant absence of the beta-F-1 antigen (a framework epitope present on the T-cell receptor beta chain) is seen in 23 percent of post-thymic T-cell lymphomas (73). In hepatosplenic T-cell lymphoma, the gamma/delta rather than the alpha/beta T-cell receptor is expressed (24).

Most post-thymic T-cell lymphomas express a CD4+/CD8- mature helper cell phenotype (8,31,75,100,103). This is particularly true for adult T-cell leukemia/lymphoma where a mature helper cell phenotype is invariably found (39). Approximately 20 percent of cases express a CD4-/

CD8+ cytotoxic/suppressor phenotype. Assessment of the ratio of CD4+ to CD8+ cells is not diagnostically useful since in histologically benign conditions, this ratio can vary from less than 10:1 to 1:10 (74). About one sixth of cases express a CD4-/CD8- phenotype and rare cases are CD4+/CD8+ (103). While these latter two phenotypes are normal in stages of thymic differentiation of T cells, they are abnormal in mature T-cell populations outside the thymus. Furthermore, these lymphomas uniformly lack expression of CD1, a marker of thymic differentiation, and also lack terminal deoxynucleotidyl transferase (TdT).

None of the immunologic methods discussed above provides a test for clonality, such as the identification of light chain restriction for the diagnosis of B-cell lymphoma. Such a test might be possible using a battery of 20 to 30 monoclonal antibodies, each directed against the different variable region proteins of the beta-T-cell receptor (19). Presumably, in reactive conditions, each individual antibody would recognize occasional positive cells, while in lymphoma, one antibody would label the neoplastic cells. However, a complete set of these antibodies is not yet available for this application.

Post-thymic T-cell lymphomas occasionally express other antigens. They may express CD30, particularly in those lymphomas with the morphologic features of anaplastic large cell lymphoma (86). The neoplastic cells of anaplastic large cell lymphoma also commonly express epithelial membrane antigen and the interleukin-2 receptor, CD25 (21). CD25 expression is also characteristic of human adult T-cell leukemia/ lymphoma (52), although some HTLV-1–negative cases also express this antigen. Intestinal T-cell lymphoma characteristically expresses CD103, an antigen present on normal mucosa-associated T-cells (84). A subset of post-thymic T-cell lymphomas expresses the neural cell adhesion molecule (NCAM) CD56 (46,113). CD56-positive cases exhibit a striking predilection for unusual anatomic sites of involvement, including the central nervous system, muscle, gastrointestinal tract, nasopharynx, skin, and lungs. There is also a significantly lower expression of CD3 and CD5 compared to CD56-negative cases. Although expression of CD56 could be construed as evidence for natural killer cell differentiation, there is little evidence of expression of other natural killer cell antigens, such as CD16 and CD57, in these CD56-positive cases. However, a high incidence of the natural killer cell–associated antigen CD16 has been reported in angiocentric T-cell lymphomas occurring in the nasal and paranasal regions (64). Post-thymic T-cell lymphomas occasionally express a B-lineage marker, particularly CD37, a phenomenon that may be used for diagnostic purposes (74).

A small subset of peripheral T-cell lymphomas expresses S-100 protein, probably corresponding to a normal minor subset of T cells (95). These cases often express CD3 and CD56 (113) and usually occur in young patients who present with systemic symptoms, splenomegaly, and cytopenia in the presence of insignificant lymphadenopathy. The disease course is highly aggressive and patients die within a few months of diagnosis (15,113). Histologically, the neoplastic lymphoid cells (medium to large) are often localized to the sinusoids of lymph nodes and liver; splenic involvement is localized mostly to the red pulp.

One pitfall in the immunologic diagnosis of post-thymic T-cell lymphoma is the entity of T-cell–rich B-cell lymphoma (see chapter 9) (59,78). T cells predominate in these lesions and may commonly represent over 90 percent of the lymphocytes. Nonetheless, the neoplastic element is the B-cell component, proved by genotypic studies or by careful immunohistochemistry, often best performed in paraffin sections.

Molecular and Cytogenetic Findings. Most post-thymic T-cell lymphomas, including variants of post-thymic T-cell lymphoma such as adult T-cell lymphoma/leukemia, T-cell lymphoma with a high content of epithelioid histiocytes, and AILD-like lymphoma, possess clonal rearrangements of the beta-T-cell receptor gene (25,26,48,66,107,108). However, some post-thymic T-cell lymphomas, including many angiocentric T-cell lymphomas, particularly those occurring in the sinonasal tract and nasopharynx, show a germline configuration for the beta-T-cell receptor gene (61,105). Some of the latter cases have clonal rearrangement of the gamma- or delta-T-cell receptor genes (98,105); others are seen to be clonal by the demonstration of a single episomal configuration of the Epstein-Barr viral terminal repeat (61).

Approximately 10 percent of post-thymic T-cell lymphomas show clonal rearrangements of the immunoglobulin heavy chain gene in addition to clonal rearrangements of the beta-T-cell receptor gene (72). Although two cases reportedly showed clonal rearrangements of the kappa light chain gene (80), reevaluation of one of these cases has revealed a B- and not T-cell immunophenotype (Weiss LM, unpublished observations, 1992).

The karyotypes of post-thymic T-cell lymphomas tend to be complex, with many different nonrecurring structural chromosomal abnormalities (27,53,54). The sites of the T-cell receptor genes, particularly 14q11-13, are among the most commonly disrupted in T-cell lymphomas, however, the overall frequency of their involvement is low (approximately 5 percent). Abnormalities of the long arm of chromosome 6 and both arms of chromosome 1 are more commonly associated with T-cell non-Hodgkin's lymphoma but some of these correlations may not be statistically significant due to the small number of cases analyzed (67). There are only minor reported cytogenetic differences between HTLV-1–positive and –negative lymphomas.

Differential Diagnosis. Post-thymic T-cell lymphomas may be confused with a wide variety of lesions, including reactive conditions, B-cell lymphoma, Hodgkin's disease, and true histiocytic neoplasms. The differential diagnosis of post-thymic T-cell lymphoma and Hodgkin's disease is discussed in chapter 14, histiocytic neoplasms in chapter 18, and mycosis fungoides in chapter 12.

Reactive Conditions. Post-thymic T-cell lymphomas may be difficult to distinguish from benign paracortical hyperplasia. Both may show a polymorphous population of small and large lymphoid cells, with scattered neutrophils, eosinophils, histiocytes, and plasma cells. To establish a histologic diagnosis of lymphoma, focus should be on the cytologic atypia of the lymphoid cells: a spectrum of atypical cells or areas with a monomorphic proliferation of medium to large lymphoid cells is probably a malignant lymphoma. However, some T-cell lymphomas lack overt cytologic atypia; immunohistochemical studies to look for an aberrant immunophenotype or gene rearrangement studies may be helpful in these borderline cases.

Differentiating between AILD and AILD-like lymphomas has already been discussed.

T-cell lymphoma with a high content of epithelioid histiocytes may be confused with granulomatous disorders such as infection and sarcoidosis. However, well-formed granulomas are not seen in lymphoma, and Langhans giant cells are infrequent. In addition, necrosis is rare in T-cell lymphoma with a high content of epithelioid histiocytes, and is found in areas with large numbers of neoplastic cells, not in the areas of the epithelioid histiocytes.

Wegener's granulomatosis may be confused with angiocentric immunoproliferative lesions involving the lung and upper respiratory tract, since both diseases affect vessel walls and are associated with necrosis. Wegener's granulomatosis lacks cellular atypia, distinguishing it from grade II or III angiocentric immunoproliferative lesions. In addition, Langhans-type giant cells, areas of palisaded histiocytes, or even well-formed granulomas are often present in Wegener's granulomatosis, features absent in angiocentric immunoproliferative lesions.

B-Cell Lymphoma. Despite the characteristic histologic features of post-thymic T-cell lymphoma, there are no pathognomonic features, and thus no absolute way to determine B or T phenotype in the absence of phenotyping or other special studies. The definitive identification of a true follicular component would provide histo-

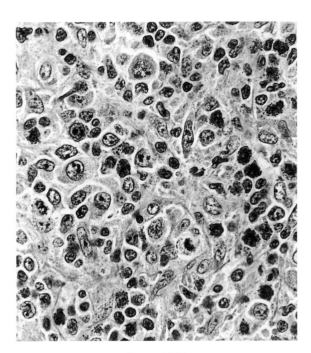

Figure 13-24
B-CELL LYMPHOMA MIMICKING
POST-THYMIC T-CELL LYMPHOMA
The diffuse effacement of architecture and mixed cell population closely mimics a T-cell lymphoma. The atypical cells of this case were positive for CD20 and negative for CD43.

logic evidence for a B-cell derivation, since T-cell lymphomas are never truly follicular. However, B-cell lymphomas may simulate T-cell lymphomas and vice versa, and even expert hematopathologists cannot reliably distinguish between the two (fig. 13-24) (41). It had been hypothesized that neoplastic cells with highly irregular cerebriform or hyperlobate nuclear outlines indicate a T lineage, however, B-cell lymphomas with cerebriform nuclei have been described (11), and the majority of hyperlobate lymphomas mark as B and not T lineage (17,68,110). Lymphomas with a high content of epithelioid histiocytes may be B lineage, and are particularly common in B-cell lymphoplasmacytic/lymphoplasmacytoid immunocytoma (70). Furthermore, B-lineage angiocentric lymphomas have also been reported. Therefore, although the characteristic histologic features described in this chapter can suggest a possible T lineage, confirmation requires immunophenotyping or other special studies.

Treatment. Since most patients with post-thymic T-cell lymphoma present in high-stage disease, most patients receive aggressive combination chemotherapy. The usual regimens are those used for diffuse large cell lymphoma. Some low-stage patients have been initially treated with radiotherapy or surgery, with chemotherapy reserved for salvage after relapse.

Prognosis. The survival rates for post-thymic T-cell lymphoma patients vary among the largest reported series (30,35,50,57,87,100). Generally, the median survival ranges from 10 to 30 months. Stage has been shown to be a better prognostic indicator than morphologic subtype (65): patients with low-stage disease do much better than those with stage III or IV. In addition, patients with primary noncutaneous disease do worse than patients with primary cutaneous disease. Patients with HTLV-1 infection have a particularly poor prognosis, with a median survival less than 1 year (9). Several studies have suggested that patients with post-thymic T-cell lymphomas composed of small cells or a mixture of small and large cells do better than those with lymphomas composed primarily of large cells (75,100); however, other studies

have not confirmed these observations or have reported the reverse (35,101). Limited data suggest that treated low-grade lymphomas of the updated Kiel classification (AILD-like, T zone, malignant lymphoma with a high content of epithelioid histiocytes) do better than the high-grade types (immunoblastic, pleomorphic) (62, 91,94). Patients with a mediastinal presentation have a relatively poor prognosis (75).

An unresolved question is whether post-thymic T-cell lymphomas have a worse clinical outcome than diffuse B-cell lymphomas of comparable morphology. Several studies have shown a worse prognosis for T-cell lymphomas (57,92), while others show a similar survival for the two groups (20,50,82, 87). Most of the studies concluding a worse prognosis for T-cell lymphoma have spanned a long period and have used "first" or "second-generation" chemotherapy, while most of the studies finding no difference in prognosis have used more aggressive chemotherapeutic regimens such as m-BACOD. Therefore, it may be that any difference in survival between post-thymic T-cell lymphoma and B-cell diffuse large cell lymphoma can be minimized by the use of aggressive chemotherapy.

REFERENCES

1. Abruzzo LV, Schmidt K, Weiss LM, et al. B-cell lymphoma complicating angioimmunoblastic lymphadenopathy: a case with oligoclonal gene rearrangements associated with Epstein-Barr virus. Blood 1993;82:241–6.
2. Anagnostopoulos I, Hummel M, Finn T, et al. Heterogeneous Epstein-Barr virus infection patterns in peripheral T-cell lymphoma of angioimmunoblastic lymphadenopathy type. Blood 1992;80:1806–12.
3. Arber DA, Weiss LM. CD15: a review. Appl Immunohistochem 1993:1:17–30.
4. _____, Weiss LM. CD43: a review. Appl Immunohistochem 1993:1:88–96.
5. _____, Weiss LM, Albujar PF, Chen YY, Jaffe ES. Nasal lymphomas in Peru: high incidence of T-cell immunophenotype and Epstein-Barr virus infection. Am J Surg Pathol 1993;17:392–99.
6. Blattner WA, Blayney DW, Robert-Guroff M, et al. Epidemiology of human T-cell leukemia/lymphoma virus (HTLV). J Infect Dis 1983;147:406–16.
7. Blayney DW, Blattner WA, Robert-Guroff M, et al. The human T-cell leukemia-lymphoma virus in the southeastern United States. JAMA 1983;250:1048–52.
8. Borowitz MJ, Reichert TA, Brynes RK, et al. The phenotypic diversity of peripheral T-cell lymphomas: the Southeastern Cancer Study Group experience. Hum Pathol 1986;17:567–74.
8a. Brunning RD, McKenna RW. Tumors of the bone marrow. Atlas of Tumor Pathology, 3rd Series, Fascicle 9. Washington, D.C.: Armed Forces Insititute of Pathology, 1994.
9. Bunn PA, Schecter GP, Jaffe E, et al. Clinical course of retrovirus-associated adult T-cell lymphoma in the United States. N Engl J Med 1983;309:257–64.
10. Burke JS, Butler JJ. Malignant lymphoma with a high content of epithelioid histiocytes (Lennert's lymphoma). Am J Clin Pathol 1976;66:1–9.
11. _____, Warnke RA, Connors JM, Beckstead JH. Diffuse malignant lymphoma with cerebriform nuclei: a B-cell lymphoma studied with monoclonal antibodies. Am J Clin Pathol 1985;83:753–9.
12. Cabeadas JM, Isaacson PG. Phenotyping of T-cell lymphomas in paraffin sections–which antibodies? Histopathology 1991;19:419–24.
13. Catovsky D, Greaves MF, Rose M, et al. Adult T-cell lymphoma-leukaemia in Blacks from the West Indies. Lancet 1982;1:639–43.

14. Chan JK, Ng CS, Lau WH, Lo ST: Most nasal/nasopharyngeal lymphomas are peripheral T-cell neoplasms. Am J Surg Pathol 1987;11:418–29.

15. _____, Ng CS, Chu YC, Wong KF. S-100 protein-positive sinusoidal large cell lymphoma. Hum Pathol 1987;18:756–9.

16. _____, Ng CS, Ngan KC, Hui PK, Lo ST, Lau WH. Angiocentric T-cell lymphoma of the skin. An aggressive lymphoma distinct from mycosis fungoides. Am J Surg Pathol 1988;12:861–76.

17. _____, Ng CS, Tung S. Multilobated B-cell lymphoma, a variant of centroblastic lymphoma. Report of four cases. Histopathology 1986;10:601–12.

18. Chott A, Dragosics B, Radaszkiewicz T. Peripheral T-cell lymphomas of the intestine. Am J Pathol 1992;141: 1361–71.

19. Clark DM, Boylston AW, Hall PA, Carrel S. Antibodies to T cell antigen receptor beta chain families detect monoclonal T cell proliferation. Lancet 1986;2:835–7.

20. Cossman J, Jaffe ES, Fisher RI. Immunologic phenotypes of diffuse, aggressive non-Hodgkin's lymphomas. Correlations with clinical features. Cancer 1984;54:1310–7.

21. Delsol G, Al Saati T, Gatter KC, et al. Coexpression of epithelial membrane antigen (EMA), Ki-1, and interleukin-2 receptor by anaplastic large cell lymphomas. Diagnostic value in so-called malignant histiocytosis. Am J Pathol 1988;130:59–70.

22. DeRemee RA, Weiland LH, McDonald TJ. Polymorphic reticulosis, lymphomatoid granulomatosis. Two diseases or one? Mayo Clin Proc 1978;53:634–40.

23. Falini B, Pileri S, De Solas I, et al. Peripheral T-cell lymphomas associated with hemophagocytic syndrome. Blood 1990;75:434–44.

24. Farcet JP, Gaulard P, Marolleau JP, et al. Hepatosplenic T-cell lymphoma: sinusal/sinusoidal localization of malignant cells expressing the T-cell receptor δ-γ. Blood 1990;75:2213–9.

25. Feller AC, Griesser H, Mak TW, Lennert K. Lymphoepithelioid lymphoma (Lennert's lymphoma) is a monoclonal proliferation of helper/inducer T cells. Blood 1986;68:663–7.

26. _____, Griesser H, von Schilling CV, et al. Clonal gene rearrangement patterns correlate with immunophenotype and clinical parameters in patients with angioimmunoblastic lymphadenopathy. Am J Pathol 1988;133:549–56.

27. Fifth International Workshop on Chromosomes in Leukemia-Lymphoma. Correlation of chromosome abnormalities with histologic and immunologic characteristics in non-Hodgkin's lymphoma and adult T cell leukemia-lymphoma. Blood 1987;70:1554–64.

28. Frizzera G, Moran EM, Rappaport H. Angioimmunoblastic lymphadenopathy with dysproteinaemia. Lancet 1974;1:1070–3.

29. _____, Moran EM, Rappaport H. Angioimmunoblastic lymphadenopathy. Diagnosis and clinical course. Am J Med 1975;59:803–18.

30. Greer JP, York JC, Cousar JB, et al. Peripheral T-cell lymphoma: a clinicopathologic study of 42 cases. J Clin Oncol 1984;2:788–98.

31. Grogan TM, Fielder K, Rangel C, et al. Peripheral T-cell lymphoma. Aggressive disease with heterogenous immunotypes. Am J Clin Pathol 1985;83:279–88.

32. _____, Richter LC, Payne CM, Rangel CS. Signet-ring cell lymphoma of T-cell origin. An immunocytochemical and ultrastructural study relating giant vacuole formation to cytoplasmic sequestration of surface membrane. Am J Surg Pathol 1985;9:684–92.

32a. Guinee DG Jr, Jaffe E, Kingma D, et al. Pulmonary lymphomatoid granulomatosis: evidence for a proliferation of Epstein-Barr virus infected B-lymphocytes with a prominent T-cell component and vasculitis. Am J Surg Pathol 1994;18:753–64.

33. Harabuchi Y, Yamanaka N, Kataura A, et al. Epstein-Barr virus in nasal T-cell lymphomas in patients with lethal midline granuloma. Lancet 1990;335:128–30.

34. Hastrup N, Hamilton-Dutoit S, Ralfkiaer E, Pallesen G. Peripheral T-cell lymphomas: an evaluation of reproducibility of the updated Kiel classification. Histopathology 1991;18:99–105.

35. Horning SJ, Weiss LM, Crabtree GS, Warnke RA. Clinical and phenotypic diversity of T cell lymphomas. Blood 1986;67:1578–82.

36. Isaacson PG, O'Connor NT, Spencer J, et al. Malignant histiocytosis of the intestine: a T-cell lymphoma. Lancet 1985;2:688–91.

37. _____, Wright DH. Malignant histiocytosis of the intestine. Hum Pathol 1978;9:661–77.

38. Jaffe ES. Post-thymic lymphoid neoplasia. In: Jaffe ES, ed. Surgical pathology of the lymph nodes and related organs. Philadelphia: WB Saunders, 1985:218–48.

39. _____, Blattner WA, Blayney DW, et al. The pathologic spectrum of adult T-cell leukemia/lymphoma in the United States. Human T-cell leukemia/lymphoma virus-associated lymphoid malignancies. Am J Surg Pathol 1984;8:263–75.

40. _____, Costa J, Fauci AS, Cossman J, Tsokos M. Malignant lymphoma and erythrophagocytosis simulating malignant histiocytosis. Am J Med 1983;75:741–9.

41. _____, Strauchen JA, Berard CW. Predictability of immunologic phenotype by morphologic criteria in diffuse aggressive non-Hodgkin's lymphomas. Am J Clin Pathol 1982;77:46–9.

42. Jones JF, Shurin S, Abramowsky C, et al. T-cell lymphomas containing Epstein-Barr viral DNA in patients with chronic Epstein-Barr virus infections. N Engl J Med 1988;318:733–41.

43. Kadin ME, Kamoun M, Lamberg J. Erythrophagocytic Tγ lymphoma. A clinicopathologic entity resembling malignant histiocytosis. N Engl J Med 1981;304:648–53.

44. Kassel SH, Echevarria RA, Guzzo FP. Midline malignant reticulosis (so-called lethal midline granuloma). Cancer 1969;23:920–35.

45. Katzenstein AL, Carrington CB, Liebow AA. Lymphomatoid granulomatosis. A clinicopathologic study of 152 cases. Cancer 1979;43:360–73.

46. Kern WF, Spier CM, Hanneman EH, Miller TP, Matzner M, Grogan TM. Neural cell adhesion molecule-positive peripheral T-cell lymphoma: a rare variant with a propensity for unusual sites of involvement. Blood 1992;79:2432–7.

47. Kim H, Jacobs C, Warnke RA, Dorfman RF. Malignant lymphoma with high content of epithelioid histiocytes. A distinct clinicopathologic entity and a form of so-called "Lennert's lymphoma." Cancer 1978;41:620–35.

48. Knowles DM. Immunophenotypic and antigen receptor gene rearrangement analysis in T cell neoplasia. Am J Pathol 1989;134:761–85.

49. _____, Halper JP. Human T-cell malignancies: correlative clinical, histopathogic, immunologic, and cytochemical analysis of 23 cases. Am J Pathol 1982;106:187–203.

50. Kwak LW, Wilson M, Weiss LM, et al. Similar outcome of treatment of B-cell and T-cell diffuse large-cell lymphomas: the Stanford experience. J Clin Oncol 1991;9:1426–31.

51. Lennert K, Feller AC. Histopathology of non-Hodgkin's lymphomas (based on the updated Kiel classification). 2nd ed. Berlin: Springer-Verlag, 1992:165–261.

52. _____, Kikuchi M, Sato E, et al. HTLV-positive and -negative T-cell lymphomas. Morphological and immuno-histochemical differences between European and HTLV–positive Japanese T-cell lymphomas. Int J Cancer 1985;35:65-72.

53. Levine EG, Arthur DC, Gajl-Peczalska KJ, et al. Correlations between immunological phenotype and karyotype in malignant lymphoma. Cancer Res 1986;46:6481–8.

54. _____, Bloomfield CD. Cytogenetics of non-Hodgkin's lymphoma. Monogr Natl Cancer Inst 1990;10:7–12.

55. Liebow AA, Carrington CB, Friedman PJ. Lymphomatoid granulomatosis. Hum Pathol 1972;3:457-558.

56. Lipford EH Jr, Margolick JB, Longo DL, Fauci AS, Jaffe ES. Angiocentric immunoproliferative lesions: a clinicopathologic spectrum of post-thymic T-cell proliferations. Blood 1988;72:1674–81.

57. Lippman SM, Miller TP, Spier CM, Slymen DJ, Grogan TM. The prognostic significance of the immunotype in diffuse large-cell lymphoma: a comparative study of the T-cell and B-cell phenotype. Blood 1988;72:436–41.

58. Lukes RJ, Tindle BH. Immunoblastic lymphadenopathy. A hyperimmune entity resembling Hodgkin's disease. N Engl J Med 1975;292:1–8.

59. Macon WR, Williams ME, Greer JP, Stein RS, Collins RD, Cousar JB. T-cell-rich B-cell lymphomas. A clinicopathologic study of 19 cases. Am J Surg Pathol 1992;16:351–63.

60. Medeiros LJ, Jaffe ES, Chen YY, Weiss LM. Localization of Epstein-Barr viral genomes in angiocentric immunoproliferative lesions. Am J Surg Pathol 1992;6:439–47.

61. _____, Peiper SC, Elwood L, Yano T, Raffeld M, Jaffe ES. Angiocentric immunoproliferative lesions: a molecular analysis of eight cases. Hum Pathol 1990;22:1150–7.

62. Nakamura S, Suchi T. A clinicopathologic study of node-based, low-grade, peripheral T-cell lymphoma: angioimmunoblastic lymphoma, T-zone lymphoma, and lymphoepithelioid lymphoma. Cancer 1991;67:2566–78.

63. Nathwani BN, Rappaport H, Moran EM, Pangalis GA, Kim H. Malignant lymphoma arising in angioimmunoblastic lymphadenopathy. Cancer 1978;41:578–606.

64. Ng CS, Chan JK, Lo ST. Expression of natural killer cell markers in non-Hodgkin's lymphomas. Hum Pathol 1987;18:1257–62.

65. Noorduyn LA, van der Valk P, van Heerde P, et al. Stage is a better prognostic indicator than morphologic subtype in primary noncutaneous T-cell lymphoma. Am J Clin Pathol 1990;93:49–57.

66. O'Connor NT, Crick JA, Wainscoat JS, et al. Evidence for monoclonal T lymphocyte proliferation in angioimmunoblastic lymphadenopathy. J Clin Pathol 1986;39:1229–32.

67. Offit K, Chaganti RS. Chromosomal aberrations in non-Hodgkin's lymphoma. Biologic and clinical correlations. Hematol Oncol Clin North Am 1991;5:853–69.

68. O'Hara CJ, Said JW, Pinkus GS. Non-Hodgkin's lymphoma, multilobated B-cell type: report of nine cases with immunohistochemical and immunoultrastructural evidence for a follicular center cell derivation. Hum Pathol 1986;17:593–9.

69. Patsouris E, Noël H, Lennert K. Angioimmunoblastic lymphadenopathy-type of T-cell lymphoma with a high content of epithelioid cells. Histopathology and comparison with lymphoepithelioid cell lymphoma. Am J Surg Pathol 1989;13:262–75.

70. _____, Noël H, Lennert K. Lymphoplasmacytic/lymphoplasmacytoid immunocytoma with a high content of epithelioid cells. Histologic and immunohistochemical findings. Am J Surg Pathol 1990;14:660–70.

71. _____, Noël H, Lennert K. Histological and immunohistological findings in lymphoepithelioid cell lymphoma (Lennert's lymphoma). Am J Surg Pathol 1988;12:341–50.

72. Pelicci PG, Knowles DM II, Dalla Favera R. Lymphoid tumors displaying rearrangements of both immunoglobulin and T cell receptor genes. J Exp Med 1985;162:1015–24.

73. Picker LJ, Brenner MB, Weiss LM, Smith SD, Warnke RA. Discordant expression of CD3 and T-cell receptor beta-chain antigens in T-lineage lymphomas. Am J Pathol 1987;129:434–40.

74. _____, Weiss LM, Medeiros LJ, Wood GS, Warnke RA. Immunophenotypic criteria for the diagnosis of non-Hodgkin's lymphoma. Am J Pathol 1987;128:181–201.

75. Pinkus GS, O'Hara CJ, Said JW. Peripheral/post-thymic T-cell lymphomas: a spectrum of disease. Clinical, pathologic, and immunologic features of 78 cases. Cancer 1990;65:971–98.

76. _____, Said JW, Hargreaves H. Malignant lymphoma T-cell type. A distinct morphologic variant with large multilobated nuclei, with a report of four cases. Am J Clin Pathol 1979;72:540–50.

77. _____, Thomas P, Said JW. Leu-M1–a marker for Reed-Sternberg cells in Hodgkin's disease. An immunoperoxidase study of paraffin-embedded tissues. Am J Pathol 1985;119:244–52.

78. Ramsey AD, Smith WJ, Isaacson PG. T-cell-rich B-cell lymphoma. Am J Surg Pathol 1988;12:433–43.

79. Saldana MJ, Patchefsky AS, Israel HI, Atkinson GW. Pulmonary angiitis and granulomatosis. The relationship between histologic features, organ involvement, and response to treatment. Hum Pathol 1977;8:391–409.

80. Sheibani K, Wu A, Ben-Ezra J, Stroup R, Rappaport H, Winberg C. Rearrangement of κ-chain and T-cell receptor β-chain genes in malignant lymphomas of "T-cell" phenotype. Am J Pathol 1987;129:201–7.

81. Shimoyama M. Minato K, Saito H, et al. Immunoblastic lymphadenopathy (IBL)-like T-cell lymphoma. Jpn J Clin Oncol 1979;9(Suppl):347–56.

82. Shipp MA, Harrington DP, Klatt MM, et al. Identification of major prognostic subgroups of patients with large-cell lymphoma treated with m-BACOD or M-BACOD. Ann Intern Med 1986;104:757–65.

83. Simrell CR, Margolick JB, Crabtree GR, Cossman J, Fauci AS, Jaffe ES. Lymphokine-induced phagocytosis in angiocentric immunoproliferative lesions (AIL) and malignant lymphoma arising in AIL. Blood 1985;65:1469–76.

84. Spencer J, Cerf-Bensussan N, Jarry A, et al. Enteropathy-associated T-cell lymphoma (malignant histiocytosis of the intestine) is recognized by a monoclonal antibody (HML-1) that defines a membrane molecule on human mucosal lymphocytes. Am J Pathol 1988;132:1–5.

85. Stansfeld AG, Diebold J, Noel H, et al. Updated Kiel classification for lymphomas [Letter]. Lancet 1988; 1:292–3.

86. Stein H, Mason DY, Gerdes J, et al. The expression of the Hodgkin's disease associated antigen Ki-1 in reactive and neoplastic tissue: evidence that Reed-Sternberg cells and histiocytic malignancies are derived from activated lymphoid cells. Blood 1985;66:848–58.

87. Stein RS, Greer JP, Flexner JM, et al. Large-cell lymphomas: clinical and prognostic features. J Clin Oncol 1990;8:1370–9.

88. Strickler JG, Weiss LM, Copenhaver CM, et al. Monoclonal antibodies reactive in routinely processed tissue sections of malignant lymphoma, with emphasis on T-cell lymphomas. Hum Pathol 1987;18:808–14.

89. Stroup RM, Burke JS, Sheibani K, Ben-Ezra J, Brownell M, Winberg CD. Splenic involvement by aggressive malignant lymphomas of B-cell and T-cell types. A morphologic and immunophenotypic study. Cancer 1992;69:413–20.

90. Su IJ, Hsieh HC, Lin KH, et al. Aggressive peripheral T-cell lymphomas containing Epstein-Barr viral DNA: a clinicopathologic and molecular analysis. Blood 1991;77:799–808.

91. Suchi T, Lennert K, Tu LY, et al. Histopathology and immunohistochemistry of peripheral T cell lymphomas: a proposal for their classification. J Clin Pathol 1987;40:995–1015.

92. Sweet DL, Collins RD, Stein RS, Ultmann JE. Prognostic significance of the Lukes and Collins classification in patients treated with COMLA. Cancer Treat Rep 1982;66:1107–11.

93. Tajima K, Kuroishi T. Estimation of rate of incidence rate of ATL among ATLV (HTLV-1) carriers in Kyushu, Japan. Jpn J Clin Oncol 1985;15:423–30.

94. Takagi N, Nakamura S, Ueda R, et al. A phenotypic and genotypic study of three node-based, low-grade peripheral T-cell lymphomas: angioimmunoblastic lymphoma, T-zone lymphoma and lymphoepithelioid lymphoma. Cancer 1992;69:2571–82.

95. Takahashi K, Yoshino T, Hayashi K, Sonobe H, Ohtsuki Y. S-100 beta positive human T lymphocytes: their characteristics and behavior under normal and pathologic conditions. Blood 1987;70:214–20.

96. The Non-Hodgkin's Lymphoma Pathologic Classification Project. National Cancer Institute sponsored study of classifications of non-Hodgkin's lymphomas. Summary and description of a working formulation for clinical usage. Cancer 1982;49:2112–35.

97. Uchiyama T, Yodoi J, Sagawa K, Takatsuki K, Uchino H. Adult T-cell leukemia: clinical and hematologic features of 16 cases. Blood 1977;50:481–92.

98. van Krieken JH, Elwood L, Andrade RE, Jaffe ES, Cossman J, Medeiros LJ. Rearrangement of the T-cell delta chain gene in T-cell lymphoma with a mature phenotype. Am J Pathol 1991;139:161–8.

99. Waldron JA, Leech JH, Glick AD, Flexner JM, Collins RD. Malignant lymphoma of peripheral T-lymphocyte origin: immunologic, pathologic, and clinical features in six patients. Cancer 1977;40:1604–17.

100. Weis JW, Winter MW, Phyliky RL, Banks PM. Peripheral T-cell lymphomas: histologic, immunohistologic, and clinical characterization. Mayo Clin Proc 1986;61:411–26.

101. Weisenburger DD, Linder J, Armitage JO. Peripheral T-cell lymphoma: a clinicopathologic study of 42 cases. Hematol Oncol 1987;5:175–87.

102. Weiss LM, Arber DA, Chang KL. CD45: a review. Appl Immunohistochem 1993;1:166–81.

103. _____, Crabtree GS, Rouse RV, Warnke RA. Morphologic and immunologic characterization of 50 peripheral T cell lymphomas. Am J Pathol 1985; 118:316–24.

104. _____, Gaffey MJ, Chen,YY, Frierson HF Jr. Frequency of Epstein-Barr viral DNA in "Western" sinonasal and Waldeyer's ring non-Hodgkin's lymphomas. Am J Surg Pathol 1992;16:156–62.

105. _____, Picker LJ, Grogan TM, Warnke RA, Sklar J. Absence of clonal beta and gamma T-cell receptor gene rearrangements in a subset of peripheral T-cell lymphomas. Am J Pathol 1988;130:436–42.

106. _____, Jaffe ES, Liu XF, Chen YY, Shibata D, Medeiros LJ. Detection and localization of Epstein-Barr viral genomes in angioimmunoblastic lymphadenopathy and angioimmunoblastic lymphadenopathy-like lymphoma. Blood 1992;79:1789–95.

107. _____, Sklar J. T cell neoplasms. In: Cossman J, ed. Molecular genetics in cancer diagnosis. New York: Elsevier, 1990:203–22.

108. _____, Strickler JG, Dorfman RF, Horning SJ, Warnke RA, Sklar J. Clonal T-cell populations in angioimmunoblastic lymphadenopathy and angioimmunoblastic lymphadenopathy-like cell lymphoma. Am J Pathol 1986;122:392–7.

109. _____, Wood GS, Dorfman RF. T cell signet ring cell lymphoma. A histologic, ultrastructural, and immunohistochemical study of two cases. Am J Surg Pathol 1985;9:273–80.

110. Weiss RL, Kjeldsberg CR, Colby TV, Marty J. Multilobated B cell lymphomas. A study of 7 cases. Hematol Oncol 1985;3:79–86.

111. Wieczorek R, Burke JS, Knowles DM. Leu-M1 antigen expression in T-cell neoplasia. Am J Pathol 1985; 121:374–80.

112. _____, Burke JS, Knowles DM II. Leu-M1 antigen expression in T-cell neoplasia. Am J Pathol 1985; 121:374–80.

113. Wong KF, Chan JK, Ng CS, Lee KC, Tsang WY, Cheung MM. CD56 (NKH1)-positive hematolymphoid malignancies: an aggressive neoplasm featuring frequent cutaneous/mucosal involvement, cytoplasmic azurophilic granules, and angiocentricity. Hum Pathol 1991;23:798–804.

14

CLASSIC HODGKIN'S DISEASE

Hodgkin's disease, a neoplastic proliferation of Reed-Sternberg cells and variants (Hodgkin cells), represents a unique cellular population whose normal counterpart has not yet been identified (if it exists at all), although the most recent evidence suggests a lymphoid origin. The Reed-Sternberg cells and variants comprise only a minority of the cellular elements; the neoplasm is diagnosed both by identification of these cells as well as the presence of a characteristic background infiltrate of host cells. Because the appearance of the Reed-Sternberg cells and variants, and the background infiltrate may vary widely, Hodgkin's disease is histologically diverse and simulates other lymphomas as well as reactive conditions.

Recognizing this wide histologic variation, investigators have attempted to subdivide Hodgkin's disease into groups that may have biologic and clinicopathologic meaning. Jackson and Parker (50) were among the first to propose a classification for Hodgkin's disease, introducing the subgroups of paragranuloma, granuloma, and sarcoma. Paragranuloma cases have a proliferation of normal lymphocytes, among which Reed-Sternberg cells are present as single cells or in small groups; granuloma cases contain numerous Reed-Sternberg cells together with a mixed infiltrate of lymphocytes, plasma cells, eosinophils and histiocytes, and fibrosis is frequent; sarcoma cases have a predominance of highly atypical neoplastic cells with only a few lymphocytes, eosinophils, and plasma cells. Although this classification scheme had prognostic value, it was clinically ineffective since most cases fit into the category of granuloma. In 1966 Lukes and Butler (72) introduced another classification system, splitting paragranuloma into the new subgroups of lymphocytic and/or histiocytic (L&H) nodular and diffuse types; splitting granuloma into nodular sclerosis and mixed types; and splitting sarcoma into diffuse fibrosis and reticular types. In an effort to simplify the latter classification, a conference held in Rye, New York, combined L&H nodular and diffuse types into a new category of lymphocyte predominance,

retained the category of nodular sclerosis, renamed the mixed category as mixed cellularity, and combined the diffuse fibrosis and reticular subgroups into the new category of lymphocyte depletion (71). The Rye classification has achieved widespread acceptance among both pathologists and clinicians. However, recent research indicates that nodular lymphocyte predominance (L&H) Hodgkin's disease (NLPHD) may be a disease entity distinct from the other types, with a unique biology and clinical course (78). For this reason, NLPHD is addressed in a separate chapter.

Definition. Classic Hodgkin's disease is a neoplasm composed of Reed-Sternberg cells and variants (Hodgkin cells) in an appropriate background of variable numbers of small lymphocytes, eosinophils, histiocytes, plasma cells, neutrophils, and fibroblasts.

Incidence. Hodgkin's disease represents approximately 20 to 30 percent of all lymphomas. About 8,000 cases were diagnosed in the United States in 1993, with an overall annual incidence of about 3 to 4 per 100,000 population (10). In contrast to non-Hodgkin's lymphomas, the incidence does not appear to be significantly increasing over time. There is an approximate 1.5 to 1 male to female ratio; the sex ratio is highest in children, but is also relatively high in the older age group as opposed to the 15- to 34-year-old bracket (76). The male predominance is seen in all histologic subtypes except nodular sclerosis. Hodgkin's disease is more common in whites than nonwhites (75).

The epidemiology of Hodgkin's disease has been comprehensively reviewed in a book by Kaplan (58) and an article by Grufferman (43). Three distinct forms have been identified by epidemiologic studies: a childhood form (0 to 14 years) common in developing countries, a young adult form (14 to 40 years) common in developed countries, and an older adult form (55 to 74 years), occurring in both groups (43). There is a bimodal age-specific incidence curve in most economically developed countries, including the United States, with a peak at 15 to 40 years and a second peak late in life (75). In the United States, there has been a decrease in the incidence of childhood Hodgkin's disease and a concomitant rise in incidence in young adults (45). The bimodal distribution is not seen in all developed countries: in Japan, for example, the peak in young adulthood is absent (2). In poorly developed countries, there is a high incidence of Hodgkin's disease in children, a relatively low incidence in the 15- to 40-year age group, and a peak later in life similar to developed countries (23). Disease incidence varies among different countries, with a relatively high incidence in the Netherlands, Denmark, and Israel, and a low incidence in Japan and Australia, particularly in the younger ages (129,94). The United States has a relatively high incidence rate (129).

Using the data summarized above, Correa and O'Conor (23) delineated several epidemiologic patterns for Hodgkin's disease: 1) developing countries: characterized by a predominance of mixed cellularity or lymphocyte depletion histology, with a high incidence in male children, low incidence in the third decade, and a second peak of high incidence in the older age groups; 2) developed countries, particularly in the urban regions: characterized by predominance of nodular sclerosis histology, with a high incidence in young adults and a low incidence in children; 3) rural areas of developed countries: characterized by histologies and incidence patterns intermediate to those seen in developing countries and urban areas of developed countries; and 4) the Orient: a relatively low incidence in all age groups.

Occasional clusters of Hodgkin's disease have been reported, but it is not clear whether this represents anything more than a chance occurrence. Numerous studies have examined the correlation between human leukocyte antigens (HLAs), but no striking findings have emerged (59). There does seem to be a low association of Hodgkin's disease with A1, B5, B18, B27, and DR5 antigens (92). There is also no consensus as to whether there is an increased incidence of Hodgkin's disease in relatives of Hodgkin's patients. Gutensohn and colleagues (47) reported that the risk of Hodgkin's disease is inversely related to number of siblings; it was later suggested that social class in childhood may be an important factor in explaining these results (45). Some studies have suggested that educational

level tends to be higher in patients with Hodgkin's disease than in the general population (19,63); others have suggested that persons employed in wood-related industries have an increased risk of disease, but the data is not clear (43). There does not appear to be an increased incidence in human immunodeficiency virus (HIV)–infected patients, although there is a higher proportion of the mixed cellularity subtype (99).

Recent studies on the possible etiology of Hodgkin's disease have focused on the Epstein-Barr virus (EBV). Patients with a history of infectious mononucleosis have a two to four times higher disease incidence than those without such a history (46). In addition, more patients with Hodgkin's disease than expected have higher titers of antibody against EBV capsid antigen (34). Furthermore, patients with Hodgkin's disease have an altered antibody pattern to EBV prior to diagnosis (83). EBV genomes have been identified within the Reed-Sternberg cells of Hodgkin's disease in up to 40 to 50 percent of cases (122, 123). In EBV-positive cases, Hodgkin cells express EBV latent membrane protein-1, a protein that has transforming potential in transfection assays (87). EBV is most commonly found in the mixed cellularity subtype, and in patients under 15 and over 50 years (51,87,123). A very high incidence of EBV-positive Hodgkin's disease was identified in Peru (13) and in HIV-infected individuals (48). However, at least 50 percent of cases of typical Hodgkin's disease show no evidence of EBV, even when highly sensitive detection methods are employed, implying that the virus is probably not of etiologic significance in all cases. The precise role of EBV in Hodgkin's disease has not yet been elucidated, but its presence in a high percentage of cases suggests an important role in pathogenesis. Human herpes virus-6 was identified in tissues involved by Hodgkin's disease in 3 of 25 cases in one study that used the polymerase chain reaction; however, it has not been determined whether the Hodgkin cells or the reactive cells were actually harboring the virus (114). No other viruses have been consistently identified in tissues affected by Hodgkin's disease to date.

Natural History and Clinical Features. Most patients present with a mass (58). In approximately 90 percent of cases, the disease first manifests in a lymph node (117): approximately 75 percent of these occur in the cervical region,

15 percent in the axillary region, and 10 percent in the inguinal region. Lymph node enlargement is usually slow and painless, and the node may be large before it is noticed. Some patients experience pain in involved lymph nodes after ingestion of alcohol.

A few patients present with symptoms of specific organ system involvement such as superior vena caval syndrome (although less commonly than those with lymphoblastic lymphoma or large cell non-Hodgkin's lymphoma), hypertrophic osteoarthropathy due to mediastinal involvement, bone pain due to bone involvement, neurologic disturbances due to spinal cord compression, or ascites or lower extremity edema due to compression of the inferior vena cava (58). Asymptomatic patients are most often diagnosed as a result of mediastinal lymphadenopathy seen on a routine radiographic examination.

There are several sites commonly involved by non-Hodgkin's lymphomas that are rarely involved in Hodgkin's disease (58). Hodgkin's disease rarely involves the palatine tonsil or Waldeyer's ring. When these areas are affected, it is usually of mixed cellularity type and secondary to extensive local lymph node involvement from the upper cervical and preauricular regions. Similarly, for unknown reasons, Hodgkin's disease rarely primarily involves the mesenteric, hypogastric, midline presacral, epitrochlear, or popliteal lymph nodes. Involvement of visceral organs (including liver and spleen), skin, and bone is almost always secondary to involvement of adjacent lymph nodes and contiguous organs, although rare cases of Hodgkin's disease primary in these sites have been described. Involvement of unusual sites at presentation may be more common in HIV-infected patients; these patients also have a tendency to present at a higher stage (99).

Constitutional symptoms occur in approximately 25 percent of patients (58). These B symptoms consist of fever higher than 38°C for 3 consecutive days, drenching night sweats, or unexplained loss of more than 10 percent of body weight within the preceding 6 months (67). The fever usually fluctuates on a daily basis, rising to up to 40 to 41°C during the late afternoon and evening and falling to normal or even subnormal levels during the early morning hours. Night sweats are a result of the nocturnal defervescence of fever. Rarely, the fever cycles over a period of 1 to 2 weeks, the so-called Pel-Ebstein fever. This phenomenon is usually restricted to patients with far advanced disease. Pruritis may also occur, and is usually generalized and severe.

One study reported that patients with lymphocyte depletion Hodgkin's disease may have characteristic clinical features: usually elderly patients presenting with systemic symptoms with a selective involvement of abdominal organs, retroperitoneal lymph nodes, and bone marrow, and a relative sparing of peripheral lymph nodes (84). Another group, however, found that these patients present similarly to those with other types of Hodgkin's disease (8); still another group concluded that both presentations occur (40).

Patients with Hodgkin's disease have defects in cellular immunity. Lymphocytopenia is common, and there is a functional defect in T lymphocytes (65). As a consequence, there is an increased susceptibility to certain types of bacterial, fungal, and viral infections, and a decreased capacity for delayed hypersensitivity reactions. In contrast to the impairment in T-cell function, there is little evidence to suggest a functional impairment of B lymphocytes.

The comprehensive studies of Kaplan and colleagues (58) have demonstrated beyond a doubt that Hodgkin's disease spreads in a nonrandom and highly predictable manner via lymphatic channels to contiguous lymph node chains and other structures. For example, since axillary lymph nodes are contiguous via direct lymphatic channels with ipsilateral infraclavicular, supraclavicular, and low cervical lymph nodes, but not with contralateral counterparts of these nodes, Hodgkin's disease occurring in axillary lymph nodes spreads to the former, but not directly to the latter, lymph nodes. Similarly, spread from supraclavicular and infraclavicular to mediastinal lymph nodes, and from there to pulmonary hilar lymph nodes, and finally to the lung is a normal sequence. Spread to subdiaphragmatic lumbar para-aortic lymph nodes generally occurs from involved supraclavicular, infraclavicular, and lower cervical lymph nodes; spread to the splenic hilar lymph nodes and spleen occurs from involved lumbar para-aortic lymph nodes. The liver is rarely involved in the absence of splenic involvement, and bone marrow involvement is also almost always associated with splenic involvement.

Table 14-1

ANN ARBOR STAGING CLASSIFICATION FOR HODGKIN'S DISEASE*
(as modified at Cotswolds)

Stage I	Involvement of a single lymph node region (I) or a single extralymphatic organ or site (I_E)
Stage II	Involvement of two or more lymph node regions on the same side of the diaphragm (II) or localized involvement of an extralymphatic organ or site (II_E)
Stage III	Involvement of lymph node regions on both sides of the diaphragm (III) or localized involvement of an extralymphatic organ or site (III_E) or spleen (III_S) or both (III_{SE}) III_1: With or without splenic hilar, celiac, or portal nodes III_2: With para-aortic, iliac, or mesenteric nodes
Stage IV	Diffuse or disseminated involvement of one or more extralymphatic organs with or without associated lymph node involvement.

*A = asymptomatic; B = fever >38° previous month, sweats previous month, weight loss >10 percent of body weight previous 6 months; X = bulk (>10 cm for lymph node, >1/3 of internal transverse diameter of thorax at >5/6 on a posteroanterior chest radiograph).

Certain modes of spread are more commonly associated with particular subtypes of Hodgkin's disease. Thus, the nodular sclerosing subtype is more often associated with lower cervical-super-clavicular-anterior mediastinal lymph nodes, while the mixed cellularity and lymphocyte depletion subtypes show comparatively less involvement of mediastinal and pulmonary hilar lymph nodes, but more involvement of the spleen.

In addition to spreading along lymphatic channels, Hodgkin's disease may spread by direct extension from lymph node to adjacent tissues. It is by this route that skin or skeletal muscle involvement usually occurs. Hematogenous dissemination may occur, either by direct invasion of veins or via the thoracic duct.

The Ann Arbor Staging classification for Hodgkin's disease, modified at Cotswolds, England (Table 14-1), takes into account the contiguous spread of Hodgkin's disease, and has proven to be a very effective staging system (67). Application of this staging system to individual patients requires extensive evaluative procedures, including biopsy, history, physical examination, clinical laboratory evaluation, and numerous radiologic studies. Chest X ray, and thoracic and abdominal/pelvic computerized tomography (CT) studies are almost always employed; bipedal lymphangiogram and gallium scans are used in some centers. Pathologic staging, in addition to the initial diagnostic biopsy, often includes bilateral bone marrow biopsies and biopsy of any clinically suspicious sites. Surgical laparotomy including splenectomy, lymph node sampling, and liver biopsy had been widely advocated in the past, but is used less frequently now due to the increased ability of other studies to obtain necessary data, the efficacy of current therapies, and postsurgical complications, including an increased incidence of infection and the small but definite increased risk of leukemia in patients who have undergone splenectomy. When a splenectomy is performed for staging purposes, it must be carefully examined, since involvement may be focal (32). The spleen should be breadloafed at 3-mm intervals, the number of gross nodules recorded, and sections taken from these areas. In addition, the splenic hilum should be carefully examined for lymph nodes.

Untreated, Hodgkin's disease progresses inexorably to more sites, with massive infiltration of the involved sites. Autopsy reveals confluent, nodular masses, distributed along the major lymph node groups (58,127). Extensive involvement of the spleen, liver, and bone marrow is usually seen, and dissemination to other organs such as lung, pancreas, kidney, and adrenals is also common. Many patients with Hodgkin's disease die of infectious complications, often bacterial (20).

Gross Anatomic Findings. Involved lymph nodes are enlarged, and vary from soft to hard, depending on the amount of fibrosis present. In nodular sclerosing Hodgkin's disease, distinct demarcation into nodules may be appreciated (fig. 14-1), but even in cases of mixed cellularity disease, a vague nodularity may be seen (fig. 14-2).

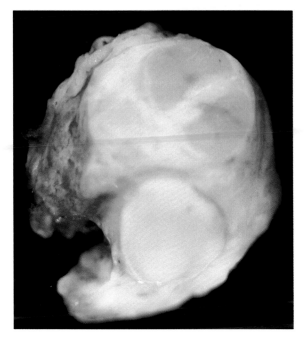

Figure 14-1
HODGKIN'S DISEASE
The lymph node parenchyma shows distinct separation into nodules by fibrous bands in this case of the nodular sclerosing subtype.

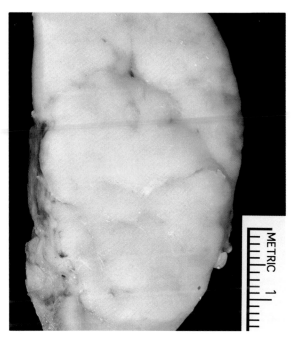

Figure 14-2
HODGKIN'S DISEASE
A vague nodularity is seen in this lymph node from a case of the mixed cellularity subtype.

In advanced cases, several lymph nodes may become matted together, due to pericapsular fibrosis. Involved spleens may be of normal weight or moderately enlarged. The cut surface usually contains discrete nodules, ranging from one to innumerable. Additional details of splenic involvement are given in chapter 20. Liver involvement manifests as white nodules, centered in the portal region.

Microscopic Findings. The diagnosis of Hodgkin's disease is established by the identification of the neoplastic elements, the Reed-Sternberg cells and variants (collectively called Hodgkin cells), in the appropriate milieu of reactive cells. Hodgkin cells are large, measuring between 20 and 50 µm or more in diameter (fig. 14-3). They generally have abundant acidophilic, amphophilic, or slightly basophilic cytoplasm, without a pale zone in the region of the Golgi apparatus such as is typically seen in immunoblasts. The nucleus is large and often bilobate or multilobate, or binucleate or multinucleate (figs. 14-4–14-6). Typically, the nuclear membrane is thickened. The chromatin pattern is usually vesicular, but with retention

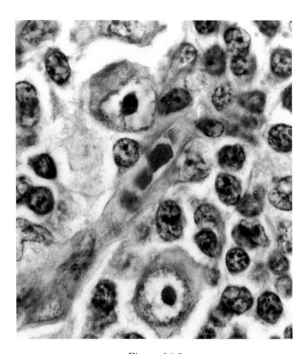

Figure 14-3
HODGKIN'S DISEASE
Two typical uninucleated Hodgkin cells are seen, in a background of small lymphocytes.

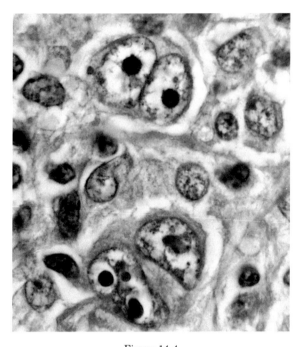

Figure 14-4
HODGKIN'S DISEASE
Binucleated diagnostic Reed-Sternberg cells are seen in this field.

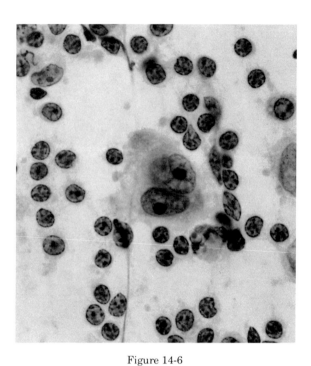

Figure 14-6
HODGKIN'S DISEASE
Hodgkin cells may often be easily identified in fine needle aspiration biopsies or in touch preparations.

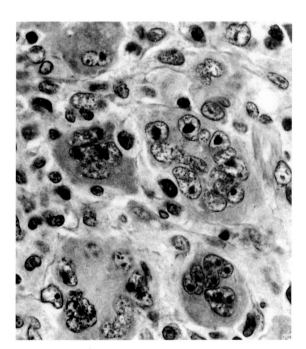

Figure 14-5
HODGKIN'S DISEASE
Multilobated nuclei or multinucleated cells are seen, with many of the lobes or nuclei possessing a prominent nucleolus.

of some coarse chromatin scattered throughout the nucleus. However, chromatin is absent around nucleoli, leaving a perinucleolar halo. There is usually one nucleolus to each nuclear lobe, prominent in size, rounded in contour, and highly eosinophilic, reminiscent of viral inclusion bodies. The diagnostic Reed-Sternberg cell has at least a bilobed nucleus, and each lobe has a prominent nucleolus. Many regard the presence of this specific cell as the sine qua non for the diagnosis of Hodgkin's disease. However, diagnostic Reed-Sternberg cells are rare in some cases (such as in occasional cases of otherwise classic nodular sclerosis Hodgkin's disease), difficult to identify due to technical factors, or may be lacking entirely (such as in small samples). Conversely, cells resembling diagnostic Reed-Sternberg cells may be observed in diseases mimicking Hodgkin's disease. In cases with few or absent diagnostic Reed-Sternberg cells, ancillary studies, such as immunohistochemistry, may be helpful.

The appearance of Hodgkin cells varies. The cells of nodular sclerosis Hodgkin's disease have multilobated nuclei, generally with smaller lobes

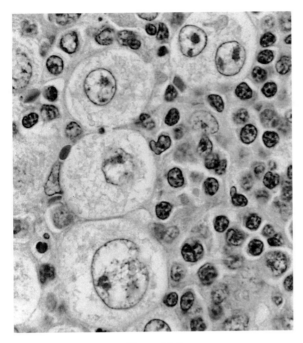

Figure 14-7
HODGKIN'S DISEASE
Several lacunar variants are seen, with multilobated nuclei with irregular outlines and artificial retraction of the cytoplasm, creating a clear space around the cells.

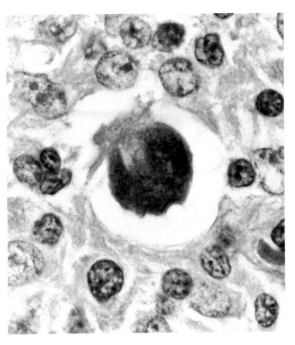

Figure 14-8
HODGKIN'S DISEASE
A "mummified" cell is seen, with pyknotic chromatin and two barely discernable nucleoli.

which contain less prominent nucleoli than seen in other Hodgkin cells (fig. 14-7). The cytoplasm is abundant and amphophilic, and, in formalin-fixed tissues often shows retraction close to the nuclear membrane so that the nucleus seems to be in a clear space or lacuna. These cells have been termed lacunar cells, however, this retraction space is artifactual, and is absent or seen to a lesser extent in tissues fixed in metal-based fixatives such as B5.

Some Hodgkin cells are seen in a state of partial degeneration. The cytoplasm becomes contracted and more eosinophilic than usual, and the nuclei become pyknotic, although nucleoli are still evident (fig. 14-8). These cells are termed "mummified" Reed-Sternberg variants. Occasionally, Hodgkin cells have highly pleomorphic nuclear features, with increased nuclear size, hyperchromatism, and highly irregular nuclear outlines and lobes (fig. 14-9).

The background cells, while not a part of the neoplastic proliferation, are almost as important as the Hodgkin cells in the histopathologic recognition of the disease and account for the bulk

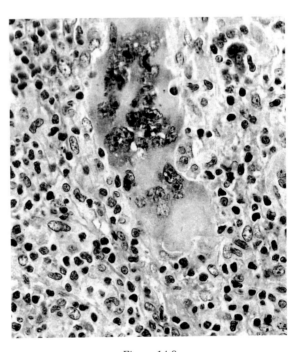

Figure 14-9
HODGKIN'S DISEASE
A highly pleomorphic Hodgkin cell is seen. Without the presence of other more characteristic cells in other fields of this biopsy, this cell could not be correctly identified. Note, however, the background of small lymphocytes.

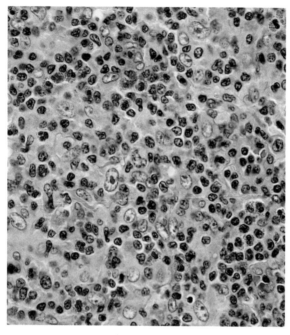

Figure 14-10
MIXED CELLULARITY HODGKIN'S DISEASE
The characteristic background infiltrate of reactive cells is seen.

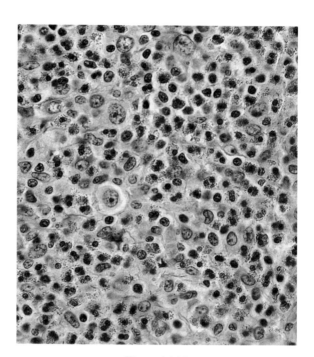

Figure 14-12
HODGKIN'S DISEASE
This case has numerous eosinophils.

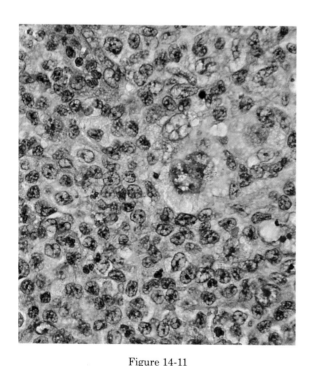

Figure 14-11
HODGKIN'S DISEASE
A Hodgkin's cell is seen in the midst of monocytoid B cells.
(Courtesy of Dr. Bharat Nathwani, Los Angeles, CA.)

of the gross mass. The background cells always make up the more abundant cellular component of Hodgkin tissues. Typically, Hodgkin cells comprise less than 1 percent of the cellular elements; in cases with abnormally large numbers of these cells, they usually comprise less than 10 percent of the cells in the tissue. The background cells are composed of lymphocytes, eosinophils, histiocytes, plasma cells, neutrophils, and fibroblasts (fig. 14-10). The majority of the lymphocytes are small, round, and regular, although occasional immunoblasts may be seen. Rarely, Hodgkin cells can be found in a background of monocytoid B-cell clusters (fig. 14-11) (80). Eosinophils vary widely in number from case to case. Occasionally, they are numerous, with the formation of eosinophilic microabcesses (fig. 14-12). The number and morphology of histiocytes also vary from case to case. The histiocytes may have an epithelioid appearance, and occasionally, well-formed granulomas may be seen (fig. 14-13). Rarely, Hodgkin's disease may be so rich in foamy histiocytes that xanthogranulomatous inflammation or a lipid storage disease is mimicked (fig. 14-14) (119). Plasma cells are often seen scattered about in Hodgkin's disease, but usually do not form sheets.

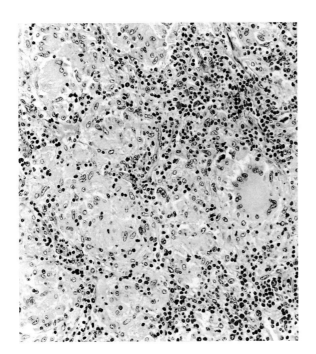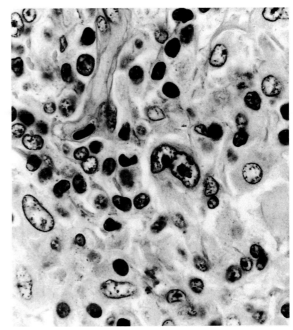

Figure 14-13
HODGKIN'S DISEASE
Left: Numerous noncaseating granulomas are present.
Right: Note the Hodgkin cell in the very center of the field.

Neutrophils are usually not found in large numbers but are occasionally numerous; their presence has been correlated with B symptoms. Fibroblasts are usually not a conspicuous feature of the infiltrate, although occasional exceptions occur (see below under variants).

As discussed, the conference panel at Rye, New York, divided Hodgkin's disease into four subtypes based on histologic appearance (71). The optimal time for histologic classification is at the evaluation of the initial biopsy, preferably of a lymph node. The effects of therapy may modify the histologic picture, while subtyping in extranodal tissues is often difficult and potentially misleading. The features of nodular sclerosis, lymphocyte predominance (excluding L&H Hodgkin's disease, nodular type), lymphocyte depletion, and mixed cellularity Hodgkin's disease are discussed.

Subtypes. *Nodular Sclerosis.* Approximately 40 to 70 percent of Hodgkin's disease is of the nodular sclerosis subtype. This histologic subtype is characterized by the formation of abundant collagen organized in broad bands that divide the lymphoid infiltrate into nodules (fig. 14-15) (72). The collagen is mature and fibroblast-poor,

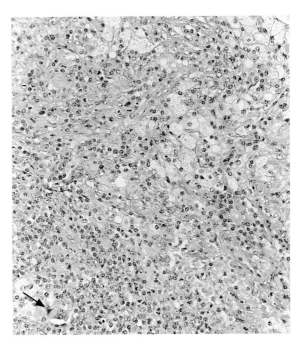

Figure 14-14
HODGKIN'S DISEASE
There are abundant foamy histiocytes. A Hodgkin cell is seen at the arrow.

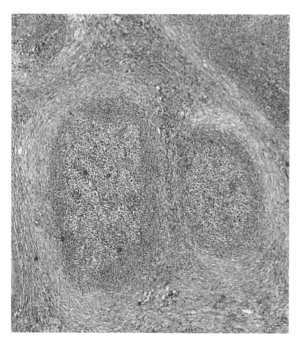

Figure 14-15
NODULAR SCLEROSING HODGKIN'S DISEASE
Fibrous bands divide the lymph node into nodules.

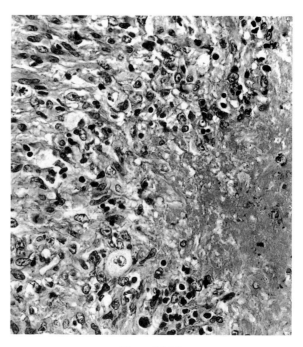

Figure 14-16
NODULAR SCLEROSING HODGKIN'S DISEASE
Necrosis is found in the center of this nodule. Several lacunar cells are present at the edge of the necrosis.

and may be demonstrated by examination for birefringence. It generally extends from a thickened capsule, following blood vessels into the interior of the lymph node. The fibrosing process may be focal, limited to only one area of the lymph node, or, in advanced cases, may interconnect with other bands, and progress to complete sclerosis of the enclosed lymphoid nodules. The presence of even focal bands of fibrosis warrants classification as nodular sclerosis, regardless of the histologic appearance in the remainder of the lymph node. The nodules of lymphoid tissue delineated by the broad bands may contain a wide range of Hodgkin cells, small lymphocytes, and other reactive cells. Eosinophils are often numerous in this subtype. The lacunar variant is usually the most common Hodgkin cell found in this histologic subtype, and its recognition helps establish the diagnosis of nodular sclerosis. Diagnostic Reed-Sternberg cells may be difficult to identify. There may be occasional necrosis in the center of the nodules, particularly when the lacunar cells form cellular aggregates (fig. 14-16). Rarely, the Hodgkin cells may be spindled, resembling sarcoma.

Because nodular sclerosis encompasses so many cases, some investigators have attempted to further subdivide this subtype. The British National Lymphoma Investigation (74) proposed two grades. Cases are classified as grade II if 1) more than 25 percent of the cellular nodules show reticular or pleomorphic lymphocyte depletion; 2) more than 80 percent of the cellular nodules show the fibrohistiocytic variant of lymphocyte depletion; or 3) more than 25 percent of the nodules contain numerous bizarre and highly anaplastic-appearing Hodgkin cells without depletion of lymphocytes. All cases of nodular sclerosis that do not fulfill these criteria are classified as grade I. Although this group has claimed that the grades are easy to distinguish, others have not agreed.

Lymphocyte Predominance. It is likely that this category of Hodgkin's disease contains two discrete entities: cases closely related to classic Hodgkin's disease, representing the end of the spectrum of mixed cellularity in which Hodgkin cells are relatively infrequent and might be expected to exhibit the phenotype associated with classic Hodgkin's disease, and cases closely related to nodular lymphocyte predominance in which

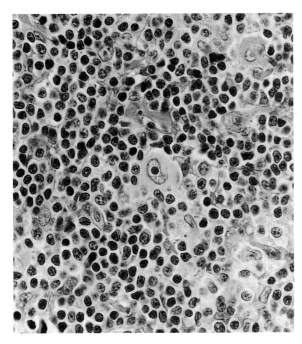

Figure 14-17
LYMPHOCYTE PREDOMINANCE
HODGKIN'S DISEASE
Only rare Hodgkin cells were identified in this case. The
majority of the infiltrate consists of small, round lymphocytes.

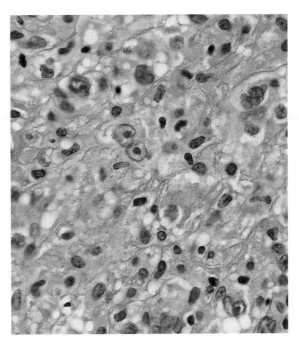

Figure 14-18
LYMPHOCYTE DEPLETION HODGKIN'S DISEASE
Diffuse fibrosis is seen and a diagnostic Reed-Sternberg
cell is present.

nodularity is minimal or absent. If L&H
Hodgkin's disease is not included, lymphocyte predominance becomes a relatively small subgroup,
comprising less than 5 percent of cases of Hodgkin's disease. Some hematopathologists recommend designating these cases as lymphocyte-rich
classic Hodgkin's disease. There are two critical
features for the diagnosis of this subtype: the rarity
of Hodgkin cells and the absence of fibrous bands
(diagnostic of nodular sclerosis) (fig. 14-17) (72).
The number of Hodgkin cells allowable in this
subtype has never been quantified, although
these cells must be rare and difficult to find; a
greater number of Hodgkin cells would classify a
case as mixed cellularity. The lymph node architecture is diffusely effaced in lymphocyte predominance, but the capsule is generally intact.
Small lymphocytes generally dominate the reactive element, although, contrary to what the
name of the subtype might imply, the predominance of lymphocytes is not the defining feature.
Histiocytes are variable in number; eosinophils
are generally few in number.

Lymphocyte Depletion. Although there are two
subcategories within lymphocyte depletion, diffuse fibrosis and reticular (72), both are rare, and
this subgroup comprises less than 5 percent of
cases of Hodgkin's disease. The incidence has decreased in recent years, as immunologic and other
studies have shown than many cases previously
thought to be lymphocyte depletion Hodgkin's disease are actually pleomorphic non-Hodgkin's lymphomas (57). In the diffuse fibrosis subcategory,
there is diffuse effacement of architecture, although the capsule is generally intact. The distinctive feature of this variant is the presence of a
disorderly reticulin fibrosis which tends to envelop individual cells (fig. 14-18). Broad bands of
collagen are absent; their presence would mandate
classification as nodular sclerosis. The overall cellularity is low, and diagnostic Reed-Sternberg cells
may be rare. In the reticular variant, diffuse effacement of architecture is seen. The key feature here
is the presence of numerous or highly pleomorphic Hodgkin cells (fig. 14-19). This subtype is
easily confused with non-Hodgkin's lymphoma.
Variable amounts of nonbirefringent collagen

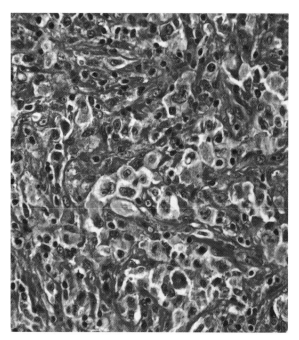

Figure 14-19
LYMPHOCYTE DEPLETION HODGKIN'S DISEASE
Numerous Hodgkin cells are seen, in a background of fibrosis.

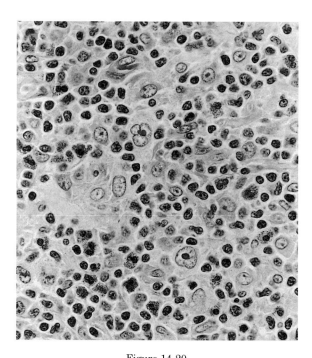

Figure 14-20
MIXED CELLULARITY HODGKIN'S DISEASE
Diffuse effacement of architecture is seen, without fibrotic bands. A mixed infiltrate, with several Hodgkin cells, is evident.

may be present, possibly indicating an overlap with the diffuse fibrosis form.

Mixed Cellularity. Approximately 20 to 50 percent of cases of Hodgkin's disease are of mixed cellularity. This subtype is histologically intermediate between the lymphocyte predominance and lymphocyte depletion subtypes. The lymph node architecture is usually diffusely obliterated, although partial involvement is common. The lymph node capsule is usually not breached. The cellularity is widely variable and necrosis is not often a prominent feature, although it may be focally present. Hodgkin cells, both mononuclear and multinuclear, are usually easy to identify (fig. 14-20). The background cells may vary widely from case to case, but generally consist of a mixture of cell types, often with numerous histiocytes and eosinophils.

Hodgkin's Disease, Unclassifiable. As originally defined by Lukes and Butler (72), the category of mixed cellularity served as a "wastebasket" category for cases that did not fit any other histologic subtype and, therefore, was essentially a diagnosis of exclusion. Currently most patholo-

gists use the category, Hodgkin's disease, unclassifiable, when subclassification is in doubt or cannot be evaluated, as in small biopsies. This designation enables the category of mixed cellularity to remain as homogeneous as possible.

Histologic Findings of Recurrent Disease. The histologic appearance of Hodgkin's disease is impressively maintained in relapse biopsies, particularly when the relapse occurs at untreated sites (22). Most cases show the same histologic subtype in the initial relapse specimen as had been seen in the initial biopsy. In addition, when an unusual histologic pattern, such as extensive necrosis or a prominent histiocytic component, is present in the initial biopsy, the same characteristic is often again present in the relapse specimen. Progression from one subtype to another, from lymphocyte predominance to mixed cellularity, or from mixed cellularity to lymphocyte depletion, occurs in a few cases (72). It also appears that nodular sclerosis can be followed by another subtype: cases of nodular sclerosis progressing to mixed cellularity have been reported. Independent of any change in histologic subtype,

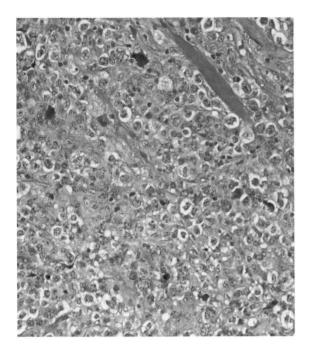

Figure 14-21
RECURRENT HODGKIN'S DISEASE
Sheets of Hodgkin cells are seen.

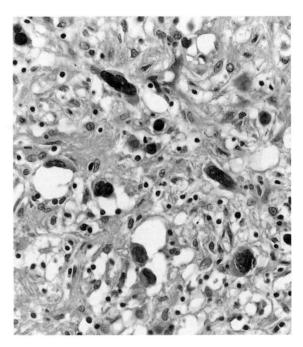

Figure 14-22
HODGKIN'S DISEASE AT AUTOPSY
Pleomorphic Hodgkin cells are present, with a relative paucity of small lymphocytes.

eosinophils, histiocytes, and Hodgkin cells tend to increase in number in relapse biopsies as compared to initial biopsies, while the lymphocytes and reactive follicles tend to decrease in number (22). When relapse occurs at a treated site, there is less propensity for retention of the original histologic appearance (31). Often, there is a marked increase in the number of Hodgkin cells, with an increase in nuclear atypia and a marked decrease in the number of small lymphocytes (fig. 14-21).

At autopsy, Hodgkin's disease shows a wide histologic variation. While in some patients, the classic patterns seen in lymph node biopsies are maintained, in others, sheets of Hodgkin cells are seen, an appearance that simulates non-Hodgkin's lymphoma (20). Most cases of nodular sclerosis lose their nodularity and sclerosis by the time of autopsy. Compared to the initial biopsy, a decrease in lymphocytes and eosinophils and an increase in the number of Hodgkin cells are seen, often with a much greater degree of nuclear atypia (fig. 14-22). In addition, there is a high incidence of vascular invasion, dissemination of disease to noncontiguous sites, and involvement of extranodal sites (42).

Successfully treated Hodgkin's disease usually shows hyalinized scars at the disease sites (20). These scars are relatively acellular, containing only fibroblasts and scattered lymphocytes (fig. 14-23). They may approximate the size of the once active lesion, and thus masquerade as residual disease. In some sites, the scars contain amorphous eosinophilic necrotic debris surrounded by a poorly cellular fibrous rim, resembling an old granuloma. Other pathologic changes seen in treated patients include radiation- and chemotherapy-related effects: fibrosis and atrophy in multiple organs, including lung, gastrointestinal tract, liver, kidney, thyroid, gonads, bone marrow, and other sites. In addition, second malignancies may occur, including acute nonlymphocytic leukemia and non-Hodgkin's lymphoma (9,60).

Criteria for Extranodal Involvement. Clearly identifiable Hodgkin cells, whether documented histologically or immunohistochemically, found in the characteristic cellular environment of Hodgkin's disease, should be regarded as evidence of involvement by Hodgkin's disease (fig. 14-24) (93). Extranodal Hodgkin's disease is

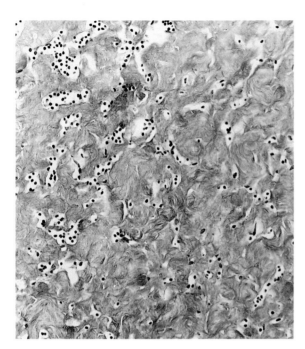

Figure 14-23
SUCCESSFULLY TREATED HODGKIN'S DISEASE
There is a fibrous scar with scattered small lymphocytes. No Hodgkin cells are seen.

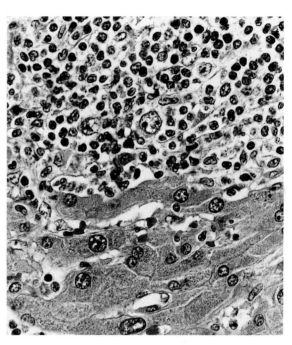

Figure 14-25
LIVER HIGHLY SUGGESTIVE OF
INVOLVEMENT BY HODGKIN'S DISEASE
The two large cells present in this field are suggestive of Hodgkin cells. Serial levels of the paraffin block or immunohistochemical studies may be useful for confirmation.

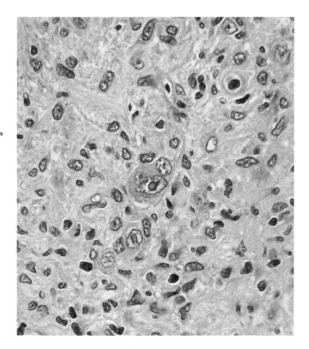

Figure 14-24
BONE MARROW INVOLVED BY HODGKIN'S DISEASE
A clearly identifiable Hodgkin cell is present in the appropriate cellular milieu.

best not subtyped. Cells suggestive of Reed-Sternberg cells, found in the appropriate cellular background of Hodgkin's disease, should be regarded as possible Hodgkin's disease (fig. 14-25). These histologic findings should prompt initiation of additional studies for confirmation (additional sections, serial levels, immunohistochemical studies). In bone marrow biopsies, a background of focal fibrosis is particularly suspicious for Hodgkin's disease (fig. 14-26). In the liver, focal involvement is invariably seen in the portal triads, while in the spleen, the white pulp is first involved, forming discrete nodules that are usually evident on gross examination. If the tissue examined is small, such as in a liver or bone marrow biopsy, consideration should be given to serial sectioning. A nonspecific lymphoid infiltrate without the presence of large atypical cells should not be considered suggestive of Hodgkin's disease, since such infiltrates may be commonly found in uninvolved tissues, particularly the liver, in patients with Hodgkin's disease (64). One exception to the above guidelines is the

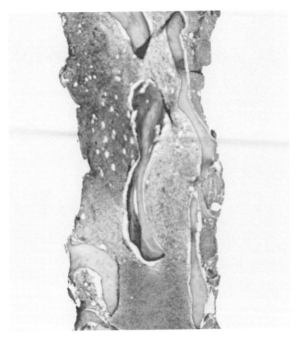

Figure 14-26
BONE MARROW INVOLVEMENT
BY HODGKIN'S DISEASE
Note the focus of fibrosis at the bottom.

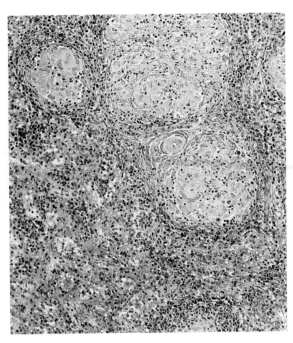

Figure 14-27
SPLEEN WITH NONCASEATING GRANULOMAS
No evidence of Hodgkin's disease was found in this spleen.

evaluation of skin biopsies. Cells closely simulating Hodgkin cells in the appropriate cellular background may be seen in lymphomatoid papulosis, a lesion that may occur in patients with Hodgkin's disease. However, Hodgkin's disease virtually never involves the skin unless adjacent structures or draining lymph nodes are involved.

Occasionally, isolated sarcoid-like granulomas can be found in extranodal sites, unassociated with Hodgkin cells or other evidence of Hodgkin's disease (fig. 14-27) (53). In the absence of such evidence, granulomas should not be interpreted as evidence of involvement by Hodgkin's disease, and should not influence the pathologic stage.

Histologic Variants. *Cellular Phase of Nodular Sclerosis.* This variant of Hodgkin's disease consists of prominent nodules containing lacunar cells, similar to typical cases of nodular sclerosis, but in contrast to the latter, there is scant or absent surrounding collagen bands (fig. 14-28) (72). Some investigators favor classification as nodular sclerosis, since histologic features classic for nodular sclerosis may become apparent in sequential biopsies (22,54,108). Others favor classification as mixed cellularity, since

Figure 14-28
CELLULAR PHASE OF NODULAR SCLEROSIS
Note the nodular architecture, but the absence of bands of collagen.

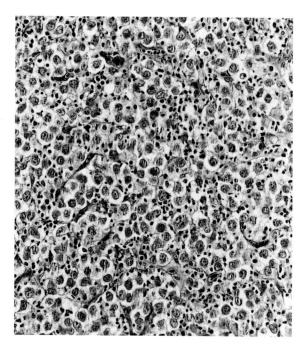

Figure 14-29
SYNCYTIAL VARIANT OF NODULAR SCLEROSIS
Sheets of Hodgkin cells are seen.

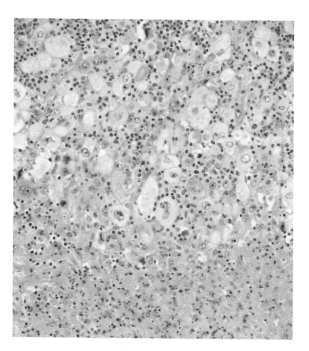

Figure 14-30
SYNCYTIAL VARIANT OF NODULAR SCLEROSIS
Numerous lacunar cells rim a focus of necrosis.

this diagnosis may be more reproducible (70). Clinical studies of a small number of cases demonstrate some clinical features and overall survival similar to mixed cellularity but a relapse-free survival similar to nodular sclerosis (21).

Syncytial Variant of Nodular Sclerosis. In this variant, numerous Hodgkin cells are found in sheets and cohesive clusters (fig. 14-29) (106). The sheets may have a central necrosis rimmed by Hodgkin cells (fig. 14-30). Occasionally, the Hodgkin cells are markedly pleomorphic and atypical. These lesions are usually classified as grade II according to the British National Lymphoma Investigation system (74). In a small biopsy, the histologic findings may simulate non-Hodgkin's lymphoma, carcinoma, or malignant melanoma; however, in a large biopsy other areas generally show foci more typical of nodular sclerosis Hodgkin's disease. If the biopsy is small, application of special studies, such as immunohistochemistry, may be essential to establish the diagnosis. Broad bands of collagen surrounding atypical cells indicates the nodular sclerosis subtype rather than lymphocyte depletion. The syncytial variant has not been demonstrated to have a poorer prognosis than other cases of nodular sclerosis.

Interfollicular Hodgkin's Disease. This variant is characterized by florid reactive hyperplasia which overshadows involvement of the interfollicular zones by Hodgkin's disease (fig. 14-31) (29). It represents a peculiar pattern of focal involvement of lymph nodes and does not constitute a classic subtype equivalent to the categories of Lukes and Butler. Its importance rests in its recognition as Hodgkin's disease, and not as a benign process. Usually, other involved lymph nodes, when sampled, show typical features of one or another of the classic subtypes; in the absence of such evidence, use of the category "unclassified" is appropriate. Study of a small number of cases has revealed no prognostic significance to the interfollicular pattern of involvement (29).

Fibroblastic Variant of Hodgkin's Disease. In a large study of Hodgkin's disease, it was noted that rare cases had areas of increased numbers of fibroblasts without thick collagen deposition (fig. 14-32) (21). This fibroblastic proliferation, most commonly seen in nodular sclerosis, may be so intense that the Hodgkin cells become obscured, and a diagnosis of sarcoma, particularly malignant fibrous histiocytoma, may be considered. According to the British National

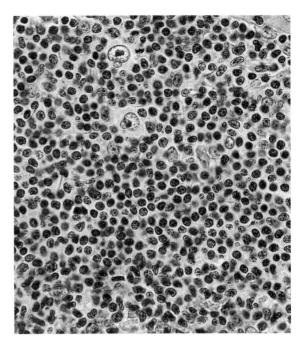

Figure 14-31
INTERFOLLICULAR HODGKIN'S DISEASE
Left: There are reactive follicles with expansion of the interfollicular region.
Right: Hodgkin cells are seen.

Lymphoma Investigation (72), cases showing a prominent fibrohistiocytic pattern (greater than 80 percent) are classified as grade II. The diagnosis can be established if attention is focused on the Hodgkin cells; special studies, including immunohistochemistry, may aid in their identification. Preliminary studies have suggested that Hodgkin's disease with a significant fibroblastic component may have a shorter relapse-free survival period than other types of Hodgkin's disease (21).

Ultrastructural Findings. Electron microscopic studies of Hodgkin cells reveal large nuclei with uniformly dispersed chromatin (fig. 14-33) (39). Nucleoli are very prominent and occupy a central position within the nucleus. Well-developed nucleolonemata are seen. The cytoplasm is abundant and usually contains great numbers of polyribosomes. Golgi regions are often composed of numerous vesicles, and variable numbers of medium-sized mitochondria are seen. Lysosomal granules are not present. The ultrastructural features are not diagnostic, and are similar to those of transformed lymphocytes.

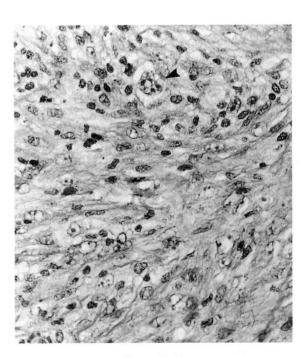

Figure 14-32
FIBROBLASTIC HODGKIN'S DISEASE
A Hodgkin cell (at arrow) is seen in the context of a fibroblastic proliferation. Confirmation of this cell as a Hodgkin cell by immunohistochemistry would be helpful in this case.

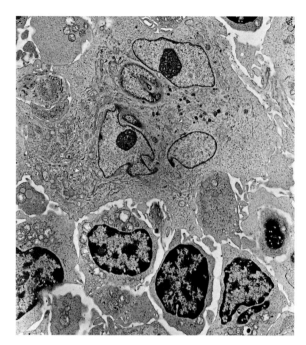

Figure 14-33
HODGKIN'S DISEASE

A multinucleated Hodgkin cell is seen, surrounded by several small lymphocytes (X2200). (Electron micrograph courtesy of Dr. Dominic V. Spagnolo, Perth, Western Australia.)

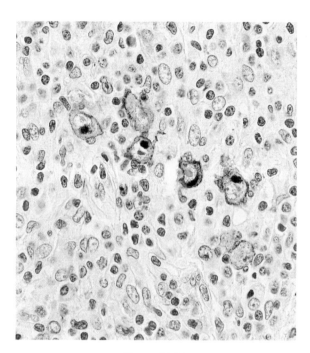

Figure 14-34
HODGKIN'S DISEASE

Note the membranous and cytoplasmic pattern of staining of this paraffin section with a CD15 antibody, with accentuation of staining in a paranuclear "dot."

Immunologic Findings. The immunology of Hodgkin's disease is a controversial topic, with different laboratories reporting divergent results, possibly as a result of variable technical procedures, antibodies, case material, and diagnostic criteria. In paraffin-embedded tissues, the Hodgkin cells express CD15 in over 80 percent of cases (fig. 14-34) (6). The pattern may be paranuclear, cytoplasmic, membranous, or a combination of the three. CD45RB (leukocyte common antigen), and CD45RO and CD43 (T-lineage–related antigens) are expressed in less than 10 percent of cases; CD20 (L26, B-lineage antigen) stains in 10 to 20 percent of cases (fig. 14-35) (7,17,33,79,98,107,121,130); CD30 (Ki-1) expression, as recognized by the monoclonal antibody BerH2, is found in about 90 percent of cases, although this percentage varies with the methodology used and the particular fixative employed (14,17,98); CD40, a protein expressed on B cells and related to nerve growth factor receptor, is found in approximately 70 percent of cases (85); and CD74 positivity is seen in most cases (101). Hodgkin cells stain for restin, an interme-

diate filament–associated protein, in about 80 percent of cases, a finding shared by anaplastic large cell lymphoma but not other non-Hodgkin's lymphomas (26). In addition to case-to-case variation in the immunophenotype of Hodgkin cells, the immunophenotype may vary between simultaneous biopsies from different involved sites as well as between serial biopsies taken over time from the same site (18).

The lectins peanut agglutinin and *Bauhinia purpurea* react with Hodgkin cells (15,49,81,97): peanut agglutinin in approximately 60 percent of cases (49,97), while one study reported *Bauhinia purpurea* positive in 97 percent of cases (97). Both of these lectins are generally negative in non-Hodgkin's lymphoma, although *Bauhinia purpurea* staining may be seen in anaplastic large cell lymphoma (15).

Hodgkin cells demonstrate a greater range of antigen expression in frozen sections or in tissues prepared using special methods, such as plastic embedding and paraformaldehyde-lysine-periodate fixation (1,12,35,49,55,98,104). With the greater sensitivity that these methodologies allow,

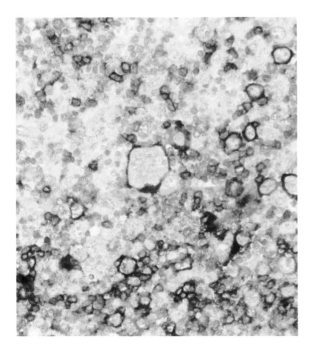

Figure 14-35
HODGKIN'S DISEASE
In a subset of cases, CD20 may stain Hodgkin cells.

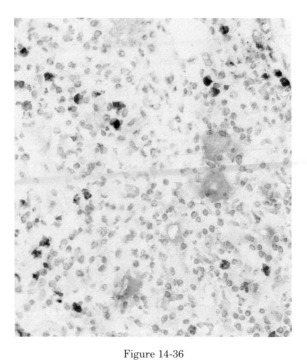

Figure 14-36
HODGKIN'S DISEASE
Staining of Hodgkin cells is seen in this frozen section using an anti-CD25 antibody.

a larger number of cases exhibit reactivity for one or more pan-T- or pan-B-cell antigens, including the framework antigen of the T-cell receptor beta chain (25). Often, however, only some of the Hodgkin cells stain for a given antigen (98). Hodgkin cells have detectable immunoglobulin of the IgG class (111). However, it is polyclonal within a given cell, and most likely represents passive uptake via the Fc receptor rather than active synthesis (56). Hodgkin cells also express HLA-DR, CD25 (the interleukin-2 receptor), and CD71 (the transferrin receptor) (fig. 14-36). The small lymphocytes in Hodgkin's disease are mostly T lymphocytes, and usually CD4-positive T-helper cells (88). In addition, cells with the phenotype of dendritic cells and macrophages can be identified. Two distinct patterns of follicular dendritic cells have been demonstrated: in about half the cases of nodular sclerosis and one fifth of the cases of mixed cellularity, there are expanded and disrupted networks of follicular dendritic cells, with Hodgkin cells and epithelioid histiocytes found between the follicular dendritic cell processes (3,4); in the other cases, follicular dendritic cells are rare or lacking.

Molecular and Cytogenetic Findings. The results of antigen receptor gene rearrangement studies are controversial (122). In most cases, there are not enough Hodgkin cells for any clonal rearrangements to be detected by Southern blot hybridization (125). Therefore, a germline configuration for immunoglobulin heavy and light chain genes and the beta-T-cell receptor gene is found in most cases. Some studies suggest that as the number of Hodgkin cells increases, whether in vivo (selecting recurrences with large numbers of Hodgkin cells) or in vitro (enriching for such cells), the percentage of cases with detectable clonal immunoglobulin gene rearrangements increases (109,124). Some studies, however, have not confirmed this observation, while still others find a high percentage of cases with clonal rearrangements of T-cell receptor genes (41). When clonal rearrangements of either the immunoglobulin or T-cell receptor genes are found, the intensity of the rearranged bands is almost always faint.

Cytogenetic studies have been hindered by the difficulty of growing Hodgkin cells in culture and the rarity of the malignant cells in tissue biopsies (95). A recent review of the literature reported only 40 well-documented cases studied cytogenetically with banding techniques (112). No consistent, recurring chromosomal aberrations were identified, although the karyotypes were generally hyperdiploid with structural abnormalities. In one study, the most common breakpoints were at 11q23, 14q32, 6q11-21, and 8q22-24, all sites at or near proto-oncogenes or key genes where breakpoints in other hematopoietic neoplasms are known to occur (11). Another study found a high incidence of structural abnormalities involving chromosomal regions 12p11-13, 13p11-13, 3q68-28, 6q15-16, and 7q31-35 (113). When compared with T-cell lymphomas, only defects on the short arms of chromosomes 12 and 13 were statistically more frequent in Hodgkin's disease (113). A more recent study confirms the frequent involvement of 14q32 but infrequent presence of t(14;18) (91).

To circumvent the difficulties in cytogenetic analysis, some investigators have used Southern blot analysis and the polymerase chain reaction (PCR) to characterize possible genomic alterations in Hodgkin cells. Several studies have assessed the prevalence of t(14;18), which juxtaposes the *bcl*-2 proto-oncogene with the joining region of the immunoglobulin heavy chain gene (see fig. 3-9). The t(14,18) cannot be detected in Hodgkin's disease by Southern blot analysis (126). In one report, PCR analysis showed that 32 percent of unselected Hodgkin tissues contained (14;18) breakpoint DNA (103). Although a few studies have shown similar findings, others have not confirmed these observations (61,69,98, 122). Overexpression of the *bcl*-2 protein, a hallmark of t(14;18), is not a general feature of Hodgkin cells, although it appears to be frequently but not exclusively associated with rare cases of Hodgkin's disease that arise in patients with concurrent or antecedent follicular non-Hodgkin's lymphoma (61). The prevalence and significance of t(14;18) in Hodgkin's disease remain controversial particularly in light of its detection at low levels by PCR in floridly reactive tonsillar tissue (66) (see chapter 6).

Abnormalities of the p53 tumor suppressor gene have been reported. Using monoclonal or polyclonal antibodies, Hodgkin cells have been shown to overexpress p53 protein, which is nor-

mally undetectable using standard immunocytochemical techniques (30,44). More recently, p53 gene mutation has been demonstrated in Hodgkin cells using single cell PCR analyses (115). Thus far, no prognostic significance has been found for these alterations.

Differential Diagnosis. Because the range of histologic appearances of Hodgkin's disease is so wide, it is not surprising that the histologic differential diagnosis is enormous. Nonhematopoietic malignancies, non-Hodgkin's lymphomas, and benign lymphadenopathies may be easily confused with Hodgkin's disease.

Carcinoma and Malignant Melanoma. At times, the metastases of carcinoma and malignant melanoma manifest as isolated single cells in lymph nodes and thus simulate Hodgkin's disease. Undifferentiated nasopharyngeal carcinoma may be particularly difficult to distinguish from Hodgkin's disease, as it often presents in a lymph node with an occult primary, and may be associated with large numbers of eosinophils, plasma cells, and areas of sclerosis. Cells within lymph node sinuses are a very common feature of metastatic carcinoma and melanoma, but an unusual feature for Hodgkin's disease. In carcinoma, the chromatin is usually vesicular and often with a single nucleolus which is often smaller and less eosinophilic than the nucleolus found in Hodgkin cells, and the nuclei are generally uniform from one cell to another. In malignant melanoma, the cytoplasm is usually more abundant and more eosinophilic than in Hodgkin cells, and nuclear pseudoinclusions are often found. In both carcinoma and melanoma, the cytoplasm may show evidence of phagocytosis of granulocytes, a feature not associated with Hodgkin's disease. Occasionally, the differential diagnosis may be impossible to resolve by histologic examination alone. Immunohistochemical studies for keratin in carcinoma, and S-100 protein and HMB-45 in melanoma should clarify the diagnostic dilemma in most cases. One should keep in mind that a variety of nonhematopoietic tumors such as adenocarcinoma may express CD15 (100).

Non-Hodgkin's Lymphomas. Several types of non-Hodgkin's lymphoma are easily confused histologically with Hodgkin's disease.

Post-Thymic T-Cell Lymphoma. Post-thymic T-cell lymphomas usually show diffuse effacement of lymph node architecture and are often composed of a mixture of cell types, including eosinophils, histiocytes, and plasma cells, and thus closely mimic Hodgkin's disease. In addition, these lymphomas may contain large cells with prominent nucleoli, bands of sclerosis, and numerous epithelioid histiocytes (Lennert's lymphoma), simulating Hodgkin's disease. The clinical history may be the first clue to the diagnosis of post-thymic T-cell lymphoma, as these patients generally are older, tend to have generalized lymphadenopathy rather than present with a single mass, and are more likely to have B symptoms. The key to the histologic distinction of this entity and Hodgkin's disease is the recognition of a spectrum of cytologically atypical cells ranging from small to medium to large in the former neoplasm (fig. 14-37). In Hodgkin's disease, there should be no range of atypia, just an abrupt difference between the reactive small, round lymphocytes and the neoplastic Hodgkin cells. Other features favoring Hodgkin's disease are the presence of partial lymph node involvement, areas of focal necrosis rimmed by atypical cells, and true noncaseating granulomas. In contrast, the presence of large numbers of mitotic figures would favor the diagnosis of post-thymic T-cell lymphoma (86).

In occasional cases, particularly those in which the histologic preparations are suboptimal, distinction between post-thymic T-cell lymphoma and Hodgkin's disease may be difficult or impossible. In these cases, immunohistochemical or immunogenotypic studies are useful. In paraffin sections, CD15, CD45RB, CD45RO, CD43, and CD30 can be used in combination (17). The value of CD15 is controversial, since its positivity varies widely in post-thymic T-cell lymphomas (6): some find a low percentage of positivity, with a finely granular, cytoplasmic pattern in a minority of cells, distinguishable from Hodgkin's disease (89); others find a high rate of positivity in a pattern identical to that seen in Hodgkin's disease (100,128). Absence of CD45RB expression is found in only 10 percent of non-Hodgkin's lymphomas, and absence of CD45RO and CD43 expression is seen in less than 10 percent of T-cell lymphomas. CD30 expression is seen in about 90 percent of cases of Hodgkin's disease, but less than 10 percent of cases of non-Hodgkin's lymphoma. CD40 may represent another potentially useful marker, as it is found on Hodgkin cells in 70 percent of cases, but is only weakly present

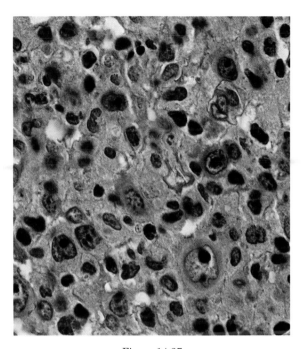

Figure 14-37
POST-THYMIC T-CELL LYMPHOMA
Although a Hodgkin-like cell is present, note the range of atypia among the other cells.

on the neoplastic cells of non-Hodgkin's lymphoma in 13 percent of cases (85). In view of the above data, reliance on the results of panels of antibodies is highly recommended.

In frozen sections, the neoplastic cells of post-thymic T-cell lymphoma generally express several pan-T-cell antigens, although aberrant absence of one or more is common. In Hodgkin's disease, the majority of the small lymphocytes express a normal T-cell phenotype, while the Hodgkin cells either do not express pan-T-cell antigens or only express one or two T-cell markers and often express them in a minority of the cells.

The presence of a distinct clonal rearrangement of the beta-T-cell receptor gene favors a diagnosis of post-thymic T-cell lymphoma, but the absence of this rearrangement or the presence of a small clonal population should be interpreted with care, as a proportion of T-cell lymphomas may lack T-cell gene rearrangements, and the presence of small clonal T-cell populations have been reported in Hodgkin's disease.

Anaplastic Large Cell Lymphoma. Anaplastic large cell lymphoma may also be easily confused with Hodgkin's disease. The neoplastic cells of

297

this lymphoma cytologically resemble Hodgkin cells and may be distributed among reactive cells in a pattern similar to Hodgkin's disease. Again, the clinical history is helpful, as anaplastic large cell lymphoma is common in children, an age group unusual (although still possible) for Hodgkin's disease; often involves the inguinal region, a site unusual (although again still possible) for Hodgkin's disease; and is often associated with skin lesions. Histologically, many cases of anaplastic large cell lymphoma demonstrate at least focal involvement of the lymph node sinuses, a rare feature for Hodgkin's disease. In addition, cells with multiple atypical nuclei arranged in a wreath-like pattern ("doughnut" cells) are often found in this lymphoma. Although plasma cells may be prominent, large numbers of eosinophils are generally not present. Histologically borderline cases do occur; similar to the situation with other post-thymic T-cell lymphomas, immunohistochemical and immunogenotypic studies may be of great use in the distinction. Although the neoplastic cells of both anaplastic large cell lymphoma and Hodgkin's disease express CD30, use of CD45RB, CD43, CD45RO, and CD15 allows diagnosis in most cases (the first three antigens often found in anaplastic large cell lymphoma and the last antigen in Hodgkin's disease). In addition, the neoplastic cells of anaplastic large cell lymphoma are often positive for epithelial membrane antigen, an antigen infrequently expressed in classic Hodgkin's disease.

Leoncini and colleagues (62) have called attention to a possible overlap between anaplastic large cell lymphoma and Hodgkin's disease in a few cases. A controversial proposal, these investigators have noted a continuous spectrum of nuclear profiles, immunophenotypes, and immunogenotypes between the two lymphomas; thus, some cases may be difficult to firmly diagnose as either anaplastic large cell lymphoma or Hodgkin's disease.

B-Cell Large Cell Lymphoma. Less commonly, B-cell lymphomas may also be confused with Hodgkin's disease. This is often a problem in the mediastinum where both nodular sclerosing Hodgkin's disease and primary B-cell sclerosing large cell lymphoma are common, and where only small biopsies are obtained through mediastinoscopy. Another problem in histologic differential diagnosis exists with T-cell–rich and histiocyte-rich B-cell lymphoma, where the neoplastic B cells are in the minority and reactive T lymphocytes or histocytes form the bulk of the infiltrate, similar to Hodgkin's disease (27,77). Special studies may be necessary to differentiate these unusual cases. B-cell immunoblastic lymphoma may contain cells indistinguishable from Reed-Sternberg cells. However, in these lymphomas, the number of Reed-Sternberg and Hodgkin cells is often paradoxically more numerous than in Hodgkin's disease. Often, the neoplastic cells possess a more basophilic cytoplasm with a clearing in the area of the Golgi apparatus. The methyl-green pyronin stain demonstrates intense pyrinophilia in the cytoplasm of B immunoblasts.

In paraffin sections, B-cell lymphomas almost always express CD45RB and CD20, and are positive for CD15 in only 5 percent of cases. While CD20 positivity may be found in up to 20 percent of cases of Hodgkin's disease, application of a panel of antibodies allows separation in most cases, since Hodgkin's cells are usually CD45RB negative and CD15 positive in paraffin sections. CD74, an antigen present on Hodgkin cells, is also seen in most B-cell lymphomas, limiting the utility of this antigen.

In frozen sections, B-cell lymphoma may be distinguished from Hodgkin's disease by the demonstration of immunoglobulins with monoclonal light chain restriction. In B-cell lymphomas that lack immunoglobulin expression, the demonstration of several pan-B-cell markers such as CD20, CD19, and CD22 in all or virtually all of the neoplastic cells should differentiate these cases from Hodgkin's disease, which, with the exception of CD20, generally only shows positivity for B-lineage markers, and when present, in a minority of the Hodgkin cells (98).

The presence of a sizable rearrangement of the immunoglobulin genes constitutes strong support for the diagnosis of B-cell lymphoma. However, faint rearrangements of these genes have been reported in Hodgkin's disease, particularly in cases with large numbers of Hodgkin cells (124).

Small Lymphocytic Lymphoma. This may be easily confused with lymphocyte predominance Hodgkin's disease. A young age favors Hodgkin's disease, while both lymphomas occur in older patients. Histologically, the prolymphocytes of small lymphocytic lymphoma simulate Hodgkin cells. A mixture of cell types, including eosinophils, favors Hodgkin's disease, while a spectrum of cells from small lymphocytes to prolymphocytes and a tendency for the larger cells to cluster into pseudofollicles favors small lymphocytic lymphoma. Rare cases of small lymphocytic lymphoma with Hodgkin-like cells have been described; in some cases these cells have the phenotypic, virologic, and biologic properties of Hodgkin cells and may represent composite lymphoma (82).

Viral Lymphadenitis, Including Infectious Mononucleosis. Usually, the biggest problem in distinguishing viral lymphadenitis from any malignant process, including Hodgkin's disease, is failure to consider it in the histologic differential diagnosis. The clinical history is important. For example, a tonsillar biopsy in a young individual should at once raise suspicion of acute infectious mononucleosis, and, even before examination of a histologic section, makes Hodgkin's disease an unlikely diagnosis, since the latter rarely presents at this site. The presence of an atypical lymphocytosis in the peripheral blood would also favor a viral etiology.

It is well known that Reed-Sternberg–like cells may be present in viral lymphadenitis. However, there are many other histologic findings that enable differentiation from Hodgkin's disease (16, 102). First, the overall lymph node architecture is usually preserved in viral lymphadenitis, with highly reactive germinal centers. The paracortical region, although usually expanded, often has a mottled appearance due to the presence of many immunoblasts evenly scattered about, in contrast to the relatively uneven distribution of Hodgkin cells. The sinuses are usually patent, and sometimes expanded by reactive monocytoid B cells. The cellular features are also different than those of Hodgkin's disease. The background cells show a maturation sequence of small lymphocytes and mature plasma cells, to plasmacytoid lymphocytes, to plasmacytoid immunoblasts (fig. 14-38). The number of immunoblasts in viral lymphadenitis is usually greater than the number of Hodgkin cells in Hodgkin's disease. However, in both, the immunoblasts may cluster around foci of necrosis.

Cat Scratch Disease and Other Necrotizing Granulomatous Disorders. In cat scratch disease, lymphogranuloma venereum, and other similar diseases, necrotizing granulomatous in-

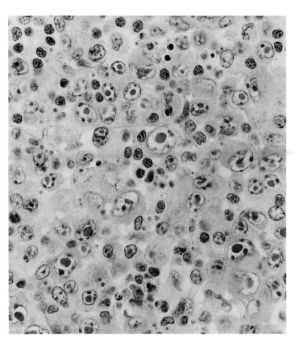

Figure 14-38
EPSTEIN-BARR VIRUS–ASSOCIATED INFECTIOUS MONONUCLEOSIS

A heterogeneous population is present, including cells mimicking Hodgkin cells. However, the spectrum of cell types and the extensive apoptosis present would not be found in Hodgkin's disease.

flammation is present. This sometimes manifests as stellate areas of necrosis, rimmed by epithelioid histocytes (fig. 14-39). In Hodgkin's disease, particularly the nodular sclerosis subtype, foci of stellate necrosis may be also present, some of which may be surrounded by epithelioid histiocytes. The periphery of the necrotic foci should be carefully examined, as Hodgkin cells are usually present, at least focally, at the edges of the necrosis in Hodgkin's disease; these cells may easily be mistaken for epithelioid histiocytes unless specifically sought.

Treatment. Hodgkin's disease is generally treated by radiation therapy, multidrug chemotherapy, or both (118). Bone marrow transplantation, a new therapy for Hodgkin's disease, is used for a select group of patients (5,52). Early stage (stage I and II) Hodgkin's disease is generally treated with radiation therapy alone (118). The dose of radiation is usually around 4,000 cGy, and is usually delivered to the neck, chest, and axilla (mantle field) and the para-aortic

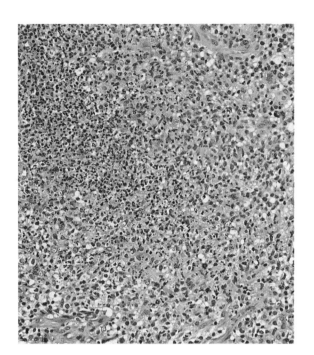 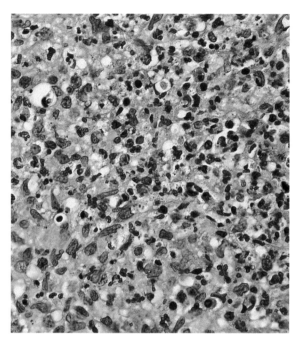

Figure 14-39
NECROTIZING GRANULOMATOUS LYMPHADENITIS
Left: A microabscess is seen.
Right: The microabscess is rimmed by histiocytes; however, Hodgkin cells are absent.

nodes and spleen (abdominal field). In some patients, particularly when fertility is not an issue, total nodal irradiation is used, with the addition of a pelvic field. Combined modality treatment (radiation therapy and multidrug chemotherapy) is usually used for patients with low stage disease with massive mediastinal involvement, although some centers are using combined modality or even chemotherapy alone in patients who have only been clinically staged and who do not have massive mediastinal disease. Higher stage disease is generally treated with combination chemotherapy, usually consisting of mechlorethamine, vincristine, procarbazine, and prednisone (MOPP) or doxorubicin, bleomycin, vinblastine, and dacarbazine (ABVD) (68). Some centers add radiation therapy, particularly to sites of bulky involvement.

If disease persists after radiation therapy multidrug chemotherapy may provide cure. Relapse after chemotherapy has a worse prognosis, particularly if it has occurred within the first year of treatment; it may be treated with additional chemotherapy using either the same or a different regimen of drugs. In general, only half of the patients who relapse achieve a durable second remission. High-dose chemotherapy (with or without radiotherapy) with autologous bone marrow transplantation, allogeneic bone marrow transplantation, or autologous peripheral blood stem-cell transplantation all have potential to become the treatment of choice for relapsed Hodgkin's disease. The data concerning these regimens are not complete, but 3- to 4-year disease-free survival rates of 35 to 50 percent have been reported (5).

Potential complications of treatment are numerous and include acute toxicity, the development of second malignancies, sterility, hypothyroidism, pulmonary fibrosis, pericarditis, accelerated atherosclerosis, infections, and avascular necrosis of bone. A wide variety of second malignancies may occur, most notably acute non-lymphocytic leukemia, but also non-Hodgkin's lymphoma, common carcinomas (including colon, breast, and lung), and sarcomas (110,116).

Prognosis. Untreated, Hodgkin's disease has a 5-year survival rate of less than 5 percent (120). However, properly treated, the overall survival rate is currently approximately 75 percent. Stage is by far the most important determinant of prognosis. Patients with stage I disease have a 5-year disease-free survival rate up to 90 percent; those with stage II disease, 75 to 90 percent; those with stage III disease, 50 to 85 percent; while those with stage IV disease, 40 to 65 percent. Other clinical factors such as age (older patients do worse), race (blacks have a uniformly poorer prognosis than whites), presence of a large mediastinal mass (greater than one third of the maximum intrathoracic diameter), presence of multiple nodules in the spleen, presence of multiple extranodal sites of involvement, decreased hematocrit, elevated levels of lactate dehydrogenase, increased erythrocyte sedimentation rate (105), increased beta-2-microglobulin (28), and elevated serum levels of CD30 and soluble CD25 may also have a negative impact on survival in high-stage patients (38,90). Treatment-related factors, such as dose of chemotherapy or type of radiation therapy, may also significantly affect survival (68). Pregnancy has no documented impact on the natural course of Hodgkin's disease (120).

The impact of histologic subclassification on prognosis has been greatly muted, primarily due the current effective treatment regimens (24),

but also because of the recognition of many cases previously diagnosed as lymphocyte depletion as non-Hodgkin's lymphoma and separation of the subgroup of nodular lymphocyte predominance from the rest of Hodgkin's disease. Several studies have shown a modest decrease in survival in nodular sclerosis Hodgkin's disease grade II as compared to grade I (37,74). Similarly, it has been shown that patients with nodular sclerosis grade I who relapse have a more successful salvage than those with grade II (37). Since cases of the syncytial variant of nodular sclerosing Hodgkin's disease meet the histologic criteria for nodular sclerosis grade II, it may be implied that these cases may also share a slightly worse prognosis, although large numbers of patients with syncytial variant have not been specifically studied for prognostic significance. The presence of noncaseating granulomas may be associated with a slightly better prognosis within a given stage (96), and cases with extensive networks of follicular dendritic cells have a favorable prognosis compared to those with only rare or absent follicular dendritic cells (4). To date, no outcome differences have been found between Epstein-Barr virus–positive and –negative Hodgkin's disease (36).

REFERENCES

1. Agnarsson BA, Kadin ME. The immunophenotype of Reed-Sternberg cells. A study of 50 cases of Hodgkin's disease using fixed frozen tissues. Cancer 1989;63:2083–7.

2. Akazaki K, Wakasa H. Frequency of lymphoreticular tumors and leukemias in Japan. JNCI 1974;52:339–43.

3. Alavaikko MJ, Hansmann ML, Nebendahl C, Parwaresch MR, Lennert K. Follicular dendritic cells in Hodgkin's disease. Am J Clin Pathol 1991;95:194–200.

4. Alavaikko MJ, Blanco G, Aine R, et al. Follicular dendritic cells have prognostic relevance in Hodgkin's disease. Am J Clin Pathol 1994;101:761–7.

5. Anderson JE, Litzow MR, Appelbaum FR, et al. Allogeneic, syngeneic, and autologous marrow transplantation for Hodgkin's disease: the 21-year Seattle experience. J Clin Oncol 1993;11:2342–50.

6. Arber DA, Weiss LM. CD15: a review. Appl Immunohistochem 1993;1:17–30.

7. _____, Weiss LM. CD43: a review. Appl Immunohistochem 1993;1:88–96.

8. Bearman RM, Pangalis GA, Rappaport H. Hodgkin's disease, lymphocyte depletion type. A clinicopathologic study of 39 patients. Cancer 1978;41:293–302.

9. Bookman MA, Longo DL. Concomitant illness in patients treated for Hodgkin's disease. Cancer Treat Rev 1986;13:77–111.

10. Boring CC, Squires TS, Tong T. Cancer statistics, 1993. Ca Cancer J Clin 1993;43:7–26.

11. Cabanillas F, Pathak S, Trujillo J, et al. Cytogenetic features of Hodgkin's disease suggest possible origin from a lymphocyte. Blood 1988;71:1615–7.

12. Casey TT, Olson SJ, Cousar JB, Collins RD. Immunophenotypes of Reed-Sternberg cells: a study of 19 cases of Hodgkin's disease in plastic-embedded sections. Blood 1989;74:2624–8.

13. Chang KL, Albujar PF, Chen YY, Johnson RM, Weiss LM. High prevalence of Epstein-Barr virus in the Reed-Sternberg cells of Hodgkin's disease occurring in Peru. Blood 1993;83;496–501.

14. _____, Arber DA, Weiss LM. CD30: a review. Appl Immunohistochem 1993;1:244–55.

15. _____, Curtis CM, Momose H, Lopategui J, Weiss LM. Sensitivity and specificity of Bauhinia purpurea as a paraffin section marker for the Reed-Sternberg cells of Hodgkin's disease. Appl Immunohistochem 1993;1:208–12.

16. Childs CC, Parham DM, Berard CW. Infectious mononucleosis. The spectrum of morphologic changes simulating lymphoma in lymph nodes and tonsils. Am J Surg Pathol 1987;11:122–32.

17. Chittal SM, Caverivière P, Schwarting R, et al. Monoclonal antibodies in the diagnosis of Hodgkin's disease. The search for a rational panel. Am J Surg Pathol 1988;12:9–21.

18. Chu WS, Abbondanzo SL, Frizzera G. Inconsistency of the immunophenotype of Reed-Sternberg cells in simultaneous and consecutive specimens from the same patients. A paraffin section evaluation in 56 patients. Am J Pathol 1992;141:11–7.

19. Cohen BM, Smetana HF, Miller RW. Hodgkin's disease: long survival in a study of 388 World War II army cases. Cancer 1964;17:856–66.

20. Colby TV, Hoppe RT, Warnke RA. Hodgkin's disease at autopsy: 1972-1977. Cancer 1981;47:1852–62.

21. _____, Hoppe RT, Warnke RA. Hodgkin's disease: a clinicopathologic study of 659 cases. Cancer 1982;49:1848–58.

22. _____, Warnke RA. The histology of the initial relapse of Hodgkin's disease. Cancer 1980;45:289–92.

23. Correa P, O'Conor GT. Epidemiologic patterns of Hodgkin's disease. Int J Cancer 1971;8:192–201.

24. Culine S, Henry-Amar M, Diebold J, et al. Relationship of histological subtypes to prognosis in early stage Hodgkin's disease: a review of 312 cases in a controlled clinical trial. The Group Pierre et Marie Currie. Eur J Cancer Clin Oncol 1989;25:551–6.

25. Dallenbach FE, Stein H. Expression of T-cell-receptor β chain in Reed-Sternberg cells. Lancet 1989;2:828–30.

26. Delabie J, Shipman R, Bruggen J, et al. Expression of the novel intermediate filament-associated protein restin in Hodgkin's disease and anaplastic large-cell lymphoma. Blood 1992;80:2891–6.

27. _____, Vandenberghe E, Kennes C, et al. Histiocyte-rich B-cell lymphoma. A distinct clinicopathologic entity possibly related to lymphocyte predominant Hodgkin's disease, paragranuloma subtype. Am J Surg Pathol 1992;16:37–48.

28. Dimopoulos MA, Cabanillas F, Lee JJ, et al. Prognostic role of serum beta2-microglobulin in Hodgkin's disease. J Clin Oncol 1993;11:1108–11.

29. Doggett RS, Colby TV, Dorfman RF. Interfollicular Hodgkin's disease. Am J Surg Pathol 1983;7:145–9.

30. Doglioni C, Pelosio P, Mombello A, Scarpa A, Chilosi M. Immunohistochemical evidence of abnormal expression of the antioncogene-encoded p53 phosphoprotein in Hodgkin's disease and CD30+ anaplastic lymphomas. Hematol Pathol 1991;5:67–73.

31. Dolginow D, Colby TV. Recurrent Hodgkin's disease in treated sites. Cancer 1981;48:1124–6.

32. Dorfman RF, Colby TV. The pathologist's role in management of patients with Hodgkin's disease. Cancer Treat Rep 1982;66:675–80.

33. _____, Gatter KC, Pulford KAF, Mason DY. An evaluation of the utility of anti-granulocyte and anti-leukocyte monoclonal antibodies in the diagnosis of Hodgkin's disease. Am J Pathol 1986;123:508–19.

34. Evans AS, Gutensohn NM. A population-based case-control study of EBV and other viral antibodies among persons with Hodgkin's disease and their siblings. Int J Cancer 1984;34:149–57.

35. Falini B, Stein H, Pileri S, et al. Expression of lymphoid-associated antigens on Hodgkin's and Reed-Sternberg cells of Hodgkin's disease. An immunocytochemical study on lymph node cytospins using monoclonal antibodies. Histopathology 1987;11:1229–42.

36. Fellbaum C, Hansmann ML, Niedermeyer H, et al. Influence of Epstein-Barr virus genomes on patient survival in Hodgkin's disease. Am J Clin Pathol 1992;98:319–23.

37. Ferry JA, Linggood RM, Convery KM, Efird JT, Eliseo R, Harris NL. Hodgkin disease, nodular sclerosis type. Implications of histologic subclassification. Cancer 1993;71:457–63.

38. Gause A, Roschansky V, Tschiersch A, et al. Low serum interleukin-2 receptor levels correlate with a good prognosis in patients with Hodgkin's lymphoma. Ann Oncol 1991;2(Suppl 2):43–7.

39. Glick AD, Leech JH, Flexner JM, Collins RD. Ultrastructural study of Reed-Sternberg cells. Comparison with transformed lymphocytes and histiocytes. Am J Pathol 1976;85:195–208.

40. Greer JP, Kinney MC, Cousar JB, et al. Lymphocyte-depleted Hodgkin's disease. Clinicopathologic review of 25 patients. Am J Med 1986;81:208–14.

41. Griesser H, Feller AC, Mak TW, Lennert K. Clonal rearrangements of T-cell receptor and immunoglobulin genes and immunophenotypic antigen expression in different subclasses of Hodgkin's disease. Int J Cancer 1987;40:157–60.

42. Grogan TM Berard CW, Steinhorn SC, et al. Changing patterns of Hodgkin's disease at autopsy: a 25-year experience at the National Cancer Institute, 1953-1978. Cancer Treat Rep 1982;66:653–65.

43. Grufferman S, Delzell E. Epidemiology of Hodgkin's disease. Epidemiol Rev 1984;6:76–106.

44. Gupta RK, Norton AJ, Thompson IW, Lister TA, Bodmer JG. p53 expression in Reed-Sternberg cells of Hodgkin's disease. Br J Cancer 1992;66:649–52.

45. Gutensohn N, Cole P. Epidemiology of Hodgkin's disease in the young. Int J Cancer 1977;19:595–604.

46. _____, Cole P. Childhood social environment and Hodgkin's disease. N Engl J Med 1981;304:135–40.

47. _____, Li FP, Johnson RE, Cole P. Hodgkin's disease, tonsillectomy and family size. N Engl J Med 1975;292:22–5.

48. Herndier BG, Sanchez HC, Chang KL, Chen YY, Weiss LM. High prevalence of Epstein-Barr virus in the Reed-Sternberg cells of HIV-associated Hodgkin's disease. Am J Pathol 1993;142:1073–9.

49. Hsu SM, Yang K, Jaffe ES. Phenotypic expression of Hodgkin's and Reed-Sternberg cells in Hodgkin's disease. Am J Pathol 1985;118:209–17.

50. Jackson H Jr, Parker F Jr. Hodgkin's disease. I. General considerations. N Engl J Med 1944;230:1–8.

51. Jarrett RF, Gallagher A, Jones DB, et al. Detection of Epstein-Barr virus genomes in Hodgkin's disease: relation to age. J Clin Pathol 1991;44:844–8.

52. Jones RJ, Piantadosi S, Mann RB, et al. High-dose cytotoxic therapy and bone marrow transplantation for relapsed Hodgkin's disease. J Clin Oncol 1990;8:527–37.

53. Kadin ME, Donaldson SS, Dorfman RF. Isolated granulomas in Hodgkin's disease. N Engl J Med 1970;283:859–61.

54. _____, Glatstein E, Dorfman RF. Clinicopathologic studies of 117 untreated patients subjected to laparotomy for the staging of Hodgkin's disease. Cancer 1971;27:1277–94.

55. _____, Muramoto L, Said J. Expression of T-cell antigens on Reed-Sternberg cells in a subset of patients with nodular sclerosing and mixed cellularity Hodgkin's disease. Am J Pathol 1988;130:345–53.

56. _____, Stites DP, Levy R, Warnke R. Exogenous immunoglobulin and the macrophage origin of Reed-Sternberg cells in Hodgkin's disease. N Engl J Med 1978;299:1208–14.

57. Kant JA, Hubbard SM, Longo DL, Simon RM, DeVita VT, Jaffe ES. The pathologic and clinical heterogeneity of lymphocyte-depleted Hodgkin's disease. J Clin Oncol 1986;4:284–94.

58. Kaplan HS. Hodgkin's disease. 2nd ed. Cambridge: Harvard University Press, 1980.

59. Kissmeyer-Nielsen F, Kjerbye KE, Lamm LU. HL-A in Hodgkin's disease. III. A prospective study. Transplant Rev 1975;22:168–74.

60. Krikorian JG, Burke JS, Rosenberg SA, Kaplan HS. Occurrence of non-Hodgkin's lymphoma after therapy for Hodgkin's disease. N Engl J Med 1979;300:452–8.

61. LeBrun DP, Ngan BY, Weiss LM, Huie P, Warnke RA, Cleary ML. The bcl-2 oncogene in Hodgkin's disease arising in the setting of follicular non-Hodgkin's lymphoma. Blood 1994;83:223–30.

62. Leoncini L, del Vecchio MT, Kraft R, et al. Hodgkin's disease and CD30-positive anaplastic large cell lymphomas–a continuous spectrum of malignant disorders. A quantitive morphometric and immunohistologic study. Am J Pathol 1990;137:1047–57.

63. Leshan L, Marvin S, Lyerly O. Some evidence of a relationship between Hodgkin's disease and intelligence. Arch Gen Psychiat 1959;1:477–9.

64. Leslie KO, Colby TV. Hepatic parenchymal lymphoid aggregates in Hodgkin's disease. Hum Pathol 1984; 15:808–9.

65. Levy R, Kaplan HS. Impaired lymphocyte function in untreated Hodgkin's disease. N Eng J Med 1974;290:181–6.

66. Limpens J, de Jong D, van Krieken JH, et al. Bcl-2/JH rearrangements in benign lymphoid tissues with follicular hyperplasia. Oncogene 1991;6:2271–6.

67. Lister TA, Crowther D, Sutcliffe SB, et al. Report of a committee convened to discuss the evaluation and staging of patients with Hodgkin's disease: Cotswolds meeting. J Clin Oncol 1989;7:1630–6.

68. Longo DL, Young RC, Wesley M, et al. Twenty years of MOPP therapy for Hodgkin's disease. J Clin Oncol 1986;4:1295–306.

69. Louie DC, Kant JA, Brooks JJ, Reed JC. Absence of t(14;18) major and minor breakpoints and of bcl-2 protein overproduction in Reed-Sternberg cells of Hodgkin's disease. Am J Pathol 1991;139:1231–7.

70. Lukes RJ. Criteria for involvement of lymph node, bone marrow, spleen, and liver in Hodgkin's disease. Cancer Res 1971;31:1755–67.

71. _____, Craver LF, Hall TC, Rappaport H, Rubin P. Report of the nomenclature committee. Cancer Res 1966;26:1311.

72. _____, Butler JJ. The pathology and nomenclature of Hodgkin's disease. Cancer Res 1966;26:1063–83.

73. _____, Butler JJ, Hicks EB. Natural history of Hodgkin's disease as related to its pathologic picture. Cancer 1966;19:317–44.

74. MacLennan KA, Bennett MH, Tu A, et al. Relationship of histopathologic features to survival and relapse in nodular sclerosing Hodgkin's disease. A study of 1659 patients. Cancer 1989;64:1686–93.

75. MacMahon B. Epidemiological evidence on the nature of Hodgkin's disease. Cancer 1957;10:1045–54.

76. _____. Epidemiology of Hodgkin's disease. Cancer Res 1966;26:1189–200.

77. Macon WR, Williams ME, Greer JP, Stein RS, Collins RD, Cousar JB. T-cell-rich B-cell lymphomas. A clinicopathologic study of 19 cases. Am J Surg Pathol 1992;16:351–63.

78. Mason DY, Banks PM, Chan J, et al. Nodular lymphocyte predominance Hodgkin's disease. A distinct clinicopathological entity. Am J Surg Pathol 1994;18:526–30.

79. Medeiros LJ, Weiss LM, Warnke RA, Dorfman RF. Utility of combining antigranulocyte with antileukocyte antibodies in differentiating Hodgkin's disease from non-Hodgkin's lymphoma. Cancer 1988;62:2475–81.

80. Mohrmann RL, Nathwani BN, Brynes RK, Sheibani K. Hodgkin's disease occurring in monocytoid B-cell clusters. Am J Clin Pathol 1991;95:802–8.

81. Möller P. Peanut lectin: a useful tool for detecting Hodgkin cells in paraffin sections. Virchows Arch [A] 1982;396:313–7.

82. Momose H, Jaffe ES, Shin SS, Chen YY, Weiss LM. Chronic lymphocytic leukemia/small lymphocytic lymphocytic lymphoma with Reed-Sternberg-like cells and possible transformation to Hodgkin's disease. Mediation by Epstein-Barr virus. Am J Surg Pathol 1992;16:859–67.

83. Mueller N, Evans A, Harris NL, et al. Hodgkin's disease and Epstein-Barr virus. Altered antibody pattern before diagnosis. N Engl J Med 1989;320:689–95.

84. Neiman RS, Rosen PJ, Lukes RJ. Lymphocyte-depletion Hodgkin's disease. A clinicopathological entity. N Engl J Med 1973;288:751–5.

85. O'Grady JT, Stewart S, Lowrey J, Howie SE, Krajewski AS. CD40 expression in Hodgkin's disease. Am J Pathol 1994;144:21–6.

86. Osborne BM, Uthman MO, Butler JJ, McLaughlin P. Differentiation of T-cell lymphoma from Hodgkin's disease. Mitotic rate and S-phase analysis. Am J Clin Pathol 1990;93:227–32.

87. Pallesen G, Hamilton-Dutoit SJ, Rowe M, Young LS. Expression of Epstein-Barr virus latent gene products in tumour cells of Hodgkin's disease. Lancet 1991;337:320–2.

88. Pinkus GS, Barbuto D, Said JW, Churchill WH. Lymphocyte subpopulations of lymph nodes and spleens in Hodgkin's disease. Cancer 1978;42:1270–9.

89. _____, Thomas P, Said JW. Leu-M1–a marker for Reed-Sternberg cells in Hodgkin's disease. An immunoperoxidase study of paraffin-embedded tissues. Am J Pathol 1985;119:244–52.

90. Pizzolo G, Vinante F, Chilosi M, et al. Serum levels of soluble CD30 molecule (Ki-1 antigen) in Hodgkin's disease: relationship with disease activity and clinical stage. Br J Haematol 1990;75:282–4.

91. Poppema S, Kaleta J, Hepperle B. Chromosomal abnormalities in patients with Hodgkin's disease. Evidence for frequent involvement of the 14q chromosomal region but infrequent bcl-2 gene rearrangement in Reed-Sternberg cells. JNCI 1992;84:1789–93.

92. Pražák J, Hermanská Z. Study of HLA antigens in patients with Hodgkin's disease. Eur J Haematol 1989;43:50–3.

93. Rappaport H, Berard CW, Butler JJ, Dorfman RF, Lukes RJ, Thomas LB. Report of the Committee on Histopathological Criteria Contributing to Staging of Hodgkin's Disease. Cancer Res 1971;31:1864–5.

94. Robinson E. The occurrence of malignant lymphoma in Israel. Harefuah 1966;71:339–40.

95. Rowley JD. Chromosomes in Hodgkin's disease. Cancer Treat Rep 1982;66:639–43.

96. Sacks EL, Donaldson SS, Gordon J, Dorfman RF. Epithelioid granulomas associated with Hodgkin's disease. Clinical correlations in 55 previously untreated patients. Cancer 1978;41:562–7.

97. Sarker AB, Akagi T, Jeon HJ, et al. Bauhinia purpurea—a new paraffin section marker for Reed-Sternberg cells of Hodgkin's disease. A comparison with Leu-M1 (CD15), LN2 (CD74), peanut agglutinin, and Ber-H2 (CD30). Am J Pathol 1992;141:19–23.

98. Schmid C, Pan L, Diss T, Isaacson PG. Expression of B-cell antigens by Hodgkin's and Reed-Sternberg cells in Hodgkin's disease. Am J Pathol 1991;139:701–7.

99. Schoeppel SL, Hoppe RT, Dorfman RF, et al. Hodgkin's disease in homosexual men with generalized lymphadenopathy. Ann Intern Med 1985;102:68–70.

100. Sheibani K, Battifora H, Burke JS, Rappaport H. Leu-M1 antigen in human neoplasms. An immunohistologic study of 400 cases. Am J Surg Pathol 1986;10:227–36.

101. Sherrod AE, Felder B, Levy N, et al. Immunohistologic identification of phenotypic antigens associated wtih Hodgkin and Reed-Sternberg cells. A paraffin section study. Cancer 1986;57:2135–40.

102. Shin SS, Berry GJ, Weiss LM. Infectious mononucleosis. Diagnosis by in situ hybridization in two cases with atypical features. Am J Surg Pathol 1991;15:625–31.

103. Stetler-Stevenson M, Crush-Stanton S, Cossman J. Involvement of the bcl-2 gene in Hodgkin's disease. J Natl Cancer Inst 1990;82:855–8.

104. Strauchen JA, Dimitriu-Bona A. Immunopathology of Hodgkin's disease. Characterization of Reed-Sternberg cells with monoclonal antibodies. Am J Pathol 1986;123:293–300.

105. Straus DJ, Gaynor JJ, Myers J, et al. Prognostic factors among 185 adults with newly diagnosed advanced Hodgkin's disase treated with alternating potentially noncross-resistant chemotherapy and intermediate-dose radiation therapy. J Clin Oncol 1990;8:1173–86.

106. Strickler JG, Michie SA, Warnke RA, Dorfman RF. The "syncytial variant" of nodular sclerosing Hodgkin's disease. Am J Surg Pathol 1986;10:470–7.

107. _____, Weiss LM, Copenhaver CM, et al. Monoclonal antibodies reactive in routinely processed tissue sections of malignant lymphoma, with emphasis on T-cell lymphomas. Hum Pathol 1987;18:808–14.

108. Strum SB, Rappaport H. Interrelations of the histologic types of Hodgkin's disease. Arch Pathol 1971;91:127–34.

109. Sundeen J, Lipford E, Uppenkamp M, et al. Rearranged antigen receptor genes in Hodgkin's disease. Blood 1987;70:96–103.

110. Swerdlow AJ, Douglas AJ, Hodson GV, et al. Risk of second primary cancers after Hodgkin's disease by type of treatment: analysis of 2846 patients in the British National Lymphoma Investigation. Brit Med J. 1992;304:1137–43.

111. Taylor CR. The nature of Reed-Sternberg cells and other malignant "reticulum" cells. Lancet 1974;2:802–7.

112. Thangavelu M, Le Beau MM. Chromosomal abnormalities in Hodgkin's disase. Hematol Oncol Clin North Am 1989;3:221–36.

113. Tilly H, Bastard C, Delastre T, et al. Cytogenetic studies in untreated Hodgkin's disease. Blood 1991;77:1298–304.

114. Torelli G, Marasca R, Luppi M, et al. Human herpesvirus-6 in human lymphomas: identification of specific sequences in Hodgkin's lymphomas by polymerase chain reaction. Blood 1991;77:2251–8.

115. Trumper LH, Brady G, Bagg A, et al. Single-cell analysis of Hodgkin's and Reed-Sternberg cells: molecular heterogeneity of gene expression and p53 mutations. Blood 1993;81:3097–115.

116. Tucker MA, Coleman CN, Cox RS, et al. Risk of second cancers after treatment for Hodgkin's disease. N Engl J Med 1988;318:76–81.

117. Ultmann JE, Moran EM. Clinical course and complications in Hodgkin's disease. Arch Intern Med 1973;131:332–53.

118. Urba WJ, Longo DL. Hodgkin's disease. N Engl J Med 1992;326:678–87.

119. Variakojis D, Strum SB, Rappaport H. The foamy macrophages in Hodgkin's disease. Arch Pathol 1972;93:453–6.

120. Weinshel EL, Peterson BA. Hodgkin's disease. Ca Cancer J Clin 1993;43:327–46.

121. Weiss LM, Arber DA, Chang KL. CD45: a review. Appl Immunohistochem 1993;1:166–181.

122. _____, Chang KL. Molecular biologic studies of Hodgkin's disease. Semin Diagn Pathol 1992;9:272–8.

123. _____, Chen YY, Liu XF, Shibata D. Epstein-Barr virus and Hodgkin's disease. A correlative in situ hybridization and polymerase chain reaction study. Am J Pathol 1991;139:1259–65.

124. _____, Strickler JG, Hu E, Warnke RA, Sklar J. Immunoglobulin gene rearrangements in Hodgkin's disease. Hum Pathol 1986;17:1009–14.

125. _____, Warnke RA, Sklar J. Clonal antigen receptor gene rearrangements and Epstein-Barr viral DNA in tissues of Hodgkin's disease. Hematol Oncol 1988;6:233–8.

126. _____, Warnke RA, Sklar J, Cleary ML. Molecular analysis of the t(14;18) chromosomal translocation in malignant lymphomas. N Engl J Med 1987;317:1185–9.

127. Westling P. Studies of the prognosis in Hodgkin's disease. Acta Radiol. 1965;245(Suppl.):5–125.

128. Wieczorek R, Burke JS, Knowles DM II. Leu-M1 antigen expression in T-cell neoplasia. Am J Pathol 1985;121:374–80.

129. World Health Organization. Mortality from Hodgkin's disease and from leukaemia and aleukaemia. WHO Epidemiol and Vital Statist Rep 1955;8:81–114.

130. Zukerberg LR, Collins AB, Ferry JA, Harris NL. Coexpression of CD15 and CD20 by Reed-Sternberg cells in Hodgkin's disease. Am J Pathol 1991;139:475–83.

15

NODULAR LYMPHOCYTE PREDOMINANCE (L&H) HODGKIN'S DISEASE (NODULAR PARAGRANULOMA)

Definition. Nodular lymphocyte predominance (lymphocytic and histiocytic/L&H) Hodgkin's disease (NLPHD) is a nodular proliferation of small lymphocytes, histiocytes, and characteristic large cells with multilobated nuclei, termed L&H cells. There is a strong trend not to require the presence of diagnostic Reed-Sternberg cells for the diagnosis, as it is doubtful if they or other Hodgkin's cells, as defined in chapter 14, truly occur in this disease (25,49). It has not been definitively established whether nodular lymphocyte predominance represents a true neoplasm or a peculiar reactive process. This entity is also known as nodular paragranuloma.

Incidence. Nodular lymphocyte predominance accounts for approximately 2 to 6 percent of cases of Hodgkin's disease (20,23). There is a male to female ratio of approximately 2.5 to 1 (17,36). It occurs in all age groups, with a peak in the fourth decade of life. This peak is due to an increase in the frequency in men between the ages of 30 and 40 years, while the incidence in females is about the same in all age groups (36). With the exception of progressive transformation of germinal centers, there are no known associated lesions or diseases (17). There is no predilection for nodular lymphocyte predominance for any particular occupational group.

Natural History and Clinical Features. Patients usually present with isolated lymphadenopathy of long duration. In approximately two thirds of patients, the lymphadenopathy is present for greater than 3 months; in about 5 percent of patients, it has been present for greater than 10 years (17). Occasionally, there is a history of prior reactive follicular hyperplasia, often with progressive transformation of germinal centers (4,35). However, there is no definite evidence that the presence of progressive transformation of germinal centers in a lymph node biopsy predisposes to subsequent development of NLPHD (29). Cervical, axillary, and inguinal lymph nodes are most often involved, para-aortic and iliac lymph nodes are sometimes involved, while mediastinal or mesenteric lymph nodes are rarely involved

(17,36). B symptoms are uncommon. Approximately 50 percent of patients are Ann Arbor stage I at diagnosis, 20 percent are stage II, 20 percent are stage III, and 10 percent are stage IV. Splenic involvement is seen in about 15 percent of patients and liver involvement in about 10 percent. Bone marrow involvement or involvement of other visceral organs is rare. The erythrocyte sedimentation rate is elevated in 43 percent of patients, but other laboratory tests are usually normal.

Several studies have found that patients with NLPHD generally have a very slow disease course, irrespective of treatment (17,37). Patients tend to have single or multiple relapses, independent of stage or treatment and equally distributed up to 10 years after initial therapy, unusual behavior for classic Hodgkin's disease (37,38). Other investigations have found no significant differences between the natural history of this entity and classic Hodgkin's disease (3).

Relapses are usually local or regional, but in one third of patients, the relapse is nonregional or the disease is generalized (17). There is no correlation between treatment and site of recurrence. In addition, patients may develop lymphadenopathy with histologic features of progressive transformation of germinal centers, with or without evidence of coexisting NLPHD (4,35).

Transformation into another subtype of Hodgkin's disease has been reported, but there is a greater tendency (1 to 10 percent of cases) for transformation to a B-, or much less commonly, T- lineage non-Hodgkin's lymphoma of large cell type (16,26). Some lymphomas may coexist with nodular lymphocyte predominance (5,43); in one study, there was a predilection for the axillary lymph nodes, a high rate of occurrence in blacks, and an excellent survival without development of disseminated disease (43).

Histologic Findings. The diagnosis of NLPHD is established by the identification of the characteristic L&H cells in the background of a nodular proliferation of small lymphocytes and histiocytes (22,23,35). L&H cells are large, with large nuclei and usually scant cytoplasm (fig. 15-1). The nuclei

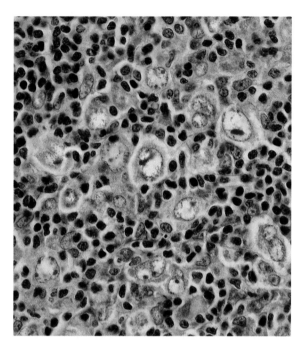

Figure 15-1
NODULAR LYMPHOCYTE PREDOMINANCE (L&H)
Numerous L&H cells are seen in this field.

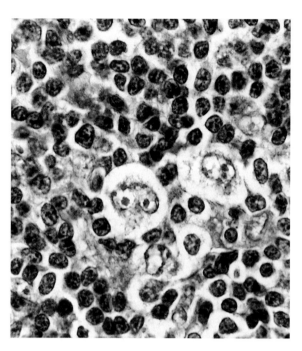

Figure 15-3
NODULAR LYMPHOCYTE PREDOMINANCE (L&H)
A cell resembling a diagnostic Reed-Sternberg cell is seen.

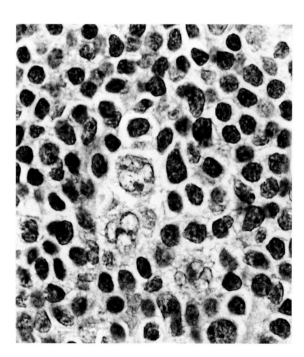

Figure 15-2
NODULAR LYMPHOCYTE PREDOMINANCE (L&H)
Three L&H cells with highly irregular nuclear contours
are seen in a background of small lymphocytes.

are often multilobated, often to such an extreme that they also have been termed "popcorn" cells (fig. 15-2). The chromatin is usually vesicular, with a thin nuclear envelope; the nucleoli are generally medium sized, and smaller than those seen in the Reed-Sternberg cell variants of other types of Hodgkin's disease. Some L&H cells may be multinucleated and may contain large nucleoli; it is these cells that can closely simulate or be indistinguishable from the diagnostic Reed-Sternberg cells of classic Hodgkin's disease (fig. 15-3).

At low magnification, the lymph node architecture usually shows focal obliteration, with a rim of uninvolved or hyperplastic lymphoid tissue. Occasionally, reactive follicular hyperplasia with progressive transformation of germinal centers is seen adjacent to the lesion. Large nodules are found within the involved areas, usually larger than the follicles seen in benign lymph node cortex or follicular lymphoma (fig. 15-4). A reticulin stain is useful in demonstrating the nodularity by showing compression of the reticulin in the internodular areas; however, portions of the lesion may show diffuse architectural

Figure 15-4
NODULAR LYMPHOCYTE PREDOMINANCE (L&H)
Nodules larger than those typically seen in follicular lymphoma are present.

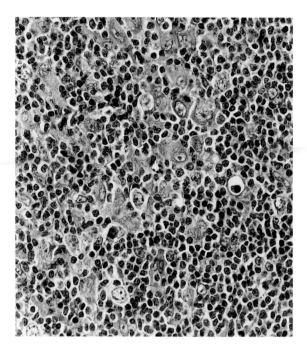

Figure 15-5
NODULAR LYMPHOCYTE PREDOMINANCE (L&H)
The characteristic background of small lymphocytes and epithelioid histiocytes is seen.

effacement. The nodules are composed of a mixture of small lymphocytes, epithelioid histiocytes, and L&H cells, with small lymphocytes generally predominating (fig. 15-5). This mixture of cell types can impart a mottled appearance to the nodules. The proportion of epithelioid histiocytes and L&H cells within the nodules varies from case to case and may even vary from nodule to nodule within the same case; occasionally, large numbers of L&H cells may be present (fig. 15-6). Rarely, polykaryocytes are found. Eosinophils, neutrophils, and plasma cells are uncommon within the nodules. Epithelioid histiocytes and L&H cells may also be found at the margins of the nodules; the former may be prominent enough to create a "wreath" around the nodules (fig. 15-7). The intervening paracortex is often compressed, and is composed primarily of small lymphocytes with scattered plasma cells; eosinophils and neutrophils are generally sparse throughout the lymph node.

Occasional cases may show minimal or absent nodularity at low magnification, and have been termed *diffuse lymphocyte predominance (L&H)* or *diffuse paragranuloma* by some (fig. 15-8) (15,

28). These cases lack typical Hodgkin's cells, but possess L&H cells with their characteristic phenotype (see below), and often occur in patients with a previous history of NLPHD. Although the clinical behavior of these cases may be similar to that of NLPHD, clinical studies have not yet been reported.

Immunologic Findings. L&H cells show a characteristic phenotype distinct from the Hodgkin's cells of classic Hodgkin's disease (6,8,10, 14,30,31,45). They have numerous features consistent with a B-cell lineage and express the pan-B markers CD19, CD20, CD22, CD74, CDw75, and CD45RA (fig. 15-9). In contrast to Hodgkin's cells, L&H cells are positive for leukocyte common antigen (CD45RB) (fig. 15-10). They lack most T-lineage markers, but one study reported expression of cytoplasmic CD3 in three of nine cases (7). The L&H cells may express CD30 or epithelial membrane antigen (6,42). They generally lack CD15 expression, although positivity may be obtained after pretreatment with neuraminidase (18).

The expression of immunoglobulin by L&H cells is controversial. Although J chain, a protein associated with immunoglobulin synthesis, can

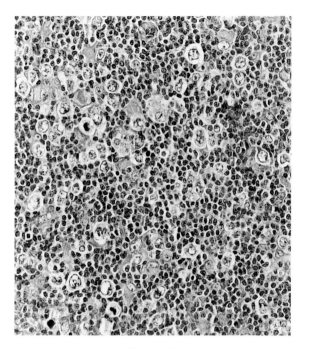

Figure 15-6
NODULAR LYMPHOCYTE PREDOMINANCE (L&H)
Large numbers of L&H cells are present in this case.

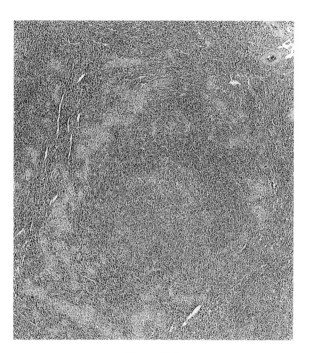

Figure 15-7
NODULAR LYMPHOCYTE PREDOMINANCE (L&H)
A "wreath" of epithelioid histiocytes is seen around this nodule.

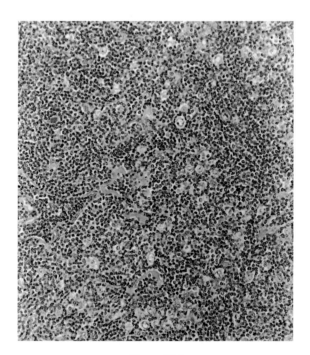

Figure 15-8
DIFFUSE LYMPHOCYTE PREDOMINANCE (L&H)
Although a vague nodularity may be still appreciated, a diffuse scattering of L&H cells is seen.

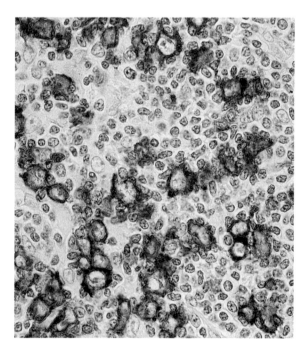

Figure 15-9
NODULAR LYMPHOCYTE PREDOMINANCE (L&H)
Positivity of the L&H cells for CD20 is seen.

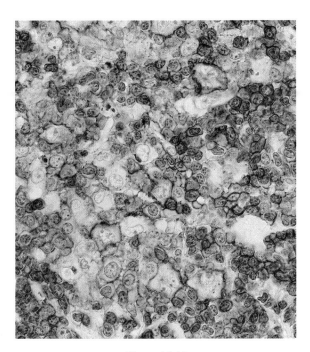

Figure 15-10
NODULAR LYMPHOCYTE PREDOMINANCE (L&H)
Positivity of the L&H cells for CD45RB is seen.

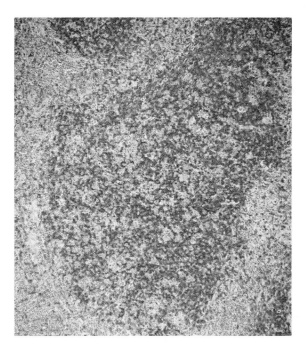

Figure 15-11
NODULAR LYMPHOCYTE PREDOMINANCE (L&H)
The nodules are composed primarily of B lymphocytes.

be demonstrated (41,42,25), most investigators have not found clear expression of immunoglobulin heavy or light chains (27,30,42). One group has claimed a polyclonal or multiclonal pattern of light chain expression (34,45) while another has found exclusively kappa light chain restriction (41); however, two studies have failed to demonstrate evidence of light chain mRNA expression within the L&H cells (27,39). One study found expression of IgD immunoglobulin heavy chain in the L&H cells (45).

Most small lymphocytes within the nodules are mature B lymphocytes, and are polyclonal (fig. 15-11) (8,34,45). They express membrane IgM and IgD, identical to the B lymphocytes of the mantle zone of normal follicles. In addition, the nodules contain numerous follicular dendritic cells, as indicated by staining for CD21, CD35, and a monoclonal antibody specific for follicular dendritic cells, R4/23, implying that the nodules represent altered germinal centers (1,34,45). However, in contrast to normal germinal centers, the follicular dendritic cell processes are more separated, and surround L&H cells and epithelioid histiocytes (2). Scattered T cells can also be identified in the nodules; they are usually of

helper phenotype. In addition to possessing the normal pan-T markers, many T cells expressing CD57 can be identified, particularly those T cells that appear to "rosette" around L&H cells (fig. 5-12) (19,33,45). The function of this cell population in this disease is not clear. Normal CD57-expressing T cells are present in the light zones of germinal centers, suggesting that they play a role in B-cell differentiation toward memory cells (32).

In diffuse lymphocyte predominance, the antigen profile for the L&H cells is identical to that seen in the nodular variant, with expression of leukocyte common antigen and B-lineage markers, and absence of CD15 expression. The two variants differ in pattern of follicular dendritic cells (15). Whereas follicular dendritic cells are arranged in sharply defined meshworks in the follicles in the nodular variant, they are either absent or present in a diffuse, ill-defined meshwork, usually of small size, in the diffuse variant. In addition, more T cells and fewer B cells are present in the diffuse variant.

Molecular and Cytogenetic Findings. Cases of NLPHD lack evidence of either clonal immunoglobulin gene rearrangements or *bcl*-2 rearrangements by Southern blot and polymerase chain

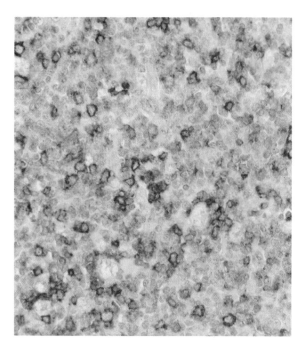

Figure 15-12
NODULAR LYMPHOCYTE PREDOMINANCE (L&H)
Many of the small lymphocytes within the nodules are positive for CD57. Note the "wreath" of CD57-positive cells present around the L&H cells.

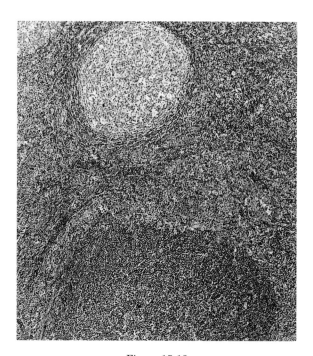

Figure 15-13
PROGRESSIVE TRANSFORMATION
OF GERMINAL CENTERS
A reactive follicle is seen at top, while a progressively transformed follicle is seen at bottom.

reaction studies (21,40,47,48). There have been no extensive cytogenetic studies of NLPHD. Most cases studied to date lack evidence of the Epstein-Barr viral genome within the L&H cells (46).

Differential Diagnosis. *Progressive Transformation of Germinal Centers (PTGC).* This is a pattern of reactive follicular hyperplasia in which occasional secondary follicles become larger, the borderline between the germinal center and the lymphocytes of the mantle zone becomes indefinable, and germinal center cells become fewer, resulting in the formation of large nodules of small lymphocytes scattered among other reactive secondary follicles (fig. 15-13). It most frequently occurs in young males presenting with an asymptomatic, solitary, enlarged lymph node (11,29). The progressively transformed germinal centers are usually found in lymph nodes having florid reactive hyperplasia; architectural effacement is not seen. This is in contrast to nodular lymphocyte predominance in which there is at least focal architectural effacement by the nodules. The most crucial distinction between the two lesions, however, is in the

definitive identification of the characteristic L&H cells in NLPHD. A lymph node showing all the characteristic features of nodular lymphocyte predominance, yet lacking L&H cells, should be regarded as suspicious for, but not diagnostic of, NLPHD. In addition, a lymph node showing all the characteristic features of progressive transformation of germinal centers, yet having one or more nodules containing L&H cells should be regarded as progressive transformation of germinal centers with probable coexisting nodular lymphocyte predominance. Immunostaining for CD20 may be useful in highlighting the L&H cells, but they should be distinguished from B immunoblasts, which also stain for CD20.

Classic Hodgkin's Disease. Many cases of classic Hodgkin's disease have a vaguely nodular pattern, and this may even be a prominent finding in the cellular phase of nodular sclerosis. Conversely, some cases of lymphocyte predominance may have only a focal nodular appearance or may lack nodularity completely (diffuse lymphocyte predominance). Thus, the key distinguishing feature between lymphocyte predominance (L&H) and classic Hodgkin's disease is the character of the atypical cells: L&H cells in the former and classic Hodgkin's cells in the latter. L&H cells usually have less prominent nucleoli, thinner nuclear envelopes, and less cytoplasm than classic Hodgkin's cells. However, some L&H cells closely resemble Hodgkin's cells, and rare cells resemble Reed-Sternberg cells. This has led to confusion between the two diseases for many years. In addition, lacunar variants may lack prominent nucleoli and thick nuclear envelopes, and the retraction of their cytoplasm may preclude evaluation of the amount of the cytoplasm, thus simulating L&H cells. If more than rare cells approximating classic Hodgkin's cells are identified in a lymph node biopsy, the diagnosis of lymphocyte predominance (L&H) should be questioned.

Because of the immunophenotypic differences between L&H cells and other Hodgkin's cells, immunohistochemistry may be essential for accurate diagnosis in borderline cases. The use of paraffin-reactive antibodies directed against CD45RB (leukocyte common antigen), CD15 antigen, and a B- and T-lineage–associated marker (e.g., CD20 and CD43) should resolve most diagnostic problems. L&H cells are usually CD45RB+, CD15-, CD20+, and CD43-, while classic Hodgkin cells are usually CD45RB-, CD15+, CD20-, and CD43-. Exceptions to typical staining patterns occur; therefore, it is important to rely on the results of a battery of stains rather than one single antibody. The most common overlap in the staining profile of these two entities is the expression of CD20 by classic Hodgkin's cells in about 10 to 20 percent of cases. In this circumstance, the addition of B-cell marker CD45RA may be useful. A positive reaction in the large atypical cells strongly favors NLPHD, although the absence of reactivity does not rule this out since this marker is less sensitive in detecting B-lineage cells (12). CD57 reactivity of small lymphocytes may also help to distinguish NLPHD from classic Hodgkin's disease, as numerous CD57 lymphocytes are usually found in the nodules of the former disease, often ringing the L&H cells, while they are infrequent in the latter (19).

Rare cases in which classic Hodgkin's disease has either predated, followed, or coexisted with lesions histologically typical of NLPHD have been reported (12,16,26). In these cases, the morphologic features were typical for each disease at each site, with the exception of one biopsy in which cells with features of classic Hodgkin's cells and L&H cells coexisted (fig. 17-8). Phenotypic profiles remained distinct for all cases studied. These cases suggest that there may still be some histogenetic relationship between NLPHD and classic Hodgkin's disease.

Follicular Lymphoma. The age of the patient may be helpful in distinguishing this and NLPHD, since follicular lymphoma is rare under the age of 30 years. In follicular lymphoma, the lymph node architecture usually shows complete obliteration by a nodular process, while in NLPHD there is often a rim of uninvolved cortex. In addition, the nodules of follicular lymphoma are generally smaller than those of NLPHD. The floral variant of follicular lymphoma (see chapter 6) may be confused with NLPHD, since it may contain large, irregularly shaped follicles closely resembling the nodules of NLPHD or PTGC (13). In addition, the follicles may sometimes contain occasional pleomorphic large cells. However, the nodules in NLPHD are still almost always larger than those in the floral variant of follicular lymphoma. Cytologically, the nodules of follicular lymphoma, including the floral variant, are composed predominantly of atypical cells, and not the small, regular lymphocytes that are found within the nodules of NLPHD. In difficult cases, immunohistochemical studies may be of use, as more CD57-positive cells are seen in nodular lymphocyte predominance (19).

Large Cell Lymphoma. Some cases of NLPHD may contain large numbers of L&H cells, even to the extent of forming clusters. When the large, atypical cells form sheets, especially outside the nodules, transformation to large cell lymphoma may have occurred (fig. 15-14). However, it is not clear from the literature whether these cases of large cell lymphoma behave like ordinary intermediate grade non-Hodgkin's lymphoma; the available data suggests that the prognosis of large cell lymphoma arising in a background of nodular L&H Hodgkin's disease may be quite good (43). These large cell lymphomas are usually of B-cell type, lack *bcl*-2 expression, and are EBV negative (14). Rare lymphomas of T-cell type have also been seen complicating nodular lymphocyte predominance.

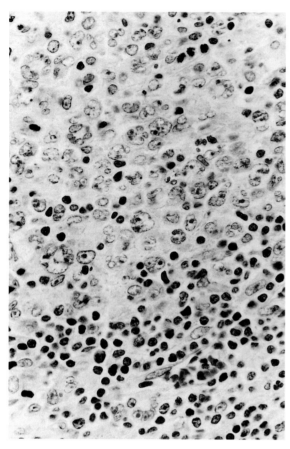

Figure 15-14
NODULAR LYMPHOCYTE PREDOMINANCE (L&H)
IN TRANSITION TO DIFFUSE
LARGE CELL LYMPHOMA

In this case, sheets of L&H cells are present in the internodular areas, indicating transition to diffuse large cell lymphoma.

Histiocyte- and T-Cell–Rich B-Cell Lymphoma. Delabie and colleagues (9) described a series of lymphoma cases called histiocyte-rich B-cell lymphoma in which the prominent reactive histiocytic component obscured the malignant B-cell population. The involved lymph nodes showed a mixed nodular and diffuse effacement by an infiltrate composed of reactive lymphocytes and numerous histiocytes obscuring a tumor population composed of variably sized scattered cells with irregular or multilobated vesicular nuclei. The histiocytes were generally nonepithelioid, in contrast to the frequent epithelioid histiocytes in nodular lymphocyte predominance. All presented with stage IVB disease with splenomegaly, and followed an aggressive

clinical course, although the age and sex distribution and the propensity to progress to a diffuse large cell lymphoma were similar to nodular lymphocyte predominance. Hansmann and colleagues (17) have noted a poor outcome for patients with nodular lymphocyte predominance in stage IV or with splenic involvement. At this time, it is not clear whether there is a relationship between histiocyte-rich B-cell lymphoma and nodular lymphocyte predominance; it is likely that in the past at least some cases were diagnosed as high-stage NLPHD.

T-cell–rich B-cell lymphomas are unusual non-Hodgkin's lymphomas that show diffuse effacement by an infiltrate with a predominance of reactive T cells and a minority of neoplastic B cells (24). Although these lymphomas are more commonly confused with peripheral T-cell lymphoma and other types of Hodgkin's disease, some cases mimic diffuse lymphocyte predominance. The complete absence of nodularity and the presence of clustering of tumor cells into small groups in a case otherwise suspicious for lymphocyte predominance should raise concern for T-cell–rich B-cell lymphoma. Immunophenotypic studies may be useful in distinguishing the two. Although the large atypical cells may share an identical phenotype, greater numbers of CD57-positive cells are found in NLPHD, often forming a ring around the L&H cells. Molecular studies are also useful for diagnosis: for example, it has been shown that cases of T-cell–rich B-cell lymphoma generally have detectable immunoglobulin gene rearrangements (24).

Treatment. Since cases of nodular lymphocyte predominance Hodgkin's disease have historically been included in clinical trials of classic Hodgkin's disease, it is not clear what the proper treatment should be. Lymphocyte predominance treated by standard Hodgkin's disease therapies tends to relapse, and the site of relapse is independent of treatment type (17,37). Anecdotal observation of untreated cases suggests that aggressive treatment may not be necessary, particularly for patients with low-stage disease.

Prognosis. The overall prognosis for patients with NLPHD is excellent, despite the frequent relapses. Patients with stage I to III disease without splenic involvement have about the same probability of survival as the general population (17). Patients with higher stage disease, including those with splenic involvement, have a worse prognosis. There is about a 60 percent survival for stage IV patients; death usually occurs within the first year after diagnosis. The probability of survival decreases with increasing age. While some studies have shown that, within the category of lymphocyte predominance, the presence of a nodular architecture is a significant predictor of relapse-free survival (37), this has not been seen in other studies (3,44).

REFERENCES

1. Abdulaziz Z, Mason DY, Stein H, Gatter KC, Nash JR. An immunohistological study of the cellular constituents of Hodgkin's disease using a monoclonal antibody panel. Histopathology 1984;8:1–25.
2. Alavaikko MJ, Hansmann ML, Nebendahl C, Parwaresch MR, Lennert K. Follicular dendritic cells in Hodgkin's disease. Am J Clin Pathol 1991;95:194–200.
3. Borg-Grech A, Radford JA, Crowther D, Swindell R, Harris M. A comparative study of the nodular and diffuse variants of lymphocyte-predominant Hodgkin's disease. J Clin Oncol 1989;7:1303–9.
4. Burns BF, Colby TV, Dorfman RF. Differential diagnostic features of nodular L&H Hodgkin's disease, including progressive transformation of germinal centers. Am J Surg Pathol 1984;8:253–61.
5. Chittal SM, Alard C, Rossi JF, et al. Further phenotypic evidence that nodular, lymphocyte-predominant Hodgkin's disease is a large B-cell lymphoma in evolution. Am J Surg Pathol 1990;14:1024–35.
6. _____, Caverivière P, Schwarting R, et al. Monoclonal antibodies in the diagnosis of Hodgkin's disease. The search for a rational panel. Am J Surg Pathol 1988;12:9–21.
7. Cibull ML, Stein H, Gatter KC, Mason DY. The expression of the CD3 antigen in Hodgkin's disease. Histopathology 1989;15:597–605.
8. Coles FB, Cartun RW, Pastuszak WT. Hodgkin's disease, lymphocyte predominant type: immunoreactivity with B-cell antibodies. Mod Pathol 1988;1:274–8.
9. Delabie J, Vandenberghe E, Kennes C, et al. Histiocyte-rich B-cell lymphoma. A distinct clinicopathologic entity possibly related to lymphocyte predominant Hodgkin's disease, paragranuloma subtype. Am J Surg Pathol 1992;16:37–48.
10. Dorfman RF, Gatter KC, Pulford KA, Mason DY. An evaluation of the utility of anti-granulocyte and anti-leukocyte monoclonal antibodies in the diagnosis of Hodgkin's disease. Am J Pathol 1986;123:508–19.
11. Ferry JA, Zukerberg LR, Harris NL. Florid progressive transformation of germinal centers. A syndrome affecting young men, without early progression to nodular lymphocyte predominance Hodgkin's disease. Am J Surg Pathol 1992;16:252–8.
12. Gelb AB, Dorfman RF, Warnke RA. Coexistence of nodular lymphocyte predominant Hodgkin disease and Hodgkin's disease of the usual type. Am J Surg Pathol 1993;17:364–74.
13. Goates JJ, Kamel OW, LeBrun DP, Benharroch D, Dorfman RF. Floral variant of follicular lymphoma. Immunological and molecular studies support a neoplastic process. Am J Surg Pathol 1994;18:37–47.
14. Hansmann ML, Shibata D, Lorenzen J, Hell K, Nathwani BN, Fischer R. Incidence of Epstein-Barr virus, bcl-2 expression and chromosomal translocation t(14;18) in large cell lymphoma associated with paragranuloma (lymphocyte-predominant Hodgkin's disease). Hum Pathol 1994;25:240–3.
15. _____, Stein H, Dallenbach F, Fellbaum C. Diffuse lymphocyte-predominant Hodgkin's disease (diffuse paragranuloma). A variant of the B-cell-derived nodular type. Am J Pathol 1991;138:29–36.
16. _____, Stein H, Fellbaum C, Hui PK, Parwaresch MR, Lennert K. Nodular paragranuloma can transform into high-grade malignant lymphoma of B type. Hum Pathol 1989;20:1169–75.
17. _____, Zwingers T, Bske A, Lffler H, Lennert K. Clinical features of nodular paragranuloma (Hodgkin's disease, lymphocyte predominance type, nodular). J Cancer Res Clin Oncol 1984;108:321–30.
18. Hsu SM, Ho YS, Li PJ, et al. L&H variants of Reed-Sternberg cells express sialylated Leu M1 antigen. Am J Pathol 1986;122:199–203.
19. Kamel OW, Gelb, Shibuya RB, Warnke RA. Leu 7 (CD57) reactivity distinguishes nodular lymphocyte predominance Hodgkin's disease from nodular sclerosing Hodgkin's disase, T-cell-rich B-cell lymphoma and follicular lymphoma. Am J Pathol 1991;142:541–6.
20. Lennert K, Mohri N. Histologische Klassifizierung und Vorkommen des M. Hodgkin. Internist (Berl) 1974; 15:57–65.
21. Linden MD, Fishleder AJ, Katzin WE, Tubbs RR. Absence of B-cell or T-cell clonal expansion in nodular, lymphocyte predominance Hodgkin's disease. Human Pathol 1988;19:591–4.
22. Lukes RJ. Criteria for involvement of lymph node, bone marrow, spleen, and liver in Hodgkin's disease. Cancer Res 1971;31:1755–67
23. _____, Butler JJ, Hicks EB. Natural history of Hodgkin's disease as related to its pathologic picture. Cancer 1966;19:317–44.
24. Macon WR, Williams ME, Greer JP, Stein RS, Collins RD, Cousar JB. T-cell-rich B-cell lymphomas. A clinicopathologic study of 19 cases. Am J Surg Pathol 1992;16:351–63.
25. Mason DY, Banks PM, Chan J, et al. Nodular lymphocyte predominance Hodgkin's disease. A distinct clinicopathological entity Am J Surg Pathol 1994;18:526–30.
26. Miettinen M, Franssila KO, Saxén E. Hodgkin disease, lymphocytic predominance nodular. Increased risk for subsequent non-Hodgkin's lymphomas. Cancer 1983; 51:2293–300.

27. Momose H, Chen YY, Ben-Ezra J, Weiss LM. Nodular lymphocyte predominant Hodgkin's disease: study of immunoglobulin light chain protein and mRNA expression. Hum Pathol 1992;23:1115–9.

28. Nicholas DS, Harris S, Wright DH. Lymphocyte predominance Hodgkin's disease—an immunohistochemical study. Histopathology 1990;16:157–65.

29. Osborne BM, Butler JJ. Clinical implications of progressive transformation of germinal centers. Am J Surg Pathol 1984;8:725–33.

30. Pinkus GS, Said JW. Hodgkin's disease, lymphocyte predominance type, nodular–a distinct entity? Unique staining profile for L&H variants of Reed-Sternberg cells defined by monoclonal antibodies to leukocyte common antigen, granulocyte-specific antigen, and B-cell-specific antigen. Am J Pathol 1985;118:1–6.

31. _____, Said JW. Hodgkin's disease, lymphocyte predominance type, nodular–further evidence for a B cell derivation. L&H variants of Reed-Sternberg cells express L26, a pan B cell marker. Am J Pathol 1988;133:211–7.

32. Poppema S. Lymphocyte-predominance Hodgkin's disease. Int Rev Exp Pathol 1992;33:53–79.

33. _____. The nature of the lymphocytes surrounding Reed-Sternberg cells in nodular lymphocyte predominance and other types of Hodgkin's disease. Alberta Heritage Foundation for Medical Research and the Alberta Cancer Board. Am J Pathol 1989;13:351–7.

34. _____, Kaiserling E, Lennert K. Nodular paragranuloma and progressively transformed germinal centers. Ultrastructural and immunohistologic findings. Virchows Arch [Cell Pathol] 1979;31:211–25.

35. _____, Kaiserling E, Lennert K. Hodgkin's disease with lymphoctye predominance, nodular type (nodular paragranuloma) and progressively transformed germinal centers–a cytohistological study. Histopathology 1979;3:295–308.

36. _____, Kaiserling E, Lennert K. Epidemiology of nodular paragranuloma (Hodgkin's disease with lymphocytic predominance, nodular). J Cancer Res Clin Oncol 1979;95:57–63.

37. Regula DP Jr, Hoppe RT, Weiss LM. Nodular and diffuse types of lymphocyte predominance Hodgkin's disease. N Engl J Med 1988;318:214–9.

38. _____, Weiss LM, Warnke RA, Dorfman RF. Lymphocyte predominance Hodgkin's disease: a reappraisal based upon histological and immunophenotypical findings in relapsing cases. Histopathology 1987;11:1107–20.

39. Ruprai AK, Pringle, JH, Angel CA, Kind CN, Lauder I. Localization of immunoglobulin light chain mRNA expression in Hodgkin's disease by in situ hybridization. J Pathol 1991;164:37–40.

40. Said JW, Sassoon AF, Shintaku IP, Kurtin PJ, Pinkus GS. Absence of bcl-2 major breakpoint region and JH gene rearrangement in lymphocyte predominance Hodgkin's disease. Results of Southern blot analysis and polymerase chain reaction. Am J Pathol 1991;138:261–4.

41. Schmid C, Sargent C, Isaacson PG. L and H cells of nodular lymphocyte predominant Hodgkin's disease show immunoglobulin light chain restriction. Am J Pathol 1991;139:1281–9.

42. Stein H, Hansmann ML, Lennert K, Brandtzaeg P, Gatter KC, Mason DY. Reed-Sternberg and Hodgkin's cells in lymphocyte-predominant Hodgkin's disease of nodular subtype contain J chain. Am J Clin Pathol 1986;86:292–7.

43. Sundeen JT, Cossman J, Jaffe ES. Lymphocyte predominant Hodgkin's disease nodular subtype with coexistent large cell lymphoma. Histological progression or composite malignancy. Am J Surg Pathol 1988;12:599–606.

44. Tefferi A, Zellers RA, Banks PM, Therneau TM, Colgan JP. Clinical correlates of distinct immuophenotypic and histologic subcategories of lymphocyte-predominance Hodgkin's disease. J Clin Oncol 1990;8:1959–65.

45. Timens W, Visser L, Poppema S. Nodular lymphocyte predominance type of Hodgkin's disease is a germinal center lymphoma. Lab Invest 1986;54:457–61.

46. Weiss LM, Chen YY, Liu XF, Shibata D. Epstein-Barr virus and Hodgkin's disease. A correlative in situ hybridization and polymerase chain reaction study. Am J Pathol 1991;139:1259–65.

47. _____, Warnke RA, Sklar J: Clonal antigen receptor gene rearrangements and Epstein-Barr viral DNA in tissues of Hodgkin's disease. Hematol Oncol 1988;6:233–8.

48. _____, Warnke RA, Sklar J, Cleary ML. Molecular analysis of the t(14;18) chromosomal translocation in malignant lymphomas. N Engl J Med 1987;317:1185–9.

49. Wright DH. Lymphocyte predominance Hodgkin's disease [Letter]. N Engl J Med 1988;319:246.

◇ ◇ ◇

16

PLASMA CELL NEOPLASMS AND AMYLOIDOSIS

Plasma cells are terminally differentiated B lymphocytes with the ability to secrete immunoglobulins. The most common plasma cell neoplasm is multiple myeloma, which is a disseminated, monoclonal proliferation of plasma cells. This neoplasm, together with the related entities plasma cell leukemia and heavy chain disease, is dealt with in the Fascicle, Tumors of the Bone Marrow (7a). In this chapter, plasmacytoma and amyloid deposits in lymph node and spleen are discussed.

PLASMACYTOMA

Definition. Plasmacytoma is a local tumorous collection of monoclonal plasma cells. It can occur alone (*solitary plasmacytoma*) or in a setting of multiple myeloma (presence of plasmacytoma is a major criterion in the diagnosis of multiple myeloma) (8,29). In the Kiel classification, solitary plasmacytoma is considered a form of lymphoma (malignant lymphoma, plasmacytic) (31,32), but this category includes only examples occurring in lymph nodes or tonsils and composed entirely of mature plasma cells. In the British National Lymphoma Investigation classification, plasmacytoma is classified as diffuse lymphoma, plasma cell type. Three subtypes are recognized: well differentiated, plasmablastic, and pleomorphic (21). Solitary plasmacytoma may be viewed as a localized form of plasma cell neoplasm, and is associated with a much better prognosis than multiple myeloma (35); some authors, however, view solitary osseous plasmacytoma as an early form of multiple myeloma because of its high risk of subsequent dissemination (18,28,50).

Incidence. Solitary plasmacytoma is rare (5). In one series of 822 patients with plasma cell neoplasms, only 6.1 percent presented with solitary osseous and extramedullary plasmacytomas (28). In another series, 24 cases (8.3 percent) of solitary plasmacytoma were identified among 288 patients with plasma cell neoplasms (10).

Clinical Features. Solitary plasmacytoma is classified into two types, which differ in clinical features and behavior (7,8,12,15,17,30,52,53). *Solitary osseous plasmacytoma* is a single bone lesion on radiographs, with the histology of a plasma cell tumor but without an increase in plasma cells in a random bone marrow sample. *Extramedullary plasmacytoma* is a single plasmacytoma at an extraskeletal site; the bone marrow and skeletal radiographs are normal, aside from possible bone erosions or damage adjacent to the primary lesion; there may be regional lymph node metastasis.

A diagnosis of plasmacytoma should prompt further clinical, biochemical, hematologic, and radiologic investigations to determine whether the lesion is truly solitary or in fact a localized presentation of multiple myeloma. An M-band may or may not be detected in the serum, and the paraproteinemia can persist or disappear after resection or radiation therapy of the plasmacytoma (1,2).

The male predominance for solitary plasmacytomas (ratio of 3 to 1), is much more striking as compared with multiple myeloma (10,28). A wide age range is affected. Patients with solitary osseous plasmacytoma (median age, 50 to 60 years) are reported to be a decade younger than those with solitary extramedullary plasmacytoma (median age, 60 to 70 years) (2,7,10,12,15,28,35,50,52,53).

Solitary osseous plasmacytoma usually presents as localized pain, and there may be neurologic symptoms due to compression of spinal cord or nerve roots. The axial skeleton (vertebral bodies, pelvic bones, scapula) is more frequently affected than the appendicular skeleton. Radiologically, the tumors appear either as discrete single or multilocular osteolytic lesions (8).

Extramedullary plasmacytoma occurs most commonly in the upper aerodigestive tract (particularly paranasal sinus, nasopharynx, nose, tonsil, larynx), and presents as nasal obstruction, epistaxis, pain, dysphagia, or dyspnea (24). The tumor is sometimes multifocal (50). The regional lymph nodes are sometimes involved, and may represent the initial presentation of the plasmacytoma. Extramedullary plasmacytoma can occur in almost any organ, including the spleen (23); most cases of gastrointestinal plasmacytoma, however, have been reinterpreted as low-grade B-cell lymphoma with plasma cell differentiation (22,55).

Primary plasmacytoma of lymph node, a form of solitary extramedullary plasmacytoma, is extremely rare (1,19,26,36,53). In the Kiel Lymphoma Registry, it accounts for only 0.01 percent of lymphoma cases (31,32,36). Of 167 cases of extramedullary plasmacytoma seen at the Mayo Clinic over a 23-year period, only 15 were of primary nodal type (36). Before a diagnosis of primary plasmacytoma of lymph node is made, an extramedullary plasmacytoma must be carefully searched for in the drainage area, and evidence of systemic disease must be excluded. As with other extramedullary plasmacytomas, there is a male predominance (2 to 1). The median age is 60 years. Patients present with lymph node enlargement in the absence of systemic symptoms, most frequently in the neck, followed by the axilla. Rarely, lymphadenopathy is generalized (33). Paraproteinemia occurs in slightly less than half of the cases (36). The prognosis is favorable (1), and although some patients die from disseminated nodal disease, progression to multiple myeloma is uncommon (36).

Rarely, plasmacytoma occurs as a form of Epstein-Barr virus (EBV)–associated lymphoproliferative disorder in immunocompromised patients (34). It remains to be clarified whether EBV-positive plasmacytoma will regress on withdrawal of immunosuppressants, like other post-transplant lymphoproliferative disorders.

Microscopic Findings. The basic histologic features of plasmacytoma, whether solitary or part of multiple myeloma, are the same. There is a dense, monotonous infiltrate of plasma cells that can exhibit a broad morphologic spectrum ranging from mature-looking plasma cells to anaplastic cells; in an individual case all plasma cells usually show a similar degree of differentiation. This morphologic variation gives rise to three plasmacytoma subtypes. In the *plasmacytic type,* the plasma cells appear mature (Marschalko type plasma cells), with eccentric round nuclei, condensed coarsely clumped "clockface" chromatin, basophilic cytoplasm, and a prominent pale Golgi zone (fig. 16-1). In some cases, the plasma cells are less mature: the nuclei are larger, the chromatin is less condensed but still clumped, nucleoli can be distinct, and the cytoplasm often appears slightly less basophilic (fig. 16-2). In the *plasmablastic type,* the plasma cells appear "blastic"; they possess large vesicu-

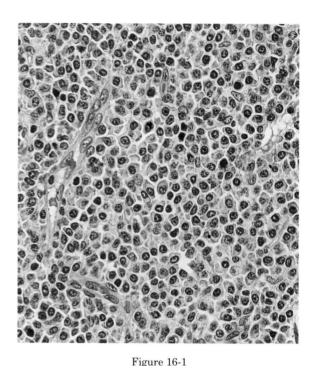

Figure 16-1
PLASMACYTOMA
This example is composed predominantly of mature-looking plasma cells.

lar nuclei, irregularly condensed chromatin, prominent central nucleoli, and a moderate rim of amphophilic to basophilic cytoplasm with a small pale Golgi zone (fig. 16-3). In the *anaplastic type,* which overlaps morphologically with the plasmablastic type, there are immature and blastic plasma cells that show significant variation in size and may have a nuclear membrane with irregular foldings (fig. 16-4). Nuclear pseudoinclusions (Dutcher bodies), cleaved nuclei, multilobated nuclei, and multinucleated forms can be seen in any plasmacytoma subtype (fig. 16-5). Mitotic counts are usually low in the plasmacytic type, but are often high in the plasmablastic and anaplastic types. Intracytoplasmic or extracellular deposits of immunoglobulin in the form of globules (Russell bodies) or crystals, which are usually periodic acid–Schiff (PAS)–positive, can occur (figs. 16-6, 16-7). Solitary or multiple clear vacuoles (signet ring cells) have rarely been reported to occur in multiple myeloma, but can potentially occur in plasmacytomas as well (9,16). Detached small fragments of cytoplasm (plasma cell bodies) are sometimes found among the neoplastic cells.

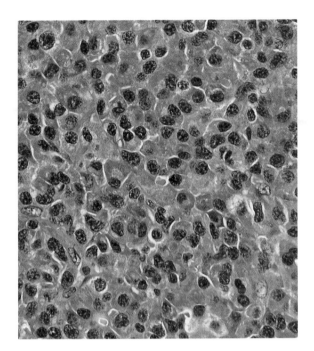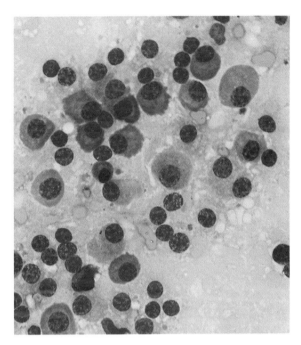

Figure 16-2
PLASMACYTOMA

Left: Compared with those illustrated in figure 16-1, the plasma cells of this example are less mature-looking, with larger nuclei, and slightly less condensed chromatin.

Right: The plasmacytic nature is best appreciated in Giemsa-stained touch preparations. Note the coarse chromatin and basophilic cytoplasm. In plasmacytoma, the cytoplasm of the neoplastic cells is often more lightly stained than the normal plasma cells.

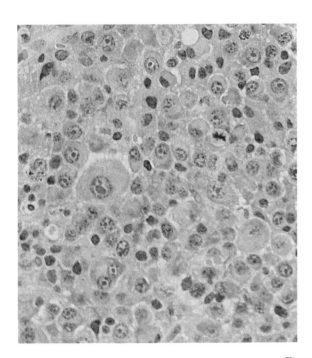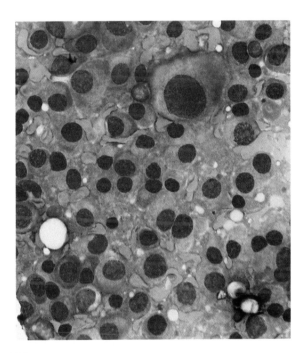

Figure 16-3
PLASMABLASTIC PLASMACYTOMA OF THE NASOPHARYNX

Left: The tumor cells possess vesicular nuclei and large nucleoli, mimicking immunoblasts, but the immunophenotype is characteristic of plasmacytoma. Plasmacytic features are evident in some smaller cells.

Right: The plasmacytic nature of this neoplasm is better appreciated in this Giemsa-stained touch preparation.

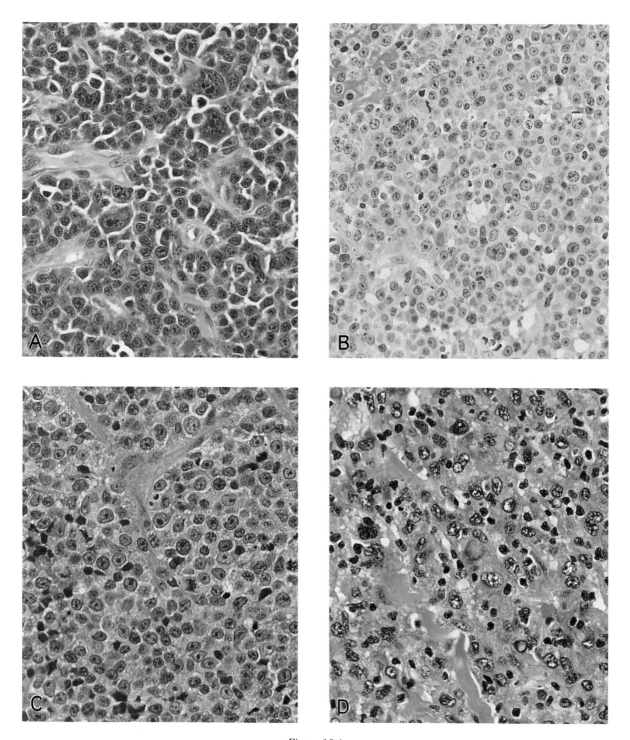

Figure 16-4
ANAPLASTIC PLASMACYTOMA, SHOWING A BROAD MORPHOLOGIC SPECTRUM

A: The neoplastic cells show striking variation in size. The plasmacytic nature of this tumor is readily appreciated from the coarsely clumped chromatin and basophilic cytoplasm.

B: This example is composed of cells with vesicular nuclei and distinct nucleoli, and distinction from large cell (immunoblastic) lymphoma may be difficult. However, a significant number of cells exhibit the coarse chromatin pattern and basophilic cytoplasm characteristic of plasma cells.

C: This example is practically indistinguishable from large cell lymphoma.

D: This example may be mistaken for an undifferentiated malignancy. The clue to diagnosis is the basophilia of the cytoplasm.

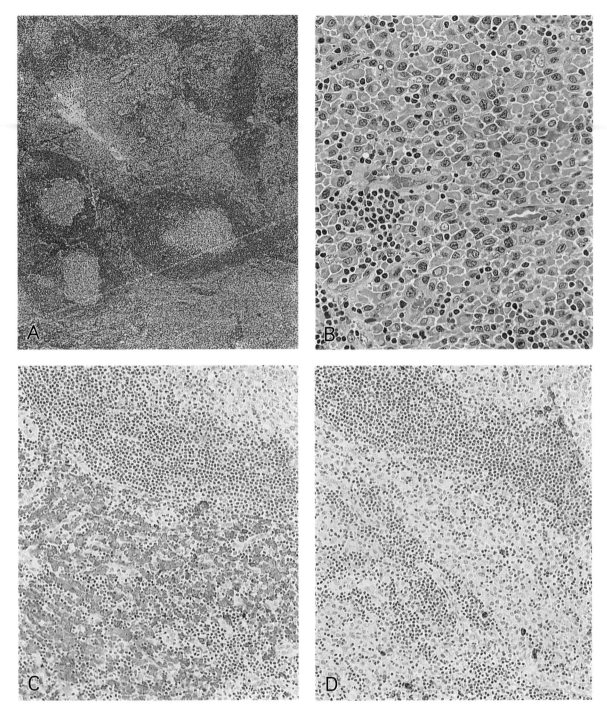

Figure 16-5

PLASMACYTOMA INVOLVING LYMPH NODE

A: There is incomplete effacement of architecture, with the neoplastic infiltrate expanding the areas between the reactive lymphoid follicles.

B: The plasma cells are atypical; occasional nuclear pseudoinclusions are seen.

C: The plasma cells show strong immunostaining for lambda light chain (brown). Occasional cells in the lymphoid follicle in the upper field are lambda positive.

D: Only occasional plasma cells, which are small, show immunostaining for kappa light chain, whereas the larger atypical plasma cells are negative, confirming that the plasma cell population is monotypic. Some cells in the lymphoid follicle in the upper field are kappa positive, indicating that this follicle is reactive (polytypic).

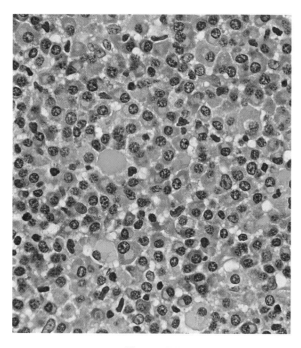

Figure 16-6
PLASMACYTOMA
Some cells contain amorphous eosinophilic globular inclusions in the cytoplasm.

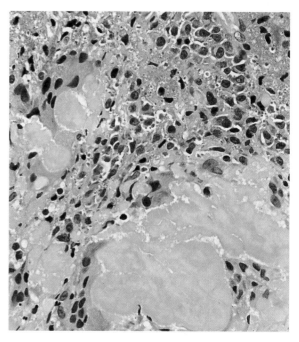

Figure 16-8
PLASMACYTOMA WITH AMYLOID DEPOSITION
Note prominence of eosinophilic, amorphous amyloid among the neoplastic plasma cells.

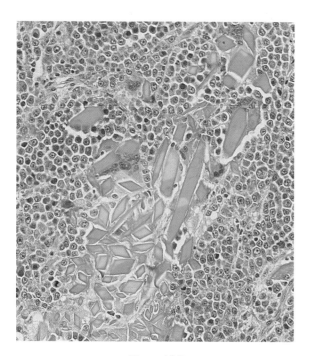

Figure 16-7
PLASMACYTOMA WITH CRYSTALLOIDS
This plasmacytoma of lymph node is associated with deposition of crystalloid material.

Amyloid or amorphous deposits of immunoglobulin, which may be accompanied by a foreign body reaction, sometimes occur within the plasmacytoma (fig. 16-8) (37). A pseudoangiomatous pattern is occasionally created by lakes of erythrocytes and plasma surrounded by neoplastic plasma cells (fig. 16-9) (32). We have observed the rare occurrence of myxoid change in a plasmacytoma of the soft tissues (fig. 16-10).

In lymph nodes involved by plasmacytoma, architectural effacement is complete or partial. There are often some residual lymphoid follicles (fig. 16-5) (31). The monotonous plasma cell population is traversed by a regular network of reticulin fibers and small blood vessels (32). Occasional sclerotic bands extend from the capsule into the parenchyma. The lymphatics can sometimes be distended by inspissated protein (32).

Immunologic Findings. The plasma cells in plasmacytoma typically show monotypic cytoplasmic immunoglobulin (usually IgG and IgA type) and lack surface immunoglobulin. The former is best demonstrated in paraffin sections. Since diffuse cytoplasmic staining for immunoglobulin may be due to passive uptake of immunoglobulin from

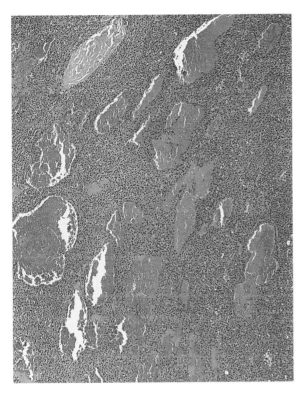

Figure 16-9
PLASMACYTOMA WITH BLOOD LAKES
Irregular blood lakes are surrounded by neoplastic plasma cells.

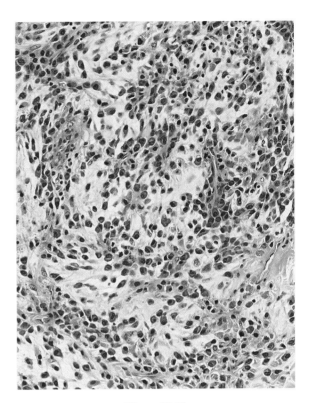

Figure 16-10
PLASMACYTOMA WITH MYXOID STROMA
Plasmacytoma of soft tissue with areas showing myxoid changes in the stroma. Some plasma cells are spindle shaped.

the interstitial fluid, only diffuse cytoplasmic staining with Golgi accentuation or Golgi staining alone provides strong evidence that the immunoglobulin being demonstrated results from endogenous synthesis (fig. 16-11). Immunoglobulin is usually not detectable in frozen sections, which are optimal for demonstration of surface but not cytoplasmic immunoglobulin. In situ hybridization for immunoglobulin mRNA is an alternative technique for specific demonstration of cellular immunoglobulin synthesis, circumventing the problem of background staining or passive absorption.

The neoplastic plasma cells, like normal plasma cells, usually lack the surface antigens normally expressed by B cells. Failure to stain for leukocyte common antigen (LCA) and B-cell surface antigens (such as CD19, CD20) is highly characteristic, although this phenomenon is more consistently observed in paraffin than frozen sections (Table 1) (47,54). On the other hand, the B-cell antigen CD79a (mb-1), which is nor-

mally expressed in plasma cells, is demonstrable in a significant proportion of cases. There is variable staining with CD38 (T10) and the plasma cell–associated markers PC-1, PC-2, and PCA-1 (3,4,39,47). The newly available antibody VS38, which detects plasma cell differentiation in routine sections, may be of help in diagnosis because all cases of plasmacytoma or myeloma studied thus far have been positive (48).

There may be staining with paraffin section–reactive T-cell markers such as CD43 and CD45RO (39). Like normal plasma cells, the neoplastic cells often stain for epithelial membrane antigen (EMA) (39,40). Rarely, cytokeratin immunoreactivity is detected (44,54).

CD56, CD10, occasional T-cell antigens (such as CD2, CD3, CD4, CD8), and myelomonocytic antigens (such as CD13, CD15) have been reported to be expressed in some cases of multiple myeloma (14,45,49). These markers can potentially be detected in plasmacytomas as well, although they have not been specifically studied on these tumors.

321

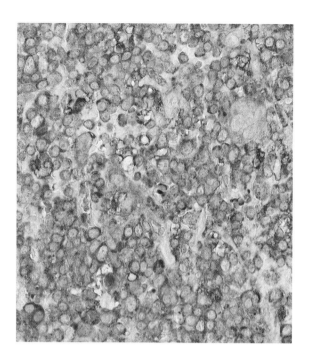 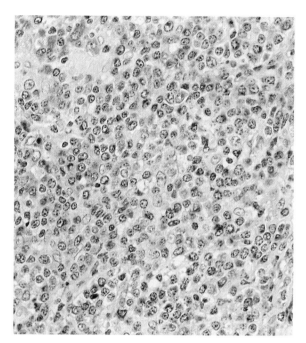

Figure 16-11
IMMUNOHISTOCHEMICAL STAINING IN PLASMACYTOMA
Left: Plasmacytoma showing diffuse cytoplasmic staining for lambda light chain, with accentuation of staining in the Golgi zone. Practically all cells show positive (monotypic) staining.
Right: Another example showing monotypic immunostaining for kappa light chain. Localization of the reaction product in the Golgi zone strongly suggests endogenous synthesis rather than passive absorption from the interstitium.

Table 16-1

IMMUNOHISTOCHEMICAL FEATURES HELPFUL FOR DISTINGUISHING PLASMACYTOMA FROM LARGE B-CELL (IMMUNOBLASTIC) LYMPHOMA

	Plasmacytoma	Immunoblastic Lymphoma
Leukocyte common antigen (CD45)	–	+
B-cell surface antigens, e.g., CD19, CD20	–	+
Epithelial membrane antigen	+	–
CD38 (T10)	+	–
Immunoglobulin type	Usually IgG or IgA	Usually IgM or IgG

– = usually negative; + = usually positive.

Differential Diagnosis. Distinction between plasmacytoma and reactive plasmacytosis may be difficult. In the latter, the plasma cells are often accompanied by many hyperplastic lymphoid follicles, and exhibit a range of differentiation from plasmablasts (uncommon) to mature forms. Some degree of nuclear atypia or immaturity can be seen in the plasma cells. Immunostaining for cytoplasmic immunoglobulin is most helpful in that light chain restriction supports a diagnosis of plasmacytoma.

The borderline between lymphoplasmacytic lymphoma (small lymphocytic lymphoma with plasmacytic features) and plasmacytoma is not always sharp. In plasmacytoma, there is a pure proliferation of plasma cells, whereas in lymphoplasmacytic lymphoma, the plasma cells are accompanied by many small lymphocytes and sometimes plasmablasts. Other low-grade B-cell lymphomas such as follicular lymphoma, lymphoma of mucosa-associated lymphoid tissue, and monocytoid B-cell lymphoma may also show plasmacytic differentiation, that is, presence of monotypic plasma cells expressing the same immunoglobulin class as the lymphoma cells (11,25,27,31,38,43,55). Although the plasma cells can occasionally be so numerous that plasmacytoma is mimicked, the identification of a significant nonplasmacytic neoplastic lymphoid component distinguishes these lymphoma types. There are unusual examples of follicular lymphoma in which large numbers of atypical plasma cells are found in the neoplastic follicles, looking like a "follicular plasmacytoma" (see fig. 6-35) (43). However, since some follicular center cells (centroblasts and centrocytes) are intermingled with the plasma cells, these cases are more appropriately interpreted as follicular center cell lymphoma with an extreme degree of plasmacytic differentiation, albeit unusual in that plasma cells occur in abundance within the follicles instead of the interfollicular regions.

The anaplastic or plasmablastic type of plasmacytoma overlaps morphologically with immunoblastic lymphoma of plasmacytoid type (46). In the former, the chromatin is more coarsely clumped (particularly on the nuclear membrane) in at least some cells, similar to the pattern observed in plasma cells. There are often some more mature-looking atypical plasma cells. Giemsa-stained touch preparations are helpful in revealing the characteristic clumped chromatin of plasma cells (fig. 16-3, left). Immunohistochemical studies are also helpful in the differential diagnosis (Table 16-1) (47).

The anaplastic type of plasmacytoma may be difficult to distinguish from undifferentiated carcinoma or melanoma. An LCA-negative/EMA-positive immunophenotype, coupled with occasional cytokeratin reactivity, may erroneously suggest carcinoma (fig. 16-4). Histologic clues to the plasmacytic nature of the tumor are the presence of coarsely clumped clock-face chromatin in some cells and striking basophilia of the cytoplasm associated with a pale Golgi zone. The

diagnosis can be confirmed by immunohistochemical demonstration of monotypic cytoplasmic immunoglobulin.

In the plasma cell variant of Castleman's disease, numerous plasma cells occur among the hyperplastic follicles, some of which may be penetrated by hyalinized blood vessels. The plasma cells are monotypic in some cases (20,41), and it has been proposed that this entity represents the nodal counterpart of benign monoclonal gammopathy (41). A diagnosis of plasmacytoma is not generally rendered if the clinicopathologic features fit a diagnosis of Castleman's disease of plasma cell variant.

Treatment and Prognosis. The prognosis of solitary plasmacytoma is much better than that of multiple myeloma, and the median survival is 7 to 9 years (28,35).

Patients with solitary osseous plasmacytoma are usually treated with radiation therapy after biopsy, curettage, or laminectomy (7). The suggested dose of radiation is 45 to 50 Gy in 4 to 5 weeks; doses lower than 45 Gy have been associated with a high incidence of local failure (17,42). Approximately 40 to 50 percent of cases progress to multiple myeloma, usually after an interval of several years (5,7,10,12,15,17,35). Relapse in the same or a separate site (usually in the axial skeleton, the site of active hematopoiesis) can occur (17,50). In one study, the overall survival was 74 percent at 5 years and 45 percent at 10 years; the 5- and 10-year disease-free survivals were 43 percent and 25 percent, respectively (17). Although no parameters satisfactorily predict the likelihood of systemic dissemination, one study suggests that nuclear immaturity and prominent nucleoli may serve such a purpose (35). One study suggests that analysis of clonality on the enriched plasma cell fraction after short-term bone marrow culture may help predict systemic disease, with a greater than 20 percent monoclonal plasma cell component strongly predicting likelihood of progression to disseminated myeloma (6). Evidence of paraproteinemia, seen in approximately half of the patients with plasmacytoma, does not influence survival (17). There are conflicting data as to whether persistence of paraproteinemia after treatment is associated with a higher risk of developing disseminated disease (12,13,17).

The prognosis of extramedullary plasmacytoma is favorable. Many patients are cured by high voltage radiotherapy, with or without surgical removal of the tumor. The risk of dissemination is lower than for solitary osseous plasmacytoma; only 10 to 20 percent of cases progress to multiple myeloma (7,35). Local or distant relapse sometimes occurs (7,8,53). When spread occurs in the bone, there is no preference for bone containing active hematopoietic tissue (50). It has been suggested that the plasmablastic or anaplastic subtype is more aggressive (24). Primary cutaneous plasmacytoma differs from other extramedullary plasmacytomas by showing a high risk of complication by multiple myeloma (51).

AMYLOID DEPOSITS IN LYMPH NODE

Definition and Clinical Features. Amyloidosis is a heterogeneous disease characterized by the deposition in tissues of an amorphous-appearing, congophilic protein which ultrastructurally is composed of nonbranching fibrils. The most common types of amyloid are composed of immunoglobulin light chain (AL) and amyloid protein A (AA). The former can be idiopathic or related to plasma cell dyscrasia, while the latter is usually secondary to chronic inflammatory diseases.

Although lymph node involvement is not uncommon in systemic amyloidosis (17 to 36 percent of cases) (58,62,64), amyloid deposits presenting as lymphadenopathy are rare (64). The term *amyloid lymphadenopathy* is sometimes applied. This usually occurs in a setting of plasmacytoma, lymphoplasmacytic lymphoma, or systemic idiopathic amyloidosis (61). The prognosis is related to the underlying disease. Isolated amyloidosis of lymph node unassociated with immunoproliferative disorders or systemic amyloidosis is even more uncommon (61,62,65,66). It occurs in adults, and usually involves several groups of lymph nodes. It is associated with a favorable outcome: of the three reported cases with follow-up information, one patient died of unrelated disease 12 years after the diagnosis, one was well at 15 months, and one was alive at 4 years but with persistent lymphadenopathy.

Microscopic Findings. Deposits of amyloid within the lymph node can have different patterns: vascular, follicular, diffuse, or a combination of the three. The blood vessels are impregnated with

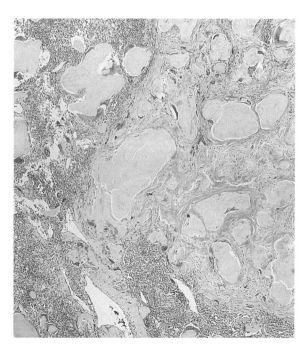

Figure 16-12
AMYLOIDOSIS OF LYMPH NODE
The irregular amorphous masses of amyloid are associated with foreign body giant cell reaction. There is also deposition of amyloid in the blood vessel wall (lower field).

amyloid in their walls, but their lumina are rarely narrowed (fig. 16-12). The lymphoid follicles can be partially or totally replaced by amyloid, resulting in amorphous round nodules (fig. 16-13). In the diffuse pattern, the amyloid is haphazardly or extensively deposited in the nodal parenchyma (fig. 16-12).

The amyloid appears as amorphous eosinophilic masses or cloud-like patches, which when stained with Congo red exhibits an orange-pink color with apple green birefringence. The amyloid deposits can be calcified, ossified, or associated with a foreign body giant cell reaction (63). Immunohistochemical studies have shown the amyloid to be composed of AL in isolated amyloidosis, idiopathic amyloidosis, and amyloidosis associated with immunoproliferative neoplasms, and composed of AA in a reactive systemic process. It has been suggested that some cases of AL type isolated amyloidosis might have an origin from a "burned out" immunoproliferative neoplasm (63). Ultrastructurally, amyloid is characterized by randomly distributed nonbranching fibrils, 7.5 nm in diameter.

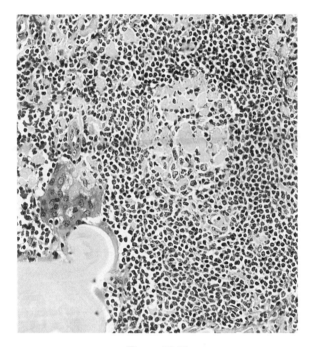

Figure 16-13
AMYLOIDOSIS OF LYMPH NODE
There is amyloid deposit within a germinal center (upper field).

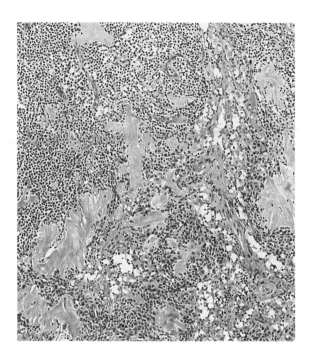

Figure 16-14
SCLEROSIS IN AN INGUINAL LYMPH NODE

There may be evidence of lymphoma or plasmacytoma in the same lymph node. Metastatic medullary thyroid carcinoma can be associated with such abundant amyloid deposits that the carcinoma is masked; careful search will reveal clusters of carcinoma cells among the amyloid.

Differential Diagnosis. Proteinaceous lymphadenopathy is a term that has been used to refer to lymph node enlargement due to deposition of acellular amorphous material with characteristic features of amyloid or other proteinaceous substances (60,68). The nonamyloid type of proteinaceous lymphadenopathy, also known as lymph node hyalinosis, occurs in association with hyperglobulinemia (including lymphoplasmacytic lymphoma), angioimmunoblastic lymphadenopathy, Hodgkin's disease, chemotherapy, radiotherapy, inflammatory reaction, or is idiopathic. The amorphous proteinaceous material (para-amyloid) appears to be an inflammatory or abnormal immune reaction product, possibly including immunoglobulin, and is PAS-positive (69). The lack of congophilia distinguishes it from amyloid.

Lymph node sclerosis may be mistaken for amyloidosis. Patchy and perivascular sclerosis is a common incidental finding in inguinal and pelvic lymph nodes, probably representing postinflammatory fibrosis (fig. 16-14). It can be distinguished from amyloid by the positive reaction with collagen stains and a lack of congophilia.

AMYLOID DEPOSITS IN SPLEEN

The spleen is commonly involved in systemic amyloidosis. The involved spleen ranges from normal size to very large. The pattern of involvement is highly variable. When the white pulp is predominantly involved, the cut surfaces of the spleen reveal discrete white nodules ("sago spleen"). When the red pulp is predominantly involved, the waxy appearance of the cut surfaces looks like lard ("lardaceous spleen") (70). An exceptional case of amyloid tumor (amyloidoma) appearing as a localized, discrete 3.5-cm tumor in the spleen of a patient with lymphoma has been reported (57).

Histologically, involvement of the white pulp initially takes the form of intercellular amyloid deposits which later coalesce to replace the white pulp (fig. 16-15). Involvement of the red pulp occurs in the walls of the splenic sinuses and

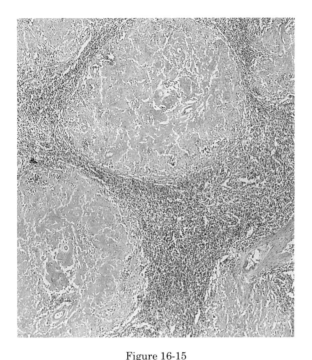

Figure 16-15
AMYLOIDOSIS OF SPLEEN
This example shows predominant deposition of amyloid in the white pulp, the "sago spleen" pattern.

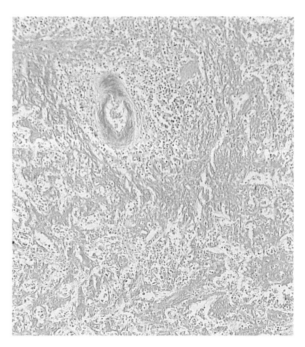

Figure 16-17
AMYLOIDOSIS OF SPLEEN
This example shows predominant red pulp involvement. Note the deposits in the blood vessel wall. (Congo red stain)

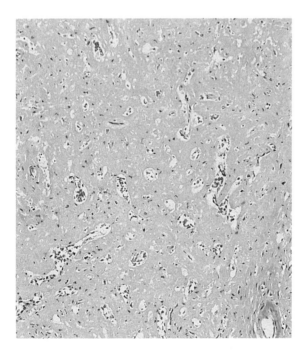

Figure 16-16
AMYLOIDOSIS OF SPLEEN
There is predominant deposition of amyloid in the red pulp. Residual sinusoids are still recognizable.

connective tissue framework; more extensive deposition results in a sieve-like matrix of amyloid with interspersed sinusoidal structures (fig. 16-16). The blood vessels are often thickened due to amyloid deposition (fig. 16-17) (67). There may be an increase in plasma cells, which are sometimes monotypic (70).

Studies correlating the chemical composition of amyloid and the pattern of splenic involvement have yielded conflicting results (56,67). Vascular involvement occurs commonly in both AL and AA amyloidosis, and can sometimes be the only involved component (particularly for AA type) (56,67). Interestingly, the spleen is always spared in the beta-2-microglobulin type of systemic amyloidosis, which occurs in patients undergoing long-term hemodialysis (59).

REFERENCES

Plasmacytoma

1. Addis BJ, Isaacson P, Billings JA. Plasmacytoma of lymph nodes. Cancer 1980;46:340–6.
2. Alexanian R. Localized and indolent myeloma. Blood 1980;56:521–5.
3. Anderson KC, Bates MP, Slaughenhoupt B, et al. A monoclonal antibody with reactivity restricted to normal and neoplastic plasma cells. J Immunol 1984;132:3172–9.
4. _____, Park E, Bates MP, et al. Antigens on human plasma cells identified by monoclonal antibodies. J Immunol 1983;130:1132–8.
5. Bataille R, Sany J. Solitary myeloma: clinical and prognostic features of a review of 114 cases. Cancer 1981;48:845–51.
6. Bezwoda WR, Gordon V, Bagg A, Mendelow B. Light chain restriction analysis of bone marrow plasma cells in patients with GSMU or "solitary" plasmacytomas: diagnostic value and correlation with clinical course. Br J Haematol 1990;74:420–3.
7. Brinch L, Hannisdal E, Abrahamsen AF, Kvaloy S, Langholm R. Extramedullary plasmacytomas and solitary plasma cell tumors of bone. Eur J Haematol 1990;44:132–5.
7a. Brunning RD, McKenna RW. Tumors of the bone marrow. 3rd Series, Fascicle 9. Washington D.C.: Armed Forces Institute of Pathology, 1994.
8. Callihan TR, Holbert JM Jr, Berard CW. Neoplasms of terminal B-cell differentiation: the morphologic basis of functional diversity. In: Sommers SC, Rosen PP, eds. Malignant lymphomas, a pathology annual monograph. Norwalk: Appleton Century Crofts, 1983:169–268.
9. Chen KT, Ma CK, Nelson JW, Padmanabhan A, Brittin GM. Clear cell myeloma. Am J Surg Pathol 1985;9:149–54.
10. Corwin J, Lindberg RD. Solitary plasmacytoma of bone versus extramedullary plasmacytoma and their relationship to multiple myeloma. Cancer 1979;43:1007–13.
11. Davis GG, York JC, Glick AD, McCurley TL, Collins RD, Cousar JB. Plasmacytic differentiation in parafollicular (monocytoid) B-cell lymphoma. A study of 12 cases. Am J Surg Pathol 1992;16:1066–74.
12. Dimopoulos MA, Goldstein J, Fuller L, Delasalle K, Alexanian R. Curability of solitary bone plasmacytoma. J Clin Oncol 1992;10:587–90.
13. _____, Moulopoulos A, Delasalle K, Alexanian R. Solitary plasmacytoma of bone and asymptomatic multiple myeloma. Hematol Oncol Clin North Am 1992;6:359–69.
14. Durie BG. The biology of multiple myeloma. Hematol Oncol 1988;6:77–81.
15. Ellis PA, Colls BM. Solitary plasmacytoma of bone: clinical features, treatment and survival. Hematol Oncol 1992;10:207–11.
16. Eyden BP, Banerjee SS. Multiple myeloma showing signet-ring cell change. Histopathology 1990;17:170–2.
17. Frassica DA, Frassica FJ, Schray MF, Sim FH, Kyle RA. Solitary plasmacytoma of bone: Mayo Clinic experience. Int J Radiat Oncol Biol Phys 1989;16:43–8.
18. Frizzera G. Castleman's disease and related disorders. Semin Diagn Pathol 1988;5:346–64.
19. Gaston EA, Dollinger MR, Strong EW, Hajdu SI. Primary plasmacytoma of lymph nodes. Lymphology 1969;2:7–15.
20. Hall PA, Donaghy M, Cotter FE, Stansfeld AG, Levison DA. An immunohistological and genotypic study of the plasma cell form of Castleman's disease. Histopathology 1989;14:333–46.
21. Henry K. Neoplastic disorders of lymphoreticular tissue. In: Henry K, Symmers WS, eds. Thymus, lymph nodes, spleen and lymphatics. Systemic pathology, 3rd ed., Vol. 7. Edinburgh: Churchill Livingstone, 1992: 611–960.
22. _____, Farrer-Brown G. Primary lymphomas of the gastrointestinal tract. I. Plasma cell tumors. Histopathology 1977;1:53–76.
23. Horny HP, Saal J, Kaiserling E. Primary splenic presentation of plasma cell dyscrasia: report of two cases. Hematol Pathol 1992;6:155–60.
24. Hyams VJ, Batsakis JG, Michaels L. Tumors of the upper respiratory tract and ear. Atlas of Tumor Pathology. 2nd series, Fascicle 25. Washington D.C.: Armed Forces Institute of Pathology, 1988:220–4.
25. Isaacson PG, Spencer J. Malignant lymphoma of mucosa-associated lymphoid tissue. Histopathology 1987;11:445–62.
26. Jansen J, Blok P. Primary plasmacytoma of lymph nodes, a case report. Acta Hematol 1979;61:100–5.
27. Keith TA, Cousar JB, Glick AD, Vogler LB, Collins RD. Plasmacytic differentiation in follicular center cell (FCC) lymphomas. Am J Clin Pathol 1985;84:283–90.
28. Knowling MA, Harwood AR, Bergsagel DE. Comparison of extramedullary plasmacytomas with solitary and multiple plasma cell tumors of bone. J Clin Oncol 1983;1:255–62.
29. Kyle RA. Diagnostic criteria of multiple myeloma. Hematol Oncol Clin North Am 1992;6:347–58.
30. Lasker JC, Bishop JO, Wilbanks JH, Lane M. Solitary myeloma of the talus bone. Cancer 1991;68:202–5.
31. Lennert K, Feller AC. Histopathology of non-Hodgkin's lymphomas (based on the updated Kiel classification). 2nd ed. Berlin: Springer-Verlag, 1992:76–114.
32. _____, Mohri N. Histopathology and diagnosis of non-Hodgkin's lymphomas. In: Lennert K, ed. Malignant lymphomas other than Hodgkin's disease, histology, cytology, ultrastructure, immunology. Berlin: Springer-Verlag, 1978:111–469.
33. Matsushima T, Murakami H, Tamura J, Sawamura M, Naruse T, Tsuchiya J. Primary plasmacytoma of generalized lymph nodes: a long survivor. Am J Hematol 1993;43:237–9.
34. Medeiros LJ, Kingma DW, Martin AW, Barker RL, Jaffe ES, Peiper SC. Epstein-Barr virus (EBV)-induced lymphoproliferative disorders (LPD) manifesting as plasmacytomas [Abstract]. Mod Pathol 1993;6:96A.
35. Meis JM, Butler JJ, Osborne BM, Ordonez NG. Solitary plasmacytomas of bone and extramedullary plasmacytomas. A clinicopathologic and immunohistochemical study. Cancer 1987;59:1475–85.
36. Menke DM, Kyle RA, Horny HP, et al. Primary lymph node plasmacytomas (plasmacytic lymphomas) [Abstract]. Mod Pathol 1993;6:96A.
37. Morinaga S, Watanabe H, Gemma A, et al. Plasmacytoma of the lung associated with nodular deposits of immunoglobulin. Am J Surg Pathol 1987;11:989–95.
38. Nizze H, Cogliatti SB, Von Schilling C, Feller AC, Lennert K. Monocytoid B-cell lymphoma: morphological variants and relationship to low-grade B-cell lymphoma of mucosa-associated lymphoid tissue. Histopathology 1991;18:403–14.

39. Petruch UR, Horny HP, Kaiserling E. Frequent expression of haemopoietic and non-haemopoietic antigens by neoplastic plasma cells: an immunohistochemical study using formalin-fixed, paraffin-embedded tissue. Histopathology 1992;20:35–40.

40. Pinkus GS, Kurtin PJ. Epithelial membrane antigen—a diagnostic discriminant in surgical pathology. Hum Pathol 1985;16:929–40.

41. Radaszkiewicz T, Hansmann ML, Lennert K. Monoclonality and polyclonality of plasma cells in Castleman's disease of the plasma cell variant. Histopathology 1989;14:11–24.

42. Salmon SE, Cassady JR. Plasma cell neoplasms. In: DeVita VT Jr, Hellman S, Rosenberg SA, eds. Cancer, principles and practice of oncology. 3rd ed. Philadelphia: JB Lippincott, 1989:1853–95.

43. Schmid U, Karow J, Lennert K. Follicular malignant non-Hodgkin's lymphoma with pronounced plasmacytic differentiation: a plasmacytoma-like lymphoma. Virchows Arch [A] 1985;405:473–81.

44. Sewell HF, Thompson WD, King DJ. IgD myeloma/immunoblastic lymphoma cells expressing cytokeratin. Br J Cancer 1986;53:695–6.

45. Spier CM, Grogan TM, Durie BG, et al. T-cell antigen-positive multiple myeloma. Blood 1990;3:302–7.

46. Strand WR, Banks PM, Kyle RA. Anaplastic plasma cell myeloma and immunoblastic lymphoma, clinical, pathologic, and immunologic comparison. Am J Med 1984;76:861–7.

47. Strickler JG, Audeh MW, Copenhaver CM, Warnke RA. Immunophenotypic differences between plasmacytoma/multiple myeloma and immunoblastic lymphoma. Cancer 1988;61:1782–6.

48. Turley H, Jones M, Erber W, Mayne K, de Waele M, Gatter K. VS38: a new monoclonal antibody for detecting plasma cell differentiation in routine sections. J Clin Pathol 1994;47:418–22.

49. Van Camp B, Durie BG, Spier C, et al. Plasma cells in multiple myeloma express a natural killer cell-associated antigen: CD56 (NKH-1; Leu-19). Blood 1990;76:377–82.

50. Wiltshaw E. The natural history of extramedullary plasmacytoma and its relation to solitary myeloma of bone and myelomatosis. Medicine 1976;55:217–38.

51. Wong KF, Chan JK, Li LP, Yau TK, Lee AW. Primary cutaneous plasmacytoma—report of two cases and review of the literature. Am J Dermatopathol 1994;16:392–7.

52. Woodruff RK, Malpas JS, White FE. Solitary plasmacytoma. II: Solitary plasmacytoma of bone. Cancer 1979;43:2344–7.

53. Woodruff RK, Whittle JM, Malpas JS. Solitary plasmacytoma. I: Extramedullary soft tissue plasmacytoma. Cancer 1979;43:2340–3.

54. Wotherspoon AC, Norton AJ, Isaacson PG. Immunoreactive cytokeratins in plasmacytomas. Histopathology 1989;14:141–50.

55. Wright DH, Isaacson PG. Gut-associated lymphoid tumours. In: Whitehead R, ed. Gastrointestinal and esophageal pathology. Edinburgh: Churchill Livingstone, 1989:643–61.

Amyloid Deposits in Lymph Node and Spleen

56. Buck FS, Koss MN. Correspondence re: splenic amyloidosis, correlations between chemical types of amyloid protein and morphological features [Letter]. Mod Pathol 1992;5:97.

57. Chen KT, Flam MS, Workman RD. Amyloid tumor of the spleen. Am J Surg Pathol 1987;11:723–5.

58. Eisen HN. Primary systemic amyloidosis. Am J Med 1946;1:144–60.

59. Gal R, Korzets A, Schwartz A, Rath-Wolfson L, Gafter U. Systemic distribution of beta 2-microglobulin-derived amyloidosis in patients who undergo long-term hemodialysis. Report of seven cases and review of the literature. Arch Pathol Lab Med 1994;118:718–21.

60. Ioachim HL. Lymph node pathology. 2nd ed. Philadelphia: J.B. Lippincott, 1994:273–8.

61. Kahn H, Strauchen JA, Gilbert HS, Fuchs A. Immunoglobulin-related amyloidosis presenting as recurrent isolated lymph node involvement. Arch Pathol Lab Med 1991;115:948–50.

62. Ko HS, Davidson JW, Pruzanski W. Amyloid lymphadenopathy [Letter]. Ann Intern Med 1976;85:763–4.

63. Krishnan J, Chu WS, Elrod JP, Frizzera G. Tumoral presentation of amyloidosis (amyloidomas) in soft tissues, a report of 14 cases. Am J Clin Pathol 1993; 100:135–44.

64. MacKenzie DH. Amyloidosis presenting as lymphadenopathy. Br Med J 1963;2:1449–50.

65. Newland JR, Linke RP, Kleinsasser O, Lennert K. Lymph node enlargement due to amyloid. Virchows Arch [A] 1983;399:233–6.

66. _____, Linke RP, Lennert K. Amyloid deposits in lymph nodes: a morphologic and immunohistochemical study. Hum Pathol 1986;17:1245–9.

67. Ohyama T, Shimokama T, Yoshikawa Y, Watanabe T. Splenic amyloidosis: correlations between chemical types of amyloid protein and morphological features. Mod Pathol 1990;3:419–22.

68. Osborne BM, Butler JJ, Mackay B. Proteinaceous lymphadenopathy with hypergammaglobulinemia. Am J Surg Pathol 1979;3:137–45.

69. Paradinas FJ. Primary and secondary immune disorders. In: Stansfeld AG, d'Ardenne AJ, eds. Lymph node biopsy interpretation. 2nd ed. Edinburgh: Churchill Livingstone, 1992;143–86.

70. Wolf BC, Neiman RS, Bennington TL. Disorders of the spleen. Major problems in pathology, Vol. 20. Philadelphia: WB Saunders, 1989:104–6.

17
HISTOLOGIC COMBINATIONS AND EVOLUTION
IN TUMORS OF THE LYMPHOID SYSTEM

One of the most intriguing aspects of the lymphomas is the variation in architectural and cellular features seen at presentation or during the disease course. Terms used to describe these changes include progression, variation, conversion, evolution, and transformation. Lymphoid tumors with two or more different histologic appearances in the same patient have been recognized for many years. In 1928, Richter (4) provided one of the most notable descriptions of this phenomenon when he described a case of "generalized reticulum cell sarcoma of lymph nodes associated with lymphatic leukemia." Thirteen years later, Warren and Picena (5) reported a link between lymphosarcoma and reticulum cell sarcoma. But it was not until 1948, when Custer and Bernhard (2) described a patient who had follicular lymphoma followed by Hodgkin's disease, that the interrelationship between Hodgkin's disease and other lymphatic tumors was illustrated. Custer (1) later recommended the term *composite lymphoma* for a lymphoma characterized by more than one histologic pattern within the same or in two different organs. More recently, Rappaport (3) reserved composite lymphoma for two distinctly different and well-demarcated types of lymphoma at a single anatomic site or tumor mass. The term *discordant lymphoma* describes two different types of lymphoma at separate anatomic sites.

The incidence of composite or discordant lymphoma varies among different types of lymphoma, depends upon the number of anatomic sites examined histologically at the time of presentation or during the course of disease, is affected by the time interval to biopsy or autopsy, and is influenced by the success or lack of success of treatment. The recent recognition that most tumors of the lymphoid system, including Hodgkin's disease, likely derive from B or T lymphocytes, and the better understanding of some of the phenotypic and genotypic features of these tumors, have led to a reassessment of the implications of such combinations. These histologic combinations as examples of tumor progression,

tumor cell differentiation, or the consequence of immunodeficiency secondary to neoplasia or treatment are described.

HISTOLOGIC COMBINATIONS AS EVIDENCE OF TUMOR PROGRESSION

Transformation of Low-Grade B-Cell Lymphoma

Histologic progression in B-lineage lymphomas is most evident in patients whose initial biopsies show features of low-grade lymphoma, for example, diffuse small lymphocytic, follicular small cleaved, or follicular mixed small cleaved and large cell lymphomas. These lymphomas typically transform to large cell type (fig. 17-1). However, they occasionally progress to lymphoblastic or small noncleaved cell lymphoma (fig. 17-2) (7,11,17,22,23). In autopsy series, up to 80 percent of follicular lymphomas show a changed architectural pattern and up to 60 percent evolve to large cell type (12,15,18,19). The incidence of progression in pattern or cell type in follicular lymphoma (documented by biopsies of relapses obtained at least 5 months after initial presentation) is lower than that reported in autopsy series (about 40 percent) (6,9,14); however, this may be affected by a variety of factors, as mentioned above. Data obtained from staging laparotomy reveal that 5 percent of patients with low-grade follicular lymphoma affecting peripheral sites have unsuspected large cell lymphoma in abdominal sites and 10 percent of patients with large cell lymphoma affecting peripheral sites have follicular lymphoma in abdominal sites (13). A lower incidence of tumor progression (about 15 percent) is reported in small lymphocytic lymphoma and chronic lymphocytic leukemia (fig. 17-3) (12,15). The clinical outcome with transformation is poor, but patients who respond to salvage chemotherapy do better (6).

Evidence for the clonal relatedness of two different histologic forms of lymphoma in the same patient comes from phenotypic studies demonstrating expression of the same immunoglobulin

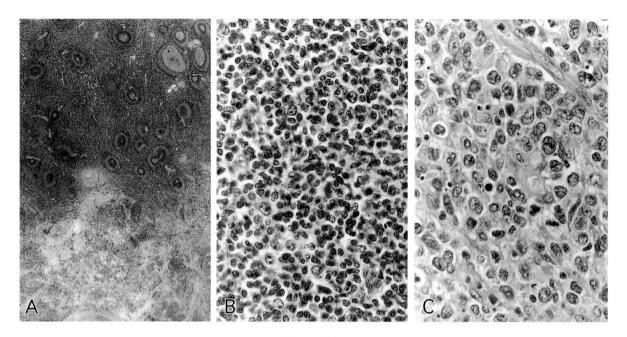

Figure 17-1
SPLEEN SHOWING BOTH FOLLICULAR SMALL CLEAVED CELL LYMPHOMA
AND DIFFUSE LARGE CELL LYMPHOMA AS EVIDENCE OF TUMOR PROGRESSION

A: The dark follicles at top are composed of small cleaved cells (illustrated in B) while the pale-staining follicles show an admixture of small cleaved and large cells (not illustrated).

C: A high magnification photomicrograph of the bottom area in A showing large cell lymphoma.

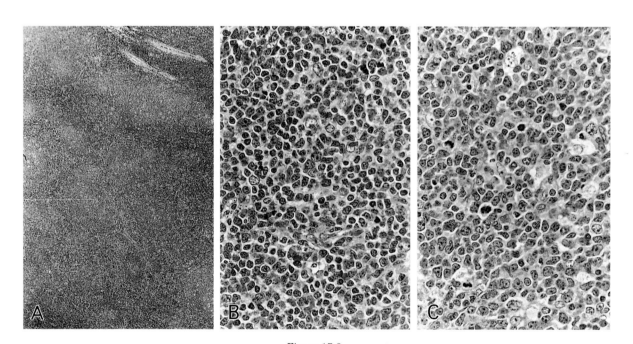

Figure 17-2
LYMPH NODE SHOWING BOTH FOLLICULAR SMALL CLEAVED CELL LYMPHOMA
AND DIFFUSE SMALL NONCLEAVED CELL LYMPHOMA AS EVIDENCE OF TUMOR PROGRESSION

A: The follicles in the central region are composed of small cleaved cells and occasional large cells (illustrated in B) while more diffuse areas near the top and bottom are composed of small noncleaved cells (illustrated in C).

C: The lymphoma cell nuclei are approximately the same size as the nuclei of the tingible body macrophages and mitotic figures are prominent. This patient had circulating lymphoma cells of both types: "buttock" cells and Burkitt's cells.

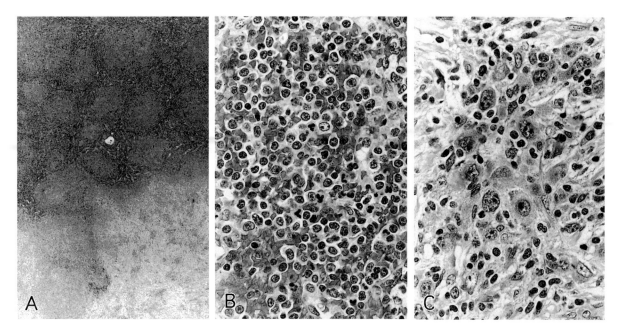

Figure 17-3
SPLEEN SHOWING BOTH SMALL LYMPHOCYTIC LYMPHOMA
AND LARGE CELL LYMPHOMA AS EVIDENCE OF TUMOR PROGRESSION

A: The pale staining area shows a large cell lymphoma with anaplastic cells (illustrated in C) while the expanded white pulp areas show large cell lymphoma rich in reactive T cells (not illustrated).

B: The red pulp contains a lambda-monotypic population of small lymphocytes (frozen section stain not illustrated).

C: Anaplastic lymphoma cells from the pale-staining focus seen in A.

light chain and heavy chain isotype in each form and, more convincingly, from molecular studies showing identical gene rearrangements in the two histologic forms (10,20,25). A subset of follicular lymphoma showed features of biclonality since there were two phenotypically and genotypically distinct populations when analyzed for antigen receptor genes (21); these cases arose from common progenitors since they shared identical t(14;18) breakpoints (8). The biclonality resulted from extensive secondary mutations of fully assembled immunoglobulin (Ig) genes in follicular lymphoma cells through the same hypermutation mechanism that increases the Ig repertoire in normal germinal center B cells (16). Many recurring genomic defects have been described in follicular lymphomas which progress to large cell lymphomas (24); molecular dissection of these defects is likely to elucidate the mechanisms of tumor progression. Histologic transformation, composite lymphomas, and apparent biclonality may all reflect the multistep nature of lymphoma pathogenesis (fig. 17-4) wherein characteristic histologic appearances

likely result from the cumulative effect of specific acquired genomic changes.

Transformation of Low-Grade T-Cell Lymphoma

Histologic variation has also been described in T-lineage lymphomas. Depending on the number of large cells required for a diagnosis of progression, the incidence of this phenomenon in autopsy studies of mycosis fungoides has varied from 6 to 33 percent (33). Biopsy series have shown a lower incidence of about 15 percent (fig. 17-5) (34). In one clinical study, the 8 percent of lymphomas that transformed were often noted in patients with advanced stage disease, nodal effacement, and erythroderma. Survival was poor in these patients (28,29). A recent study comparing patients with tumor stage mycosis fungoides, with or without progression to large cell lymphoma, did not find differences in survival from the time of biopsy of a tumor nodule; however, the survival time was shorter in patients whose lymphomas transformed (26).

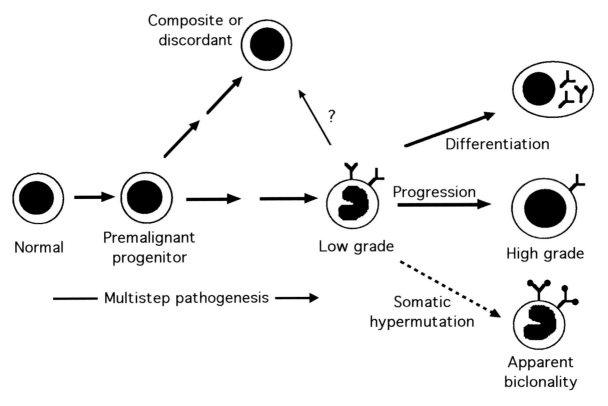

Figure 17-4

SCHEMATIC REPRESENTATION OF THE MULTISTEP PATHOGENESIS OF LYMPHOMAS

Conversion of normal lymphocytes to low-grade lymphoma cells results from the sequential accumulation of genomic changes that activate cellular proto-oncogenes or inactivate tumor suppressor genes. Premalignant progenitors may give rise to discordant or composite lymphomas due to concurrent, parallel sequences of genomic events. Genomic alterations superimposed on low-grade lymphoma cells result in histologic progression, differentiation, or composite/discordant lymphomas. Somatic hypermutation of tumor cell immunoglobulin genes may result in the appearance of biclonal lymphomas expressing surface immunoglobulin proteins with altered epitopes (rounded ends in figure).

In contrast to the small number of phenotypic abnormalities in typical mycosis fungoides, transformation is frequently associated with loss of expression of several normal T-lineage antigens together with expression of activation antigens such as CD30 (34). Recent molecular studies have demonstrated a clonal relationship between low-grade and high-grade components in a few cases (27,35).

Tumor progression in angioimmunoblastic lymphadenopathy (AILD) and AILD-like T-cell lymphoma has been well documented. Nathwani et al. (32) reported a high incidence of large cell lymphoma in follow-up biopsies from patients with AILD; however, a more recent autopsy series reported an incidence of only 13 percent (31). Recent studies have shown multiple cytogenetic defects in lymphomas from patients undergoing multiple bi-

opsies, some of which were not identified in follow-up biopsies (30). The role of Epstein-Barr virus (EBV) in this setting and in other patients with T-cell lymphoma is unclear but is discussed below.

HISTOLOGIC COMBINATIONS AS EVIDENCE OF DIFFERENTIATION

Although it has been common to view lymphomas as neoplasms composed of lymphoid cells frozen at a particular stage of differentiation, it is clear that the sequence of steps leading to lymphomagenesis interferes with differentiation, cell growth, or even programmed cell death in a variety of ways. Thus, the cells of different lymphomas may or may not resemble their presumptive normal counterparts. Furthermore, closer examination of different tumors of the lymphoid system

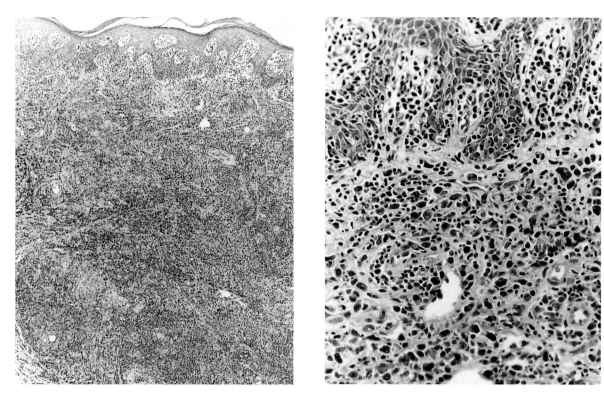

Figure 17-5
SKIN SHOWING BOTH MYCOSIS FUNGOIDES AND
LARGE CELL LYMPHOMA AS EVIDENCE OF TUMOR PROGRESSION
The tumor mass in the dermis and subcutis shows large cell lymphoma with anaplastic cells while the epidermal and very superficial dermal infiltrate is typical of mycosis fungoides.

reveals tumor components that differ to a greater or lesser extent from each other. For example, a population of monoclonal lymphocytes was identified in the peripheral blood of myeloma patients with an immunoglobulin idiotype identical to the predominant plasma cell population (44). These lymphocytes may have a phenotype resembling a mature B cell or may resemble an immature pre-B cell expressing cytoplasmic mμ chains, common acute lymphoblastic leukemia antigen (CALLA) and terminal deoxynucleotidyl transferase (TdT) (40). Although such an immature component may represent the proliferative, self-renewing population in myeloma, it may also express markers usually restricted to mature plasma cells, which complicates attempts to relate such a population to a normal stage of differentiation (40). Nevertheless, it appears that treatment directed at the immature pre-B-cell population in a patient with myeloma may have a favorable impact on survival (38).

Another example of differentiation in B-cell neoplasms is provided by a subset of follicular lymphoma that has a prominent population of plasma cells (fig. 17-6) (39,43,49). In a series of almost 200 cases of follicular lymphoma reported by Keith et al. (43), 17 (9 percent) showed large numbers of plasma cells. Based on paraffin section stains for immunoglobulin light chains, 7 patients (4 percent) had plasma cells that stained for a light chain identical to the follicular component. Three of these 7 patients had a monoclonal serum immunoglobulin of IgM isotype.

Histologic variation as a manifestation of tumor cell differentiation may explain the myriad of appearances that may be seen in low-grade lymphomas of mucosa-associated lymphoid tissues and the closely related monocytoid B-cell lymphoma. For example, such lymphomas may have varying numbers of small lymphocytes, centrocyte-like cells, monocytoid cells, plasmacytoid lymphocytes, and plasma cells (41,46).

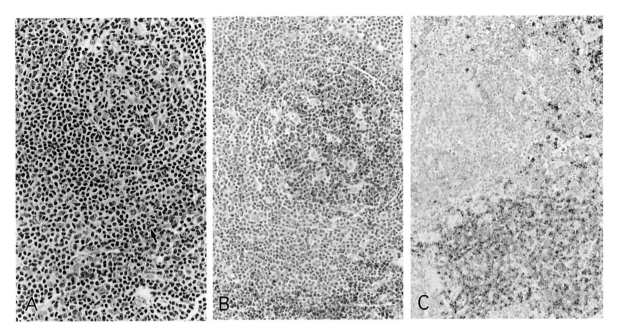

Figure 17-6
FOLLICULAR LYMPHOMA WITH DIFFERENTIATION TO PLASMA CELLS
A: The follicle at top shows an admixture of small cleaved and large cells while adjacent cells have a monocytoid appearance. The cells adjacent to the vessel at bottom represent plasmacytoid lymphocytes and plasma cells (arrow to Dutcher body).
B: Intense staining of the follicular cells for the *bcl*-2 protein suggests follicular lymphoma rather than follicular colonization by a diffuse small cell lymphoma. The adjacent monocytoid cells lack *bcl*-2 expression but the plasmacytoid cells at bottom stain for *bcl*-2.
C: Staining of the monocytoid cells, plasmacytoid cells, and plasma cells for kappa light chains confirms their neoplastic nature.

At presentation, one particular component may predominate while a different component may predominate in a follow-up biopsy. Some cases have a biphasic pattern with compartmentalization of the plasma cell component (37). In other cases, the architectural and cellular features mimic those of normal marginal zones (48). Reactive secondary follicles are frequently present in these lymphomas and may be colonized by lymphoma cells (42). Although it is tempting to interpret unusual combinations of follicular lymphoma and monocytoid B-cell lymphoma as examples of follicular colonization, the follicular component often has the unequivocal features of follicular lymphoma, including t(14;18) and *bcl*-2 overexpression (45). Some of these cases may represent follicular lymphoma with a prominent monocytoid component as a manifestation of differentiation. These mucosa-associated low-grade lymphomas may transform to large cell lymphomas (36). Both low-grade and high-grade lymphomas of the stomach have been associated with prior infection by *Helicobacter pylori* (47).

COMBINATIONS OF HODGKIN'S DISEASE AND NON-HODGKIN'S LYMPHOMA

Nodular Lymphocyte Predominance Hodgkin's Disease and Another Lymphoma

In 1983, Miettinen et al. (67) described the development of diffuse large cell lymphoma in patients with the nodular form of lymphocyte predominance Hodgkin's disease (NLPHD). In this retrospective review of 51 cases with relatively long-term clinical follow-up, 5 such cases were identified. Since only one patient had been treated for lymphoma, therapy was eliminated as a cause of the large cell lymphoma. Mixed cellularity Hodgkin's disease was seen in 2 other patients. Hodgkin's sarcoma (immunoblastic lymphoma) following untreated NLPHD had been previously illustrated by Poppema in 1979 (69). Numerous examples of this association have now been reported, including cases of "composite" large cell lymphoma and NLPHD (fig. 17-7) (52,58,60,73). The recognition of the B-cell

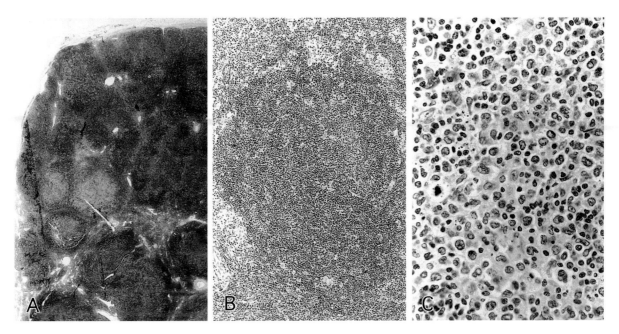

Figure 17-7
LYMPH NODE SHOWING BOTH NODULAR LYMPHOCYTE PREDOMINANCE
HODGKIN'S DISEASE AND LARGE CELL LYMPHOMA
A: The darkly stained nodules at top and bottom show a predominance of small lymphocytes with some of the nodules ringed by clusters of epithelioid histiocytes (illustrated in B).
C: The pale-staining nodules of A and diffuse areas (not illustrated) show a predominance of large cells.

nature of NLPHD has led to the suggestion that such examples represent tumor progression, transformation, or evolution. Nevertheless, the clonality of NLPHD remains controversial and few of the cases of large cell lymphoma complicating NLPHD have been studied extensively. Large cell lymphomas that arise at the same site as the NLPHD respond well to local therapy (73). As a further complication to understanding the nature of this association, a few cases of T-cell lymphoma and usual Hodgkin's disease have been described in association with NLPHD (fig. 17-8) (56,61).

Classic Hodgkin's Disease and B-Cell Lymphoma and Leukemia

In a 1948 study of 255 biopsies, Custer and Bernhard described 4 cases of Hodgkin's disease associated with follicular lymphoma; they found 3 more cases in an autopsy series of 129 patients (53). In 1974, Kim and Dorfman (63) described three patients with Hodgkin's disease in whom staging laparotomy disclosed intra-abdominal involvement by follicular lymphoma; one patient also had a focus of follicular lymphoma in the initial biopsy. In a subsequent study of 20 com-

posite lymphomas, 6 represented classic Hodgkin's disease in combination with non-Hodgkin's lymphoma (5 follicular lymphomas and 1 diffuse large cell lymphoma) (64). Recent studies of composite cases that include phenotyping describe an antigenic profile in the Hodgkin's component typical of classic Hodgkin's disease (fig. 17-9) (57,59). Hodgkin's disease has also been reported in patients with a prior diagnosis of non-Hodgkin's lymphoma, particularly the follicular subtypes (76). The immunophenotype of tumor giant cells in these patients is typical of classic Hodgkin's disease (76). EBV has not been identified in the follicular component of the composite cases or in the follicular cases that antedate a diagnosis of Hodgkin's disease (65). However, EBV has been found in both components of composite Hodgkin's disease and diffuse mixed or large cell lymphoma (65).

Recent molecular studies have also suggested a possible pathogenetic link between follicular lymphoma and Hodgkin's disease. One study reported a high incidence of t(14;18) in Hodgkin tissues using polymerase chain reaction methodology (72), but this has not been confirmed by other

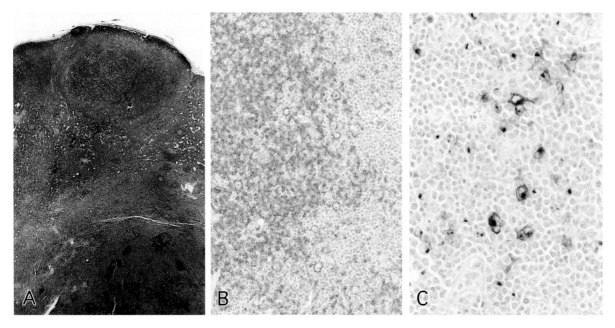

Figure 17-8
LYMPH NODE SHOWING BOTH NODULAR LYMPHOCYTE PREDOMINANCE HODGKIN'S DISEASE
AND INTERFOLLICULAR HODGKIN'S DISEASE OF THE CLASSIC TYPE

A: The nodule at top shows features of NLPHD while the interfollicular infiltrate at bottom shows features of classic Hodgkin's disease.

B: The small lymphocytes and L&H cells stain for CD20 with antibody L26 while the classic Hodgkin cells do not (not illustrated).

C: The classic Hodgkin cells stain for CD15 with antibody LeuM1 while the L&H cells do not (not illustrated).

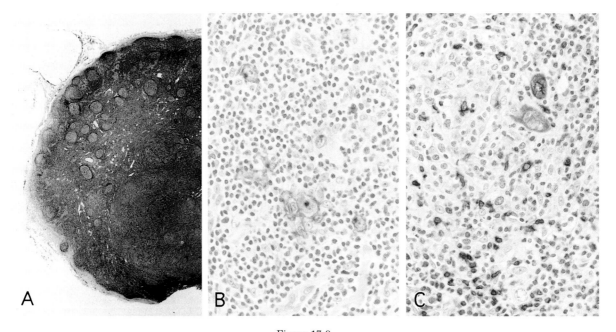

Figure 17-9
LYMPH NODE SHOWING BOTH FOLLICULAR SMALL CLEAVED CELL LYMPHOMA
AND MIXED CELLULARITY HODGKIN'S DISEASE

A: The follicles are composed of small cleaved cells while the larger nodule at right shows features of Hodgkin's disease.

B: The Hodgkin cells stain for CD15 and have other phenotypic findings of classic Hodgkin's disease. The follicles of lymphoma express the *bcl*-2 protein (not illustrated).

C: A few normal-appearing follicles contain a few small cleaved lymphoma cells and Hodgkin cells which strongly express the *bcl*-2 protein. Relapse occurred 1 year later at this same site following chemotherapy; the biopsy showed evidence of only Hodgkin's disease.

investigators (74). Another study reported a lower incidence of t(14;18) in Hodgkin tissues (2 of 32 cases) and showed that its presence correlated with a prior history of follicular lymphoma (66). In one patient, the same t(14;18) breakpoint was found in the Hodgkin biopsy as was found in the follicular lymphoma biopsy 8 years before. This study reported an additional eight cases without molecular studies in which follicular lymphoma preceded or coexisted with Hodgkin's disease. Overexpression of the *bcl*-2 protein was demonstrated in the Hodgkin cells in all cases, leading to the hypothesis that a small proportion of Hodgkin's disease arises in patients with follicular lymphoma through molecular events superimposed on a t(14;18) translocation. Unlike many cases of Hodgkin's disease, EBV was not identified in these cases (66). Although Hodgkin's disease and follicular lymphoma are two of the most prevalent lymphoma subtypes, their coincidence appears to be more frequent than would be expected at random, but convincing evidence of common progenitor cells remains elusive.

Hodgkin's disease has also been described in association with chronic lymphocytic leukemia (CLL)/small lymphocytic lymphoma (63). Although the Hodgkin-type cells in these cases were initially thought to represent a manifestation of progression or transformation, some cases also have the inflammatory cell background and tumor cell phenotype typical of classic Hodgkin's disease (50,75). Relapse biopsies sometimes show histologic and phenotypic features of Hodgkin's disease rather than CLL (62). EBV has been demonstrated in such cases (68).

Classic Hodgkin's Disease and T-Cell Lymphoma

Cases of Hodgkin's disease in association with mycosis fungoides have been reported for many years. However, such cases were usually attributed to misdiagnosis until the more recent description and illustration of convincing combinations supported by appropriate studies (51,55, 70,71). Although there have been few phenotypic studies of such cases, a recent report of a single patient described the identical T-cell receptor alpha chain gene rearrangement in separate biopsies showing Hodgkin's disease or mycosis fungoides (54). In this case, as in the majority of cases of Hodgkin's disease associated with B-cell lymphoma or leukemia, the low-grade B- or T-

lymphoproliferative disorder often preceded the development of Hodgkin's disease.

HISTOLOGIC COMBINATIONS AS EVIDENCE OF IMMUNODEFICIENCY

The occurrence of non-Hodgkin's lymphoma following therapy for Hodgkin's disease was reported more than a decade ago (83). Although persistent immunodeficiency secondary to Hodgkin's disease was considered, this uncommon late complication primarily developed in patients treated with both radiation and chemotherapy (83,85). In addition, many of the lymphomas were high-grade small noncleaved cell, a subtype that occurs frequently in other conditions of immunodeficiency: following organ transplantation or particularly following human immunodeficiency virus (HIV) infection (84,86). EBV has been localized to tumor cells in a few of these treatment-related lymphomas (82). A large British study identified 22 patients with non-Hodgkin's lymphoma in a cohort of 3,033 patients treated for Hodgkin's disease. These patients developed various types of non-Hodgkin's lymphomas and tended to have evidence of immunosuppression prior to treatment as evidenced by low lymphocyte counts, advanced stage, and systemic symptoms (77). Furthermore, non-Hodgkin's lymphoma of the brain, which commonly occurs in the setting of immunosuppression, has also been reported following treatment for Hodgkin's disease (78). A short time interval to the development of non-Hodgkin's lymphoma in one patient made a treatment effect unlikely (78).

Rare occurrences of both B-cell and T-cell lymphomas in the same patient have suggested the possibility of neoplasia in a common progenitor cell or the possibility of underlying immunodeficiency (79,81). One patient appeared to have two different B-cell and T-cell clones at different time points during the course of her disease (81). One of the clonal T-cell proliferations closely resembled mixed cellularity Hodgkin's disease. These lymphomas followed a difficult to characterize autoimmune disorder that included features of eosinophilic fasciitis. EBV was recently identified in the various lymphomas (unpublished). In addition, EBV was identified in both the Hodgkin's and non-Hodgkin's lymphomas which developed in a patient infected with HIV (80).

REFERENCES

Historical Aspects of Histologic Combinations

1. Custer RP. Pitfalls in the diagnosis of lymphoma and leukemia from the pathologist's point of view. 2nd National Cancer Conference. New York: American Cancer Society, 1954:554–7.
2. _____, Bernhard WG. The interrelationship of Hodgkin's disease and other lymphatic tumors. Am J Med Sci 1948;216:625–42.
3. Rappaport H. Tumors of the hematopoietic system. In: Atlas of Tumor Pathology, 1st Series, Fascicle 8. Washington, DC: Armed Forces Institute of Pathology, 1966.
4. Richter MN. Generalized reticular cell sarcoma of lymph nodes, associated with lymphatic leukemia. Am J Pathol 1928;4:285–92.
5. Warren S, Picena JP. Reticulum cell sarcoma of lymph nodes. Am J Pathol 1941;17:385–94.

Transformation of Low-Grade B-Cell Lymphoma

6. Acker B, Hoppe RT, Colby TV, Cox RS, Kaplan HS, Rosenberg SA. Histologic conversion in the non-Hodgkin's lymphomas. J Clin Oncol 1983;1:11–6.
7. Aventin A, Mecucci C, Guanyabens C, et al. Variant t(2;18) translocation in a Burkitt conversion of follicular lymphoma. Br J Haematol 1990;74:367–9.
8. Cleary ML, Galili N, Trela M, Levy R, Sklar J. Single cell origin of bigenotypic and biphenotypic B cell proliferations in human follicular lymphomas. J Exp Med 1988;167:582–97.
9. Cullen MH, Lister TA, Brearley RI, Shand WS, Stansfeld AG. Histological transformation of non-Hodgkin's lymphoma. A prospective study. Cancer 1979;44:645–51.
10. de Jong D, Voetdijk BM, van Ommen GJ, Kluin PM. Alterations in immunoglobulin genes reveal the origin and evolution of monotypic and bitypic B cell lymphomas. Am J Pathol 1989;134:1233–42.
11. _____, Voetdijk BM, Beverstock GC, van Ommen GJ, Willemze R, Kluin PM. Activation of the c-myc oncogene in a precursor-B-cell blast crisis of follicular lymphoma, presenting as composite lymphoma. N Eng J Med 1988;318:1373–8.
12. Garvin AJ, Simon RM, Osborne CK, Merrell J, Young RC, Berard CW. An autopsy study of histologic progression in non-Hodgkin's lymphomas. 192 cases from the National Cancer Institute. Cancer 1983;52:393–8.
13. Goffinet DR, Warnke R, Dunnick NR, et al. Clinical and surgical (laparotomy) evaluation of patients with non-Hodgkin's lymphomas. Cancer Treat Rep 1977;61:981–92.
14. Hubbard SM, Chabner BA, DeVita VT Jr, et al. Histologic progression in non-Hodgkin's lymphomas. Blood 1982;59:258–64.
15. Lennert K, Stein H, Mohri N, Kaiserling E, Hermelink HK. Malignant lymphomas other than Hodgkin's disease: histology, cytology, ultrastructure, immunology. New York: Springer-Verlag, 1978.
16. Levy S, Mendel E, Kon S, Avnur Z, Levy R. Mutational hot spots in Ig V region genes of human follicular lymphomas. J Exp Med 1988;168:475–89.
17. Mintzer DM, Andreeff M, Filippa DA, Jhanwar SC, Chaganti RS, Koziner B. Progression of nodular poorly differentiated lymphocytic lymphoma to Burkitt's-like lymphoma. Blood 1984;64:415–21.
18. Rappaport H, Winter WJ, Hicks EB. Follicular lymphoma. A re-evaluation of its position in the scheme of malignant lymphoma based on a survey of 253 cases. Cancer 1956;9:792–821.
19. Risdall R, Hoppe RT, Warnke R. Non-Hodgkin's lymphoma: a study of the evolution of the disease based upon 92 autopsied cases. Cancer 1979;44:529–42.
20. Siegelman MH, Cleary ML, Warnke R, Sklar J. Frequent biclonality and immunoglobulin gene alterations among B-cell lymphomas that show multiple histologic forms. J Exp Med 1985;161:850–63.
21. Sklar J, Cleary M, Thielemans K, Gralow J, Warnke R, Levy R. Biclonal B-cell lymphoma. N Engl J Med 1984;311:20–7.
22. Thangavelu M, Olopade O, Beckman E, et al. Clinical, morphologic, and cytogenetic characteristics of patients with lymphoid malignancies characterized by both t(14;18)(q32;q21) and t(8;14)(q24;q32) or t(8;22)(q24;q11). Genes Chromosom Cancer 1990;2:147–58.
23. Weiss LM, Warnke RA. Follicular lymphoma with blastic conversion: a report of two cases with confirmation by immunoperoxidase studies on bone marrow sections. Am J Clin Pathol 1985;83:681–6.
24. Yunis JJ, Frizzera G, Oken MM, McKenna J, Theologides A, Arnesen M. Multiple recurrent genomic defects in follicular lymphoma. A possible model for cancer. N Engl J Med 1987;316:79–84.
25. Zelenetz AD, Chen TT, Levy R. Histologic transformation of follicular lymphoma to diffuse lymphoma represents tumor progression by a single malignant B cell. J Exp Med 1991;173:197–207.

Transformation of Low-Grade T-Cell Lymphoma

26. Cerroni L, Rieger E, Hodl S, Kerl H. Clinicopathologic and immunologic features associated with transformation of mycosis fungoides to large-cell lymphoma. Am J Surg Pathol 1992;16:543–52.
27. Davis TH, Morton CC, Miller-Cassman R, Balk SP, Kadin ME. Hodgkin's disease, lymphomatoid papulosis, and cutaneous T-cell lymphoma derived from a common T-cell clone. N Engl J Med 1992;326:1115–22.
28. Dmitrovsky E, Matthews MJ, Bunn PA, et al. Cytologic transformation in cutaneous T cell lymphoma: a clinicopathologic entity associated with poor prognosis. J Clin Oncol 1987;5:208–15.
29. Greer JP, Salhany KE, Cousar JB, et al. Clinical features associated with transformation of cerebriform T-cell lymphoma to a large cell process. Hematol Oncol 1990;8:215–27.

30. Kaneko Y, Maseki N, Sakurai M, et al. Characteristic karyotypic pattern in T-cell lymphoproliferative disorders with reactive angioimmunoblastic lymphadenopathy with dysproteinemia-type features. Blood 1988;72:413–21.
31. Knecht H, Schwarze EW, Lennert K. Histological, immunohistological and autopsy findings in lymphogranulomatosis X (including angio-immunoblastic lymphadenopathy). Virchows Arch [A] 1985;406:105–24.
32. Nathwani BN, Rappaport H, Moran EM, Pangalis GA, Kim H. Malignant lymphoma arising in angioimmunoblastic lymphadenopathy. Cancer 1978;41:578–606.

33. Rappaport H, Thomas LB. Mycosis fungoides: the pathology of extracutaneous involvement. Cancer 1974;34:1198–229.
34. Salhany KE, Cousar JB, Greer JP, Casey TT, Fields JP, Collins RD. Transformation of cutaneous T cell lymphoma to large cell lymphoma. A clinicopathologic and immunologic study. Am J Pathol 1988;132:265–77.
35. Wood GS, Bahler DW, Hoppe RT, Warnke RA, Sklar JL, Levy R. Transformation of mycosis fungoides: t-cell receptor beta gene analysis demonstrates a common clonal origin for plaque-type mycosis fungoides and CD30+ large cell lymphoma. J Invest Dermatol 1993;101:296–300.

Histologic Combinations as Evidence of Differentiation

36. Chan JK, Ng CS, Isaacson PG. Relationship between high-grade lymphoma and low-grade B-cell mucosa-associated lymphoid tissue lymphoma (MALToma) of the stomach. Am J Pathol 1990;136:1153–64.
37. Chetty R, Close PM, Timme AH, Willcox PA, Forder MD. Primary biphasic lymphoplasmacytic lymphoma of the lung. A mucosa-associated lymphoid tissue lymphoma with compartmentalization of plasma cells in the lung and lymph nodes. Cancer 1992;69:1124–9.
38. Epstein J, Barlogie B, Katzmann J, Alexanian R. Phenotypic heterogeneity in aneuploid multiple myeloma indicates pre-B cell involvement. Blood 1988;71:861–5.
39. Frizzera G, Anaya JS, Banks PM. Neoplastic plasma cells in follicular lymphomas. Clinical and pathologic findings in six cases. Virchows Arch [A] 1986;409:149–62.
40. Grogan TM, Spier CM. The B-cell immunoproliferative disorders including multiple myeloma and amyloidosis. In: Knowles DM II, ed. Neoplastic hematopathology. Baltimore: Williams & Wilkins, 1992.
41. Isaacson PG. Lymphomas of mucosa-associated lymphoid tissue (MALT). Histopathology 1990;16:617–9.
42. _____, Wotherspoon AC, Diss T, Pan LX. Follicular colonization in B-cell lymphoma of mucosa-associated lymphoid tissue. Am J Surg Pathol 1991;15:819–28.
43. Keith TA, Cousar JB, Glick AD, Vogler LB, Collins RD. Plasmacytic differentiation in follicular center cell (FCC) lymphomas. Am J Clin Pathol 1985;84:283–90.

44. Kubagawa H, Vogler LB, Capra JD, Conrad ME, Lawton AR, Cooper MD. Studies on the clonal origin of multiple myeloma. Use of individually specific (idiotypic) antibodies to trace the oncogenic event to its earliest point of expression in B-cell differentiation. J Exp Med 1979;150:792–807.
45. Ngan BY, Warnke RA, Wilson M, Takagi K, Cleary ML, Dorfman RF. Monocytoid B-cell lymphoma: a study of 36 cases. Hum Pathol 1991;22:409–21.
46. Nizze H, Cogliatti SB, von Schilling C, Feller AC, Lennert K. Monocytoid B-cell lymphoma: morphological variants and relationship to low-grade B-cell lymphoma of the mucosa-associated lymphoid tissue. Histopathology 1991;18:403–14.
47. Parsonnet J, Hansen S, Rodriguez L, et al. Helicobacter pylori infection and gastric lymphoma. N Engl J Med 1994;330:1267–71.
48. Schmid C, Kirkham N, Diss T, Isaacson PG. Splenic marginal zone cell lymphoma. Am J Surg Pathol 1992;16:455–66.
49. Schmid U, Karow J, Lennert K. Follicular malignant non-Hodgkin's lymphoma with pronounced plasmacytic differentiation: a plasmacytoma–like lymphoma. Virchows Arch [A] 1985;405:473–81.

Combinations of Hodgkin's Disease and Non-Hodgkin's Lymphoma

50. Brecher M, Banks PM. Hodgkin's disease variant of Richter's syndrome. Report of eight cases. Am J Clin Pathol 1990;93:333–9.
51. Chan WC, Greim ML, Grozea PN, Freel RJ, Variakojis D. Mycosis fungoides and Hodgkin's disease occurring in the same patient. Report of three cases. Cancer 1979;44:1408–13.
52. Chittal SM, Alard C, Rossi JF, et al. Further phenotypic evidence that nodular, lymphocyte-predominant Hodgkin's disease is a large B-cell lymphoma in evolution. Am J Surg Pathol 1990;14:1024–35.
53. _____, Bernhard WG. The interrelationship of Hodgkin's disease and other lymphatic tumors. Am J Med Sci 1948;216:625–42.
54. Davis TH, Morton CC, Miller-Cassman R, Balk SP, Kadin ME. Hodgkin's disease, lymphomatoid papulosis, and cutaneous T-cell lymphoma derived from a common T-cell clone. N Engl J Med 1992;326:1115–22.

55. Donald D, Green JA, White J. Mycosis fungoides associated with nodular sclerosing Hodgkin's disease. Cancer 1980;46:2505–8.
56. Gelb AB, Dorfman RF, Warnke RA. Coexistence of nodular lymphocyte predominance Hodgkin's disease and Hodgkin's disease of the usual type. Am J Surg Pathol 1993;17:364–74.
57. Gonzalez CL, Medeiros LJ, Jaffe ES. Composite lymphoma. A clinicopathologic analysis of nine patients with Hodgkin's disease and B-cell non-Hodgkin's lymphoma. Am J Clin Pathol 1991;96:81–9.
58. Grossman DM, Hanson CA, Schnitzer B. Simultaneous lymphocyte predominant Hodgkin's disease and large-cell lymphoma. Am J Surg Pathol 1991;15:668–76.
59. Hansmann ML, Fellbaum C, Hui PK, Lennert K. Morphological and immunohistochemical investigation of non-Hodgkin's lymphoma combined with Hodgkin's disease. Histopathology 1989;15:35–48.

60. _____, Stein H, Fellbaum C, Hui PK, Parwaresch MR, Lennert K. Nodular paragranuloma can transform into high-grade malignant lymphoma of B type. Hum Pathol 1989;20:1169–75.

61. Harris NL. The relationship between Hodgkin's disease and non-Hodgkin's lymphoma. Semin Diagn Pathol 1992;9:304–10.

62. Jaffe ES, Zarate-Osorno A, Medeiros J. The interrelationship of Hodgkin's disease and non-Hodgkin's lymphomas—lessons learned from composite and sequential malignancies. Semin Diagn Pathol 1992;9:297–303.

63. Kim H, Dorfman RF. Morphological studies of 84 untreated patients subjected to laparotomy for the staging of non-Hodgkin's lymphomas. Cancer 1974;33:657–74.

64. _____, Hendrickson MR, Dorfman RF. Composite lymphomas. Cancer 1977;40:959–76.

65. Kingma DW, Medeiros LJ, Barletta J, et al. Epstein-Barr virus is infrequently identified in non-Hodgkin's lymphomas associated with Hodgkin's disease. Am J Surg Pathol 1994;18:48–61.

66. LeBrun DP, Ngan BY, Weiss LM, Warnke RA, Cleary ML. The bcl-2 oncogene in the origin of Hodgkin's disease arising in the setting of follicular non-Hodgkin's lymphoma. Blood 1994;83:223–30.

67. Miettinen M, Franssila KO, Saxen E. Hodgkin's disease, lymphocytic predominance nodular. Increased risk for subsequent non-Hodgkin's lymphomas. Cancer 1983;51:2293–300.

68. Momose H, Jaffe ES, Shin SS, Chen YY, Weiss LM. Chronic lymphocytic leukemia/small lymphocytic lymphoma with Reed-Sternberg-like cells and possible transformation to Hodgkin's disease. Mediation by Epstein-Barr virus. Am J Surg Pathol 1992;16:859–67.

69. Poppema S, Kaiserling E, Lennert K. Hodgkin's disease with lymphocytic predominance, nodular type (nodular paragranuloma) and progressively transformed germinal centres–a cytohistological study. Histopathol 1979;3:295–308.

70. Rappaport H, Thomas LB. Mycosis fungoides: the pathology of extracutaneous involvement. Cancer 1974;34:1198–229.

71. Scheen SR III, Banks PM, Winkelmann RK. Morphologic heterogeneity of malignant lymphomas developing in mycosis fungoides. Mayo Clin Proc 1984;59:95–106.

72. Stetler-Stevenson M, Crush-Stanton S, Cossman J. Involvement of the bcl-2 gene in Hodgkin's disease. JNCI 1990;82:855–8.

73. Sundeen JT, Cossman J, Jaffe ES. Lymphocyte predominant Hodgkin's disease nodular subtype with coexistent large cell lymphoma. Histological progression or composite malignancy? Am J Surg Pathol 1988;12:599–606.

74. Weiss LM, Chang KL. Molecular biologic studies of Hodgkin's disease. Semin Diagn Pathol 1992;9:272–8.

75. Williams J, Schned A, Cotelingam JD, Jaffe ES. Chronic lymphocytic leukemia with coexistent Hodgkin's disease. Implications for the origin of the Reed-Sternberg cell. Am J Surg Pathol 1991;15:33–42.

76. Zarate OA, Medeiros LJ, Kingma DW, Longo DL, Jaffe ES. Hodgkin's disease following non-Hodgkin's lymphoma. A clinicopathologic and immunophenotypic study of nine cases. Am J Surg Pathol 1993;17:123–32.

Histologic Combinations as Evidence of Immunodeficiency

77. Bennett MH, MacLennan KA, Vaughan Hudson G, Vaughan Hudson B. Non-Hodgkin's lymphoma arising in patients treated for Hodgkin's disease in the BNLI: a 20-year experience. British National Lymphoma Investigation. Ann Oncol 1991;2(Suppl 2):83–92.

78. Davenport RD, O'Donnell LR, Schnitzer B, McKeever PE. Non-Hodgkin's lymphoma of the brain after Hodgkin's disease. An immunohistochemical study. Cancer 1991;67:440–3.

79. Deane M, Amlot P, Pappas H, Norton JD. Independent clonal origin of T- and B-cell clones in a composite lymphoma. Leuk Res 1991;15:811–7.

80. Guarner J, del Rio C, Hendrix L, Unger ER. Composite Hodgkin's and non-Hodgkin's lymphoma in a patient with acquired immune deficiency syndrome. In-situ demonstration of Epstein-Barr virus. Cancer 1990;66:796–800.

81. Hu E, Weiss LM, Warnke R, Sklar J. Non-Hodgkin's lymphoma containing both B and T-cell clones. Blood 1987;70:287–92.

82. Kingma DW, Medeiros LJ, Barletta J, et al. Epstein-Barr virus is infrequently identified in non-Hodgkin's lymphomas associated with Hodgkin's disease. Am J Surg Pathol 1994;18:48–61.

83. Krikorian JG, Burke JS, Rosenberg SA, Kaplan HS. Occurrence of non-Hodgkin's lymphoma after therapy for Hodgkin's disease. N Eng J Med 1979;300:452–8.

84. Travis LB, Gonzalez CL, Hankey BF, Jaffe ES. Hodgkin's disease following non-Hodgkin's lymphoma. Cancer 1992;69:2337–42.

85. Tucker MA, Coleman CN, Cox RS, Varghese A, Rosenberg SA. Risk of second cancers after treatment for Hodgkin's disease. N Engl J Med 1988;318:76–81.

86. Zarate OA, Medeiros LJ, Longo DL, Jaffe ES. Non-Hodgkin's lymphomas arising in patients successfully treated for Hodgkin's disease. A clinical, histologic, and immunophenotypic study of 14 cases. Am J Surg Pathol 1992;16:885–95.

❖❖❖

18
HISTIOCYTIC AND DENDRITIC CELL PROLIFERATIONS

LANGERHANS' CELL HISTIOCYTOSIS

Definition. Langerhans' cell histiocytosis is a clonal proliferative disorder of Langerhans cells. Synonyms include *histiocytosis X* and *Langerhans' cell granulomatosis*. The disease manifests as three main, although sometimes overlapping, clinical syndromes: unifocal disease (solitary eosinophilic granuloma), multifocal unisystem disease (many cases of what had been previously designated Hand-Schüller-Christian syndrome), and multifocal multisystem disease (many cases of what had been previously designated Letterer-Siwe syndrome).

Incidence. Langerhans' cell histiocytosis is a rare disease that affects males twice as often as females and occurs primarily in children. The age at presentation varies with the clinical syndrome: the median age of presentation with multifocal multisystem disease is less than 3 years (12); the age of presentation with multifocal unisystem disease is somewhat older; and unifocal disease most commonly occurs in older children and adolescents. Adults, when affected, usually have unifocal disease; nonetheless, all three clinical syndromes have been reported to occur in all age groups.

Langerhans' cell histiocytosis occurs more often in northern European Caucasians than in Hispanics, and rarely occurs in blacks (34). No known environmental factors are associated with its occurrence, with the exception that isolated Langerhans' cell histiocytosis of the lung is particularly common in active cigarette smokers (7,11). There is also a high prevalence of pulmonary and extrapulmonary neoplasms in patients with pulmonary Langerhans' cell histiocytosis; cigarette smoking may be the common denominator (30).

The possibility of an infectious agent as an etiologic factor has been extensively investigated. One group found evidence of human herpesvirus 6 in lesions of Langerhans' cell histiocytosis (18). However, another group failed to confirm this finding, nor did they find molecular evidence of seven other viruses, including the Epstein-Barr virus, in a study of 50 cases (19).

Natural History and Clinical Features. In multifocal multisystem disease, a wide variety of sites may be involved. The skin, bone, and lymph nodes are the most commonly involved sites at presentation, and liver, spleen, lung, and mucosal involvement often develop during the disease course. Skin involvement usually manifests as a generalized erythematous scaling or eczematoid rash. Bony lesions are as common as skin lesions, with the skull, sella turcica, sphenoid bone, maxilla, mandible, and bones of the upper extremity most often affected (8). The bony lesions are lytic, and may be asymptomatic or painful. Manifestations include fever, anemia, and thrombocytopenia. Diabetes insipidus may occur, and is usually due to bony lesions of the sella turcica. Multifocal unisystem disease usually manifests as multiple bone lesions.

Unifocal unisystem disease usually presents in the bone as a painful solitary lytic lesion in the skull, femur, rib, mandible, vertebral body, or pelvis (14). When isolated lung involvement occurs, patients present with cough, dyspnea, chest pain, fever, hemoptysis, or weight loss. The chest radiograph may show a nodular, reticulonodular, interstitial, alveolar, or cystic pattern (16). Laboratory studies generally show no abnormalities other than deficits in pulmonary function. It is still not clear whether isolated involvement of the lung truly represents a form of Langerhans' cell histiocytosis or, rather, a peculiar reactive process. Other sites of localized disease that have been reported include lymph node, thymus, and soft tissue (29,32). Patients with isolated lymph node involvement are usually afebrile, with sometimes painful lymphadenopathy, which is often in the cervical or inguinal region (21).

The Histiocyte Society has recommended a uniform pathologic staging system, listed in Table 18-1, to standardize description of disease extent (9).

The course of the disease is generally related to the number of affected organs at presentation, especially if involvement is associated with organ dysfunction, but may be highly variable from case to case. A unifocal unisystem lesion

Table 18-1

PATHOLOGIC STAGING OF LANGERHANS' CELL HISTIOCYTOSIS
(HISTIOCYTE SOCIETY)

A. Bone only or bone with involvement of first echelon lymph nodes in drainage field (osteolymphatic disease) and/or contiguous soft tissue involvement.

    A1. Monostotic

    A2. Monostotic with osteolymphatic disease

    A3. Monostotic with contiguous soft tissue involvement

    A4. Polyostotic

    A5. Polyostotic with osteolymphatic disease

    A6. Polyostotic with contiguous soft tissue involvement

B. Skin and/or other squamous mucous membranes only or with involvement of related superficial lymph nodes.

    B1. Nodular disease: neonatal period without nodal disease

    B2. Nodular disease: neonatal period with nodal disease

    B3. Multiple nodules or diffuse maculopapular disease without nodal disease

    B4. Multiple nodules or diffuse maculopapular disease with nodal disease

C. Soft tissue and viscera only excluding above and multisystem disease. Specify tissue involved, e.g., lung, lymph node, brain.

D. Multisystem disease with any combination of above. Specify each organ/tissue involved, e.g., skin, bone marrow, bone.

---

may rapidly progress to multisystem involvement, or multisystem involvement may undergo spontaneous regression, albeit rarely (5). The rate of progression of disease may also vary widely. In general, however, patients with unifocal unisystem disease develop disseminated disease in fewer than 10 percent of cases. Death, when it occurs, generally results from intercurrent infection or as a consequence of extensive bone marrow involvement.

Microscopic Findings. Although lesions vary in their histologic appearance, the diagnosis of Langerhans' cell histiocytosis is established by the definitive identification of proliferating Langerhans' cells. Langerhans' cells are mononuclear cells approximately 12 to 15 μm in diameter (fig. 18-1). The cytoplasm is generally eosinophilic and moderate in amount. The nucleus has a characteristic folded, indented, grooved, contorted, or lobulated appearance, generally with inconspicuous nucleoli. The nuclear membrane is thin, and the chromatin is fine (fig. 18-2). Although cytologic atypia may be present in some cases, the nuclei are usually cytologically benign in appearance. The mitotic activity varies widely from lesion to lesion, and

ranges from 0 to 25 mitotic figures per 10 high-power fields, with a median of 2 (25).

The Langerhans' cells are usually present in a mixed background of eosinophils, mononuclear and multinuclear histiocytes, neutrophils, and small lymphocytes (fig. 18-3). Early lesions tend to be highly cellular, with large numbers of Langerhans cells and eosinophils (fig. 18-4), while older lesions have more histiocytes, often with foamy cytoplasm, and fewer eosinophils (fig. 18-5). In very late lesions, fibrosis may dominate, Langerhans' cells may be difficult to identify, and the predominant elements may be histiocytes, lymphocytes, and plasma cells (fig. 18-6). Necrosis is occasionally present, particularly in the center of clusters of eosinophils, as eosinophilic microabscesses (fig. 18-7). Areas of necrosis, eosinophils, and multinucleated histiocytes are usually more numerous in bone lesions than in skin, lung, or lymph node lesions (fig. 18-8) (23).

Lymph nodes are involved by Langerhans' cell histiocytosis in several ways. The involved lymph node may drain a site of bone (osteolymphatic) or skin disease; unless there are superimposed dermatopathic changes (present in the paracortical areas), the affected lymph nodes are generally small

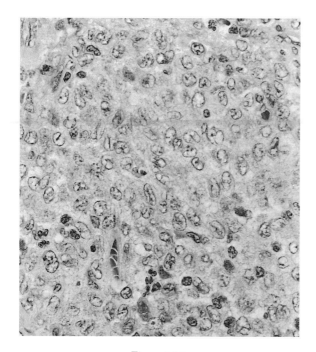

Figure 18-1
LANGERHANS' CELL HISTIOCYTOSIS
The proliferating cells have relatively bland nuclei, often with folds or clefts.

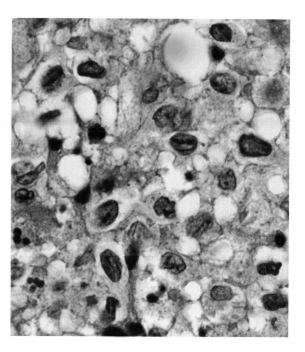

Figure 18-2
LANGERHANS' CELL HISTIOCYTOSIS
Note the bland cytologic features with fine chromatin.

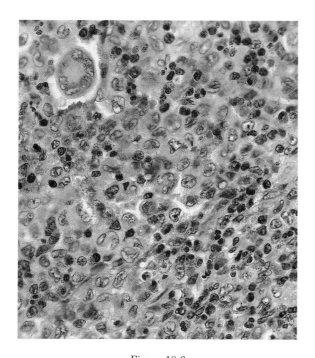

Figure 18-3
LANGERHANS' CELL HISTIOCYTOSIS
A mixed infiltrate of Langerhans' cells, eosinophils, histiocytes, and multinucleated giant cells is present.

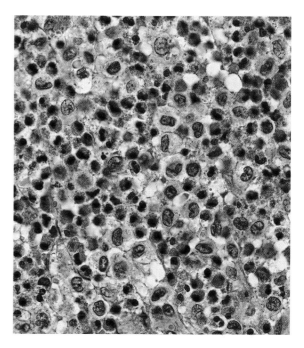

Figure 18-4
LANGERHANS' CELL HISTIOCYTOSIS
This lesion consists almost entirely of Langerhans' cells and eosinophils, and presumably represents an early lesion.

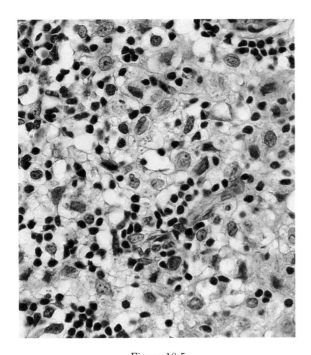

Figure 18-5
LANGERHANS' CELL HISTIOCYTOSIS
Lymphocytes and histiocytes dominate this lesion, although Langerhans' cells still can be identified.

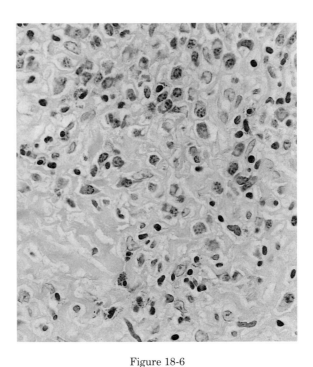

Figure 18-6
LANGERHANS' CELL HISTIOCYTOSIS
This lesion is highly fibrotic, and contains numerous plasma cells, fibroblasts, lymphocytes, and histiocytes. It presumably represents a late lesion. Langerhans' cells are difficult to identify in this particular field.

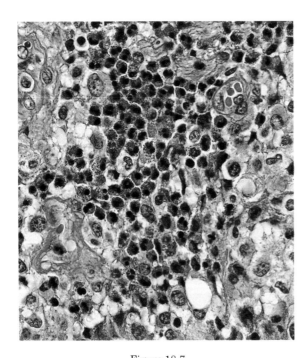

Figure 18-7
LANGERHANS' CELL HISTIOCYTOSIS
An eosinophilic abscess is seen among proliferating Langerhans' cells.

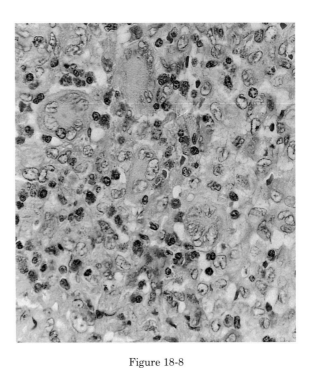

Figure 18-8
LANGERHANS' CELL HISTIOCYTOSIS
Multinucleated giant cells dominate the histologic appearance of this bone lesion.

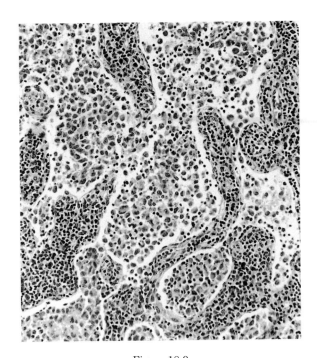

Figure 18-9
LANGERHANS' CELL HISTIOCYTOSIS
The sinuses of this lymph node are distended by prolif-
erating Langerhans cells and eosinophils.

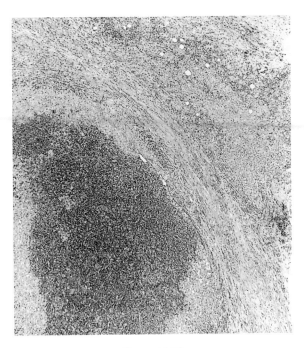

Figure 18-10
LANGERHANS' CELL HISTIOCYTOSIS
In addition to involvement of the sinuses, extensive
perinodal infiltration is present.

and show focal involvement of the sinuses by
Langerhans' cell histiocytosis. Another type of involvement is seen within the context of multisystem
disease or as a primary site of unifocal unisystem
disease. Again, the lymph nodes almost always
show a sinusoidal pattern of involvement, often with
marked distention of the sinuses (fig. 18-9). The
process often extends into the perinodal tissues (fig.
18-10) (21). The overall lymph node architecture is
generally retained, although partial or even complete effacement of architecture may be seen in
advanced cases (fig. 18-11). A rare manifestation is
the presence of a focus of Langerhans' cell histiocytosis adjacent to a malignant lymphoma, occurring in either non-Hodgkin's lymphoma or
Hodgkin's disease (6,22). In this instance, the lesion is usually small, located adjacent to the lymphoma, and is not present in a sinusoidal location
(fig. 18-12). Rarely, Langerhans' cell histiocytosis
subsequently develops at other sites (22).

In the spleen, Langerhans' cell histiocytosis
generally involves the red pulp first (fig. 18-13).
In advanced cases, encroachment of the white
pulp may occur, although complete obliteration
of splenic architecture is rare.

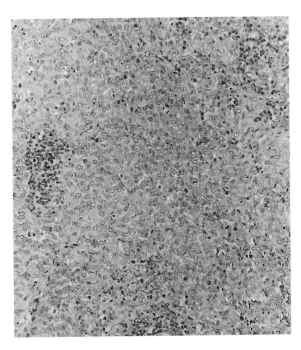

Figure 18-11
LANGERHANS' CELL HISTIOCYTOSIS
The lymph node architecture is effaced.

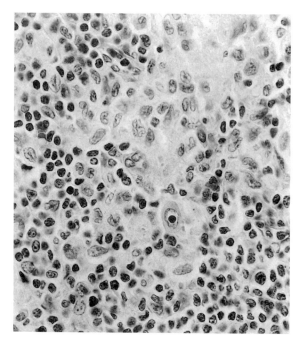

Figure 18-12
HODGKIN'S DISEASE WITH COEXISTENT
LANGERHANS' CELL HISTIOCYTOSIS
A Hodgkin cell is seen adjacent to a focus of Langerhans' cells.

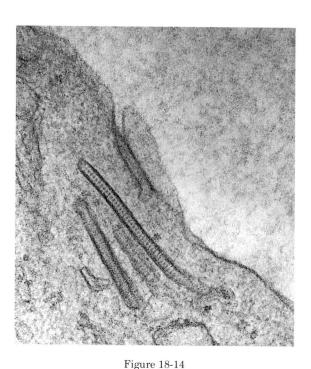

Figure 18-14
LANGERHANS' CELL HISTIOCYTOSIS
Several Birbeck granules are present in this Langerhans'
cell. (X39,000) (Electron micrograph courtesy of Dr. Dominic
V. Spagnolo, Perth, Western Australia.)

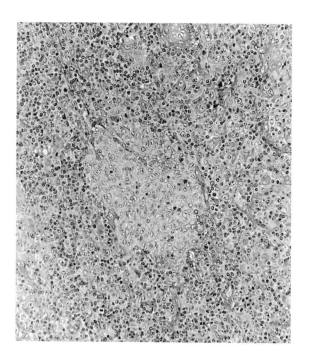

Figure 18-13
LANGERHANS' CELL HISTIOCYTOSIS
INVOLVING SPLEEN
This case shows a diffuse infiltration of the red pulp along
with formation of discrete nodules of Langerhans' cells. The
white pulp is atrophic.

On ultrastructural examination, the neoplastic Langerhans' cells have the features of their benign counterparts. The cells have an irregularly shaped nucleus, cytoplasm with variable numbers of lysosomes, irregular plasma membranes, and lack cell junctions. Pathognomonic of Langerhans' cells is the presence of Birbeck granules (fig. 18-14). These organelles are racket- or rod-shaped structures about 200 to 400 nm long and 33 nm wide, with an osmiophilic core and a double outer sheath. Birbeck granules can generally be identified in every lesion (23), but the percentage of cells containing the granules varies from case to case (20).

Malignant Langerhans' Cell Histiocytosis. Rare cases of Langerhans' cell histiocytosis contain Langerhans' cells with frankly malignant cytologic features (fig. 18-15). These cases show a male preponderance, a predilection for multisystem involvement, and a rapidly progressive clinical course (4,35). It is not yet clear whether this phenomenon represents a distinctive clinicopathologic entity or the extreme end of the morphologic and clinical spectrum of ordinary

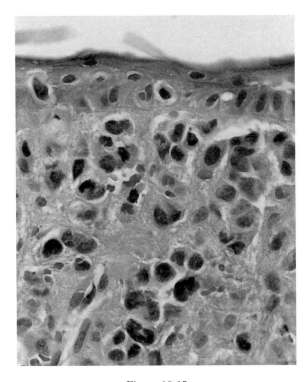

Figure 18-15
MALIGNANT LANGERHANS' CELL HISTIOCYTOSIS
Cytologically atypical cells are seen in this skin biopsy. The atypical cells had the phenotypic and ultrastructural characteristics of Langerhans' cells. (Photomicrograph courtesy of Dr. Gary S. Wood, Cleveland, OH.)

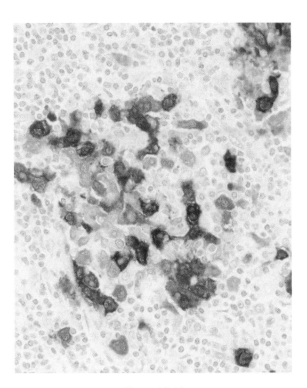

Figure 18-16
LANGERHANS' CELL HISTIOCYTOSIS: STAINING FOR S-100 PROTEIN IN PARAFFIN SECTIONS
Cytoplasmic staining of the proliferating Langerhans' cells is seen.

Langerhans' cell histiocytosis, since cases with malignant cytologic features that pursue a benign clinical course have also been described (4).

Enzyme Histochemical, Immunophenotypic, and Molecular Findings. The enzyme histochemical and immunophenotypic profile of the Langerhans' cells of Langerhans' cell histiocytosis is generally that of benign Langerhans' cells, although neoplastic Langerhans' cells exhibit cell-to-cell variability in some cases (3). Similar to histiocytes and other dendritic cells, the Langerhans' cells exhibit alpha-naphthyl acetate esterase (with variable inhibition by sodium fluoride), alpha-naphthyl butyrate esterase, acid phosphatase (not tartrate resistant), and, characteristically, adenosine triphosphatase activity (3). The cells are negative for 5'-nucleotidase, peroxidase, chloroacetate esterase, and beta-glucuronidase.

In paraffin sections, the Langerhans' cells express S-100 protein in virtually all cases (fig. 18-16), and express vimentin, CD74, and HLA-DR in greater than 80 percent of cases (1). The

cells are also positive for peanut agglutinin lectin (10). A significant proportion of cells express the macrophage-associated antigen CD68 in a granular cytoplasmic pattern of variable intensity (13). In addition, Langerhans' cells show a granular cytoplasmic staining reaction with antiplacental alkaline phosphatase in a majority of cases. They generally do not express CD45RA, CD45RB, CDw75, alpha-1-antitrypsin, epithelial membrane antigen, and CD15, although CD15 reactivity may be seen after removal of sialic acid residues (28). A few cells may be immunoreactive with lysozyme and alpha-1-antichymotrypsin (26).

In frozen sections, Langerhans' cells are positive for CD45 but negative for CD45RA, CD45RB, and CD45RO (3,36). In addition, they express CD1, CD4, CD11b (C3bi), CD11c, CD14, CD16, CD25 (IL-2 receptor), CDw32, CD71 (transferrin receptor), and HLA-A, -B, -C, and -DR, and lack expression of most B- and T-cell lineage markers (3,24, 27). CD1 is the most useful frozen section marker since other histiocytic and dendritic cells lack this marker; CD1 expression is limited to reactive and neoplastic Langerhans' cells, immature thymocytes, and T-lymphoblastic neoplasms. The Langerhans cells of Langerhans' cell histiocytosis, but not normal Langerhans cells, may also be positive for cytoplasmic CD2 and CD3 (13). The histiocytes, foamy histiocytes, and multinucleated cells, which may be observed in Langerhans' cell histiocytosis, mark as histiocytes and do not possess the antigens characteristic of Langerhans' cells, although it has been speculated that at least some of these cells may arise through maturation of neoplastic Langerhans' cells (26).

Molecular studies of the patterns of X-chromosome inactivation in the X-linked androgen-receptor gene, using the polymerase chain reaction, have shown that Langerhans' cell histiocytosis is a monoclonal proliferation; lesions that were studied included multifocal multisystem disease, multifocal unisystem disease, and unifocal disease (33). Molecular hybridization studies have shown a germline configuration for the immunoglobulin heavy chain and alpha-, beta-, and gamma-T-cell receptor genes (33). The cytogenetics of this disorder have not yet been elucidated.

Differential Diagnosis. The Writing Group of the Histiocyte Society has adopted tentative diagnostic criteria for Langerhans' cell histiocytosis (37). They recommend that only a "presumptive diagnosis" is warranted when the typical histologic findings are present, without confirmation by special studies. They apply the term "diagnosis" when the typical histologic features are present along with positivity with two or more of the following markers: adenosine triphosphatase, S-100 protein, alpha-D-mannosidase, and peanut lectin agglutinin. They recommend that a "definitive diagnosis" is established only when the typical histology is present and either Birbeck granules are found by electron microscopy or CD1 is identified by immunohistochemistry. We disagree with the strictness of these criteria, and believe that a definitive diagnosis of Langerhans' cell histiocytosis can be established from histopathology alone if the histologic findings are sufficiently characteristic.

The differential diagnosis of Langerhans' cell histiocytosis varies depending on the organ involved. In involved lymph nodes, diseases that show a sinusoidal pattern of involvement are part of the differential diagnosis, such as metastatic

neoplasms, sinusoidal malignant lymphoma, sinus histiocytosis with massive lymphadenopathy, and benign sinusoidal hyperplasia. Langerhans' cell histiocytosis generally lacks the frankly malignant features of metastatic malignant neoplasms and sinusoidal malignant lymphoma. The proliferating cells of sinus histiocytosis with massive lymphadenopathy generally have a round nucleus with a vesicular chromatin pattern and a more prominent nucleolus, more abundant cytoplasm with evidence of phagocytosis, and are usually accompanied by many plasma cells, an unusual feature for Langerhans' cell histiocytosis. Langerhans' cell histiocytosis can be distinguished from benign sinusoidal hyperplasia by the distinctive folded nucleus that characterizes the Langerhans' cells as well as the usual accompanying eosinophils.

Dermatopathic lymphadenopathy may contain large numbers of Langerhans' cells (31). In that condition, however, the proliferating cells, which also include numerous melanin-containing histiocytes and interdigitating dendritic cells, are present in the paracortical region and not the sinuses, as is the case in Langerhans' cell histiocytosis (fig. 18-17).

Treatment. Treatment includes surgery, radiation therapy, and chemotherapy; at the present time, immunotherapy with thymic extract remains experimental. Patients with unifocal unisystem disease are generally treated with surgical resection, if possible, and residual disease is treated by radiation therapy. Patients with multifocal unisystem disease are treated in the same manner by many clinicians. Chemotherapy is often reserved for multisystem disease. Both combination and single agent chemotherapy regimens are used.

Prognosis. As discussed previously, the prognosis in Langerhans' cell histiocytosis is most dependent on the pattern of organ involvement (17). There is a good correlation between the number of organ systems involved and the overall prognosis, particularly if objective signs of organ dysfunction are present (12,15). Thus, the overall survival is greater than 95 percent in patients with unifocal unisystem disease, but drops to 75 percent when two organs are affected, and continues to drop with increasing numbers of affected organ systems. The proposed clinical staging systems take these factors

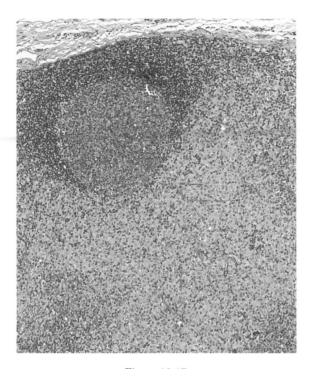

Figure 18-17
DERMATOPATHIC LYMPHADENOPATHY
The proliferating cells expand the paracortex and do not preferentially involve the sinuses.

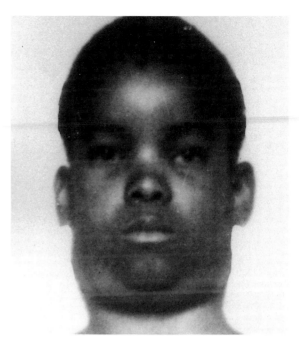

Figure 18-18
SINUS HISTIOCYTOSIS WITH MASSIVE LYMPHADENOPATHY
First case of sinus histiocytosis with massive lymphadenopathy encountered by the author (RFD) in 1960 at the South African Institute for Medical Research in Johannesburg. Bilateral cervical lymphadenopathy is clearly evident. (Fig. 1 from Rosai J, Dorfman RF. Sinus histiocytosis with massive lymphadenopathy. A newly recognized benign clinicopathological entity. Arch Pathol 1969;87:63–70.)

into account. For example, in the Lahey system, points are assigned for involvement of each of the following: skin, liver (as assessed by organ dysfunction), spleen, lung (as assessed by organ dysfunction), pituitary (diabetes insipidus), skeleton, hematopoietic system (anemia leukopenia, or thrombocytopenia), and lymph nodes (17). The influence of age is still controversial. Some believe that age under 2 years is an adverse prognostic variable (15), while others believe that age has no effect independent of the pattern of organ involvement. Favorable response to initial chemotherapy is associated with improved survival and overall disease control (15). The elderly may have a relatively poor outcome (2).

Evaluation of histologic features is not generally helpful in determining prognosis. Neither nuclear atypia nor mitotic rate correlate with clinical outcome (25), although nuclear atypia may be more prevalent in lesions from patients with multisystem involvement. The presence of eosinophils or lymphocytes was significantly associated with a more favorable outcome in one study (25).

SINUS HISTIOCYTOSIS WITH MASSIVE LYMPHADENOPATHY (ROSAI-DORFMAN DISEASE)

Definition. Sinus histiocytosis with massive lymphadenopathy (SHML) is a rare idiopathic histiocytic proliferative disorder and a distinct clinicopathologic entity (61,62). It is currently defined by its diagnostic histopathologic features, specifically its unique histiocytes. These cells are large and contain vesicular nuclei, delicate nuclear membranes, distinct nucleoli, and voluminous pale cytoplasm, often with lymphophagocytosis. The eponym Rosai-Dorfman disease is often applied, particularly in cases of extranodal disease (48,67).

Incidence. Although the first cases were identified in South Africa (fig. 18-18) (61), SHML has a worldwide distribution (53,54,67). Because of the rarity of this disorder, exact incidence rates are difficult to ascertain. A comprehensive review of 423 patients entered in a registry of

349

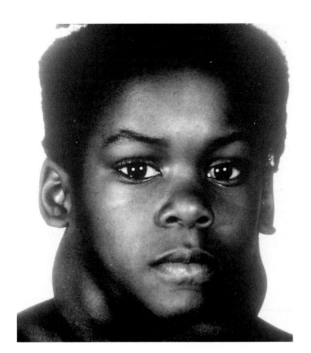
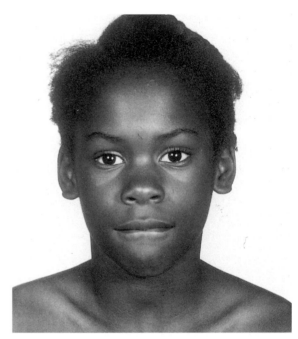

Figure 18-19
SINUS HISTIOCYTOSIS WITH MASSIVE LYMPHADENOPATHY
Left: Massive bilateral cervical lymphadenopathy in a 6-year-old West Indian child. (Fig. 1 from Rosai J, Dorfman RF. Sinus histiocytosis with massive lymphadenopathy: a pseudolymphomatous benign disorder. Analysis of 34 cases. Cancer 1972;30:1174–88.)
Right: Same patient 3 years later showing complete spontaneous regression of lymphadenopathy. (Fig. 50 from Foucar E, Rosai J, Dorfman R. Sinus histiocytosis with massive lymphadenopathy (Rosai-Dorfman disease): review of the entity. Semin Diagn Pathol 1990;7:19–73.)

cases of SHML disclosed that more than half of the cases were encountered in the United States (38.7 percent), western Europe (19.5 percent), and Africa (15.4 percent) (48).

Although initially thought to be more common in blacks from Africa and the United States (fig. 18-19), the registry contains an equal number of black and white patients, each group comprising 43.6 percent of the total, whereas a much smaller percentage are Asian or other races. Fifty-eight percent of the patients in the registry were males. Initially, the disorder was thought to have a predilection for black children living in tropical third world countries; this is no longer the case.

Case reports in the literature and those referred to the registry establish the mean age of onset at approximately 20 years, with a range from congenital to 74 years. SHML has been reported in siblings (38) and in identical twins (57).

Antibodies to human herpes virus (HHV)-6 and Epstein-Barr virus (EBV) are seen in some patients with SHML (55). Moreover, the detection of HHV-6, and to a lesser extent EBV, in involved tissues by in situ hybridization sug-

gests that these viruses may play a role in the pathogenesis of SHML (55).

Natural History and Clinical Features. As implied by the term SHML, this disorder was initially thought to originate in, and to be confined to, lymph nodes. Most cases manifest primarily with lymphadenopathy: in the registry, close to 90 percent of the patients had cervical lymphadenopathy. Involvement of many other lymph node groups has subsequently been documented (figs. 18-18, 18-19), including axillary, inguinal, mediastinal, and para-aortic nodes. It is now evident that extranodal involvement by SHML is not infrequent and 43 percent of registry cases have at least one site of extranodal SHML. Moreover, extranodal disease may be the initial and sole manifestation of the disorder (56), at times unassociated with overt lymphadenopathy (43,44). It is for such cases that the eponym Rosai-Dorfman disease is most applicable. The most common sites of extranodal disease are skin (47,64), upper respiratory tract (42), and bone (65), followed by the genitourinary system, lower respiratory tract, oral cavity, and soft tissues (figs. 18-20–18-27) (48).

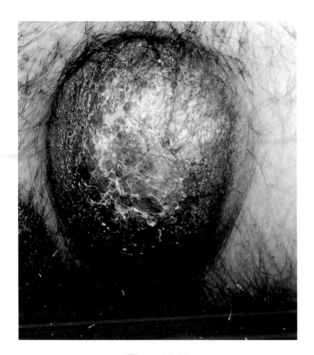

Figure 18-20
ROSAI-DORFMAN DISEASE: SKIN
Elevated plum-colored skin lesions in a 45-year-old Caucasian man, thought clinically to have mycosis fungoides.

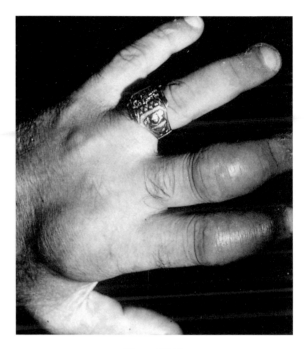

Figure 18-21
ROSAI-DORFMAN DISEASE:
SUBCUTANEOUS NODULES
Subcutaneous nodules in the hand and fingers from the same patient. These lesions responded dramatically to administration of vinblastine-loaded platelets. (Fig. 1A from Penneys NS, Ahn YS, McKinney EC, et al. Sinus histiocytosis with massive lymphadenopathy: a case with unusual skin involvement and therapeutic response to vinblastine-loaded platelets. Cancer 1982;42:1994-8.)

Although presentation with lymphadenopathy may be asymptomatic, some patients complain of pain or tenderness. A mild upper respiratory infection may precede the onset of initial or recurrent cervical adenopathy, which is usually bilateral. Approximately one quarter of patients present with fever and some may give an additional history of malaise, night sweats, and weight loss.

Laboratory studies show hematologic (46,48) and immunologic abnormalities (39,45,51). The former include anemia, characterized as mild normochromic normocytic or hypochromic microcytic. Some patients have red blood cell autoantibodies and a few develop severe and even fatal hemolytic anemia. Close to 90 percent of tested patients have an elevated erythrocyte sedimentation rate.

Immunologic studies show that 90 percent of patients have polyclonal hypergammaglobulinemia. Rare patients are positive for rheumatoid factor or antinuclear antibody, and have a positive lupus erythematosus cell preparation test. Of nine patients tested, seven showed a reversal of the CD4/CD8 ratio of circulating lymphocytes.

Additional clinical manifestations relate specifically to extranodal sites of disease: proptosis associated with orbital masses (43); central nervous system manifestations reflecting intracranial or spinal nerve lesions (44); ureteral obstruction secondary to involvement of the kidneys; laryngeal obstruction associated with disease of the upper respiratory tract; and cardiac symptoms reflecting valvular involvement by SHML.

Skin involvement may manifest in the form of a maculopapular rash or yellow xanthomatous lesions; large skin lesions are often elevated, reddish or bluish, and scaly (fig. 18-20). They may simulate the clinical features of mycosis fungoides. SHML involving the nasal cavity may present with nasal polyps.

Based on the clinical course of their disease, patients can be subdivided into the following categories: 1) those who undergo a complete and spontaneous remission; 2) those with recurrent

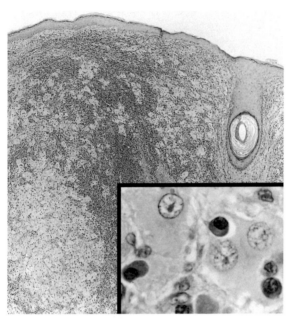

Figure 18-22
ROSAI-DORFMAN DISEASE: SKIN

Cutaneous Rosai-Dorfman disease in a 69-year-old man. The dermis is infiltrated by lymphocytes and plasma cells in addition to aggregates of typical histiocytes showing emperipolesis of plasma cells (see inset). (Courtesy of Dr. David Brown, London, England.)

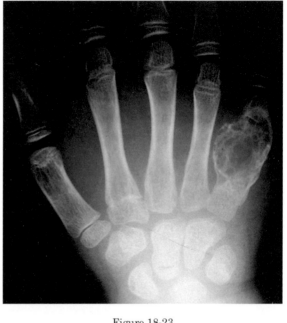

Figure 18-23
ROSAI-DORFMAN DISEASE: BONE

Radiograph shows a solitary, lytic, expansile lesion involving the fifth metacarpal of a 7-year-old boy, presenting as a painfully enlarging mass in the ulnar aspect of the right hand.

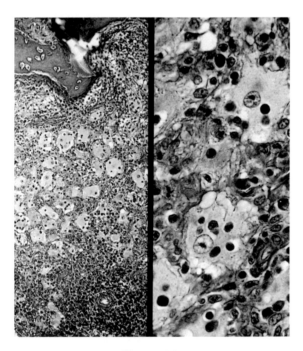

Figure 18-24
ROSAI-DORFMAN DISEASE: BONE

Hematoxylin and eosin-stained section of a bone lesion that was resected, showing numerous histiocytes demonstrating the phenomenon of emperipolesis, surrounded by many plasma cells and lymphocytes. (Courtesy of Dr. Jack Lewin, Jackson, MS.)

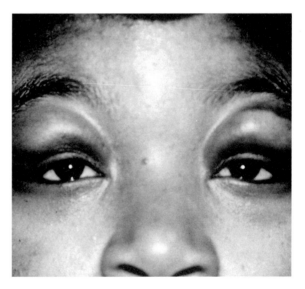

Figure 18-25
ROSAI-DORFMAN DISEASE: LACRIMAL GLANDS

Bilateral lacrimal gland involvement by SHML in an adult woman who also had cervical lymphadenopathy. (Fig. 34 from Foucar E, Rosai J, Dorfman R. Sinus histiocytosis with massive lymphadenopathy (Rosai-Dorfman disease): review of the entity. Semin Diagn Pathol 1990;7:19–73.)

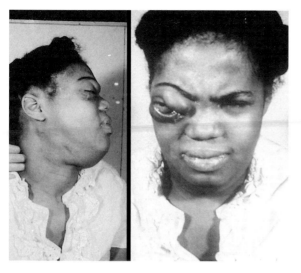

Figure 18-26
SINUS HISTIOCYTOSIS WITH MASSIVE
LYMPHADENOPATHY: ORBIT

Left: Cervical lymphadenopathy in an adult woman with SHML presenting with orbital involvement.

Right: The orbital mass was excised and the patient recovered completely. (Fig. 2 from Rosai J, Dorfman RF. Sinus histiocytosis with massive lymphadenopathy: a pseudo-lymphomatous benign disorder. Analysis of 34 cases. Cancer 1972;30:1174–88.)

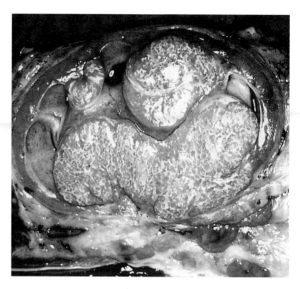

Figure 18-27
SINUS HISTIOCYTOSIS WITH MASSIVE
LYMPHADENOPATHY: KIDNEY

Involvement of the kidney by SHML. The renal masses were bright yellow and bulged above the cut surfaces. (Fig.2 from Wright DH, Richards DB. Sinus histiocytosis with massive lymphadenopathy (Rosai-Dorfman disease): a report of a case with widespread nodal and extranodal dissemination. Histopathology 1981;5:697–709.)

disease, characterized by lymphadenopathy secondary to minor upper respiratory infections; 3) those with persistent but stable disease; 4) those with progressive disease; and 5) those who die, presumably from the effects of disseminated nodal or extranodal disease. These categories are discussed further in the section on treatment and prognosis.

Macroscopic Findings. The cut surface of involved lymph nodes may be nodular or diffusely homogeneous and yellowish white. The capsule and pericapsular tissue may be thickened and fibrosed. There is extensive literature describing the manifestations of extranodal disease (48).

Microscopic Findings. *Lymph Nodes.* There is frequently capsular and pericapsular thickening and fibrosis (fig. 18-28). In the early stages of SHML, the sinusoidal architecture is well maintained (fig. 18-29). The sinuses are distended by numerous distinctive histiocytes that are characterized by extremely large, round, vesicular nuclei possessing a well-defined but delicate nuclear membrane (figs. 18-30, 18-31). Nucleoli may be single, prominent and centrally located or multiple (fig. 18-32). Rare cases may show binucleation or some nuclear atypia.

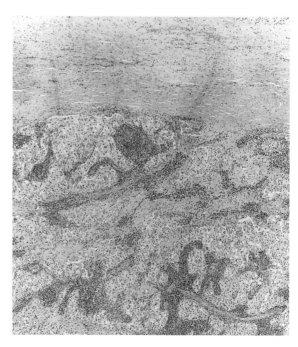

Figure 18-28
SINUS HISTIOCYTOSIS WITH MASSIVE
LYMPHADENOPATHY: LYMPH NODE

The capsule (top) of a lymph node involved by SHML is markedly thickened and fibrosed.

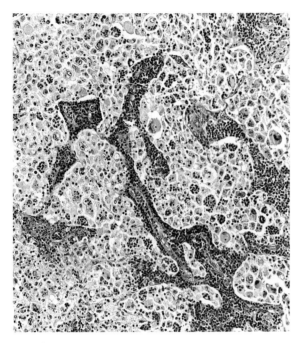

Figure 18-29
SINUS HISTIOCYTOSIS WITH MASSIVE
LYMPHADENOPATHY: LYMPH NODE

Striking distention of sinuses by characteristic histiocytes of SHML. (Figures 18-29–18-31 are from the same patient.)

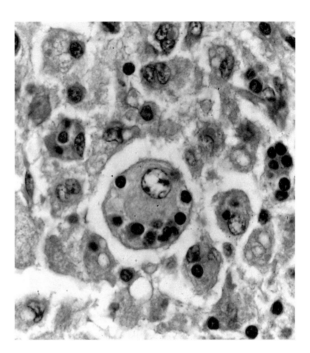

Figure 18-30
SINUS HISTIOCYTOSIS WITH MASSIVE
LYMPHADENOPATHY: LYMPH NODE

Characteristic histiocyte of SHML. The large, round, vesicular nucleus possesses a delicate nuclear membrane and prominent nucleoli. Within the pale-staining cytoplasm are well-preserved lymphocytes apparently located within cytoplasmic vacuoles (so-called lymphocytophagocytosis or emperipolesis).

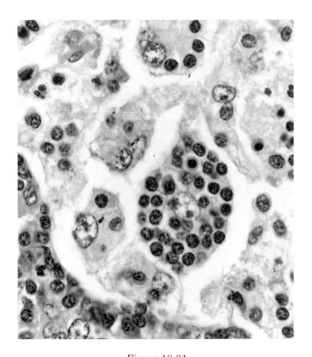

Figure 18-31
SINUS HISTIOCYTOSIS WITH MASSIVE
LYMPHADENOPATHY: LYMPH NODE

Several histiocytes show striking evidence of lymphocyte emperipolesis.

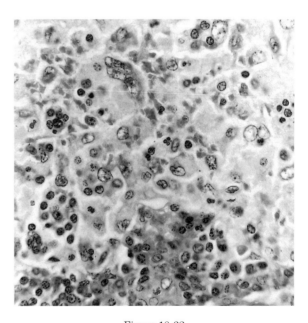

Figure 18-32
SINUS HISTIOCYTOSIS WITH MASSIVE
LYMPHADENOPATHY: LYMPH NODE

Histiocytes in this lymph node show some degree of atypia with multinucleation.

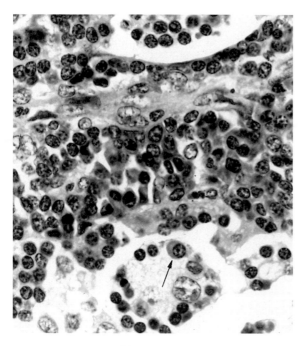

Figure 18-33
SINUS HISTIOCYTOSIS WITH MASSIVE
LYMPHADENOPATHY: LYMPH NODE
Plasma cells are prominent in the central medullary cord and
some can be seen within the cytoplasm of histiocytes (arrow).

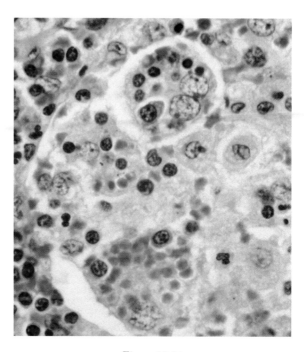

Figure 18-34
SINUS HISTIOCYTOSIS WITH MASSIVE
LYMPHADENOPATHY: LYMPH NODE
Histiocytes in this lymph node show erythrophagocytosis
in addition to emperipolesis.

The abundant pale or eosinophilic cytoplasm of
these histiocytes is often filled with apparently
intact lymphocytes, a phenomenon referred to as
lymphocytophagocytosis or emperipolesis (figs. 18-
30, 18-31, 18-33) (50). The latter term was coined
by Humble et al. (49) who noted that, when cultivated in vitro, lymphocytes have the ability to
enter and leave the cytoplasm of macrophages
without undergoing degradation. Many of the internalized lymphocytes are located within
cytoplasmic vacuoles (figs. 18-30, 18-31).

In addition to lymphocytes, intracytoplasmic
plasma cells, red blood cells, and neutrophils are
seen (figs. 18-33, 18-34). The medullary cords contain numerous plasma cells that may also be prominent within distended sinuses (fig. 18-33). Lymphoid follicles are usually not evident in lymph
nodes affected by SHML but, on occasion, reactive
germinal centers may be present in the cortex
surrounded by distended sinuses (fig. 18-35). In
patients with lymphadenopathy of long duration,
the lymph nodes may show partial or complete
effacement of normal architecture by the proliferating histiocytes, associated with numerous

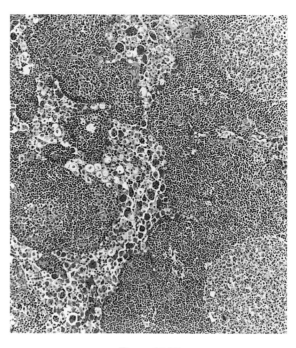

Figure 18-35
SINUS HISTIOCYTOSIS WITH MASSIVE
LYMPHADENOPATHY: LYMPH NODE
This lymph node involved by SHML shows some degree
of reactive follicular hyperplasia in the cortex.

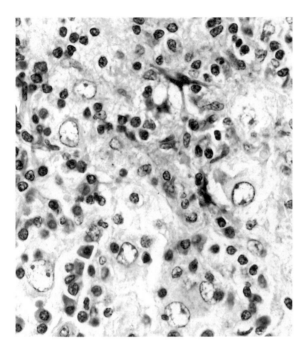

Figure 18-36
SINUS HISTIOCYTOSIS WITH MASSIVE
LYMPHADENOPATHY: LYMPH NODE

Advanced case of SHML in which the lymph node architecture was partially effaced by increased numbers of histiocytes.

plasma cells, which frequently surround and follow the lines of prominent high endothelial venules (figs. 18-36, 18-37). Clusters of foamy histiocytes with smaller nucleoli may be present (fig. 18-38). Focal aggregates of neutrophils may form microabscesses in rare instances. Suitably stained preparations have failed to identify any organisms within the above described histiocytes.

In touch preparations of lymph nodes and in fine needle aspirations stained with the Wright-Giemsa technique, the nuclei of the histiocytes are once again large but appear more variable in shape and size, and nucleoli are less prominent. Such preparations emphasize emperipolesis and the observation that many of the internalized lymphocytes lie within cytoplasmic vacuoles (fig. 18-39).

Ultrastructural studies amplify observations made with the light microscope but disclose some additional features (fig. 18-40) (63). The nuclei of the characteristically large histiocytes are more variable in size and shape, as are the nucleoli, which may be apposed to the nuclear membrane. The abundant cytoplasm contains a variety of organelles, including scattered lipid

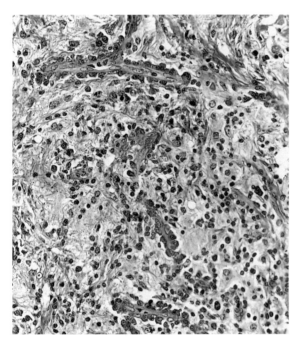

Figure 18-37
SINUS HISTIOCYTOSIS WITH MASSIVE
LYMPHADENOPATHY: LYMPH NODE

Prominent high endothelial vessels in a lymph node involved by SHML. Plasma cells characteristically aggregate around and follow the lines of these vessels.

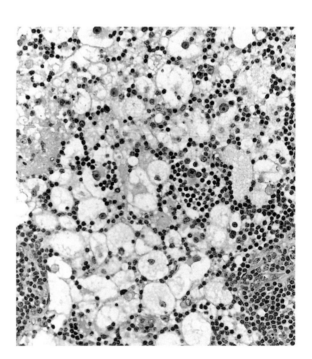

Figure 18-38
SINUS HISTIOCYTOSIS WITH MASSIVE
LYMPHADENOPATHY: LYMPH NODE

Foamy histiocytes are prominent in this lymph node involved by SHML.

droplets. Myelin figures may be evident. A prominent feature is the presence of well-preserved lymphocytes within cytoplasmic vacuoles. Some lymphocytes show degenerative changes and additional hematopoietic cells may be present within the cytoplasm. The latter cells include plasma cells, erythrocytes, and neutrophils. A distinctive ultrastructural feature of the histiocytes is the presence of numerous and complex filopodia protruding from the cell membrane. These elongated processes appear to envelop lymphocytes and may play some role in lymphocytophagocytosis or emperipolesis. Birbeck granules are not seen.

Extranodal Sites. The morphologic features of extranodal lesions recapitulate to a remarkable degree those of lymph nodes (figs. 18-41, 18-42). Dilated lymphatics filled with the characteristic histiocytes and surrounded by lymphoid tissue, including reactive germinal centers, mimic the appearance of affected lymph nodes. These lesions are often increasingly vascular in a fibrous stroma and plasma cells once again surround

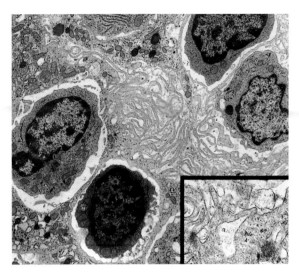

Figure 18-40
SINUS HISTIOCYTOSIS WITH MASSIVE
LYMPHADENOPATHY: LYMPH NODE

Electron micrograph of a lymph node involved by SHML clearly demonstrating the presence of lymphocytes within cytoplasmic vacuoles and the envelopment of these lymphocytes by cytoplasmic processes which may play a role in their internalization. Tactoids of fibrin are also present within the cytoplasm (inset). (Fig. 8 from Sanchez R, Sibley RK, Rosai J. The electron microscopic features of sinus histiocytosis with massive lymphadenopathy: a study of 11 cases. Ultrastruct Pathol 1981; 2:101–19.)

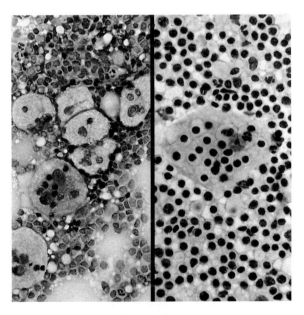

Figure 18-39
SINUS HISTIOCYTOSIS WITH
MASSIVE LYMPHADENOPATHY:
TOUCH IMPRINT OF LYMPH NODE

Touch preparations of lymph node involved by SHML.
Left: Characteristic histiocytes demonstrating emperipolesis are seen.
Right: Lymphocytes within cytoplasmic vacuoles are clearly demonstrated.

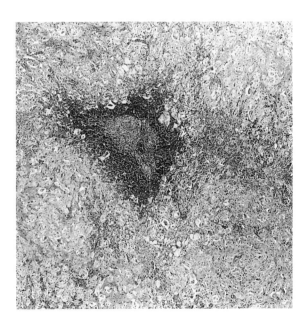

Figure 18-41
ROSAI-DORFMAN DISEASE: EXTRANODAL

Extranodal involvement by Rosai-Dorfman disease recapitulating the appearance of a lymph node. A solitary lymphoid follicle with a germinal center is seen centrally surrounded by fibrous tissue containing typical histiocytes (see fig. 18-23).

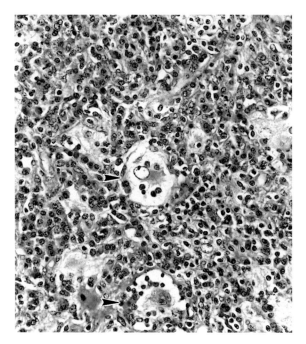

Figure 18-42
ROSAI-DORFMAN DISEASE: EXTRANODAL

Extranodal Rosai-Dorfman disease characterized by numerous plasma cells surrounding occasional histiocytes and demonstrating the phenomenon of emperipolesis (arrows).

and follow lines of these vessels. Lymphocytophagocytosis or emperipolesis may be more difficult to identify in such lesions.

Histochemical studies of nodal and extranodal lesions show activity of acid phosphatase and alpha-naphthyl acetate or alpha-butyrate esterase by the histiocytes of SHML, identical to that observed in cells of the histiocytic/monocytic series (48).

Immunologic and Molecular Genetic Findings. Immunohistochemical studies were limited in scope (40,58) until Eisen et al. (41) and Paulli et al. (59) determined the antigenic phenotype of SHML cells by using a broad panel of antibodies to macrophage/histiocyte B-cell and T-cell antigens. Both reports confirm the strong expression of S-100 protein by the histiocytes, an observation made by others (40). In our experience, this stain is very helpful in identifying the histiocytes of SHML, particularly at extranodal sites and in affected lymph nodes where the morphologic features are somewhat unusual (figs. 18-43–18-45). The above-mentioned studies further demonstrate that SHML cells express

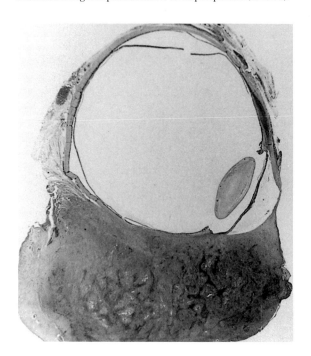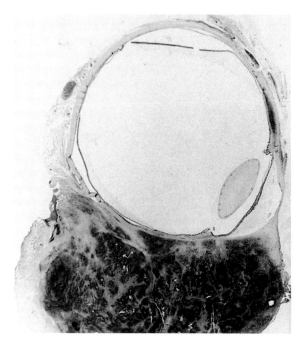

Figure 18-43
ROSAI-DORFMAN DISEASE: EYE

Left: Extranodal Rosai-Dorfman disease in a 50-year-old Nigerian man living in London. Involvement of the left orbit necessitated enucleation of the eye. The patient had multiple cutaneous and subcutaneous nodules but no palpable lymph adenopathy. (Courtesy of Dr. John Harry, London, England.)

Right: Same lesion showing strong immunoperoxidase staining for S-100 protein.

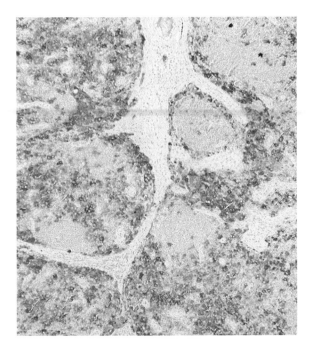

Figure 18-44
SINUS HISTIOCYTOSIS WITH MASSIVE
LYMPHADENOPATHY: LYMPH NODE
Histiocytes within sinuses of a lymph node involved by
SHML stain for S-100 protein.

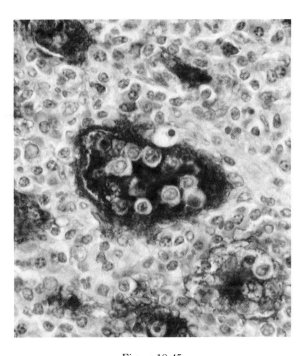

Figure 18-45
ROSAI-DORFMAN DISEASE: EXTRANODAL
These large histiocytes staining strongly for S-100 protein clearly show the presence of lymphocytes within cytoplasmic vacuoles.

pan-macrophage antigens such as CD68 (EBM11), HAM56, and CD14 (Leu-M3). The cells contain antigens functionally associated with phagocytosis (Fc receptor of IgG, complement receptor C3) and lysosomal activity (lysosome alpha-1-antichymotrypsin and alpha-1-antitrypsin). They also express antigens associated with early inflammation (Mac-387 and 27E10) and antigens commonly found on monocytes but not on tissue macrophages (OKM5 and CD15 [Leu-M1]). The cells also contain "activation" antigens, i.e., CD30 (Ki-1) and receptors for transferrin and interleukin-2. These studies provide support for the proposition that SHML cells are true, functionally activated macrophages that may be derived from circulating monocytes. SHML cells apparently do not belong to the family of dendritic cells (interdigitating dendritic cells, follicular dendritic cells, and Langerhans cells); they do not express R4/23 and CD21, antibodies strongly expressed by follicular dendritic cells. Bonetti et al. (40) maintain that Rosai-Dorfman disease is a disorder of S-100–positive, CD1-negative histiocytes, thus distinguishing SHML from

Langerhans' cell histiocytosis, since Langerhans cells express both S-100 protein and CD1. Of the three CD1a antibodies employed by Eisen et al. (41), NA34 and OKT6 (both of which are known to react with Langerhans cells) were also expressed by SHML cells in some instances. Paulli et al. (59) made similar observations in one of five cases. On the other hand, Leu-6, which has a greater specificity for Langerhans cells, was not expressed by SHML cells.

One study demonstrated a germline configuration for both the immunoglobulin heavy chain gene and the beta-T-cell receptor gene (40). To date, other molecular and genetic studies of SHML have not been reported.

Differential Diagnosis. The distinctive histiocytes of SHML that exhibit emperipolesis, their association with numerous plasma cells, and the distension of lymph node sinuses or lymphatics in extranodal sites by these cells help distinguish SHML from a variety of benign and malignant disorders in which phagocytosis of cells may be a prominent feature. The latter include melanoma and carcinoma metastatic to lymph nodes, since malignant cells have the propensity to phagocytose hematopoietic cells.

Langerhans' cell histiocytosis may manifest primarily in lymph nodes (66), with distension of sinuses by Langerhans' cells that have their own distinctive morphologic features. Their nuclei are smaller than those of SHML cells and are frequently irregular and folded with a central groove. They possess fine, dusky chromatin and inconspicuous nucleoli. Lymphocytophagocytosis or emperipolesis is not a feature of Langerhans' cells but erythrophagocytosis by sinus histiocytes accompanying these Langerhans' cells, in addition to the presence of microabscesses (usually eosinophilic) within distended sinuses, may be a prominent feature. Eosinophils, in varying numbers, are invariably associated with Langerhans' cell histiocytosis, but are not a feature of SHML. S-100 protein is also strongly expressed by Langerhans' cells, which are more likely to be CD1 positive than the histiocytes of SHML. Birbeck granules are seen in the cytoplasm of the histiocytes of Langerhans' cell histiocytosis.

SHML is distinguished from reactive sinus hyperplasia (sinus histiocytosis) by the demonstration of strong S-100 protein staining. Some dendritic cells in the medullary cords, however, may express S-100 protein.

Treatment and Prognosis. SHML manifesting with local lymph node involvement is considered a benign disorder with the propensity to regress spontaneously in most patients; however, as previously indicated, the disease may be persistent and progressive. Moreover, widespread dissemination and involvement particularly of kidney, lower respiratory tract, or liver, in association with immunologic abnormalities and anemia, presages an unfavorable prognosis: 17 of 423 patients entered in the registry died (46,48). Four of these were presumed to have died of SHML and 13 died with persistent SHML. However, the role of SHML in the cause of death is difficult to ascertain. All patients who died from or with SHML had disseminated nodal disease or involvement of many extranodal organ systems. Immunologic abnormalities that are associated with an unfavorable prognosis include autoimmune hemolytic anemia, identification of rheumatoid factor or antinuclear antibodies, or positive lupus erythematosus preparations. The association of anemia with neutrophilia, lympho-

cytopenia, and an elevated erythrocyte sedimentation rate is also associated with a poorer clinical outcome. The demonstration of immunologic abnormalities in a significant number of patients has given rise to the consideration that SHML might represent an unusual response of the hematolymphoid system to an immunologic disorder, as yet undefined.

Most patients do not require therapy other than excisional biopsy of affected tissues in order to establish the diagnosis. The large size of the lymph nodes in some patients may necessitate postoperative cosmetic surgery; other patients whose extensive disease compromises organ function may require radiation therapy and chemotherapy. The enlarged lymph nodes and extranodal lesions do not respond to antibiotic therapy and an ideal therapeutic regimen has yet to be identified. As recently indicated by Komp (52), a combination of vinca alkaloid (60), alkating agent, and corticosteroid appears to be the most beneficial chemotherapy.

FOLLICULAR DENDRITIC CELL SARCOMA

Definition. Follicular dendritic cell sarcoma is a neoplasm that shows differentiation similar to that of non-neoplastic follicular dendritic cells, which normally reside in germinal centers. Alternate names include *follicular dendritic cell tumor* and *dendritic reticulum cell tumor/sarcoma*.

Incidence and Natural History. This tumor is rare; the largest series consists of only four cases (71), and to our knowledge, approximately 16 cases have been reported (68–74). The typical presentation is of an adult man or woman with painless lymphadenopathy at one site, usually in the cervical region, although an axillary presentation has also been reported. Subsequent enlargement of other lymph nodes has been reported, but biopsy confirmation of neoplasm at the subsequent sites has not been obtained. Four cases have been reported arising within extranodal sites: one in the soft palate, one in the tonsil, and two in the intestines (69,70a). One case has been reported as a complication of hyaline-vascular Castleman's disease (68).

Recurrence may be local or at multiple sites. Only one patient died, with metastatic disease present in the liver (71).

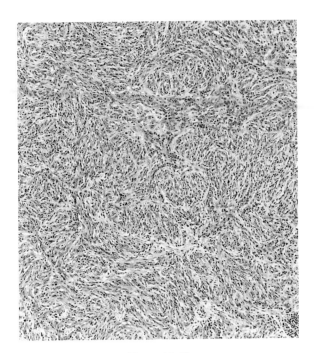

Figure 18-46
FOLLICULAR DENDRITIC CELL SARCOMA
A storiform appearance is seen.

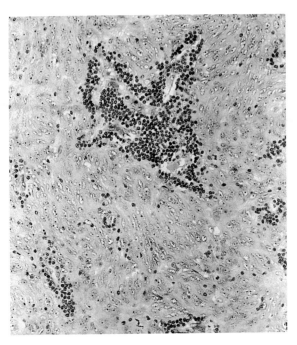

Figure 18-47
FOLLICULAR DENDRITIC CELL SARCOMA
A spindled appearance is seen, with intervening aggregates of lymphocytes.

Microscopic Findings. The lymph node architecture shows partial to complete effacement, with a sharp boundary between the neoplasm and residual lymphoid tissue. A proliferation of oval to spindled cells is seen, forming fascicles, nests, and sometimes a storiform pattern (figs. 18-46, 18-47). Occasionally, 360° whorls are formed, reminiscent of the pattern commonly observed in meningioma. The individual neoplastic cells possess oval nuclei with a relatively bland, vesicular chromatin pattern and inconspicuous nucleoli (fig. 18-48). Pseudonuclear inclusions may be present. The mitotic rate is generally low. The cytoplasm is pale to slightly eosinophilic, and does not have a fibrillar appearance on trichrome stain. Occasional multinucleated cells may be present (fig. 18-49). Small lymphocytes are usually found within the lesion, either as single cells sprinkled among the tumor cells, or as discrete collections of cells, often present in perivascular spaces. In some cases, germinal centers are occasionally found between fascicles of the neoplasm.

Electron microscopy demonstrates spindled cells with long, slender processes intertwined and connected with each other through numerous desmosomes (fig. 18-50). Lysosomes are usually

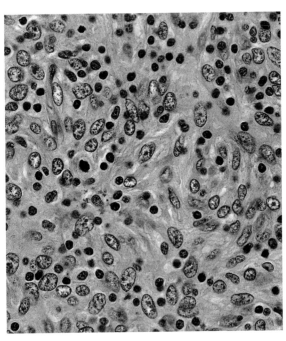

Figure 18-48
FOLLICULAR DENDRITIC CELL SARCOMA
Spindled cells with oval nuclei are present, with scattered small lymphocytes.

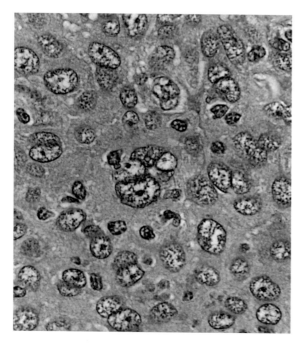

Figure 18-49
FOLLICULAR DENDRITIC CELL SARCOMA
Occasional multinucleated cells are found.

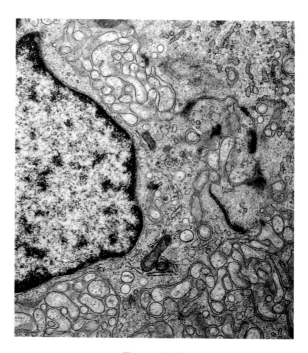

Figure 18-50
FOLLICULAR DENDRITIC CELL SARCOMA
This electron micrograph shows a cell with numerous
interdigitating processes and several cell junctions.

few. Basal lamina, tonofilaments, Birbeck granules, dense-core secretory granules, and melanosomes are uniformly absent.

Enzyme Histochemical, Immunophenotypic, and Molecular Findings. Enzyme histochemical studies performed in one case of follicular dendritic cell sarcoma revealed positivity for acid phosphatase (almost completely inhibited by tartrate), nonspecific esterase, alkaline phosphatase, and 5'-nucleotidase.

Follicular dendritic sarcoma is defined by its immunophenotype; this resembles the normal follicular dendritic cell. In paraffin sections, the neoplastic cells may be negative or equivocal for CD45RB and negative or positive for S-100 protein (71,72,74). Typically, the cells are also positive for CD35 (C3b complement receptor) and the macrophage marker CD68, and stain with monoclonal antibodies specific for follicular dendritic cells, such as R4/23. In frozen sections, the cells stain for multiple macrophage markers, the C3b and C3d receptors (CD35 and CD21, respectively) (fig. 18-51), HLA-DR, and the lymphocyte adhesion markers CD11a and CD18. They appear to express one or more B-cell lineage mark-

ers, similar to normal follicular dendritic cells, although it is uncertain whether the latter reactivity is due to synthesis rather than uptake by the cells. There is no expression of the Langerhans cell and immature T-cell marker CD1, specific T-cell lineage antigens, keratin, desmin, or the melanocyte-associated antigen HMB-45.

Two cases have been studied by molecular hybridization and have shown a germline configuration for both the immunoglobulin heavy chain gene and the beta-T-cell receptor gene (74).

Differential Diagnosis. The differential diagnosis includes all spindled lesions that occur in the lymph node. Nonhematopoietic entities such as metastatic carcinoma, metastatic malignant melanoma, and primary and metastatic sarcomas of other types may be excluded by attention to their malignant cytologic characteristics, with performance of appropriate immunohistochemical studies, if necessary. The palisaded myofibroblastoma (intranodal hemorrhagic spindle cell tumor with amianthoid fibers) is virtually always found in an inguinal lymph node, is less cellular, and does not stain with follicular dendritic cell markers. Rarely, malignant lymphoma has a spindled appearance;

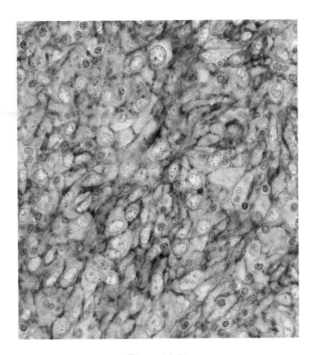

Figure 18-51
FOLLICULAR DENDRITIC CELL SARCOMA
Paraffin-section immunophenotypic studies reveal reactivity of this neoplasm for CD21.

immunohistochemical studies are important for identification of these cases. Thymoma may closely resemble follicular dendritic cell sarcoma, especially since both neoplasms may have collections of lymphocytes in perivascular spaces; the keratin reactivity of thymoma should easily differentiate it. The differentiation between follicular dendritic cell sarcoma and interdigitating dendritic cell sarcoma or an indeterminate cell tumor (see below) is primarily an immunohistochemical one, with follicular dendritic cell sarcoma expressing specific markers of differentiation. In addition, follicular dendritic cell sarcomas contain well-formed desmosomes when studied ultrastructurally. The clinical relevance of these distinctions has yet to be shown conclusively.

Treatment and Prognosis. To date, follicular dendritic cell sarcoma has been treated with local excision, sometimes followed by chemotherapy or radiotherapy. Recurrence has been independent of the type of therapy received. The one reported death due to this neoplasm followed several local recurrences.

INTERDIGITATING DENDRITIC CELL SARCOMA

Definition. Interdigitating dendritic cell sarcoma is a neoplasm that shows differentiation similar to that of non-neoplastic interdigitating dendritic cells, which normally reside in the paracortical region of the lymph node. Synonyms include *interdigitating dendritic cell tumor* and *interdigitating reticulum cell tumor/sarcoma*.

Incidence, Natural History, and Clinical Features. The neoplasm is extremely rare, with only about 20 reported cases (75–86), including one study that originally reported four cases as dendritic reticulum cell sarcoma but which we consider more likely to be the neoplasm under discussion (84). This rare lesion occurs in adults of both sexes, and usually presents in a lymph node, although presentation in extranodal sites such as the small intestine have been reported. One patient had a previous history of malignant lymphoma. Systemic symptoms such as fatigue, fever, and night sweats are occasionally present. The disease is disseminated in approximately half of cases, with involvement of numerous organs, including spleen, bone marrow, skin, liver, kidney, and lung. Local recurrence may also occur. Approximately half of patients die of disease, generally within 1 year of diagnosis.

Microscopic Findings. The histologic features of interdigitating dendritic cell sarcoma overlap both those of malignant lymphoma and follicular dendritic cell sarcoma. Some cases have histologic features identical to those described above for follicular dendritic cell sarcoma (figs. 18-52–18-54); other cases have neoplastic cells that are plumper and rounder, although spindling may be evident focally. Still other cases resemble pleomorphic large cell lymphoma with convoluted nuclei. One reported case demonstrated a spindled neoplasm in one biopsy and a more pleomorphic and less spindled neoplasm in a recurrence (85).

On ultrastructural examination, large cells are seen with interdigitating cell processes. In contrast to follicular dendritic cell sarcomas, well-formed desmosomes are not present. Basal lamina, tonofilaments, Birbeck granules, dense-core secretory granules, and melanosomes are uniformly absent.

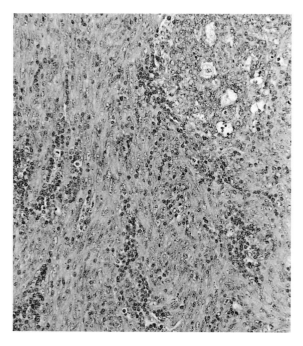

Figure 18-52
INTERDIGITATING DENDRITIC CELL SARCOMA
A spindled appearance is seen, with intervening lymphoid tissue, including a reactive germinal center. (Figures 18-52, 18-53, and 18-55 are from the same patient.)

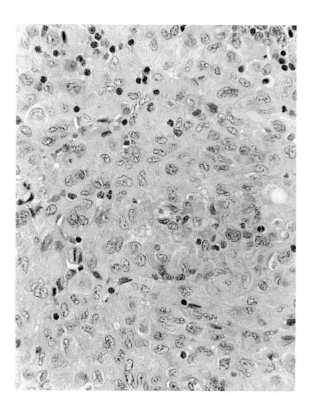

Figure 18-54
INTERDIGITATING DENDRITIC CELL SARCOMA
This case has cells with irregularly folded nuclei, reminiscent of Langerhans' cell histiocytosis.

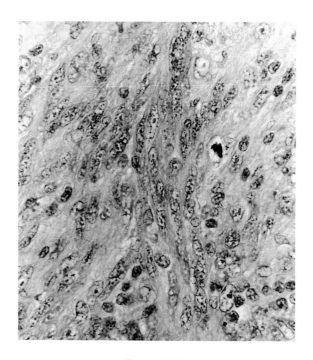

Figure 18-53
INTERDIGITATING DENDRITIC CELL SARCOMA
The cells are highly spindled in this case.

Enzyme Histochemical, Immunophenotypic, and Molecular Findings. Enzyme histochemical studies have demonstrated positivity for adenosine triphosphatase, alpha-naphthyl esterase, acid phosphatase, and 5'-nucleotidase in a majority of cases. The reactions for alkaline phosphatase, peroxidase, beta-glucuronidase, and chloroacetate esterase are negative.

Interdigitating dendritic cell sarcoma is defined by its immunophenotype, which resembles the normal interdigitating dendritic cell. In paraffin sections, the cells are positive for CD45RB, S-100 protein, and the macrophage marker CD68 (fig. 18-55) (85). In frozen sections, the cells stain for multiple macrophage markers and the lymphocyte adhesion markers CD11a and CD18. There is generally no expression of complement receptor antigens, B-cell lineage antigens, the Langerhans' cell and immature T-cell marker CD1, specific T-cell lineage antigens, specific follicular dendritic cell antigens, keratin, desmin, or the melanocyte antigen HMB-45.

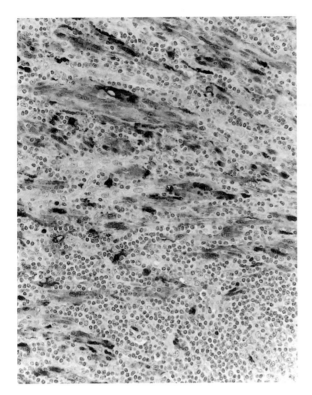

Figure 18-55
INTERDIGITATING DENDRITIC CELL SARCOMA
Positivity for S-100 protein is seen in the proliferating spindled cells.

Three cases have been studied by molecular hybridization and have shown a germline configuration for both the immunoglobulin heavy chain gene and the beta-T-cell receptor gene.

Differential Diagnosis. The differential diagnosis of interdigitating dendritic cell sarcoma is similar to the differential diagnosis given above for follicular dendritic cell sarcoma. Interdigitating dendritic cell sarcoma is distinguished from follicular dendritic cell sarcoma by the absence of desmosomes on ultrastructural examination and the absence of reactivity with monoclonal antibodies specific for follicular dendritic cells and complement receptors.

Treatment and Prognosis. Patients have been treated with local excision, usually with adjuvant radiotherapy, chemotherapy, or both; bone marrow transplant was performed for one patient. Approximately half of patients die of their disease, with no good correlation with any clinical, histologic, or treatment variables.

INDETERMINATE CELL TUMORS (PRECURSOR LANGERHANS' CELL HISTIOCYTOSIS)

Definition. An indeterminate cell tumor is a tumor showing differentiation towards indeterminate cells, a normal cell that is morphologically and antigenically similar to the Langerhans cell, but ultrastructurally lacks Birbeck granules (91,92).

Incidence, Natural History, and Clinical Features. Indeterminate cell tumors are extraordinarily rare, with very few reported cases in the literature (87–90,92,93), including one originally reported as an interdigitating reticulum cell sarcoma (89). The majority of these cases present in the skin of adults, with one or multiple lesions, although one patient presented with disseminated disease in multiple organs. Two patients had a previous history of a B-cell neoplasm (chronic lymphocytic leukemia and follicular lymphoma) and one patient had a history of mast cell leukemia. The clinical course has been variable. One patient with a skin lesion developed a metastatic lesion in a regional lymph node, the patient who presented with systemic disease subsequently died of disease; and another patient developed acute monocytic leukemia; all other patients were free of disease after treatment at last follow-up.

Microscopic Findings. The histologic examination most often reveals features similar to Langerhans' cell histiocytosis (fig. 18-56). The cytologic features of the proliferating histiocytes vary from those seen in Langerhans' cell histiocytosis to atypical forms, similar to the malignant variant of Langerhans' cell histiocytosis. The cytoplasm is abundant and pale to eosinophilic. Multinucleated and foam cells may be present.

Ultrastructural examination reveals cells similar to Langerhans cells, with the important exception that Birbeck granules cannot be identified.

Enzyme Histochemical, Immunophenotypic, and Molecular Findings. The neoplastic cells exhibit reactivity for adenosine triphosphatase, acid phosphatase (not tartrate resistant), and nonspecific esterase, and lack alkaline phosphatase, 5'-nucleotidase, peroxidase, chloroacetate esterase, beta-glucuronidase, and dipeptidylamino peptidase reactivity, consistent with normal Langerhans' cells/indeterminate cells (88,94).

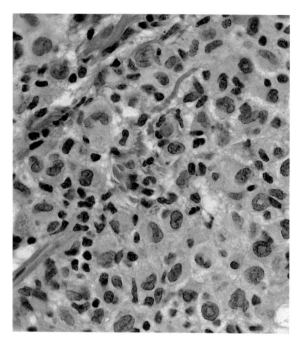

Figure 18-56
INDETERMINATE CELL TUMOR
Histologically, this neoplasm is virtually identical to Langerhans' cell histiocytosis. This case lacked Birbeck granules on ultrastructural examination. (Photomicrograph courtesy of Dr. Gary S. Wood, Cleveland, OH.)

Immunophenotypic studies show a classic Langerhans' cell/indeterminate cell phenotype: positivity for S-100 protein, CD45, CD1, and macrophage markers, and negativity for specific B- and T-cell–associated antigens. To our knowledge, no case has been studied by molecular hybridization.

Differential Diagnosis. Indeterminate cell tumors must be studied ultrastructurally and by immunophenotyping to establish the diagnosis. The tumors may be morphologically and immunologically identical to Langerhans' cell histiocytosis, but ultrastructurally lack Birbeck granules. They also express CD1, distinguishing them from follicular and interdigitating dendritic cell tumors, which lack this antigen.

Treatment and Prognosis. Most of the few reported patients have been treated with chemotherapy; one death occurred in the patient who presented with disseminated disease. Patients with one or multiple skin lesions have responded to chemotherapy; one patient who presented with an isolated skin lesion was in remission after excisional biopsy alone.

TRUE HISTIOCYTIC LYMPHOMAS (TRUE HISTIOCYTIC SARCOMAS)

Definition. The histiocytic system includes two major subsets of cells: antigen-presenting cells (dendritic cells), antigen-processing and phagocytic cells (macrophages). True histiocytic lymphomas (histiocytic sarcomas) are tumors composed of cells showing the macrophage line of differentiation (99,107). The prefix "true" is added to emphasize the distinction from "histiocytic lymphoma" which, in the Rappaport classification, is generally equivalent to large cell lymphoma of lymphoid rather than macrophage lineage according to modern terminology. Although the designation "lymphoma" may be considered inaccurate for a histiocytic neoplasm, we believe its use is justified because it has long been used to refer to the whole group of lymphoreticular neoplasms (including those of undefined lineage) and the initial histologic impression of true histiocytic lymphoma is almost always that of a lymphoma.

So-called malignant histiocytosis and plasmacytoid monocytic lymphoma are dealt with separately.

General Features. In the past, lymphomas composed of large cells were called reticulosarcoma or histiocytic lymphoma because the large cells were thought to represent histiocytes. Newer techniques have shown conclusively that almost all such cases are of B-cell or T-cell, but not histiocytic, lineage (122,123). Even cases reported as "true histiocytic lymphoma" may not be bona fide examples of such: the alleged histiocytic nature of these neoplasms is often based on immunoreactivity for lysozyme, alpha-1-antitrypsin, or alpha-1-antichymotrypsin, or on cytochemical staining for acid phosphatase or nonspecific esterase (106,108,114,118–120), markers now known to be not entirely specific for histiocytic lineage in hematolymphoid malignancies. These markers can occur in other lymphomas, in particular T-cell lymphomas (113,117).

True histiocytic lymphomas are extremely rare, accounting for less than 0.5 percent of all non-Hodgkin's lymphomas (115,116). In order to provide a proper perspective on true histiocytic lymphomas, information in the following sections is extracted only from those studies based on comprehensive immunohistochemical analyses (95–98,101,104,105,111,112,115,116).

Clinical Features. True histiocytic lymphomas occur in either sex over a wide age range, although most patients are below the age of 30 years (95–98,101,104,105,111,112,115,116). The presentation is highly variable: localized or generalized lymphadenopathy, or extranodal disease, most often in the skin (as multiple nodules), soft tissue, small intestine, and spleen (101,111, 112,116). Constitutional symptoms are common.

Microscopic Findings. The cytologic features of true histiocytic lymphoma are highly variable. The cells are large, and possess irregular, indented, pleomorphic, occasionally bizarre nuclei that are often eccentric and have fine or coarse chromatin. The nuclei can also appear grooved. There are often irregular nucleoli, either single or multiple. The cytoplasm is abundant, and is typically eosinophilic, although it can be basophilic, pale, clear, or vacuolated (fig. 18-57). Multinucleated forms are often present (fig. 18-57). Mitotic figures are readily identified. Phagocytosis of erythrocytes, leukocytes, or hemosiderin is only rarely seen (figs. 18-58, 18-59) (100,111). Foci of necrosis are common.

In lymph nodes, the pattern of infiltration can be diffuse, paracortical, sinusoidal, or patchy (figs. 18-59, 18-60). Sometimes the neoplastic cells form deceptively cohesive nodules resembling those seen in carcinoma (96). Sclerosis can be prominent (fig. 18-60). In the skin, the infiltrate is located in the dermis and is nonepidermotropic. One case has been reported to show the growth characteristics of intravascular lymphomatosis (112).

Immunologic Findings. The neoplastic cells should, by definition, lack reactivity with T-lineage (CD2, CD3, CD5, CD7) and B-lineage (CD19, CD20, CD22, CD79a) antibodies. They are often CD45 (LCA) and HLA-DR positive (111) and show variable staining with the histiocytic markers CD68, CD11c, CD13, CD14, CD15, CD32, CD33, Mac-387, and lysozyme (fig. 18-61). The minimum immunophenotypic criteria for diagnosis of true histiocytic lymphoma have not been established, but the neoplastic cells should preferably express two or more histiocytic markers in the absence of evidence of myeloid differentiation (such as chloroacetate esterase activity, myeloperoxidase activity, or myeloperoxidase immunoreactivity), since the above-listed histiocytic markers often stain myeloid cells as well. PG-M1,

an antibody directed against the macrophage-restricted form of the CD68 molecule, holds promise to be a highly specific marker reactive in paraffin sections (99).

CD4, which is normally expressed on monocytes and macrophages, is often positive in true histiocytic lymphomas. Occasional cases may express the CD30 (Ki-1) antigen (95–97,104). There is also variable staining for alpha-1-antitrypsin or alpha-1-antichymotrypsin. Many paraffin section–reactive T-cell markers (such as CD45RO and CD43), which are not entirely specific for T cells, stain true histiocytic lymphomas (109,111). Some cases may exhibit S-100 protein staining in addition, and thus display a "hybrid" immunophenotype of ordinary histiocytes and interdigitating dendritic cells (fig. 18-62) (110).

Genotypic Findings. The role of genotypic studies in the diagnosis of true histiocytic lymphoma remains undefined. While some studies report (or require) lack of rearrangements of the immunoglobulin and T-cell receptor genes (96,98, 101,104,105,115,116), other studies report the presence of such gene rearrangements (97,98, 104). It is unclear whether tumors expressing macrophage markers, lacking B-lineage/T-lineage markers, and yet showing rearrangements of the T-cell receptor or immunoglobulin gene represent true histiocytic neoplasms with aberrant gene rearrangement or T-/B-cell lymphomas with expression of histiocytic markers and aberrant loss of T-/B-lineage markers. However, to keep the entity of true histiocytic lymphoma pure, it appears justified to exclude cases showing immunoglobulin or T-cell receptor gene rearrangements.

Differential Diagnosis. Distinction of true histiocytic lymphoma from large cell lymphoma (including anaplastic large cell type) of T-cell or B-cell lineage is not possible by morphologic assessment alone, although the former should be considered whenever the tumor cells possess voluminous eosinophilic cytoplasm. Even the presence of erythrophagocytosis by the neoplastic cells is not pathognomonic, because nonhistiocytic lymphomas sometimes exhibit this phenomenon. Comprehensive immunohistochemical studies are required to substantiate the diagnosis. In addition to lack of reactivity for T-cell–and B-cell–specific markers, there should be staining with two or more monocyte/macrophage-lineage antibodies. The staining must be

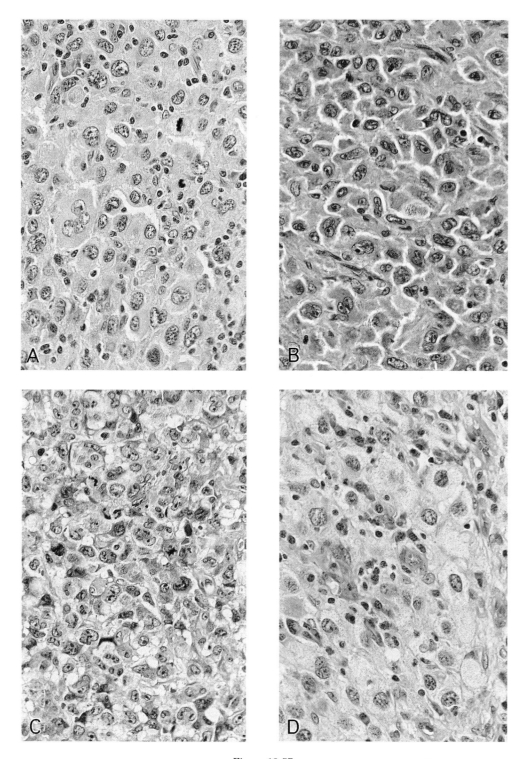

Figure 18-57
TRUE HISTIOCYTIC LYMPHOMA
Composite figure showing the varied morphology of true histiocytic lymphoma.
A: Large cells with oval or irregular nuclei and abundant eosinophilic cytoplasm. Occasional multinucleated forms are present.
B: The tumor cells exhibit grooved to contorted nuclei, delicate chromatin, and abundant eosinophilic cytoplasm.
C: This case resembles anaplastic large cell lymphoma, and shows pale-staining cytoplasm.
D: In this example, the cytoplasm is finely vacuolated ("foamy").

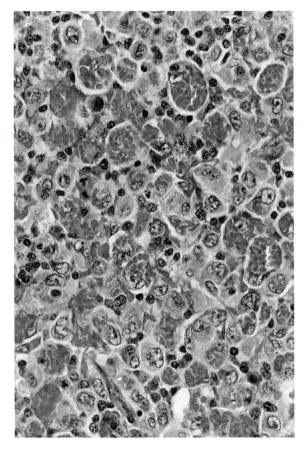

Figure 18-58
TRUE HISTIOCYTIC LYMPHOMA WITH
PROMINENT ERYTHROPHAGOCYTOSIS
This case shows prominent erythrophagocytosis, an un-
usual phenomenon in true histiocytic lymphoma.

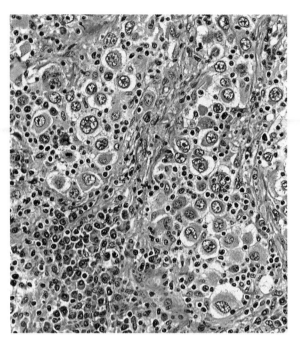

Figure 18-59
TRUE HISTIOCYTIC LYMPHOMA
This case shows sinusoidal distribution, lymphophagocytosis, and plasma cell infiltration, resulting in a resemblance to Rosai-Dorfman disease.

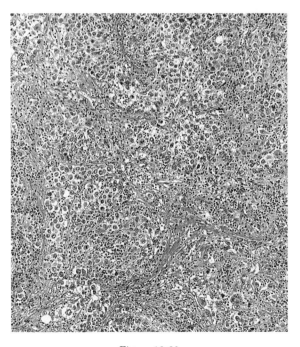

Figure 18-60
TRUE HISTIOCYTIC LYMPHOMA
This example shows extensive nodal involvement and sclerosis.

assessed on the neoplastic cells, and not on the
reactive histiocytes which not uncommonly accompany T-cell or B-cell lymphomas.

Distinction of true histiocytic lymphoma from
carcinoma or melanoma can readily be made by
immunohistochemical studies.

True histiocytic lymphoma should not be confused with malignant fibrous histiocytoma, a mesenchymal tumor unrelated to the macrophage lineage. Malignant fibrous histiocytoma typically
occurs in the deep soft tissues, pleomorphic spindly
cells are often present, and the tumor cells are not
reactive for leukocyte common antigen.

Storage diseases such as Gaucher's disease
and Niemann-Pick disease must not be mistaken for true histiocytic lymphoma. In general,
the histiocytes that accumulate in the various
storage diseases are large and possess regular

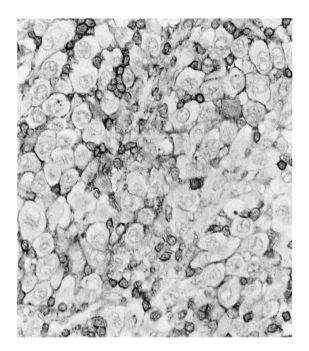 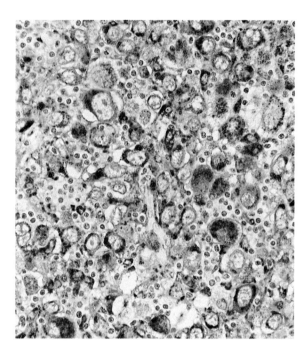

Figure 18-61
TRUE HISTIOCYTIC LYMPHOMA
Left: The large neoplastic cells show membrane staining for leukocyte common antigen (CD45RB).
Right: There is also strong staining with KP1 (CD68).

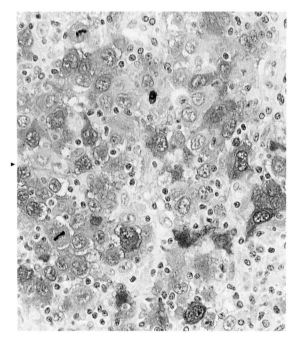

Figure 18-62
TRUE HISTIOCYTIC LYMPHOMA
This example shows immunoreactivity for S-100 protein in addition to other histiocytic markers.

nuclei with fine chromatin, although some degree of nuclear atypia is sometimes seen in Niemann-Pick disease (103,121). The histiocytes can accumulate in the spleen, lymph node, bone marrow, and other sites. The histiocytes of Gaucher's disease typically possess a central or eccentric nucleus and abundant fibrillary to striated pale cytoplasm (fig. 18-63). The histiocytes of Niemann-Pick disease possess finely vacuolated cytoplasm, but this appearance is not pathognomonic; the diagnosis has to be confirmed by biochemical or molecular studies.

Infections with *Leishmania, Mycobacterium, Histoplasma,* and *Salmonella typhi* are accompanied by a prominent accumulation of histiocytes. The histiocytes do not exhibit atypia. The diagnosis is made by demonstration of microorganisms in the histiocytes or by culture (fig. 18-64).

Treatment and Prognosis. It is unclear what the optimal treatment for true histiocytic lymphoma is, but most patients have been treated as for diffuse large cell lymphoma. Although some patients respond to chemotherapy (97,116), most do not and die from disseminated disease within 2 years (100,101,104,111,115,116).

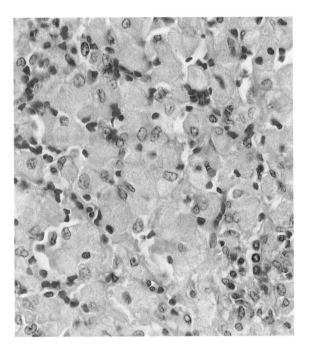

Figure 18-63
GAUCHER'S DISEASE INVOLVING SPLEEN
The histiocytes possess small, regular nuclei and abundant pale, finely striated cytoplasm.

SO-CALLED MALIGNANT HISTIOCYTOSIS

Definition. The term malignant histiocytosis was coined by Rappaport (151) for a systemic, progressive, invasive proliferation of morphologically atypical histiocytes and their precursors. Although malignant histiocytosis is widely considered to be synonymous with histiocytic medullary reticulosis, the latter includes a mixture of neoplastic and reactive conditions (132,155). The term histiocytic medullary reticulosis was coined by Scott and Robb-Smith in 1939 (156) for a clinicopathologic entity characterized histologically by abnormal histiocytes infiltrating the medullary sinuses of lymph nodes; clinically by acute onset of fever, wasting, generalized lymphadenopathy, and hepatomegaly; and terminally by jaundice, purpura, and profound cytopenia. Since precise diagnostic criteria are lacking and the disorder results from diverse pathologic conditions (132), it is advisable to drop the term histiocytic medullary reticulosis from usage.

Clinical Features. As reported in the literature, malignant histiocytosis occurs over a wide

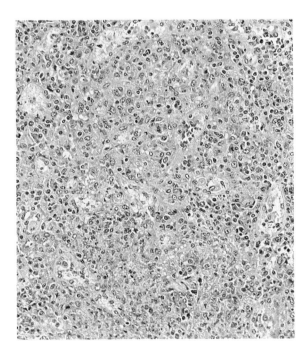

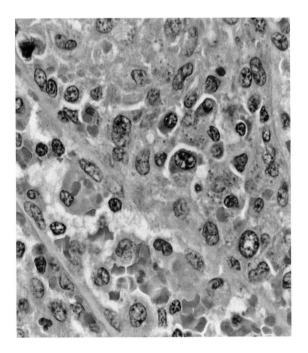

Figure 18-64
LEISHMANIASIS OF THE SPLEEN
Left: The red pulp shows marked histiocytic infiltration.
Right: *Leishmania* can be identified in the histiocytes in the form of small blue dots.

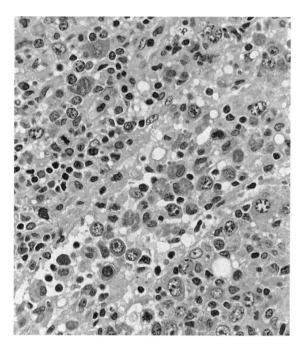

Figure 18-65
LYMPHOMA ASSOCIATED WITH REACTIVE
HEMOPHAGOCYTOSIS

Large cell lymphoma of B lineage associated with reactive histiocytes showing erythrophagocytosis. This example satisfies the diagnostic criteria of "malignant histiocytosis."

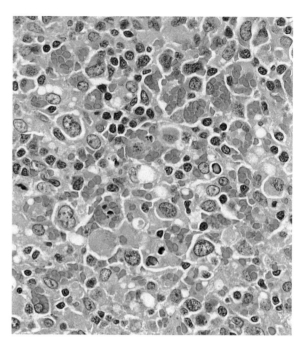

Figure 18-66
LYMPHOMA ASSOCIATED WITH REACTIVE
HEMOPHAGOCYTOSIS

Splenic large cell lymphoma of T lineage associated with a prominent component of reactive erythrophagocytic histiocytes. The nuclei of the histiocytes are much smaller than those of the lymphoma cells. The histologic features are compatible with those of "malignant histiocytosis."

age range, with a male predominance (124,163, 165). Most patients present with fever, constitutional symptoms, and hepatosplenomegaly (138, 147,157,163,170). Although lymphadenopathy is often prominent in children, it is absent or insignificant in adults. Some patients present with respiratory symptoms, neurologic complications, or skin nodules. Abdominal pain is common in children. Rarely, the initial presentation is splenomegaly alone (164).

Common laboratory findings are pancytopenia, raised erythrocyte sedimentation rate, and elevated levels of serum bilirubin, lysozyme, lactate dehydrogenase, and liver enzymes (131). The patients usually appear ill, and pleural effusion, jaundice, purpura, and profound pancytopenia are common in the terminal phase. There is usually a rapidly fatal course: median survival is less than 9 months (124,151,165), although treatment with combination chemotherapy has significantly improved the outcome (143,157,160,162,170). Cases presenting with splenomegaly or skin lesions alone have a more protracted course (130,164).

An association between malignant histiocytosis and mediastinal non seminomatous germ cell tumors occurring in young males has been recognized (129,148). Since these reported cases lack proper immunohistochemical documentation, it is unclear whether they are of true histiocytic lineage.

Pathologic Findings. As described in the literature, there is widespread involvement of the reticuloendothelial system and other organs by atypical histiocytes, which typically exhibit dispersed growth among residual lymphoreticular cells. The histiocytes often show a spectrum of differentiation, from less differentiated cells with large oval nuclei, vesicular chromatin, prominent nucleoli, and basophilic cytoplasm, to mature histiocytes with reniform nuclei, fine chromatin, and voluminous cytoplasm (figs. 18-65, 18-66). Phagocytosis of hemopoietic cells can often be seen, but is usually confined to mature histiocytes (figs. 18-65, 18-66) (124,143,151).

In lymph nodes, instead of forming monotonous sheets, the atypical cells are dispersed in the sinuses and nodal parenchyma (fig. 18-67). In the

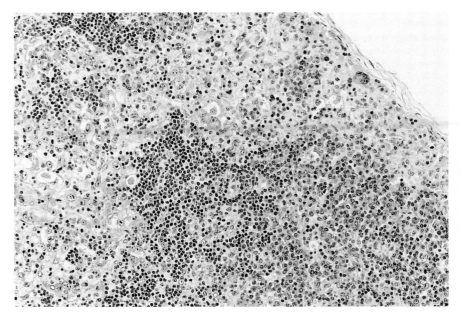

Figure 18-67
ANAPLASTIC LARGE
CELL LYMPHOMA
WITH FEATURES OF
"MALIGNANT
HISTIOCYTOSIS"
Anaplastic large cell lymphoma of T lineage involving lymph node. The large neoplastic cells are loosely dispersed in the sinusoids and paracortex, a pattern characteristic of "malignant histiocytosis."

spleen, there is predominant involvement of the red pulp, with the atypical histiocytes loosely scattered in the sinusoids and pulp cords. In the liver, both the portal tracts and sinusoids can be infiltrated. In the bone marrow, variable numbers of histiocytes occur among the hemopoietic cells, and hemophagocytosis is often prominent. Some authors have relied more on lymph node findings (165) and others more on bone marrow findings (143) to diagnose malignant histiocytosis.

Differential Diagnosis. For management purposes, it is not critical to distinguish between malignant histiocytosis and large cell lymphoma or true histiocytic lymphoma if the patient is to be given chemotherapy. However, it is most important not to mistake reactive hemophagocytic syndrome for malignant histiocytosis. The former is a benign process which may develop in association with a variety of conditions such as infection and lymphoma (128,152,154,168,169). The histiocytes that proliferate in this condition are bland-looking and lack the cytologic atypia required for the diagnosis of malignant histiocytosis (fig. 18-68). They frequently exhibit phagocytosis of erythrocytes and other hemopoietic cells (fig. 18-69).

Critical Reappraisal of the Entity "Malignant Histiocytosis." Malignant histiocytosis has traditionally been viewed as a malignant, disseminated proliferation of histiocytes. The original diagnostic criteria were formulated on morphologic grounds only, although some subsequent studies have attempted to substantiate the histiocytic nature of the cellular proliferation based on cytochemistry, immunohistochemistry, and electron microscopy (125,131,134,143,153, 163). However, reassessment of malignant histiocytosis based on monoclonal antibody studies and genotypic analyses has shown that most cases actually represent large cell lymphomas, particularly anaplastic large cell Ki-1 and postthymic T-cell types (including Tγ-erythrophagocytic lymphoma) with or without a component of reactive hemophagocytic syndrome (126, 127,137,140,159,166,167). "Malignant histiocytosis of the intestine" has also been reinterpreted as a T-cell lymphoma (enteropathy-associated T-cell lymphoma) (136). The histologic description of the primitive or poorly differentiated "histiocytes" corresponds well to that of activated lymphoid cells and immunoblasts of B-cell or T-cell lineage. Cytochemical reactions for acid phosphatase and nonspecific esterase have been demonstrated to be not unique for the histiocytic lineage among neoplasms (150,159). Neither can immunostaining for lysozyme, alpha-1-antitrypsin, and alpha-1-antichymotrypsin be considered reliable indicators of histiocytic lineage, since these markers can be expressed in T-cell and B-cell lymphomas (135,150,158). Although the chromosomal translocation involving the long arm of chromosome 5, usually in the form

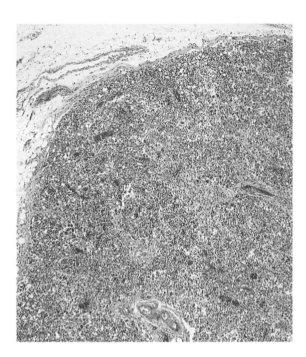
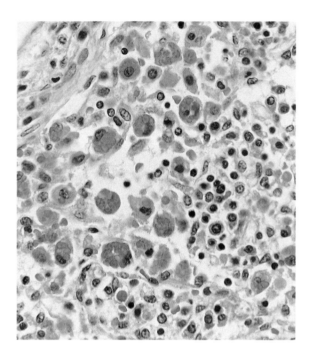

Figure 18-68
REACTIVE HEMOPHAGOCYTOSIS IN LYMPH NODE
Left: The sinusoids are packed with histiocytes, and the parenchyma shows lymphocyte depletion.
Right: The histiocytes possess regular, bland-looking nuclei. Many are engorged with phagocytosed erythrocytes.

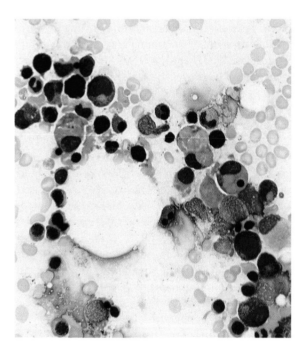

Figure 18-69
BONE MARROW IN REACTIVE
HEMOPHAGOCYTIC SYNDROME
Histiocytes showing prominent phagocytosis of hemopoietic elements (red cells, normoblasts, platelets) are increased. These histiocytes possess bland-looking nuclei and
lack distinct nucleoli. (Giemsa stain)

of t(2;5), has been considered to be characteristic
of some cases of malignant histiocytosis (139,
145–147), reassessment has shown that all these
cases express the Ki-1 (CD30) antigen and are
reclassifiable as anaplastic or nonanaplastic
large cell Ki-1 lymphoma (144).

Malignant histiocytosis is more appropriately
viewed as a syndrome, rather than a single disease
entity, that can result from a variety of hematolymphoid malignancies. As far as possible, each
case should be classified according to the current
terminology, such as "anaplastic large cell Ki-1
lymphoma" or "post-thymic T-cell lymphoma associated with reactive hemophagocytic syndrome."
Depending on individual preference, the phrase
"consistent with so-called malignant histiocytosis"
may be appended. Malignant histiocytosis of true
histiocytic lineage is exceptionally rare, and should
be diagnosed only after comprehensive immunohistochemical analyses using monoclonal antibodies reactive with T cells, B cells, and monocytes/
macrophages (133,141,142,161). The diagnosis is
preferably supported by genotypic demonstration
of a germline configuration of the immunoglobulin
and T-cell receptor genes. Malignant histiocytosis

Table 18-2

IMMUNOHISTOCHEMICAL PROFILE OF PLASMACYTOID MONOCYTES*

	Fresh/Frozen Tissues	Paraffin Sections
T-cell–associated markers	CD2–, CD3–, CD5–, CD8–, CD4+	CD45RO–, CD3–, CD43+
B-cell–associated markers	CD19–, CD20–, CD22–	CD20–, CD45RA+, CD74 (LN2) +, CD75 (LN1) –/+
Myelomonocytic markers	CD68+, CD36+, CD14–/+, CD15–/+	CD68+, Mac387–, lysozyme–
Others	CD25–, CD45+, CD71+, HLA-DR+	CD45RB+

* Plasmacytoid monocytic lymphoma shows an identical immunophenotype with the following exceptions: CD2 sometimes positive; CD5 often positive; CD75 often negative.

of true histiocytic type and true histiocytic lymphoma probably represent different manifestations of the same disease process, with the former showing disseminated and dispersed growth of histiocytes, and the latter showing more localized mass-forming lesions. However, a study suggests that the neoplastic histiocytes of bona fide malignant histiocytosis differ from those of true histiocytic lymphoma in that the monocyte markers CD11b, CD11c, and CD14 are commonly expressed, and are thus related more to monocytes and free histiocytes than fixed histiocytes (149). Further studies are required to clarify this issue. Some cases of malignant histiocytosis are alleged to be biphenotypic, that is, expressing both macrophage and T-cell markers (150). Some cases are also reported to express CD30 antigen and overlap with CD30-positive anaplastic large cell lymphoma (147).

PLASMACYTOID MONOCYTIC LYMPHOMA (SO-CALLED PLASMACYTOID T-CELL LYMPHOMA)

Definition. Plasmacytoid monocytic lymphoma (plasmacytoid T-cell lymphoma) is a tumorous proliferation of cells showing cytologic features of plasmacytoid monocytes (so-called plasmacytoid T cells).

Cytology and Nature of Plasmacytoid Monocytes. T-associated plasma cells (lymphoblasts) were first characterized in 1958 by Lennert and Remmele (188,189). They were so named because of their morphologic resemblance to plasma cells, including the presence of a well-developed rough endoplasmic reticulum and Golgi apparatus ultrastructurally. These cells

were subsequently renamed plasmacytoid T cells because they were believed to represent a form of T cell serving a secretory function (195). Since recent immunohistochemical studies have shown these cells to be more related to the myelomonocytic than T-cell lineage, the designations plasmacytoid monocyte and plasmacytoid T-zone cell have been proposed (172,177,181,183).

Plasmacytoid monocytes can occur in a wide variety of reactive lymphoid proliferations, and inconsistently in some hematolymphoid malignancies such as Hodgkin's disease, mycosis fungoides, and acute lymphoblastic leukemia (174,176,178–182,184,186,192,194,195). They are particularly common in Castleman's disease (hyaline vascular type) and Kikuchi's necrotizing lymphadenitis. The cells form small violaceous cellular clusters in the paracortex, although they can also occur singly (fig. 18-70A). They are medium-sized, and possess round or slightly folded nuclei, fine chromatin, small nucleoli, and an eccentric rim of amphophilic cytoplasm (fig. 18-70B). A pale paranuclear zone is lacking. The cytoplasm appears grey-blue with Giemsa stain. The many interspersed pyknotic nuclei aid in their recognition at medium magnification. In some larger cell clusters, tingible body macrophages may be present.

Immunohistochemically, plasmacytoid monocytes do not stain with B-lineage or T-lineage specific markers. The only T-cell–associated marker they stain with is CD4, which, however, is also known to stain histiocytes. In addition, they stain with a variety of histiocytic markers, such as CD68 and CD36 (Table 18-2; fig. 18-70C) (174,177,178,180,181,183,184,186,192).

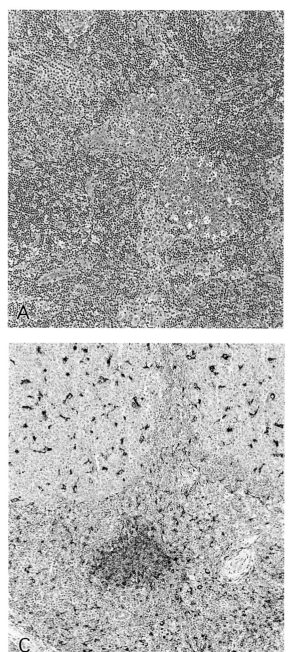

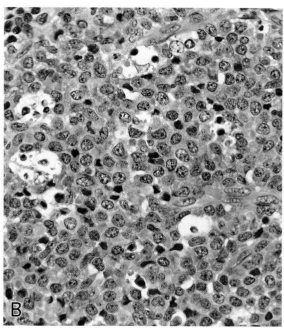

Figure 18-70
PLASMACYTOID MONOCYTES
IN A REACTIVE LYMPH NODE
A: Plasmacytoid monocytes occur as violaceous clusters in the paracortex; note the prominent karyorrhexis. Two reactive lymphoid follicles are seen in the upper field.
B: Plasmacytoid monocytes are medium-sized cells with violaceous cytoplasm.
C: The plasmacytoid monocytes are best highlighted by immunostaining with CD68 (center). The tingible body macrophages in the lymphoid follicles (upper field) are also stained by CD68.

Natural History and Clinical Features. Patients with plasmacytoid monocytic lymphoma are usually elderly and present with systemic symptoms such as fatigue and weight loss (171,173,178,185,187,190,191,193). Most have generalized lymphadenopathy and hepatosplenomegaly. At the time of diagnosis, or shortly thereafter, the patients are also found to have myelomonocytic leukemia. Despite chemotherapy, death from leukemia occurs within months.

A case reported as acute leukemia/lymphoma of plasmacytoid T-cell lymphoma (175) does not appear to be a typical example of plasmacytoid monocytic lymphoma, either in terms of clinical features, immunophenotype (CD2 positive), or genotype (presence of T-cell receptor gene rearrangement).

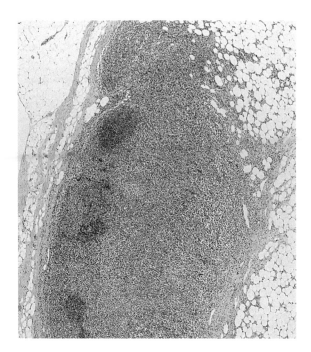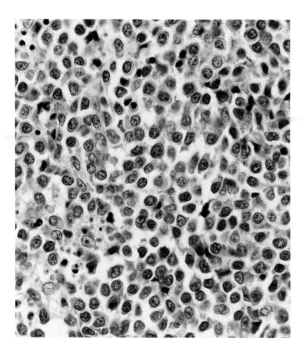

Figure 18-71
PLASMACYTOID MONOCYTIC LYMPHOMA
Left: The lymph node is almost totally replaced by a monotonous infiltrate.
Right: The infiltrate comprises medium-sized cells with eccentric nuclei, fine chromatin, and a definite rim of amphophilic cytoplasm.
(Courtesy of Dr. F. Facchetti, Brescia, Italy.)

Microscopic Findings. The lymph nodes show diffuse or paracortical infiltration by uniform, medium-sized cells in the form of diffuse sheets, nodules, or smaller aggregates. These cells possess round or ovoid nuclei that are often eccentrically located. The chromatin is dispersed or clumped, and nucleoli are inconspicuous. The cytoplasm is amphophilic and moderate in amount (figs. 18-71, 18-72). Mitotic figures are sparse. There are often scattered pyknotic cells with occasional interspersed tingible body macrophages.

In lymph nodes that are also involved by the myelomonocytic leukemic process, there are aggregates of cells with indented or twisted nuclei, delicate chromatin, and abundant cytoplasm (171, 178). Immature myeloid cells (promyelocytes and myelocytes), neutrophils, and megakaryocytes can also be seen (fig. 18-72, right) (171).

Immunophenotypic and Genotypic Findings. Plasmacytoid monocytic lymphoma stains for CD4 and various histiocytic markers (such as CD68 and CD36); it frequently expresses CD5 although this antigen is absent on normal plasmacytoid monocytes (Table 18-2) (171,173,178,

185,187,190,191). Immunohistochemical analyses should always be performed to confirm the diagnosis, and to distinguish it from lymphoplasmacytoid lymphoma (see fig. 18-67). Except for one reported case, which is probably a different entity (175), no rearrangements of the T-cell receptor or immunoglobulin gene have been seen.

The Nature of Plasmacytoid Monocytes in Plasmacytoid Monocytic Lymphoma. It is currently unclear whether the plasmacytoid monocytes observed in plasmacytoid monocytic lymphoma are neoplastic or reactive. Conclusive clonal markers are so far lacking. The aberrant immunophenotype (additional expression of CD5 antigen) appears to support a neoplastic nature. The consistent association with myelomonocytic leukemia as well as the documented myelomonocytic nature of plasmacytoid monocytes suggest that the plasmacytoid monocytes may belong to the same neoplastic clone as the leukemic process (fig. 18-73) (178). In a broad sense, perhaps plasmacytoid monocytic lymphoma can be viewed as a peculiar form of granulocytic sarcoma (171).

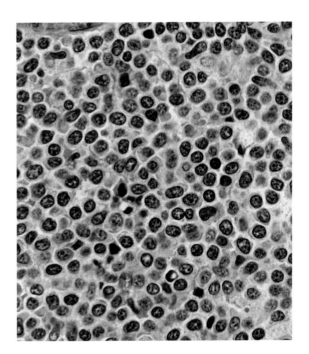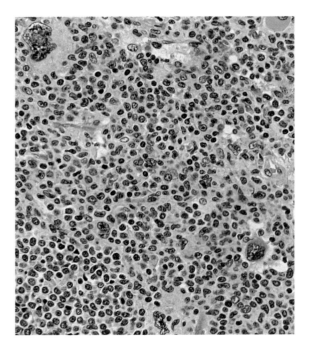

Figure 18-72
PLASMACYTOID MONOCYTIC LYMPHOMA

Left: This example strongly mimics lymphoplasmacytoid lymphoma because of the condensed nuclear chromatin and amphophilic cytoplasm.

Right: The interspersed myelocytes and megakaryocytes provide evidence of the presence of an associated myeloproliferative disorder. (Courtesy of Dr. Wing C. Chan, Omaha, NE.) (Figures 18-72 and 18-73 are from the same case.)

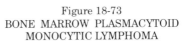

Figure 18-73
BONE MARROW PLASMACYTOID MONOCYTIC LYMPHOMA

Bone marrow biopsy from a patient with plasmacytoid monocytic lymphoma. The high cellularity, increase in megakaryocytes, and increase in myeloid cells are compatible with a diagnosis of myeloproliferative disease. (Courtesy of Dr. Wing C. Chan, Omaha, NE.)

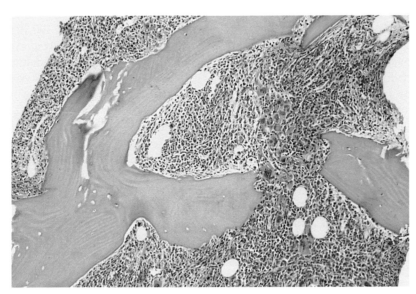

On the other hand, since the plasmacytoid monocytes are sharply compartmentalized from the myelomonocytic leukemic cells, with no transitional forms, the plasmacytoid monocytes sometimes regress rather than continue to expand (185), and an identical infiltrate of plasmacytoid monocytes can occur in lineage-unrelated leukemias (such as acute lymphoblastic leukemia) (178). Thus the possibility remains that the plasmacytoid monocytes are merely reactive.

REFERENCES

Langerhans' Cell Histiocytosis

1. Azumi N, Sheibani K, Swartz WG, Stroup RM, Rappaport H. Antigenic phenotype of Langerhans' cell histiocytosis: an immunohistochemical study demonstrating the value of LN-2, LN-3 and vimentin. Hum Pathol 1988;19:1376–82.
2. Bartholdy N, Thommesen P. Histiocytosis X. VII. Prognostic significance of skull lesions. Acta Radiol Oncology 1983;22:125–7.
3. Beckstead JH, Wood GS, Turner RR. Histiocytosis X cells and Langerhans' cells: enzyme histochemical and immunologic similarities. Hum Pathol 1984;15:826–33.
4. Ben-Ezra J, Bailey A, Azumi N, et al. Malignant histiocytosis X. A distinct clinicopathologic entity. Cancer 1991;68:1050–60.
5. Broadbent V, Pritchard J, Davies EG, et al. Spontaneous remission of multi-system histiocytosis X. Lancet 1984;1:253–4.
6. Burns BF, Colby TV, Dorfman RD. Langerhans' cell granulomatosis (histiocytosis X) associated with malignant lymphomas. Am J Surg Pathol 1983;7:529–33.
7. Colby TV, Lombard C. Histiocytosis X in the lung. Hum Pathol 1983;14:847–56.
8. Enriquez P, Dahlin DC, Hayles AB, Henderson ED. Histiocytosis X: a clinical study. Mayo Clin Proc 1967;42:88–99.
9. Favara BE, Jaffe R. Pathology of Langerhans' cell histiocytosis. Hematol Oncol Clin North Am 1987;1:75–97.
10. _____, McCarthy RC, Mierau GW. Histiocytosis X. Hum Pathol 1983;14:663–76.
11. Friedman PJ, Liebow AA, Sokoloff J. Eosinophilic granuloma of lung. Clinical aspects of primary pulmonary histiocytosis in the adult. Medicine (Baltimore) 1981;60:385–96.
12. Greenberger JS, Crocker AC, Vawter G, Jaffe N, Cassady JR. Results of treatment of 127 patients with systemic histiocytosis (Letterer-Siwe syndrome, Schuller-Christian syndrome and multifocal eosinophilic granuloma). Medicine 1981;60:311–38.
13. Hage C, Willman CL, Favara BE, Isaacson PG. Langerhans' cell histiocytosis (histiocytosis X): immunophenotype and growth fraction. Hum Pathol 1993;24:840–5.
14. Hartman KS. Histiocytosis X: a review of 114 cases with oral involvement. Oral Surg Oral Med Oral Pathol 1980;49:38–54.
15. Komp DM, Herson J, Starling KA, Vietti TJ, Hvizdala E. A staging system for histiocytosis X: a Southwest Oncology Group Study. Cancer 1981;47:798–800.
16. LaCronique J, Roth C, Battesti JP, Basset F, Chretien J. Chest radiological features of pulmonary histiocytosis X: a report based on 50 adult cases. Thorax 1982;37:104–9.
17. Lahey ME. Prognostic factors in histiocytosis X. Am J Pediatr Hematol Oncol 1981;3:57–60.
18. Leahy MA, Knejei SM, Friedmanash M, et al. Human herpesvirus 6 is present in lesions of Langerhans' cell histiocytosis. J Invest Dermatol 1993;101:642–5.
19. McClain K, Jin H, Gresik V, Favara B. Langerhans' cell histiocytosis—lack of viral etiology. Am J Hematol 1994;47:16–20.
20. Mierau GW, Favara BE, Brenman JM. Electron microscopy in histiocytosis X. Ultrastruct Pathol 1982; 3:137–42.
21. Motoi M, Helbron D, Kaiserling E, Lennert K. Eosinophilic granuloma of lymph nodes–a variant of histiocytosis X. Histopathology 1980;4:585–606.
22. Neumann MP, Frizzera G. The coexistence of Langerhans' cell granulomatosis and malignant lymphoma may take different forms: report of seven cases with a review of the literature. Hum Pathol 1986;17:1060–5.
23. Nezelof C, Frileux-Herbet F, Cronier-Sachot J. Disseminated histiocytosis X: analysis of prognostic factors based on a retrospective study of 50 cases. Cancer 1979;44:1824–38.
24. Ornvold K, Ralfkiaer E, Carstensen H. Immunohistochemical study of the abnormal cells in Langerhans' cell histiocytosis (histiocytosis X). Virchows Arch [A] 1990;416:403–10.
25. Risdall RJ, Dehner LP, Duray P, Kobrinsky N, Robison L, Nesbit ME Jr. Histiocytosis X (Langerhans' cell histiocytosis). Prognostic role of histopathology. Arch Pathol Lab Med 1983;107:59–63.
26. Ruco LP, Pulford KAF, Mason DY, et al. Expression of macrophage-associated antigens in tissues involved by Langerhans' cell histiocytosis (histiocytosis X). Am J Clin Pathol 1989;92:273–9.
27. _____, Remotti D, Monardo F, et al. Letterer-Siwe disease: immunohistochemical evidence for a proliferative disorder involving immature cells of Langerhans' lineage. Virchows Arch [A] 1988;413:239–47.
28. Santamaria M, Llamas L, Ree HJ, et al. Expression of sialylated Leu-M1 antigen in histiocytosis X. Am J Clin Pathol 1988;89:211–6.
29. Siegal GP, Dehner LP, Rosai J. Histiocytosis X (Langerhans' cell granulomatosis) of the thymus. A clinicopathologic study of four childhood cases. Am J Surg Pathol 1985;9:117–24.
30. Tomashefski JF, Khiyami A, Kleinerman J. Neoplasms associated with pulmonary eosinophilic granuloma. Arch Pathol Lab Med 1991;115:499–506.
31. Weiss LM, Beckstead JH, Warnke RA, Wood GS. Leu-6-expressing cells in lymph nodes: dendritic cells phenotypically similar to interdigitating cells. Hum Pathol 1986;17:179–84.
32. Williams JW, Dorfman RF. Lymphadenopathy as the initial manifestation of histiocytosis X. Am J Surg Pathol 1979;3:405–21.
33. Willman CL, Busque L, Griffith BB, et al. Langerhans'-cell histiocytosis (histiocytosis X)—a clonal proliferative disease. N Engl J Med 1994;331:154–60.
34. Winkelmann RK. The skin in histiocytosis X. Mayo Clin Proc 1969;44:535–48.
35. Wood C, Wood GS, Deneau DG, Oseroff A, Beckstead JH, Malin J. Malignant histiocytosis X. Report of a rapidly fatal case in an elderly man. Cancer 1984;54:347–52.
36. Wood GS, Freudenthal PS, Edinger A, Steinman RM, Warnke RA. CD45 epitope mapping of human CD1a+ dendritic cells and peripheral blood dendritic cells. Am J Pathol 1991;138:1451–9.
37. Writing Group of the Histiocyte Society. Histiocytosis syndromes in children. Lancet 1987;1:208–9.

Sinus Histiocytosis with Massive Lymphadenopathy (Rosai-Dorfman Disease)

38. Bankaci M, Morris RF, Stool SE, et al. Sinus histiocytosis with massive lymphadenopathy. Report of its occurrence in two siblings with retropharyngeal involvement in both. Ann Otol Rhinol Laryngol 1978;87(3 Pt 1):327–31.

39. Becroft DM, Dix MR, Gillman JC, MacGregor BJ. Benign sinus histiocytosis with massive lymphadenopathy: transient immunological defects in a child with mediastinal involvement. J Clin Pathol 1973;26:463–69.

40. Bonetti F, Chilosi M, Menestrina F, et al. Immunohistochemical analysis of Rosai-Dorfman histiocytosis. A disease of S-100 + CD1- histiocytes. Virchows Arch [A] 1987;411:129–35.

41. Eisen RN, Buckley PJ, Rosai J. Immunophenotypic characterization of sinus histiocytosis with massive lymphadenopathy (Rosai-Dorfman disease). Semin Diagn Pathol 1990;7:74–82.

42. Foucar E, Rosai J, Dorfman RF. Sinus histiocytosis with massive lymphadenopathy: ear, nose, and throat manifestations. Arch Otolaryngol 1978;104:687–93.

43. _____, Rosai J, Dorfman RF. The ophthalmologic manifestations of sinus histiocytosis with massive lymphadenopathy. Am J Ophthalmol 1979;87:354–67.

44. _____, Rosai J, Dorfman RF, Brynes RK. The neurologic manifestations of sinus histiocytosis with massive lymphadenopathy. Neurology 1982;32:365–70.

45. _____, Rosai J, Dorfman RF, Eyman JM. Immunological abnormalities and their significance in sinus histiocytosis with massive lymphadenopathy. Am J Clin Pathol 1984;82:515–25.

46. _____, Rosai J, Dorfman RF. Sinus histiocytosis with massive lymphadenopathy. An analysis of 14 deaths occurring in a patient registry. Cancer 1984;54:1834–40.

47. _____, Rosai J, Dorfman RF. Sinus histiocytosis with massive lymphadenopathy. Current status and future directions. Arch Dermatol 1988;124:1211–14.

48. _____, Rosai J, Dorfman R. Sinus histiocytosis with massive lymphadenopathy (Rosai-Dorfman disease). Review of the entity. Semin Diagn Pathol 1990;7:19–73.

49. Humble JG, Jayne WHW, Pulvertaft RJV. Biological interaction between lymphocytes and other cells. Br J Haematol 1956;2:283–94.

50. Ioachim HL. Emperipolesis of lymphoid cells in mixed cultures. Lab Invest 1965;14:1784–94.

51. Karpas A, Worman C, Arno J, Naginton J. Sinus histiocytosis with massive lymphadenopathy: virological, immunological, and morphologic studies. Br J Haematol 1980;45:195–200.

52. Komp DM. The treatment of sinus histiocytosis with massive lymphadenopathy (Rosai-Dorfman disease). Semin Diagn Pathology 1990;7:83–6.

53. Lampert F, Lennert K. Sinus histiocytosis with massive lymphadenopathy: fifteen new cases. Cancer 1976;37:783–89.

54. Lennert K, Niedorf HR, Blumcke S, Hardmeier T. Lymphadenitis with massive hemophagocytic sinus histiocytosis. Virchows Arch [Cell Pathol] 1972;10:14–29.

55. Levine PH, Jahan N, Murari P, Manak M, Jaffe ES. Detection of human herpesvirus 6 in tissues involved by sinus histiocytosis with massive lymphadenopathy (Rosai-Dorfman disease). J Infect Dis 1992;166:291–5.

56. Lewin JR, Das SK, Blumenthal BI, D'Cruz C, Patel RB, Howell GE. Osseous pseudotumor. The sole manifestation of sinus histiocytosis with massive lymphadenopathy. Am J Clin Pathol 1985;84:547–50.

57. Marsh WL Jr, McCarrick JP, Harlan DM. Sinus histiocytosis with massive lymphadenopathy. Occurrence in identical twins with retroperitoneal disease. Arch Pathol Lab Med 1988;112:298–301.

58. Miettinen M, Paljakka P, Haveri P, Saxen E. Sinus histiocytosis with massive lymphadenopathy. A nodal and extranodal proliferation of S-100 positive histiocytes? Am J Clin Pathol 1987;88:270–7.

59. Paulli M, Rosso R, Kindl S, et al. Immunophenotypic characterization of the cell infiltrate in five cases of sinus histiocytosis with massive lymphadenopathy (Rosai-Dorfman disease). Hum Pathol 1992;647–54.

60. Penneys NS, Ahn YS, McKinney EC, et al. Sinus histiocytosis with massive lymphadenopathy: a case with unusual skin involvement and therapeutic response to vinblastin-loaded platelets. Cancer 1982;49:1994–8.

61. Rosai J, Dorfman RF. Sinus histiocytosis with massive lymphadenopathy. A newly recognized benign clinicopathological entity. Arch Pathol 1969;87:63–70.

62. _____, Dorfman RF. Sinus histiocytosis with massive lymphadenopathy: a pseudolymphomatous benign disorder. Analysis of 34 cases. Cancer 1972;30:1174–88.

63. Sanchez R, Sibley RK, Rosai J, et al. The electron microscopic features of sinus histiocytosis with massive lymphadenopathy: a study of 11 cases. Ultrastruct Pathol 1981;2:101–19.

64. Thawerani H, Sanchez RL, Rosai J, Dorfman RF. The cutaneous manifestations of sinus histiocytosis with massive lymphadenopathy. Arch Dermatol 1978;114:191–7.

65. Walker PD, Rosai J, Dorfman RF. The osseous manifestations of sinus histiocytosis with massive lymphadenopathy. Am J Clin Pathol 1981;75:131–9.

66. Williams JW, Dorfman RF. Lymphadenopathy as the initial manifestation of histiocytosis X. Am J Surg Pathol 1979;3:405–21.

67. Wright DH, Richards DB. Sinus histiocytosis with massive lymphadenopathy (Rosai-Dorfman disease): report of a case with widespread nodal and extranodal dissemination. Histopathology 1981;5:697–709.

Follicular Dendritic Cell Sarcoma

68. Chan JK, Tsang WY, Ng CS. Follicular dendritic cell tumor and vascular neoplasm complicating hyaline-vascular Castleman's disease. Am J Surg Pathol 1994;18:517–25.

69. _____, Tsang WY, Ng CS, Tang SK, Lee AW. Follicular dendritic cell tumors of the oral cavity. Am J Surg Pathol 1994;18:148–57.

70. Hollowood K, Pease C, Mackay AM, Fletcher CD. Sarcomatoid tumors of lymph nodes showing follicular dendritic cell differentiation. J Pathol 1991;163:205–16.

70a. _____, Stamp G, Zouvani I, Fletcher CD. Extranodal follicular dendritic cell sarcoma of the gastrointestinal tract. Morphologic, immunohistochemical and ultrastructural analysis of two cases. Am J Clin Pathol 1995;103:90–7.

71. Monda L, Warnke R, Rosai J. A primary lymph node malignancy with features suggestive of dendritic reticulum cell differentiation. A report of four cases. Am J Pathol 1986;122:562–72.

71a. Nguyen DT, Diamond LW, Hansmann ML, Hell K, Fischer R. Follicular dendritic cell sarcoma, identification by monoclonal antibodies in paraffin sections. Appl Immunohistochem 1994;2:60–4.

72. Pallesen G, Myhre-Jensen O. Immunophenotypic analysis of neoplastic cells in follicular dendritic cell sarcoma. Leukemia 1987;1:549–57.

73. Strickler JG, Parkin JL, Schmidt CM, Hurd DD. Primary skin malignancy with features suggestive of dendritic reticulum cell differentiation. Ultrastruct Pathol 1990;14:273–82.

74. Weiss LM, Berry GJ, Dorfman RF, et al. Spindle cell neoplasms of lymph nodes of probable reticulum cell lineage. True reticulum cell sarcoma? Am J Surg Pathol 1990;14:405–14.

Interdigitating Dendritic Cell Sarcoma

75. Feltkamp CA, van Heerde P, Feltkamp-Vroom TM, Koudstaal J. A malignant tumor arising from interdigitating cells; light microscopical, ultrastructural, immuno- and enzyme-histochemical characteristics. Virchows Arch [A] 1981;393:183–92.

76. Hammar SP, Rudolph RH, Bockus DE, Remington FL. Interdigitating reticulum cell sarcoma with unusual features. Ultrastruct Pathol 1991;15:631–45.

77. Hui PK, Feller AC, Kaiserling E, et al. Skin tumor of T accessory cells (interdigitating reticulum cells) with high content of T lymphocytes. Am J Dermatopathol 1987;9:129–37.

78. Miettinen M, Fletcher CD, Lasota J. True histiocytic lymphoma of small intestine. Analysis of two S-100 protein-positive cases with features of interdigitating reticulum cell sarcoma. Am J Clin Pathol 1993;100:285–92.

79. Nakamura S, Hara K, Suchi T, et al. Interdigitating cell sarcoma. A morphologic, immunohistologic, and enzyme-histochemical study. Cancer 1988;61:562–8.

80. Rabkin MS, Kjeldsberg CR, Hammond ME, Wittwer CT, Nathwani B. Clinical, ultrastuctural, immunohistochemical and DNA content anlaysis of lymphomas having features of interdigitating reticulum cells. Cancer 1988;61:1594–601.

81. Salisbury JR, Ramsay AD, Isaacson PG. Histiocytic lymphoma: a report of a case with an unusual phenotype. J Pathol 1985;146:99–106.

82. Turner RR, Wood GS, Beckstead JH, Colby TV, Horning SJ, Warnke RA. Histiocytic malignancies. Morphologic, immunologic and enzymatic heterogeneity. Am J Surg Pathol 1984;8:485–500.

83. van den Oord JJ, de Wolf-Peeters C, de Vos R, Thomas J, Desmet VJ. Sarcoma arising from interdigitating reticulum cells: report of a case studied with light and electron microscopy, and enzyme- and immunohistochemistry. Histopathology 1986;10:509–23.

84. Van der Valk, P, Ruiter DJ, Den Ottolander GJ, Te Velde J, Spaander PJ, Meijer CJ. Dendritic reticulum cell sarcoma? Four cases of a lymphoma probably derived from dendritic reticulum cells of the follicular compartment. Histopathology 1982;6:269–87.

85. Weiss LM, Berry GJ, Dorfman RF, et al. Spindle cell neoplasms of lymph nodes of probable reticulum cell lineage. True reticulum cell sarcoma? Am J Surg Pathol 1990;14:405–14.

86. Yamakawa M, Matsuda M, Imai Y, Arai S, Harada K, Sato T. Lymph node interdigitating cell sarcoma. A case report. Am J Clin Pathol 1992;97:139–46.

Indeterminate Cell Tumors (Precursor Langerhans' Cell Histiocytosis)

87. Berti E, Gianotti R, Alessi E. Unusual cutaneous histiocytosis expressing an intermediate immunophenotype between Langerhans' cells and dermal macrophages. Arch Dermatol 1988;124:1250–3.

88. Bonetti F, Knowles DM, Chilosi M, et al. A distinctive cutaneous malignant neoplasm expressing the Langerhans' cell phenotype. Synchronous occurrence with B-chronic lymphocytic leukemia. Cancer 1985;55:2417–25.

89. Chan WC, Zaatari G. Lymph node interdigitating cell sarcoma. Am J Clin Pathol 1986;85:739–44.

90. Kolde G, Bröcker EB. Multiple skin tumors of indeterminate cells in an adult. J Am Acad Dermatol 1986;15:591–7.

91. Murphy GF, Bhan AK, Harrist TJ, Mihm MC. In situ identification for T6-positive cells in normal human dermis by immunoelectron microscopy. Br J Dermatol 1983;423–31.

92. Segal GH, Mesa MV, Fishleder AJ, et al. Precursor Langerhans' cell histiocytosis. An unusual histiocytic proliferation in a patient with persistent non-Hodgkin lymphoma and terminal acute monocytic leukemia. Cancer 1992;70:547–53.

93. Wood GS, Haber RS: Novel histiocytoses considered in the context of histiocyte subset differentiation [editorial]. Arch Dermatol 1993;129:210–4

94. _____, Hu CH, Beckstead JH, Turner RR, Winkelmann RK. The indeterminate cell proliferative disorder: report of a case manifesting as an unusual cutaneous histiocytosis. J Dermatol Surg Oncol 1985;11:1111–9.

True Histiocytic Lymphoma

95. Andreesen R, Brugger W, Lohr GW, Bross KJ. Human macrophages can express the Hodgkin's cell-associated antigen Ki-1 (CD30). Am J Pathol 1989;134:187–92.

96. Banks PM, Metter J, Allred DC. Anaplastic large cell (Ki-1) lymphoma with histiocytic phenotype simulating carcinoma. Am J Clin Pathol 1990;94:445–52.

97. Burns BF, Cripps C, Dardick I. A case of Ki-1 large cell anaplastic lymphoma with ultrastructural features. Hum Pathol 1989;20:393–6.

98. Carbone A, Gloghini A, De Re V, Tamaro P, Boiocchi M, Volpe R. Histopathologic, immunophenotypic, and genotypic analysis of Ki-1 anaplastic large cell lymphomas that express histiocyte-associated antigens. Cancer 1990;66:2547–56.

99. Falini B, Flenghi L, Pileri S, et al. PG-M1: a new monoclonal antibody directed against a fixative-resistant epitope on the macrophage-restricted form of the CD68 molecule. Am J Pathol 1993;142:1359–72.

100. Foucar K, Foucar E. The mononuclear phagocyte and immunoregulatory effector (M-PIRE) system: evolving concepts. Semin Diagn Pathol 1990;7:4–18.
101. Franchino C, Reich C, Distenfeld A, Ubriaco A, Knowles DM. A clinicopathologically distinctive primary splenic histiocytic neoplasm. Demonstration of its histiocytic derivation by immunophenotypic and molecular genetic analysis. Am J Surg Pathol 1988;12:398–404.
102. Gastineau DA, Banks PM, Knowles DM. Primary splenic neoplasm [Letter]. Am J Surg Pathol 1989;13:989.
103. Groopman JE, Golde DW. The histiocytic disorders: a pathophysiologic analysis. Ann Intern Med 1981;94:95–107.
104. Hanson CA, Jaszcz W, Kersey JH, et al. True histiocytic lymphoma: histopathologic, immunophenotypic and genotypic analysis. Br J Hematol 1989;73:187–98.
105. Hsu SM, Ho YS, Hsu PL. Lymphomas of true histiocytic origin: expression of different phenotypes in so-called true histiocytic lymphoma and malignant histiocytosis. Am J Pathol 1991;138:1389–404.
106. Isaacson PG, O'Connor NT, Spencer J, et al. Malignant histiocytosis of the intestine: a T-cell lymphoma. Lancet 1985;2:688–91.
107. Jaffe ES. Histiocytoses of lymph nodes: biology and differential diagnosis. Semin Diagn Pathol 1988;5:376–90.
108. Kahn LB, Mir R, Selzer G. True histiocytic lymphomas and histiocyte-rich lymphomas of the gastrointestinal tract. Am J Surg Pathol 1985;9(Suppl):109–15.
109. Kamel O, Kell D, Gocke C, Warnke R. True histiocytic lymphoma: a study of 12 cases based on current definition [Abstract]. Mod Pathol 1994;7:112A.
110. Miettinen M, Fletcher CD, Lasota J. True histiocytic lymphoma of small intestine. Analysis of two S-100 protein-positive cases with features of interdigitating reticulum cell sarcoma. Am J Clin Pathol 1993;100:285–92.
111. Milchgrub S, Kamel OW, Wiley E, Vuitch F, Cleary ML, Warnke RA. Malignant histiocytic neoplasms of the small intestine. Am J Surg Pathol 1992;16:11–20.
112. O'Grady JT, Shahidullah H, Doherty VR, al-Nafussi A. Intravascular histiocytosis. Histopathology 1994;24:265–8.
113. Pallesen G. Immunophenotypic markers for characterizing malignant lymphoma, malignant histiocytosis and tumors derived from accessory cells. Cancer Rev 1987;8:1–65.
114. Pileri S, Mazza P, Rivano MT. Malignant histiocytosis (true histiocytic lymphoma), clinicopathologic study of 25 cases. Histopathology 1985;9:905–20.
115. Ralfkiaer E, Delsol G, O'Connor NT, et al. Malignant lymphomas of true histiocytic origin. A clinical, histological, immunophenotypic and genotypic study. J Pathol 1990;160:9–17.
116. Soria C, Orradre JL, Garcia-Almagro D, Martinez B, Algara P, Piris MA. True histiocytic lymphoma (monocytic sarcoma). Am J Dermatopathol 1992;14:511–7.
117. Stein H, Mason DY. Immunologic analysis of tissue sections in diagnosis of lymphoma. In: Hoffbrand AV, ed. Recent advances in hematology, No. 4. Edinburgh: Churchill Livingstone, 1985:127–69.
118. Van der Valk P, Meijer CJ, Willemze R, Van Oosterom AT, Spaander PJ, te Velde J. Histiocytic sarcoma (true histiocytic lymphoma): a clinicopathological study of 20 cases. Histopathology 1984;8:105–23.
119. _____, Meijer CJ. Histiocytic sarcoma. Clinical picture, morphology, markers, differential diagnosis. Pathol Annu 1985;20(Pt 2):1–28.
120. Van Heerde P, Feltkamp CA, Hart AA, Somers R, van Unnik JA, Vroom TM. Malignant histiocytosis and related tumours. A clinicopathologic study of 42 cases using cytological, histochemical and ultrastructural parameters. Hematol Oncol 1984;2:13–32.
121. Volk BW, Adachi M, Schneck L. The pathology of sphingolipidoses. Semin Hematol 1972;9:317–48.
122. Weiss LM, Trela MJ, Cleary ML, Turner RR, Warnke RA, Sklar J. Frequent immunoglobulin and T-cell receptor gene rearrangement in "histiocytic" neoplasms. Am J Pathol 1985;121:369–73.
123. Wong KF, Chan JK. Hemophagocytic disorders—a review. Hematol Rev 1991;5:5–37.

Malignant Histiocytosis

124. Byrne GE, Rappaport H. Malignant histiocytosis. Gann Monogr Cancer Res 1975;15:145–61.
125. Carbone A, Micheau C, Caillaud JM, Carlu C. A cytochemical and immunohistochemical approach to malignant histiocytosis. Cancer 1981;47:2862–71.
126. Cattoretti G, Villa A, Vezzoni P, Giardini R, Lombardi L, Rilke F. Malignant histiocytosis. A phenotypic and genotypic investigation. Am J Pathol 1990;136:1009–19.
127. Chan JK, Ng CS, Hui PK, Leung TW, Lo ES, Lau WH, McGuire LJ. Anaplastic large cell lymphoma. Delineation of two morphological types. Histopathology 1989;15:11–34.
128. _____, Ng CS, Law CK, Ng WF, Wong KF. Reactive hemophagocytic syndrome, a study of 7 fatal cases. Pathology 1987;19:43–50.
129. deMent SH. Association between mediastinal germ cell tumors and hematologic malignancies: an update. Hum Pathol 1990;21:699–703.
130. Dodd HJ, Stansfeld AG, Chambers TJ. Cutaneous malignant histiocytosis—a clinicopathologic review of five cases. Br J Dermatol 1985;113:455–61.
131. Ducatman BS, Wick MR, Morgan TW, Banks PM, Pierre RV. Malignant histiocytosis: a clinical, histologic, and immunohistochemical study of 20 cases. Hum Pathol 1984;15:368–77.
132. Falini B, Pileri S, De Solas I, et al. Peripheral T-cell lymphoma associated with hemophagocytic syndrome. Blood 1990;75:434–44.
133. Hsu SM, Ho YS, Hsu PL. Lymphomas of true histiocytic origin: expression of different phenotypes in so-called true histiocytic lymphoma and malignant histiocytosis. Am J Pathol 1991;138:1389–404.
134. Huhn D, Meister P. Malignant histiocytosis, morphologic and cytochemical findings. Cancer 1978;42:1341–9.
135. Isaacson PG. Histiocytic malignancy [Commentary]. Histopathology 1985;9:1007–11.
136. _____, O'Connor NT, Spencer J, et al. Malignant histiocytosis of the intestine: a T-cell lymphoma. Lancet 1985;2:688–91.
137. Ishii E, Hara T, Okamura J, Suda M, Takeuchi T, Iida K, Ueda K. Malignant histiocytosis in infants: surface marker analysis of malignant cells in two cases. Med Pediatr Oncol 1987;15:102–8.
138. Jurco S III, Starling K, Hawkins EP. Malignant histiocytosis in childhood: morphologic considerations. Hum Pathol 1983;14:1059–65.

_____, Langholm R, Godal T, Marton PF. T-zone lymphoma with predominance of 1 "plasmacytoid T cells" associated with myelomonocytic leukaemia—a distinct clinicopathologic entity. J Pathol 1986; 150:247–55.

Brubaker R, Swerdlow SH. Plasmacytoid T-cells in a reactive lymph node. Detection by flow cytometry? Am J Clin Pathol 1990;93:569–71.

Caldwell CW, Yesus YW, Loy TS, Bickel JT, Perry MC. Acute leukemia/lymphoma of plasmacytoid T-cell type. Am J Clin Pathol 1990;94:778–86.

De Vos R, de Wolf-Peeters C, Facchetti F, Desmet V. Plasmacytoid monocytes in epithelioid cell granulomas: ultrastructural and immunoelectron microscopic study. Ultrastruct Pathol 1990;14:291–302.

Facchetti F, de Wolf-Peeters C, Mason DY, Pulford K, van den Oord JJ, Desmet VJ. Plasmacytoid T cells. Immunohistochemical evidence for their mono-cyte/macrophage origin. Am J Pathol 1988;133:15–21.

_____, de Wolf-Peeters C, Kennes C, et al. Leukemia-associated lymph node infiltrates of plasmacytoid monocytes (so-called plasmacytoid T-cells), evidence for two distinct histological and immunophenotypical patterns. Am J Surg Pathol 1990;14:101–12.

_____, de Wolf-Peeters C, van den Oord JJ, Desmet VJ. Plasmacytoid T cells in a case of lympho-cytic infiltration of skin. A component of the skin-associated lymphoid tissue? J Pathol 1988;155:295–300.

_____, de Wolf-Peeters C, De Vos R, van den Oord JJ, Pulford KA, Desmet VJ. Plasmacytoid monocytes (so-called plasmacytoid T cells) in granulomatous lymphadenitis. Hum Pathol 1989;20:588–93.

_____, de Wolf-Peeters C, van den Oord VJ, de Vos R, Desmet VJ. Plasmacytoid T cells: a cell population normally present in the reactive lymph node. An immunohistochemical and electronmicroscopic study. Hum Pathol 1988;19:1085–92.

_____, de Wolf-Peeters C, van den Oord JJ, Desmet VJ. Plasmacytoid monocytes (so-called plasmacytoid T cells) in Hodgkin's disease. J Pathol 1989;158:57–66.

_____, de Wolf-Peeters C, van den Oord JJ, de Vos R, Desmet VJ. Plasmacytoid monocytes (so-called plasmacytoid T-cells) in Kikuchi's lymphadenitis. An immunohistologic study. Am J Clin Pathol 1989;92:42–50.

184. Harris NL, Bhan AK. "Plasmacytoid T cells" in Castleman's disease, immunohistologic phenotype. Am J Surg Pathol 1987;11:109–13.

185. _____, Demirjian Z. Plasmacytoid T-zone cell pro-liferation in a patient with chronic myelomonocytic leukemia. Histologic and immunohistologic character-ization. Am J Surg Pathol 1991;15:87–95.

186. Horny HP, Feller AC, Horst HA, Lennert K. Im-munocytology of plasmacytoid T cells: marker analysis indicates a unique phenotype of this enigmatic cell. Hum Pathol 1987;18:28–32.

187. Koo CH, Mason DY, Miller R, Ben-Ezra J, Sheibani K, Rappaport H. Additional evidence that "plasmacytoid T-cell lymphoma" associated with chronic myeloprolif-erative disorders is of macrophage/monocyte origin. Am J Clin Pathol 1990;93:822–7.

188. Lennert K, Kaiserling E, Muller-Hermelink HK. T-as-sociated plasma cells [Letter]. Lancet 1975;1:1031–2.

189. _____, Remmele W. Karyometrische Unter-suchungen an Lymphknotenzellen des Menschen. I. Mitt. Germinoblasten, Lymphoblasten und Lymphozyten. Acta Hematol (Basel) 1958;19:99–113.

190. Muller-Hermelink HK, Stein H, Steinmann G, Lennert K. Malignant lymphoma of plasmacytoid T-cells. Morphologic and immunologic studies characterizing a special type of T-cell. Am J Surg Pathol 1983;7:849–62.

191. Prasthofer EF, Prchal JT, Grizzle WE, Grossi CE. Plas-macytoid T-cell lymphoma associated with chronic mye-loproliferative disorder. Am J Surg Pathol 1985;9:380-7.

192. Takeshita M, Muller H, Mix D, Stutte HJ, Schmidts HL. Immuno- and enzyme histochemical characteriza-tion of "plasmacytoid T-cells" in formalin-fixed paraf-fin-embedded tissue of reactive lymph nodes. Pathol Res Pract 1991;187:848–55.

193. Thomas JO, Beiske K, Hann I, Koo C, Mason DY. Immu-nohistological diagnosis of "plasmacytoid T-cell lymphoma" in paraffin wax sections. J Clin Pathol 1991;44:632–5.

194. Toonstra J, van der Putte SC. Plasmacytoid monocytes in Jessner's lymphocytic infiltration of the skin. A valuable clue for the diagnosis. Am J Dermatopathol 1991;13:321–8.

195. Vollenweider R, Lennert K. Plasmacytoid T-cell clus-ters in non-specific lymphadenitis. Virchows Arch [Cell Pathol] 1983;44:1–14.

❖❖❖

139. Kaneko Y, Kikuchi M, Ishihara A, Abe R, Takayama S, Sakurai M. Chromosome abnormalities in malignant histiocytosis. Cancer 1985;56:144–51.

140. _____, Frizzera G, Edamura S, et al. A novel translocation, t(2;5)(p23;q35) in childhood phagocytic large T-cell lymphoma mimicking malignant histiocytosis. Blood 1989;73:806–13.

141. Kelly PM, McGovern M, Gatter KC, Theaker JM, McGee JO. EBM/11 reactivity in malignant histiocytosis. J Clin Pathol 1988;41:1305–9.

142. Koo CH, Reifel J, Kogut N, Cove JK, Rappaport H. True histiocytic malignancy associated with a malignant teratoma in a patient with 46XY gonadal dysgenesis. Am J Surg Pathol 1992;16:175–83.

143. Lampert IA, Catovsky D, Bergier N. Malignant histiocytosis: a clinicopathological study of 12 cases. Br J Haematol 1978;40:65–77.

144. Mason DY, Bastard C, Rimokh R, et al. CD30-positive large cell lymphomas ("Ki-1 lymphoma") are associated with a chromosomal translocation involving 5q35. Br J Haematol 1990;74:161–8.

145. Morgan R, Hecht BK, Sandberg AA, Hecht F, Smith SD. Chromosome 5q35 breakpoint in malignant histiocytosis [Letter]. N Engl J Med 1986;314:1322.

146. _____, Smith SD, Hecht BK, et al. Lack of involvement of the c-fms and N-myc genes by chromosomal translocation t(2;5)(p23;q35) common to malignancies with features of so-called malignant histiocytosis. Blood 1989;73:2155–64.

147. Nezelof C, Barbey S, Gogusev J, Terrier-Lacombe MJ. Malignant histiocytosis in childhood: a distinctive CD30-positive clinicopathologic entity associated with a chromosomal translocation involving 5q35. Semin Diagn Pathol 1992;9:75–89.

148. Nichols CR, Roth BJ, Heerema N, Griep J, Tricot G. Hematologic neoplasia associated with primary mediastinal germ-cell tumors. N Engl J Med 1990;322:1425–9.

149. Oka K, Mori N, Yatabe Y, Kojima M. Malignant histiocytosis. A report of three cases. Arch Pathol Lab Med 1992;116:1228–33.

150. Pallesen G. Immunophenotypic markers for characterizing malignant lymphoma, malignant histiocytosis and tumors derived from accessory cells. Cancer Rev 1987;8:1065.

151. Rappaport H. Tumors of the hematopoietic system. Atlas of Tumor Pathology. First series, Section 3, Fascicle 8. Washington D.C.: Armed Forces Institute of Pathology. 1966:48–63.

152. Reiner AP, Spivak JL. Hematophagic histiocytosis: a report of 23 new patients and a review of the literature. Medicine (Baltimore) 1988;67:369–88.

153. Risdall RJ, Brunning RD, Dehner LP, Sibley RK, McKenna RW. Malignant histiocytosis: a light- and electron-microscopic and histochemical study. Am J Surg Pathol 1980;4:439–50.

154. _____, McKenna RW, Nesbit ME, et al. Virus-associated hemophagocytic syndrome, a benign histio-

cytic proliferation distinct from m
sis. Cancer 1979;44:993–1002.

155. Robb-Smith AH. Before our time
histiocytic medullary reticulosis: a
topathology 1990;17:279–83.

156. Scott RB, Robb-Smith AH. His
reticulosis. Lancet 1939;ii:194–8.

157. Sonneveld P, van Lom K, Kappers-I
Abels J. Clinicopathological diagno
malignant histiocytosis. Br J Haema

158. Stein H, Mason DY. Immunologic
sections in diagnosis of lymphoma
ed. Recent advances in haematolog
Churchill Livingstone, 1985:127–6

159. _____, Mason DY, Gerdes J, et
the Hodgkin's disease associated an
and neoplastic lymphoid tissue: evide
berg cells and histiocytic malignanc
activated lymphoid cells. Blood 1985

160. Stein RS, Moran EM, Byrne (
histiocytosis: complete remission
chemotherapy. Cancer 1976;38:108

161. Takeshita M, Kikuchi M, Ohshima
row findings in malignant histiocy
nant lymphoma with concurrent h
drome. Leuk Lymphoma 1993;12:7

162. Tseng A Jr., Coleman CN, Cox RS,
of malignant histiocytosis. Blood 1

163. Van Heerde P, Feltkamp CA, Hart
Vonik JA, Vroom TM. Malignant h
lated tumors. A clinicopathologic
using cytological, histochemical a
parameters. Hematol Oncol 1984;2

164. Vardiman JW, Byrne GE Jr, Rapp
histiocytosis with massive splenom
atic patients: a possible chronic f
Cancer 1975;36:419–27.

165. Warnke RA, Kim H, Dorfman RF. M
sis (histiocytic medullary reticulosis
study of 29 cases. Cancer 1975;35:2

166. Weiss LM, Trela MJ, Cleary ML, 1
RA, Sklar J. Frequent immunoglo
ceptor gene rearrangements in "hist
Am J Pathol 1985;121:369–73.

167. Wilson MS, Weiss LM, Gatter KC, Ma
Warnke RA. Malignant histiocytosis
cases previously reported in 1975 base
immunophenotyping studies. Cancer

168. Wong KF, Chan JK. Hemophagocy
view. Hematol Rev 1991;5:5–37.

169. _____, Chan JK. Reactive he
drome—a clinicopathologic study o
Oriental population. Am J Med 199

170. Zucker JM, Caillaux JM, Vanel D, C
Malignant histiocytosis in childhood
therapeutic results in 22 cases. Canc

Plasmacytoid Monocytic Lymphoma

171. Baddoura FK, Hanson C, Chan WC. Plasmacytoid monocytic proliferation associated with myeloproliferative disorders. Cancer 1992;69:1457–67.

172. Beiske K, Munthe-Kaas A, Davies C I
T. Single cell studies on the immunolo
of plasmacytoid T-zone cells. Lab Inve

139. Kaneko Y, Kikuchi M, Ishihara A, Abe R, Takayama S, Sakurai M. Chromosome abnormalities in malignant histiocytosis. Cancer 1985;56:144–51.

140. _____, Frizzera G, Edamura S, et al. A novel translocation, t(2;5)(p23;q35) in childhood phagocytic large T-cell lymphoma mimicking malignant histiocytosis. Blood 1989;73:806–13.

141. Kelly PM, McGovern M, Gatter KC, Theaker JM, McGee JO. EBM/11 reactivity in malignant histiocytosis. J Clin Pathol 1988;41:1305–9.

142. Koo CH, Reifel J, Kogut N, Cove JK, Rappaport H. True histiocytic malignancy associated with a malignant teratoma in a patient with 46XY gonadal dysgenesis. Am J Surg Pathol 1992;16:175–83.

143. Lampert IA, Catovsky D, Bergier N. Malignant histiocytosis: a clinicopathological study of 12 cases. Br J Haematol 1978;40:65–77.

144. Mason DY, Bastard C, Rimokh R, et al. CD30-positive large cell lymphomas ("Ki-1 lymphoma") are associated with a chromosomal translocation involving 5q35. Br J Haematol 1990;74:161–8.

145. Morgan R, Hecht BK, Sandberg AA, Hecht F, Smith SD. Chromosome 5q35 breakpoint in malignant histiocytosis [Letter]. N Engl J Med 1986;314:1322.

146. _____, Smith SD, Hecht BK, et al. Lack of involvement of the c-fms and N-myc genes by chromosomal translocation t(2;5)(p23;q35) common to malignancies with features of so-called malignant histiocytosis. Blood 1989;73:2155–64.

147. Nezelof C, Barbey S, Gogusev J, Terrier-Lacombe MJ. Malignant histiocytosis in childhood: a distinctive CD30-positive clinicopathologic entity associated with a chromosomal translocation involving 5q35. Semin Diagn Pathol 1992;9:75–89.

148. Nichols CR, Roth BJ, Heerema N, Griep J, Tricot G. Hematologic neoplasia associated with primary mediastinal germ-cell tumors. N Engl J Med 1990;322:1425–9.

149. Oka K, Mori N, Yatabe Y, Kojima M. Malignant histiocytosis. A report of three cases. Arch Pathol Lab Med 1992;116:1228–33.

150. Pallesen G. Immunophenotypic markers for characterizing malignant lymphoma, malignant histiocytosis and tumors derived from accessory cells. Cancer Rev 1987;8:1065.

151. Rappaport H. Tumors of the hematopoietic system. Atlas of Tumor Pathology. First series, Section 3, Fascicle 8. Washington D.C.: Armed Forces Institute of Pathology. 1966:48–63.

152. Reiner AP, Spivak JL. Hematophagic histiocytosis: a report of 23 new patients and a review of the literature. Medicine (Baltimore) 1988;67:369–88.

153. Risdall RJ, Brunning RD, Dehner LP, Sibley RK, McKenna RW. Malignant histiocytosis: a light- and electron-microscopic and histochemical study. Am J Surg Pathol 1980;4:439–50.

154. _____, McKenna RW, Nesbit ME, et al. Virus-associated hemophagocytic syndrome, a benign histiocytic proliferation distinct from malignant histiocytosis. Cancer 1979;44:993–1002.

155. Robb-Smith AH. Before our time: half a century of histiocytic medullary reticulosis: a T–cell teaser? Histopathology 1990;17:279–83.

156. Scott RB, Robb-Smith AH. Histiocytic medullary reticulosis. Lancet 1939;ii:194–8.

157. Sonneveld P, van Lom K, Kappers-Klunne M, Prins ME, Abels J. Clinicopathological diagnosis and treatment of malignant histiocytosis. Br J Haematol 1990;75:511–6.

158. Stein H, Mason DY. Immunological analysis of tissue sections in diagnosis of lymphoma. In: Hoffbrand AV, ed. Recent advances in haematology. No. 4. Edinburgh: Churchill Livingstone, 1985:127–69.

159. _____, Mason DY, Gerdes J, et al. The expression of the Hodgkin's disease associated antigen Ki-1 in reactive and neoplastic lymphoid tissue: evidence that Reed-Sternberg cells and histiocytic malignancies are derived from activated lymphoid cells. Blood 1985; 66:848–58.

160. Stein RS, Moran EM, Bryne GE Jr. Malignant histiocytosis: complete remission with combination chemotherapy. Cancer 1976;38:1083–6.

161. Takeshita M, Kikuchi M, Ohshima K, et al. Bone marrow findings in malignant histiocytosis and/or malignant lymphoma with concurrent hemophagocytic syndrome. Leuk Lymphoma 1993;12:79–89.

162. Tseng A Jr., Coleman CN, Cox RS, et al. The treatment of malignant histiocytosis. Blood 1984;64:48–53.

163. Van Heerde P, Feltkamp CA, Hart AA, Somers R, Van Vonik JA, Vroom TM. Malignant histiocytosis and related tumors. A clinicopathologic study of 42 cases using cytological, histochemical and ultrastructural parameters. Hematol Oncol 1984;2:13–32.

164. Vardiman JW, Byrne GE Jr, Rappaport H. Malignant histiocytosis with massive splenomegaly in asymptomatic patients: a possible chronic form of the disease. Cancer 1975;36:419–27.

165. Warnke RA, Kim H, Dorfman RF. Malignant histiocytosis (histiocytic medullary reticulosis). A clinicopathologic study of 29 cases. Cancer 1975;35:215–30.

166. Weiss LM, Trela MJ, Cleary ML, Turner RR, Warnke RA, Sklar J. Frequent immunoglobulin and T-cell receptor gene rearrangements in "histiocytic" neoplasms. Am J Pathol 1985;121:369–73.

167. Wilson MS, Weiss LM, Gatter KC, Mason DY, Dorfman RF, Warnke RA. Malignant histiocytosis: a reassessment of cases previously reported in 1975 based on paraffin section immunophenotyping studies. Cancer 1990;66:530–6.

168. Wong KF, Chan JK. Hemophagocytic disorders—a review. Hematol Rev 1991;5:5–37.

169. _____, Chan JK. Reactive hemophagocytic syndrome—a clinicopathologic study of 40 patients in an Oriental population. Am J Med 1992;93:177–80.

170. Zucker JM, Caillaux JM, Vanel D, Gerald-Marchant R. Malignant histiocytosis in childhood, clinical study and therapeutic results in 22 cases. Cancer 1980;45:2821–9.

Plasmacytoid Monocytic Lymphoma

171. Baddoura FK, Hanson C, Chan WC. Plasmacytoid monocytic proliferation associated with myeloproliferative disorders. Cancer 1992;69:1457–67.

172. Beiske K, Munthe-Kaas A, Davies CD, Marton PF, Godal T. Single cell studies on the immunological marker profile of plasmacytoid T-zone cells. Lab Invest 1987;56:381–93.

173. _____, Langholm R, Godal T, Marton PF. T-zone lymphoma with predominance of 1 "plasmacytoid T cells" associated with myelomonocytic leukaemia—a distinct clinicopathologic entity. J Pathol 1986; 150:247–55.

174. Brubaker R, Swerdlow SH. Plasmacytoid T-cells in a reactive lymph node. Detection by flow cytometry? Am J Clin Pathol 1990;93:569–71.

175. Caldwell CW, Yesus YW, Loy TS, Bickel JT, Perry MC. Acute leukemia/lymphoma of plasmacytoid T-cell type. Am J Clin Pathol 1990;94:778–86.

176. De Vos R, de Wolf-Peeters C, Facchetti F, Desmet V. Plasmacytoid monocytes in epithelioid cell granulomas: ultrastructural and immunoelectron microscopic study. Ultrastruct Pathol 1990;14:291–302.

177. Facchetti F, de Wolf-Peeters C, Mason DY, Pulford K, van den Oord JJ, Desmet VJ. Plasmacytoid T cells. Immunohistochemical evidence for their monocyte/macrophage origin. Am J Pathol 1988;133:15–21.

178. _____, de Wolf-Peeters C, Kennes C, et al. Leukemia-associated lymph node infiltrates of plasmacytoid monocytes (so-called plasmacytoid T-cells), evidence for two distinct histological and immunophenotypical patterns. Am J Surg Pathol 1990;14:101–12.

179. _____, de Wolf-Peeters C, van den Oord JJ, Desmet VJ. Plasmacytoid T cells in a case of lymphocytic infiltration of skin. A component of the skin-associated lymphoid tissue? J Pathol 1988;155:295–300.

180. _____, de Wolf-Peeters C, De Vos R, van den Oord JJ, Pulford KA, Desmet VJ. Plasmacytoid monocytes (so-called plasmacytoid T cells) in granulomatous lymphadenitis. Hum Pathol 1989;20:588–93.

181. _____, de Wolf-Peeters C, van den Oord VJ, de Vos R, Desmet VJ. Plasmacytoid T cells: a cell population normally present in the reactive lymph node. An immunohistochemical and electronmicroscopic study. Hum Pathol 1988;19:1085–92.

182. _____, de Wolf-Peeters C, van den Oord JJ, Desmet VJ. Plasmacytoid monocytes (so-called plasmacytoid T cells) in Hodgkin's disease. J Pathol 1989;158:57–66.

183. _____, de Wolf-Peeters C, van den Oord JJ, de Vos R, Desmet VJ. Plasmacytoid monocytes (so-called plasmacytoid T-cells) in Kikuchi's lymphadenitis. An immunohistologic study. Am J Clin Pathol 1989;92:42–50.

184. Harris NL, Bhan AK. "Plasmacytoid T cells" in Castleman's disease, immunohistologic phenotype. Am J Surg Pathol 1987;11:109–13.

185. _____, Demirjian Z. Plasmacytoid T-zone cell proliferation in a patient with chronic myelomonocytic leukemia. Histologic and immunohistologic characterization. Am J Surg Pathol 1991;15:87–95.

186. Horny HP, Feller AC, Horst HA, Lennert K. Immunocytology of plasmacytoid T cells: marker analysis indicates a unique phenotype of this enigmatic cell. Hum Pathol 1987;18:28–32.

187. Koo CH, Mason DY, Miller R, Ben-Ezra J, Sheibani K, Rappaport H. Additional evidence that "plasmacytoid T-cell lymphoma" associated with chronic myeloproliferative disorders is of macrophage/monocyte origin. Am J Clin Pathol 1990;93:822–7.

188. Lennert K, Kaiserling E, Muller-Hermelink HK. T-associated plasma cells [Letter]. Lancet 1975;1:1031–2.

189. _____, Remmele W. Karyometrische Untersuchungen an Lymphknotenzellen des Menschen. I. Mitt. Germinoblasten, Lymphoblasten und Lymphozyten. Acta Hematol (Basel) 1958;19:99–113.

190. Muller-Hermelink HK, Stein H, Steinmann G, Lennert K. Malignant lymphoma of plasmacytoid T-cells. Morphologic and immunologic studies characterizing a special type of T-cell. Am J Surg Pathol 1983;7:849–62.

191. Prasthofer EF, Prchal JT, Grizzle WE, Grossi CE. Plasmacytoid T-cell lymphoma associated with chronic myeloproliferative disorder. Am J Surg Pathol 1985;9:380-7.

192. Takeshita M, Muller H, Mix D, Stutte HJ, Schmidts HL. Immuno- and enzyme histochemical characterization of "plasmacytoid T-cells" in formalin-fixed paraffin-embedded tissue of reactive lymph nodes. Pathol Res Pract 1991;187:848–55.

193. Thomas JO, Beiske K, Hann I, Koo C, Mason DY. Immunohistological diagnosis of "plasmacytoid T-cell lymphoma" in paraffin wax sections. J Clin Pathol 1991;44:632–5.

194. Toonstra J, van der Putte SC. Plasmacytoid monocytes in Jessner's lymphocytic infiltration of the skin. A valuable clue for the diagnosis. Am J Dermatopathol 1991;13:321–8.

195. Vollenweider R, Lennert K. Plasmacytoid T-cell clusters in non-specific lymphadenitis. Virchows Arch [Cell Pathol] 1983;44:1–14.

✧ ✧ ✧

19

EXTRAMEDULLARY LEUKEMIA AND MASTOCYTOSIS

LEUKEMIC INFILTRATION

Leukemia is discussed in detail in the Fascicle, Tumors of the Bone Marrow (2). This section briefly covers the histologic changes in parenchymal organs.

Both acute and chronic leukemias infiltrate lymph nodes, spleen, liver, and other organs (1–3), but histologic diagnosis of tissue involvement is rarely a problem if the history of leukemia is known.

In lymph nodes, the leukemic infiltrate causes partial or complete effacement of architecture, with predominant involvement of the medullary cords and sinuses in the early stages (figs. 19-1, 19-2). Frequently, the perinodal fibrous tissue is infiltrated, resulting in a single-file pattern (fig. 19-3).

In the liver, the sinusoids are preferentially involved, but the portal tracts can also be infil-

trated (fig. 19-4). More extensive involvement results in destruction of hepatocytes and formation of tumor nodules (fig. 19-5).

The cut surface of the spleen is typically homogeneously beefy red, with inconspicuous white pulp. The leukemic cells extensively infiltrate the red pulp, and are associated with atrophy of the white pulp (with the exception of chronic lymphocytic leukemia in which both the white and red pulp are involved) (fig. 19-6). The leukemic cells commonly infiltrate the fibrous trabeculae and walls of blood vessels (fig. 19-7); this feature strongly favors a diagnosis of neoplastic infiltrate over a reactive process, with the exception of infectious mononucleosis.

Cytologically, the infiltrates of acute lymphoblastic leukemia and chronic lymphocytic leukemia are identical to those of lymphoblastic lymphoma and small lymphocytic lymphoma,

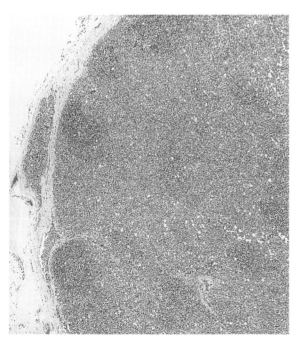

Figure 19-1
CHRONIC MYELOID LEUKEMIA
INVOLVING LYMPH NODE

There is incomplete nodal involvement, with pink-staining areas (leukemic infiltrate) alternating with blue-staining areas (residual lymphoid cells).

Figure 19-2
ACUTE MYELOID LEUKEMIA INVOLVING
LYMPH NODE (GRANULOCYTIC SARCOMA)

Patchy infiltration of lymph node, with islands of residual dark-staining small lymphocytes found among the violaceous leukemic infiltrate.

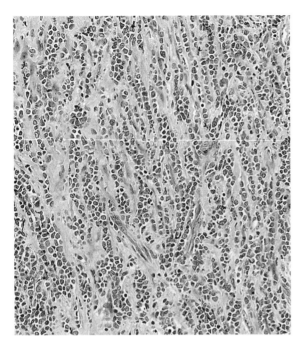

Figure 19-3
ACUTE MYELOID LEUKEMIA
INVOLVING LYMPH NODE

Acute myeloid leukemic cells infiltrate the fibrous capsule of the lymph node in a single-file pattern, attributable to insinuation of the neoplastic cells between the individual collagen fibers.

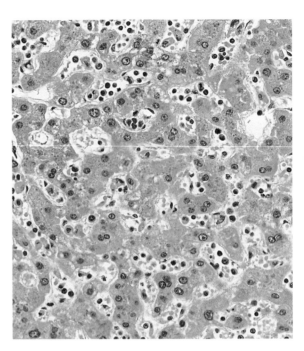

Figure 19-4
ACUTE MYELOID LEUKEMIA INVOLVING LIVER

The leukemic cells are characteristically localized in the sinusoids.

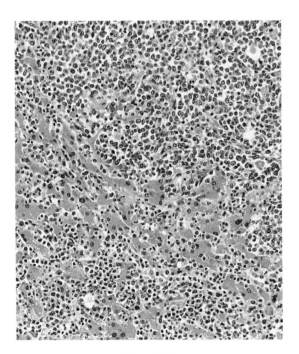

Figure 19-5
CHRONIC MYELOID LEUKEMIA WITH FOCAL
BLASTIC TRANSFORMATION IN THE LIVER

There is destruction of the liver parenchyma in addition to sinusoidal infiltration.

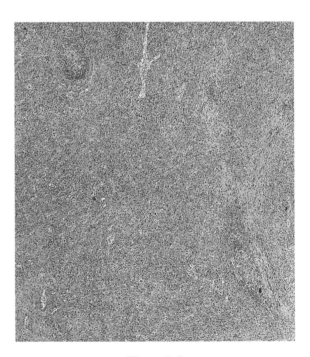

Figure 19-6
CHRONIC MYELOID LEUKEMIA
INVOLVING SPLEEN

Characteristically, there is marked infiltration of the red pulp accompanied by atrophy and loss of the white pulp.

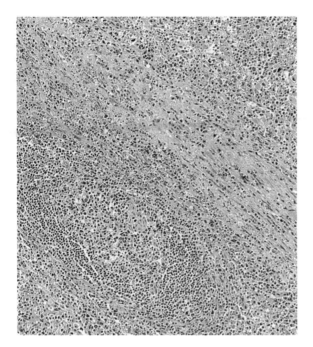

Figure 19-7
CHRONIC MYELOID LEUKEMIA
INVOLVING SPLEEN
Infiltration of the fibrous trabeculae strongly favors the
diagnosis of leukemia over agnogenic myeloid metaplasia.

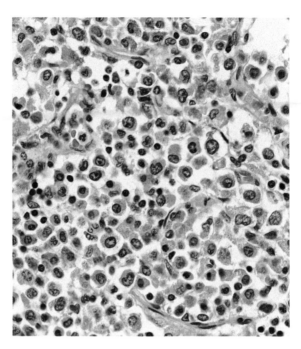

Figure 19-8
CHRONIC MYELOID LEUKEMIA
INVOLVING LYMPH NODE
The infiltrate is composed of a mixture of mature and
immature myeloid cells.

respectively. In chronic myeloid leukemia, the infiltrate consists of a mixture of mature and immature myeloid cells (fig. 19-8). In acute myeloid leukemia, there is a monotonous infiltrate of primitive myeloid cells. When a mass-forming lesion is found in an extramedullary site, application of the term *granulocytic sarcoma* is appropriate.

GRANULOCYTIC SARCOMA

Definition. Granulocytic sarcoma is a localized extramedullary tumor mass composed of primitive myeloid cells (39,43). It is also known as *myeloid sarcoma, myelosarcoma, myeloblastoma, chloroma,* or *extramedullary myeloblastic tumor* (26).

Natural History and Clinical Features. Granulocytic sarcoma occurs in a wide variety of sites, such as skin, bone, soft tissues, lymph node, gastrointestinal tract, orbit, palate, upper respiratory tract, heart, nervous system, testis, breast, female genital tract, urinary bladder, and mediastinum (4,8–12,18,20–25,30,31,36,39,45). The patients can be of any age, without sex pre-

dilection. The presenting symptoms include a mass lesion, pain, or symptoms referable to the location of the tumor (such as paralysis) (26).

There are several modes of presentation (6,9, 11,13,22,23,29,32,34–36,37–39,44,49): 1) patients have known acute myeloid leukemia, with the granulocytic sarcoma developing during active disease or as the first sign of relapse; 2) patients have a known myeloproliferative disorder or myelodysplastic syndrome, with the granulocytic sarcoma representing the first manifestation of blastic transformation; or 3) the granulocytic sarcoma develops in a previously healthy patient. It is in the last situation that the disease is most often mistaken for lymphoma; further work-up may reveal clinical or subclinical leukemia, or no evidence of leukemia at all. In the latter circumstance, with rare exceptions, leukemia almost always manifests after an interval of weeks to years (usually within 1 year) if systemic treatment is not given (26,36). In rare cases, granulocytic sarcoma may develop subsequent to T-lymphoblastic lymphoma associated with tissue and peripheral blood eosinophilia (5).

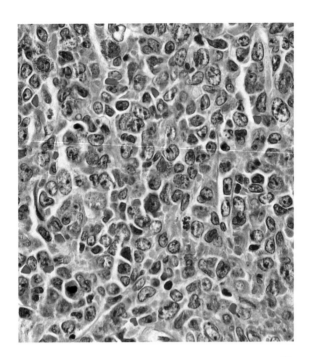 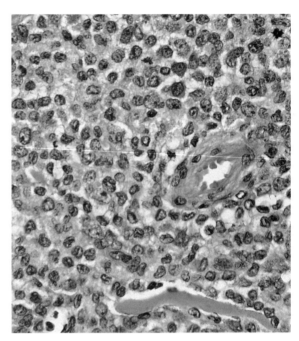

Figure 19-9
GRANULOCYTIC SARCOMA WITH INTERSPERSED EOSINOPHILIC MYELOCYTES
Left: In this testicular mass, the eosinophilic myelocytes interspersed among the blastic cells provide a strong clue to the correct diagnosis of granulocytic sarcoma rather than large cell lymphoma.
Right: In this skin tumor, the diagnosis of granulocytic sarcoma can be readily made because of the presence of eosinophilic myelocytes among the blast cells.

Gross Findings. Granulocytic sarcoma is also known as chloroma because the fresh specimen often exhibits a greenish hue (43). The green color, which is attributable to the presence of myeloperoxidase, fades on exposure to air and after formalin fixation, but can be restored by immersing the tissue in hydrogen peroxide or sodium metabisulfite (43). The absence of a greenish color, however, does not exclude the possibility of granulocytic sarcoma.

Microscopic Findings. There is a diffuse monotonous infiltrate of medium-sized or large cells, often associated with a sprinkling of eosinophilic myelocytes. The latter, although neither pathognomonic nor consistently present, provide an important clue to the diagnosis of granulocytic sarcoma (fig. 19-9) (46). The neoplastic cells have round, irregularly folded or lobated nuclei; fine or vesicular chromatin; and small to prominent nucleoli (fig. 19-10). The cytoplasm is scanty to moderate, and fine granularity can usually be seen in some cells if thinly cut sections are examined (figs. 19-10D, 19-11). Giemsa-stained touch

preparations are particularly helpful for detection of azurophilic granules or Auer rods (fig. 19-12) (12,26). However, the presence of azurophilic granules is not pathognomonic of granulocytic sarcoma, because some lymphomas have similar granules (27). Exceptionally, the neoplastic cells may assume a signet ring appearance (45). The mitotic count is variable. Some tumors are better differentiated, with recognizable promyelocytes and myelocytes, whereas many are poorly differentiated and composed predominantly of immature blastic cells (36).

There can be interspersed tingible body macrophages, imparting a "starry-sky" appearance. Infiltration of the fibrous stroma frequently creates a single-file pattern due to insinuation of the tumor cells between the collagen fibers (see fig. 19-3) and invasion of blood vessel walls is common. Rare cases show prominent sclerosis (fig. 19-13). In lymph nodes, the involvement is frequently partial, with the infiltrate concentrated in the interfollicular, sinusoidal, and perinodal regions (see fig. 19-2). A case of acute megakaryoblastic

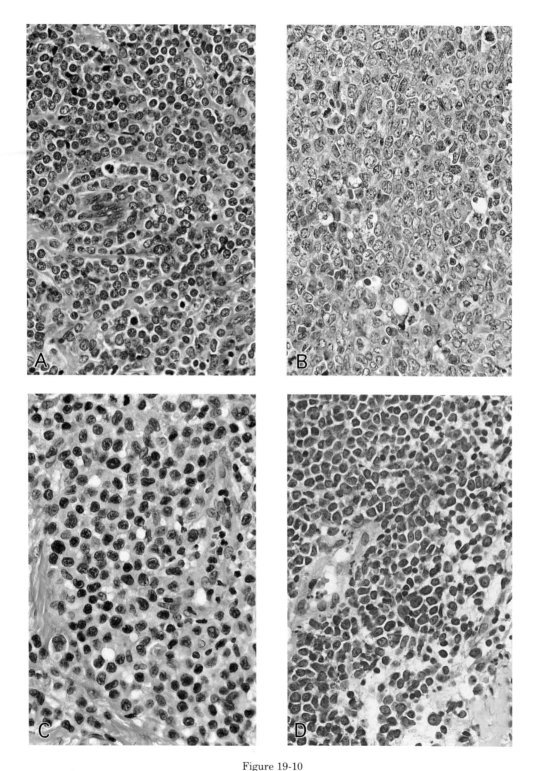

Figure 19-10
THE CYTOLOGIC SPECTRUM OF GRANULOCYTIC SARCOMA (LYMPH NODE)

A: The medium-sized cells have fine chromatin, mimicking lymphoblastic lymphoma.

B: The large blast cells may lead to a mistaken diagnosis of large cell lymphoma. There are some interspersed eosinophilic myelocytes.

C: In this example, the neoplastic cells have irregularly folded to convoluted nuclei.

D: Although this medium-sized cell infiltrate may lead to serious consideration of lymphoblastic lymphoma, the distinct nucleoli and cytoplasmic granules seen in some cells should suggest the correct diagnosis.

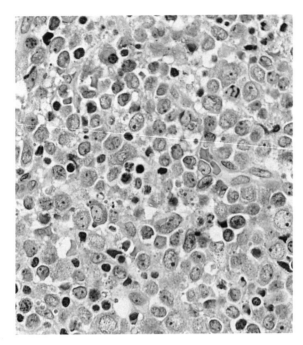

Figure 19-11
GRANULOCYTIC SARCOMA
INVOLVING THE SPINAL DURA

In this thinly cut section, granules are evident in some neoplastic cells. This neoplasm could easily be mistaken for a large cell lymphoma if attention is not paid to the cytoplasmic granules.

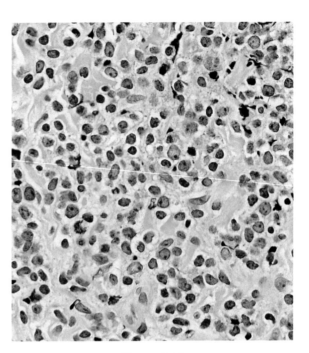

Figure 19-13
GRANULOCYTIC SARCOMA OF
THE ANTERIOR MEDIASTINUM

This example is associated with prominent sclerosis, mimicking sclerosing large B-cell lymphoma of the mediastinum.

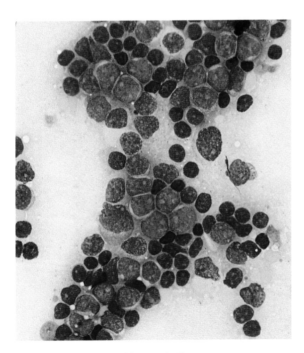

Figure 19-12
GRANULOCYTIC SARCOMA OF LYMPH NODE
Giemsa-stained touch preparation showing azurophilic granules in the cytoplasm of many neoplastic cells.

leukemia involving lymph node has been reported to show deceptively cohesive growth mimicking a carcinoma (7).

Confirmation of the diagnosis can be obtained by the Leder stain (chloroacetate esterase reaction), which is positive in about 75 percent of cases. Staining must be interpreted in myeloid precursors with nucleoli, and not on reactive granulocytes or mast cells that are present in the background (fig. 19-14). The percentage of positive cells can be very low. This stain works well on formalin-fixed paraffin-embedded tissues, but not on acid-decalcified or Zenker-fixed tissues; it works on B5-fixed tissue only if the iodine treatment step is eliminated. Lysozyme immunostain is positive in 89 percent of cases (33,39), but the frequently heavy background staining may render interpretation difficult. A combination of the Leder stain and lysozyme immunostain permits confirmation of the diagnosis of granulocytic sarcoma in almost all cases (39). Other newer antibodies (in particular antimyeloperoxidase) are also helpful for confirming the myeloid nature of the tumor.

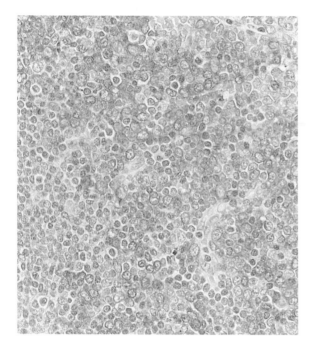

Figure 19-14
GRANULOCYTIC SARCOMA OF LYMPH NODE
Many of the myeloid precursors show positive (red) staining for chloroacetate esterase.

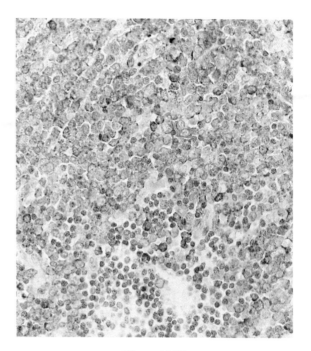

Figure 19-15
GRANULOCYTIC SARCOMA OF LYMPH NODE
The neoplastic cells immunostain (brown) with antimyeloperoxidase.

Immunologic Findings. The availability of a variety of antibodies reactive with monocytes/myeloid cells in paraffin sections (Leu-M1 [CD15], Mac-387, and KP1 [CD68]) has facilitated the diagnosis of granulocytic sarcoma (16, 17,26). However, these antibodies are not entirely specific. PG-M1 (CD68) stains only those cases with evidence of monocytic differentiation, that is, monocytic or myelomonocytic types (19). Antibodies against neutrophil elastase (NP57) and cathepsin G show high specificity for the myeloid lineage, but are not very sensitive (14,15,23, 41,42). The single most sensitive and specific antibody for detection of myeloid differentiation in paraffin sections is an antiserum against myeloperoxidase (fig. 19-15) (40,48).

Granulocytic sarcomas often stain with paraffin section–reactive T-cell markers (such as MT1 [CD43]), UCHL1 [CD45RO]), and variably with the paraffin section–reactive B-cell markers (such as L26 [CD20], MB2, LN2 [CD74]) (16,17,26); as a result, an erroneous diagnosis of lymphoma may be made if granulocytic sarcoma is not suspected and only this panel of T-cell and B-cell markers is applied. At least a proportion of cases stain with

the bone marrow progenitor cell marker CD34, but this marker can also be frequently demonstrated in acute lymphoblastic leukemia (24).

The diagnosis of erythroleukemia involving lymph node may be facilitated by the application of antihemoglobin or antiglycophorin antibodies (28). Confirmation of diagnosis of tumor-forming acute megakaryoblastic leukemia can be achieved by immunostaining with antifactor VIII–related antigen, CD31 (antiplatelet glycoprotein IIa), and CD61 (antiplatelet glycoprotein IIIa) (7).

If frozen tissues or touch preparations are available, cytochemical studies (with myeloperoxidase and Sudan black) can be performed (35). In addition, a variety of monoclonal antibodies such as antimyeloperoxidase, Leu-M5 (CD11c), MY7 (CD13), MY4 (CD14), OKM1 (CD14), Leu-M1 (CD15), and MY9 (CD33) can be applied to aid in the diagnosis.

Ultrastructural Findings. A diagnosis of granulocytic sarcoma is confirmed when electron microscopic studies show large electron-dense primary granules and less dense secondary granules. The presence of ellipsoidal crystalloid granules also supports the diagnosis (26).

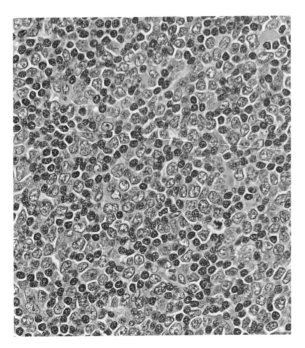

Figure 19-16
GRANULOCYTIC SARCOMA OF LYMPH NODE
Intermingling of the large blastic cells with the residual small
lymphocytes creates a pattern like diffuse mixed cell lymphoma.

Table 19-1

HISTOLOGIC CLUES FOR RECOGNITION OF GRANULOCYTIC SARCOMA

Patchy or sinusoidal lymph node involvement, associated with single-file pattern of infiltration in the capsular region

Intermingling with eosinophilic myelocytes

Fine granularity of the cytoplasm

Tumor cells appearing "odd," not conforming to the recognized categories of lymphoma

Differential Diagnosis. The diagnosis of granulocytic sarcoma is usually straightforward if the patient is known to have myeloid leukemia. However, when no such history is present or given, granulocytic sarcoma is often mistaken for non-Hodgkin's lymphoma or other tumors such as Ewing's sarcoma and Langerhans' cell histiocytosis (39,47). The occasional admixture of immature myeloid cells with lymphocytes may give a false impression of mixed cell lymphoma (fig. 19-16). The diagnosis of granulocytic sarcoma requires a high index of suspicion. The presence of certain histologic features, present in isolation or in combination, in a case of suspected lymphoma, should raise the possibility (Table 19-1). Semi-thin sections are best for appreciation of the cytoplasmic granules and the eosinophilic myelocytes. If Giemsa-stained touch preparations are available, azurophilic granules and Auer rods should be sought. Cytochemical and immunocytochemical studies can provide confirmatory evidence of myeloid differentiation.

Occasional T-cell lymphomas may be associated with an infiltrate of eosinophilic myelocytes

(46), thus mimicking granulocytic sarcoma. Therefore the diagnosis of granulocytic sarcoma should always be confirmed by histochemical or immunohistochemical studies.

Treatment and Prognosis. Although radiation therapy can effect local control of granulocytic sarcoma, it usually fails to prevent relapse or progression of disease. Patients with localized granulocytic sarcoma should therefore be treated in the same way as those with acute myeloid leukemia, and the overall prognosis is also similar (26,30). In some patients, systemic chemotherapy can successfully prevent progression to acute myeloid leukemia, and long-term survival is possible (36).

HAIRY CELL LEUKEMIA

Definition. Hairy cell leukemia, previously known as leukemic reticuloendotheliosis, is an indolent leukemia characterized by circulating cells with multiple long cytoplasmic projections (53,63). This lymphoproliferative disease is, with very rare exceptions, of B lineage.

Clinical Features. Hairy cell leukemia is dealt with in greater depth in the Fascicle, Tumors of the Bone Marrow (54). Only the salient features and histologic findings of the extramedullary sites are covered in this chapter.

Hairy cell leukemia occurs predominantly in middle-aged adults, with a male predominance. Most patients present with nonspecific symptoms such as tiredness, dyspnea on exertion, abdominal fullness, or signs of infection (55,59,61,73). Splenomegaly is common, the liver may be palpable, but lymphadenopathy is uncommon. Necrotizing vasculitis is an uncommon associated occurrence

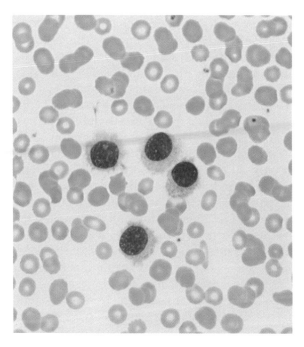

Figure 19-17
HAIRY CELL LEUKEMIA AS SEEN
IN PERIPHERAL BLOOD SMEAR
Note the abundance of pale-staining cytoplasm and hairy cell processes.

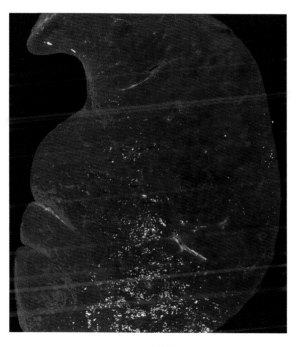

Figure 19-18
HAIRY CELL LEUKEMIA
INVOLVING SPLEEN
This enlarged spleen exhibits a homogeneous "meaty" appearance.

(68,71,80,81). Exceptionally, hairy cell leukemia is associated with a large cell lymphoma (50,99).

The peripheral blood usually shows cytopenia (especially monocytopenia) and circulating hairy cells with abundant pale cytoplasm and long villi (fig. 19-17). The nuclei of the hairy cells are round or indented, often eccentric, with fairly condensed chromatin and an inconspicuous nucleolus (89). Rare variants showing a central large nucleolus have also been described (60,67). It is often difficult to obtain a satisfactory bone marrow aspirate as a result of the increase in reticulin (55).

Gross and Microscopic Findings. The spleen is typically enlarged, often weighing over 1 kg. The cut surface is uniformly meaty red and firm (fig. 19-18). Areas of infarct are sometimes found (56). Rarely, tumor nodules are seen (76). Histologically, the red pulp cords and sinuses are diffusely expanded by a monotonous infiltrate of mononuclear cells, with atrophy and destruction of the white pulp (fig. 19-19). Often, the infiltrate is so extensive that distinction of splenic cords from sinuses is impossible. There is frequently

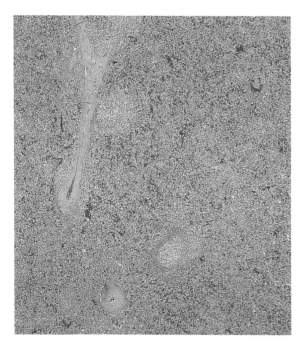

Figure 19-19
HAIRY CELL LEUKEMIA INVOLVING SPLEEN
There is extensive infiltration of the red pulp. The white pulp is atrophic.

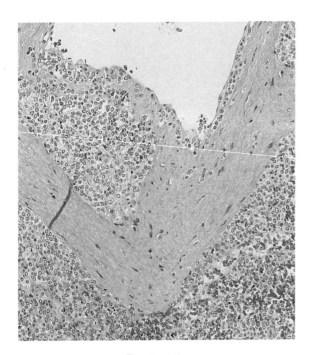

Figure 19-20
HAIRY CELL LEUKEMIA INVOLVING SPLEEN
The leukemic cells show mural and subendothelial infiltration of the blood vessel.

infiltration of the subendothelium of the trabecular veins (fig. 19-20) (57). The tumor cells possess medium-sized nuclei that are oval, reniform, or occasionally multilobated or convoluted (52,74). The nuclear chromatin is fine, and nucleoli are indistinct. Mitotic figures are sparse. The nuclei often appear widely spaced due to the presence of voluminous cytoplasm. The cytoplasm is clear (with or without interlocking cell borders), pale or lightly eosinophilic; these differences are at least in part related to fixation techniques (fig. 19-21). In toluidine blue–stained thin plastic sections, characteristic (though not pathognomonic) rod-shaped structures corresponding ultrastructurally to the ribosome-lamella complex may be detected in the cytoplasm (82). Small and large irregular blood lakes lined by the neoplastic cells (pseudosinuses) are common (fig. 19-22), and may be prominent enough to mimic a cavernous hemangioma (57). In spleens with subtle or minimal involvement by hairy cell leukemia, the infiltrate tends to be localized as small aggregates adjacent to the fibrous trabeculae or subendothelial regions of the trabecular veins (fig. 19-23) (57,58).

Lymph nodes involved by hairy cell leukemia are usually only slightly enlarged. The infiltrate begins in the B-cell regions (83), that is, in the outer cortex beneath the subcapsular sinuses, in the form of nodules or broad bands (fig. 19-24). In late phases, the capsule, trabeculae, blood vessels, and perinodal tissues can be infiltrated (83).

Histologic involvement of the liver almost always occurs, although hepatomegaly is detected in only 20 to 40 percent of patients (89). The leukemic infiltrate occurs in the sinusoids and the portal tracts. In heavily infiltrated areas, the sinusoids are often dilated and congested with erythrocytes, even to the extent of peliosis (100). When the infiltrate is mild, particularly if the "clear cell" pattern is not evident, a nonspecific inflammatory process may be mimicked.

Cytochemical Findings. Most cases of hairy cell leukemia stain for acid phosphatase, which is typically tartrate resistant. This enzyme reaction is an excellent marker of hairy cell leukemia (89), and is best demonstrated on touch preparations. It is not entirely pathognomonic, since a few cases of hairy cell leukemia (less than 5 percent) do not stain while other lymphoproliferative diseases do (89,101).

Immunophenotypic and Genotypic Findings. The immunophenotype of hairy cell leukemia is distinctive in the combined expression of B-lineage markers, histiocytic markers, and a variety of other markers (62,63,64,69,70, 75,77,84,87,98,). These include B-lineage markers (CD19, CD20, CD22, monotypic surface immunoglobulin, and the B-subset marker DBA.44); histiocytic markers (CD11c [Leu-M5] and CD68 [EBM/11, KP-1]); activation markers (CD25 [interleukin-2 receptor]); some plasma cell–associated markers (PCA-1 [but not PC-1]); and hairy cell leukemia–associated markers (HC-1, HC-2, and B-ly7 [CD103]). Although previously thought to be hairy cell leukemia–specific, B-ly7 has been found to be identical to HML1, an antibody marking intestinal intraepithelial T lymphocytes (75,86,95,97).

Hairy cell leukemia, in contrast to other chronic B-lymphoproliferative disorders, is CD5 negative; it is also CD10 negative. Some studies have reported reactivity for S-100 protein, but others have failed to reproduce this finding (88,93,96).

The B-cell nature of hairy cell leukemia has been conclusively settled by the demonstration of

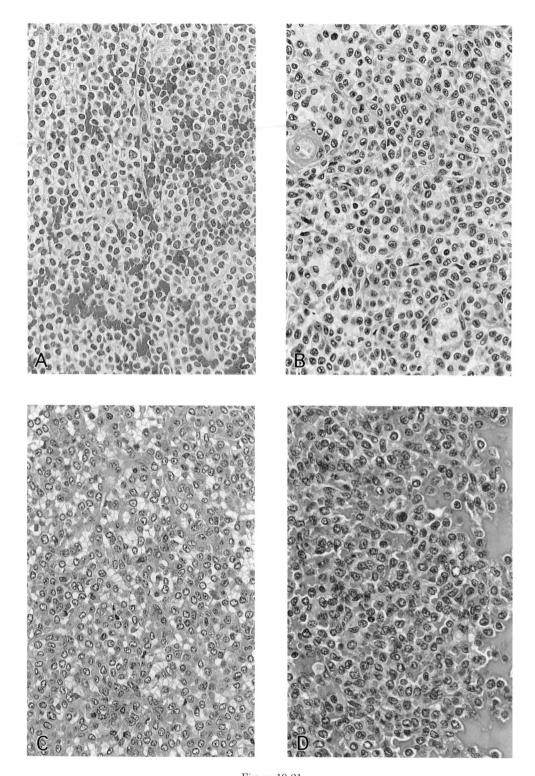

Figure 19-21
CYTOLOGIC SPECTRUM OF HAIRY CELL LEUKEMIA

A: Monotonous population of medium-sized cells with clear cytoplasm and interlocking cell borders. Some nuclei are indented.
B: The nuclei are indented or grooved, and the cytoplasm is pale.
C: The cells have regular oval nuclei and eosinophilic cytoplasm.
D: In this example, the nuclei appear slightly more crowded, that is, the cytoplasm is less abundant.

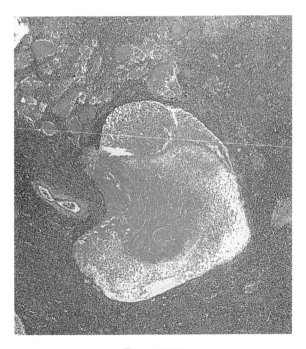

Figure 19-22
HAIRY CELL LEUKEMIA INVOLVING THE SPLEEN
Note the effacement of architecture and the blood lakes.

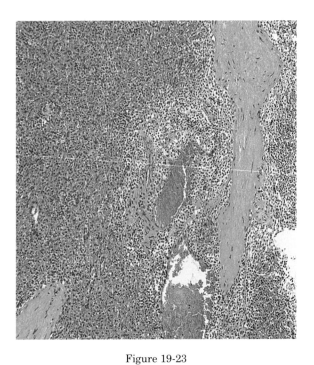

Figure 19-23
EARLY INVOLVEMENT OF SPLEEN
BY HAIRY CELL LEUKEMIA
There is predominant localization of the leukemic infiltrate around the fibrous trabeculae.

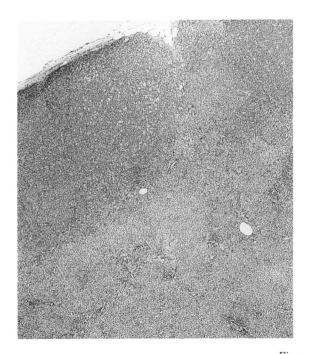

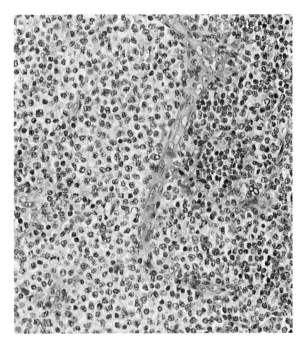

Figure 19-24
HAIRY CELL LEUKEMIA INVOLVING LYMPH NODE
Left: The nodal architecture is incompletely effaced, with some residual lymphoid tissue in the superficial cortex.
Right: The infiltrate is composed of a monotonous infiltrate of medium-sized cells with widely spaced nuclei. Residual small lymphocytes are seen in the right upper field.

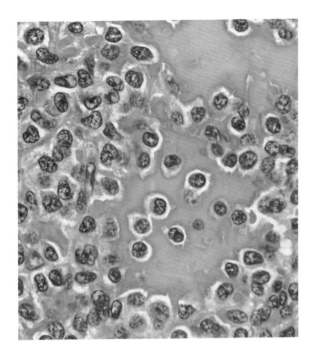

Figure 19-25
HAIRY CELL LEUKEMIA INVOLVING SPLEEN
The hairy processes are best appreciated in areas where the leukemic cells are bathed in serum; the outline of the individual cells then appears fluffy.

Table 19-2

DIFFERENTIAL DIAGNOSIS OF CLEAR CELLS IN HEMATOLYMPHOID NEOPLASMS

Hairy cell leukemia

Monocytoid B-cell lymphoma

Low-grade B-cell lymphoma of mucosa-associated lymphoid tissue

Mast cell disease (mastocytosis)

Post-thymic T-cell lymphoma

Signet ring cell lymphoma

Mediastinal large B-cell lymphoma

Diffuse large B-cell lymphoma (rare cases)

rearrangements of the heavy and light chain immunoglobulin genes (65,72,87). The normal counterpart of hairy cell leukemia is not known, but it has been suggested to correspond to a pre-plasma cell stage of B-cell differentiation (51,75,87).

Exceptional cases of hairy cell leukemia exhibiting T-lineage markers have also been reported. The human T-cell lymphotropic virus type II (HTLV-II) was originally isolated from such a case (78,94). However, a case of hairy cell leukemia alleged to be of T-cell lineage has recently been reinterpreted to represent coexistence of B-cell hairy cell leukemia and an HTLV-II–related T-cell lymphoproliferation (91,92).

Ultrastructural Findings. Characteristic, though not pathognomonic, ultrastructural findings of hairy cell leukemia are long microvilli with a broad base and ribosome-lamella complexes (59,61,66). The latter are found in approximately 50 percent of cases, and consist of a central hollow space surrounded by parallel arrays of membranes with intermingled ribosomes. Some pinocytotic vesicles and lysosomes may be found. Erythrophagocytosis is rare, even though

phagocytic activity (latex particles or bacteria) can be frequently demonstrated in vitro (66).

Differential Diagnosis. In the spleen, hairy cell leukemia can be distinguished from other low-grade lymphomas and B-cell chronic lymphocytic leukemia by the apparent wide separation of the nuclei, attributable to the abundance of cytoplasm. In areas where the neoplastic cells are bathed in serum, the cytoplasmic processes can often be appreciated as a negative image (fig. 19-25). The pattern of splenic involvement is also different: lymphoma predominantly involves the splenic white pulp and only secondarily infiltrates the red pulp (57). Although the presence of blood lakes favors a diagnosis of hairy cell leukemia, this feature is not pathognomonic.

Cytologically, it is difficult to distinguish hairy cell leukemia from monocytoid B-cell lymphoma, some post-thymic T-cell lymphomas (monomorphous medium-sized cell type), and mastocytosis (Table 19-2). However, the clinical settings of these diseases are different. Monocytoid B-cell lymphoma is often a limited-stage disease, and involvement of the blood, bone marrow, or spleen is rare. In systemic mastocytosis, skin involvement is common, but peripheral blood involvement is rare. If the cellular infiltrate is accompanied by significant numbers of eosinophils and sclerosis, the diagnosis of mastocytosis is highly likely. Cytochemical and immunohistochemical studies are most helpful in the differential diagnosis.

A disease closely mimicking hairy cell leukemia is splenic B-cell lymphoma with circulating villous lymphocytes (85). In contrast to hairy cell leukemia, monoclonal gammopathy is common, the cytoplasmic processes are usually polarized to one side of the cell, bone marrow involvement is minimal, splenic involvement occurs predominantly in the white pulp, and the neoplastic cells lack tartrate-resistant acid phosphatase activity.

Treatment and Prognosis. The clinical course of hairy cell leukemia is quite variable, with some patients dying within 2 years of diagnosis, but many surviving for 10 or more years (59). Infection is a common complication, and represents the immediate cause of death in many patients. The overall median survival is 4 to 5 years (59).

Patients with few symptoms and satisfactory hematologic indices may require no specific therapy other than close follow-up (59,63). Splenectomy, which improves the cytopenia, has been the standard treatment, but newer forms of therapy are now available. Alpha-interferon is an effective treatment and reduces the incidence of opportunistic infection, but the remissions are usually partial. 2'-deoxycoformycin, an adenosine deaminase inhibitor, produces a high complete remission rate (greater than 75 percent). Newer drugs such as 2-chlorodeoxyadenosine (an adenosine deaminase–resistant purine analogue) and fludarabine monophosphate (an adenosine nucleoside analogue) have also been reported to be effective (63,79,90).

SYSTEMIC MASTOCYTOSIS (SYSTEMIC MAST CELL DISEASE)

Definition. Systemic mastocytosis (systemic mast cell disease) is a rare disease characterized by generalized abnormal infiltration of mast cells, most notably involving the spleen, bone marrow, lymph node, liver, and sometimes other parenchymal organs; there may or may not be cutaneous involvement (urticaria pigmentosa). Currently there is no firm proof as to whether the mast cell proliferation is a clonal neoplastic disorder or an abnormal hyperplastic process (102,114). It has been suggested that some forms of cutaneous mastocytosis represent reactive hyperplasia rather than neoplastic proliferation of mast cells caused by increased production of the

Table 19-3

CLASSIFICATION OF MAST CELL DISEASE*

Nonsystemic mast cell disease

    Localized mastocytosis (solitary or multiple mast cell nevi)

    Urticaria pigmentosa (disseminated cutaneous mastocytosis)

    Mastocytosis of bone marrow

    Solitary mast cell tumor (such as lung, spleen, oral mucosa)

    Mast cell sarcoma**

Systemic mast cell disease

    Benign systemic mastocytosis (cases with skin involvement)

    Malignant mastocytosis (cases without skin involvement)

    ± myelodysplasia

    ± myeloproliferative disease

    ± mast cell leukemia

*From reference 121.
**May be associated with mast cell leukemia.

soluble form of mast cell growth factor (stem cell factor or c-kit ligand) related to increased proteolytic processing (117).

Some authors restrict the term systemic mastocytosis to cases with skin lesions, and apply the term *malignant mastocytosis* to those without (Table 19-3) (111,116,121). However, skin involvement is not always a reliable indicator of outcome: rare patients with skin lesions have a poor prognosis while occasional patients without skin lesions have indolent disease (128). Other authors use the term *benign systemic mastocytosis* for those cases with limited lesions, mild symptoms, and prolonged course, and the term *malignant systemic mastocytosis* for those with tumor mass formation, leukemia, or bone marrow failure (113). Travis et al. (125,128) proposed classifying systemic mastocytosis into four categories, irrespective of the presence or absence of skin lesions (Table 19-4): *indolent systemic mast cell disease; systemic mast cell disease with associated hematologic disorders; mast cell leukemia;* and *aggressive systemic mast cell disease.*

Table 19-4
CLASSIFICATION OF SYSTEMIC MAST CELL DISEASE*

Category	Criteria	Frequency
Indolent systemic mast cell disease	Patients with favorable prognostic factors	Most common type (50%)
Systemic mast cell disease associated with hematologic disorders	Documented systemic mast cell disease with: myelodysplastic disorders, myeloproliferative syndromes, acute leukemia, malignant lymphoma, or chronic neutropenia	35%
Mast cell leukemia	>10 percent circulating atypical mast cells at presentation, and marrow typically shows diffuse mast cell infiltrates	Rare (2%)
Aggressive systemic mast cell disease	Patients with poor prognostic factors but not meeting the criteria for mast cell leukemia or other neoplastic/dysplastic hematologic disorders	Uncommon (14%)

*From reference 128.

The last category is also known as *lymphadenopathic mastocytosis with eosinophilia* in the National Institute of Health classification scheme (118), and is characterized by prominent rapid development of lymphadenopathy, documented mastocytosis, and eosinophilia.

Clinical Features. Systemic mastocytosis occurs over a wide age range, with a mean of 60 years. There is a slight male predominance (128). The patients can present with cutaneous disease (but only about 10 percent of patients with urticaria pigmentosa have systemic mastocytosis), anaphylaxis, bone pain or fracture, gastrointestinal symptoms (abdominal pain, diarrhea, nausea, vomiting, peptic ulcer), respiratory manifestations (wheezing, dyspnea), hematologic manifestations (anemia, leukocytosis, leukopenia, thrombocytopenia, thrombocytosis, eosinophilia, monocytosis, circulating mast cells), or hepatosplenomegaly (128). Many of these symptoms are attributable to the release of histamine by mast cells. Radiographs of bone may show osteoporosis, osteolytic lesions, osteosclerosis, or mixed osteolytic/osteosclerotic lesions.

Many patients have associated solid malignancies or hematologic disorders (myelodysplastic syndrome, myeloproliferative disorders, leukemia, malignant lymphoma) (109,111,127, 130,132). Hematologic abnormalities are more often found in patients without cutaneous lesions (111). The frequent coexistence of systemic

Table 19-5
HISTOLOGIC TRIAD FOR RECOGNITION OF MAST CELL DISEASE

Clusters of pale or clear cells with oval or reniform ("monocytoid") nuclei

Eosinophils

Sclerosis

mastocytosis with dysplastic and neoplastic disorders of myeloid cells suggests that systemic mastocytosis itself may be a disorder of myeloid cells and that mast cells may be myeloid in origin (121,130). A rare association between systemic mast cell disease and mediastinal germ cell tumor has been reported, and it is postulated that cytokine secretion by the germ cell tumor may stimulate mast cell proliferation (104).

Microscopic Findings. Systemic mastocytosis is often mistaken for other lymphoreticular proliferative disorders because the granules of the mast cells are often difficult to discern in routine hematoxylin and eosin–stained sections. The major criteria for histologic diagnosis are listed in Table 19-5 (fig. 19-26). The diagnosis can be confirmed by the Giemsa, toluidine blue, or Leder (chloroacetate esterase) stain, which highlight the mast cell granules well (fig. 19-27) (115).

Leder's stain is more sensitive than the metachromatic stains, but it also stains myeloid cells and cannot be used on acid decalcified tissues (126). The more aggressive cases of systemic mastocytosis show optimal staining with toluidine blue at a higher pH (5.5 to 6.0) compared with normal mast cells or those found in urticaria pigmentosa (pH 4.0) (113,116).

In hematoxylin and eosin–stained sections, the mast cells have relatively small, oval, indented or bilobed nuclei with fine chromatin and inconspicuous nucleoli (fig. 19-28) (103,116,121, 126). They have an appreciable amount of clear to pale cytoplasm, resembling macrophages or monocytoid B cells. The density and size of the cytoplasmic granules are highly variable: in some cases the granules are readily seen, but in others they may be sparse and tiny. Mitotic figures are rarely identified. Some mast cells may be spindle shaped, resembling fibroblasts (figs. 19-28D, 19-29). The mast cell infiltrate is almost invariably accompanied by variable numbers of eosinophils and delicate sclerotic bands (figs. 19-26, 19-28D).

The bone marrow, spleen, lymph node, and liver are the organs most commonly affected in systemic mastocytosis (106). In the skin, the

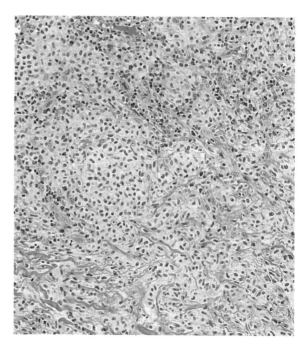

Figure 19-26
SYSTEMIC MASTOCYTOSIS
INVOLVING LYMPH NODE
The mast cells are characteristically associated with delicate collagen fibrils and eosinophils. Since they possess indented nuclei and abundant clear cytoplasm, they may be mistaken for histiocytes.

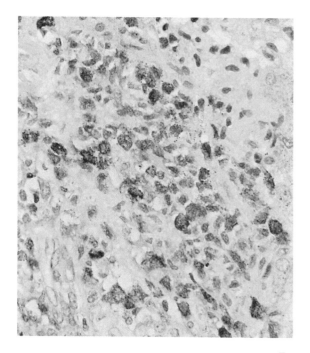

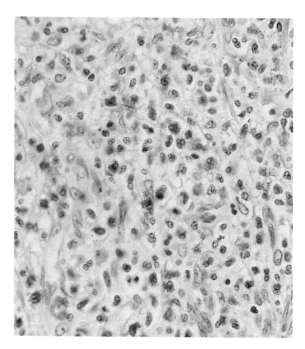

Figure 19-27
SYSTEMIC MASTOCYTOSIS
Left: The mast cell granules are well highlighted by the metachromatic staining with toluidine blue.
Right: The mast cells show weak to strong staining (red) for chloroacetate esterase.

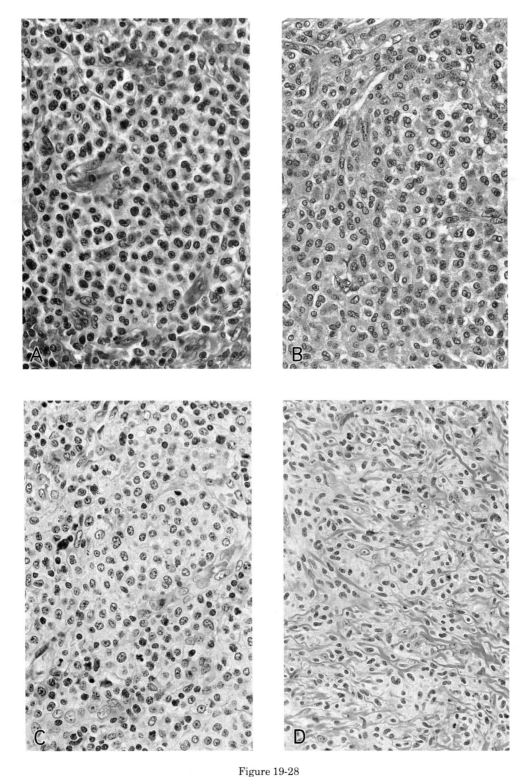

Figure 19-28
THE CYTOLOGIC SPECTRUM OF SYSTEMIC MASTOCYTOSIS
A: The mast cells have round or bilobed nuclei, and finely granular cytoplasm.
B: Most of the mast cells are bilobed and have obviously granular cytoplasm.
C: The mast cells have clear cytoplasm, and cytoplasmic granules are not evident.
D: The nuclei of the mast cells are ovoid or elongated, and the cytoplasm is clear. Note the characteristic delicate sclerosis.

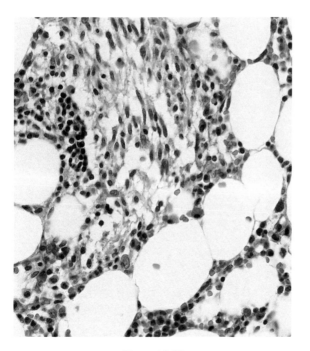

Figure 19-29
SYSTEMIC MASTOCYTOSIS
INVOLVING BONE MARROW
The mast cells have a spindly configuration.

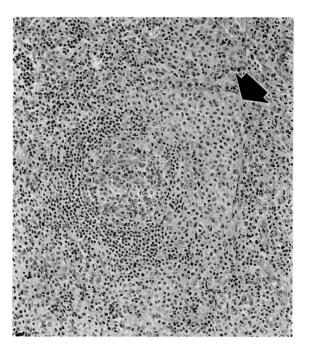

Figure 19-31
SYSTEMIC MASTOCYTOSIS
INVOLVING LYMPH NODE
There is a tendency for the mast cell infiltrate to exhibit a perifollicular distribution (arrow).

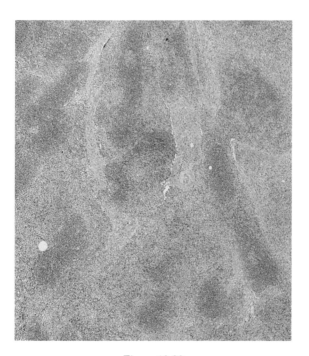

Figure 19-30
SYSTEMIC MASTOCYTOSIS
INVOLVING LYMPH NODE
The pale-staining infiltrate of mast cells occurs predominantly in an interfollicular pattern.

epidermis often shows mild acanthosis and increased pigmentation of the basal layer (120,121). Polygonal to fusiform mast cells occur in a perivascular or periadnexal location in the upper dermis, or show more diffuse and dense infiltration of the entire dermis. Eosinophils are often scattered throughout the lesion.

The mast cell infiltrate in lymph node tends to occur in a sinusoidal, paracortical, or perifollicular pattern (fig. 19-30) (103,116,121,126), but a recent study suggests that the infiltrate occurs mainly in the medullary cords and sinuses (107). The mast cells can even overrun the lymphoid follicles, creating a vague nodular pattern (fig. 19-31). Eosinophils often accompany the mast cell infiltrate, and delicate sclerosis is common. The mast cell clusters can exhibit a perivascular distribution (fig. 19-32). There can be a striking proliferation of capillaries and venules (fig. 19-33) (103,107). The capsule and perinodal soft tissue are rarely involved. For cases associated with hematologic disorders, a leukemic infiltrate is sometimes seen in the lymph node (107).

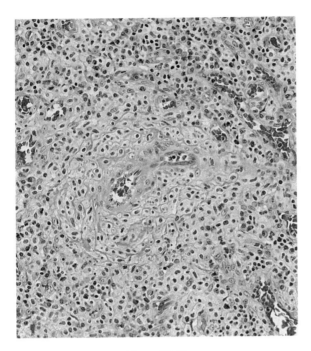

Figure 19-32
SYSTEMIC MASTOCYTOSIS
INVOLVING LYMPH NODE
The mast cell infiltrate can be centered on arterioles. Note
the characteristic sclerosis.

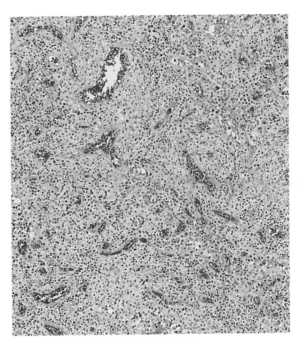

Figure 19-33
SYSTEMIC MASTOCYTOSIS
INVOLVING LYMPH NODE
The mast cell infiltrate is accompanied by a prominent
vascular proliferation.

The enlarged spleen weighs on average 500 g
(117,122), but can weigh more than 2 kg (103).
The splenic capsule is often thickened. The cut
surface reveals prominent fibrous trabeculae,
with or without small irregular nodules that
measure 1 to 2 mm (fig. 19-34) (126). Calcifica-
tions may be present. In the spleen, the involvement is usually haphazard, but the preferential
sites of localization are the marginal zone of the
white pulp and the fibrous trabeculae (figs. 19-35,
19-36). Occasionally, the mast cells diffusely infiltrate the red pulp (110). The lesion appears to evolve
towards a sclerotic phase, in which the mast cell
population becomes less inconspicuous (fig. 19-37).
Any spleen with significant unexplained sclerosis
should lead to a search for systemic mastocytosis.

Hepatomegaly is found in about 75 percent of
patients with systemic mastocytosis, but histologic
evidence of mast cell infiltration is present in only
42 percent of cases. In the liver, the mast cells are
found predominantly in aggregates in the portal
tracts, but they can also be loosely scattered
throughout the sinusoids (fig. 19-38) (106). Lymphocytes may be intermingled with the mast

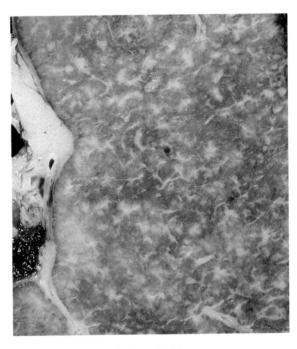

Figure 19-34
SYSTEMIC MASTOCYTOSIS INVOLVING SPLEEN
The cut surface of this enlarged spleen reveals prominent
fibrous streaks.

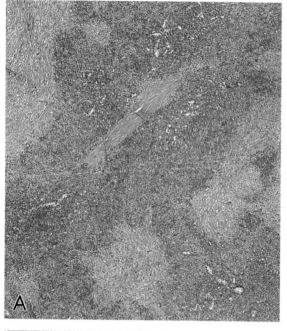
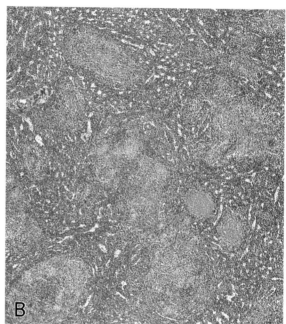
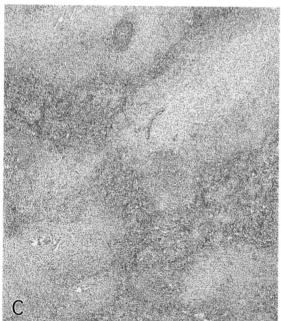

Figure 19-35
SYSTEMIC MASTOCYTOSIS INVOLVING SPLEEN
Low magnification view showing the different patterns of involvement.
A: Patchy involvement associated with sclerosis.
B: Almost exclusive localization around the Malpighian corpuscles.
C: Extensive infiltration (pale-staining areas) of the splenic parenchyma associated with minimal sclerosis.

cells. Unlike other sites of involvement, eosinophils are often sparse or absent. Periportal fibrosis, and occasionally cirrhosis, can be present.

The pattern of bone marrow involvement is highly variable. It can be subtle, taking the form of tiny "eosinophilic fibrohistiocytic lesions" composed of fusiform mast cells mixed with eosinophils and variable numbers of T and B lymphocytes (fig. 19-29) (122–124); or it can be wide- spread through-

out the bone marrow, with paratrabecular and perivascular accentuation. The accompanying fibrosis can be so extensive that agnogenic myeloid metaplasia is mimicked (103,105,109). The bony trabeculae may be widened or thinned (103).

Mast cell sarcoma, a tumefactive infiltrate of immature mast cells, is extremely rare (108). It may be the sole lesion, but has also been observed in patients with mast cell leukemia (129).

Immunologic Findings. The normal mast cells show immunoreactivity with KP1 (CD68), but not Ki-M1p, PG-M1 (CD68), HAM56, Mac-387, LN5, S-100 protein, and CD35 (112). KP1 also stains the mast cells of mastocytosis. Of interest, Ki-M1p stains nearly all cases of mastocytosis, while PG-M1 stains approximately half.

Differential Diagnosis. The major differential diagnoses include lymphoma (particularly monocytoid B-cell lymphoma and post-thymic T-cell lymphoma), hairy cell leukemia, and reactive histiocytic proliferations (Table 19-2). The associated eosinophils and sclerosis should provide a strong clue that the pale cell clusters are most likely mast cells rather than lymphoma/leukemia cells; the diagnosis can be readily confirmed by staining for mast cell granules. Electron microscopy can demonstrate the mast cell granules, which are bound by unit membrane and filled with electron-dense material (121).

Langerhans' cell histiocytosis may also enter into the differential diagnosis because of the "monocytoid" appearance of the mast cell nuclei

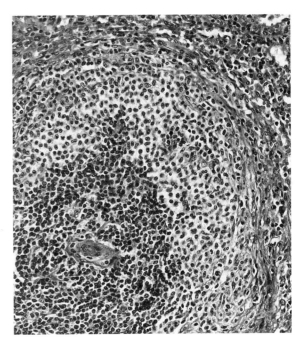

Figure 19-36
SYSTEMIC MASTOCYTOSIS INVOLVING SPLEEN
The mast cell infiltrate often exhibits a perifollicular growth pattern around the Malpighian corpuscles.

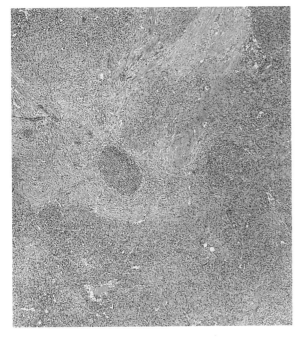
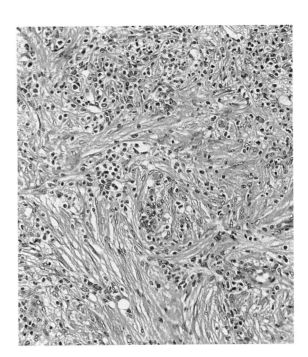

Figure 19-37
SYSTEMIC MASTOCYTOSIS INVOLVING SPLEEN
Left: In the late phase, sclerotic fibrous bands predominate.
Right: Mast cells may be difficult to identify.

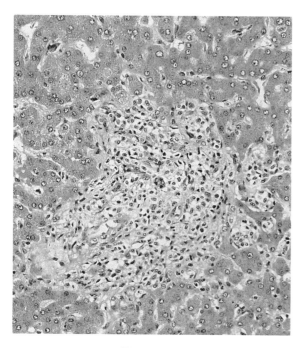

Figure 19-38
SYSTEMIC MASTOCYTOSIS INVOLVING LIVER
The infiltrate occurs predominantly in the portal tract.

and tissue eosinophilia. However, the mast cells are smaller, and the grooved nuclei and voluminous cytoplasm characteristic of Langerhans cells are lacking.

In the bone marrow, systemic mastocytosis can be distinguished from the increase in mast cells seen in various bone marrow disorders by the presence of mast cell clusters (131).

Treatment and Prognosis. The clinical course of systemic mastocytosis is variable: some cases are indolent, others are aggressive. The overall 5-year survival is 52 percent (128), with most disease-related deaths occurring in the first 3 years. Patients with the indolent form of systemic mastocytosis have an almost normal

life expectancy, although some may die from complications of the disease such as gastrointestinal bleeding or perforation. Those with aggressive systemic mastocytosis generally live only 2 to 3 years after diagnosis (118,128). For cases associated with myelodysplastic syndrome or frank leukemia, the prognosis is determined by the hematologic disorder (118). The rare mast cell leukemias are highly aggressive, with median survival less than 6 months (125,129).

Univariate analysis has revealed the following unfavorable prognostic factors: male sex, old age, constitutional symptoms, absence of skin lesions, anemia, thrombocytopenia, abnormal liver function tests, lobulated mast cell nuclei, low percentage of fat cells in the bone marrow, and associated hematologic disorders (103,121, 128,130). Multivariate analysis has identified five independent variables related to poorer survival (128): old age, male sex, low hemoglobin level, current or previous malignancy, and lobulated mast cell nuclei.

There is no effective treatment for systemic mastocytosis so far, and response to multiagent chemotherapy is unsatisfactory (128,132). A recent report suggests that interferon alpha-2b may produce satisfactory partial remission (114). Symptomatic treatment can be accomplished by an H1 antihistamine for flushing and pruritus, an H2-histamine blocker or proton pump inhibitor for gastric and duodenal manifestations, sodium cromoglycate for diarrhea and abdominal pain, and a nonsteroidal anti-inflammatory drug to block mast cell biosynthesis of prostaglandin D2 for severe flushing associated with vascular collapse unresponsive to H1 and H2 antihistamines (102,119). However, nonsteroidal anti-inflammatory drugs have to be used with caution because they lead to mast cell activation in some patients, resulting in life-threatening anaphylactic episodes (128).

REFERENCES

Leukemic Infiltration

1. Barcos M. Pathology of leukemia. In: Henderson ES, Lister TA, eds. William Dameshek and Frederick Gunz's leukemia. 5th ed. Philadelphia: W.B. Saunders, 1990:163–202.
2. Brunning RD, McKenna RW. Tumors of the bone marrow. Atlas of Tumor Pathology. 3rd Series, Fascicle 9. Washington D.C.: Armed Forces Institute of Pathology, 1994.
3. Rappaport H. Tumors of the hematopoietic System. Atlas of Tumor Pathology, 1st Series, Fascicle 8. Washington D.C.: Armed Forces Institute of Pathology, 1966.

Granulocytic Sarcoma

5. Abeler V, Kjorstad KE, Langholm R, Marton PF. Granulocytic sarcoma (chloroma) of the uterine cervix: report of two cases. Int J Gynecol Pathol 1983;2:88–92.
4. Abruzzo LV, Jaffe ES, Cotelingam JD, Whang-Peng J, Del Duca V Jr, Medeiros LJ. T-cell lymphoblastic lymphoma with eosinophilia associated with subsequent myeloid malignancy. Am J Surg Pathol 1992;16:235–45.
6. Adam LR, Angus B, Carey P, Davison EV. Cytogenetic analysis of a granulocytic sarcoma in a patient without systemic leukaemia. J Clin Pathol 1991;44:81–2.
7. Ashfaq R, Weinberg AG, Argyle CA. Acute megakaryoblastic leukemia simulating carcinoma. Am J Clin Pathol 1992;98:55–60.
8. Banerjee D, Silva E. Mediastinal mass with acute leukemia. Myeloblastoma masquerading as lymphoblastic lymphoma. Arch Pathol Lab Med 1981;105:126–9.
9. Brugo EA, Larkin E, Molina-Escobar J, Constanzi J. Primary granulocytic sarcoma of the small bowel. Cancer 1975;35:1333–40.
10. Castella A, Davey FR, Elabdawi A, Gordon GB. Granulocytic sarcoma of the hard palate: report of the first case. Hum Pathol 1984;15:1190–2.
11. Chan JK, Lau WH, Saw D. Extradural granulocytic sarcoma of the spine: a unique case of long survival after local therapy. Am J Hematol 1986;22:439–41.
12. _____, Ng CS. Diagnosis of granulocytic sarcoma [Letter]. Pathology 1987;19:317.
13. Comings DE, Fayen AW, Carter P. Myeloblastoma preceding blood and marrow evidence of acute leukemia. Cancer 1965;18:253–8.
14. Crocker J, Jenkins R, Burnett D. Immunohistochemical demonstration of leucocyte elastase in human tissues. J Clin Pathol 1984;37:1114–8.
15. _____, Jenkins R, Burnett D. Immunohistochemical localization of cathepsin G in human tissues. Am J Surg Pathol 1985;9:338–43.
16. Davey FR, Elghetany T, Kurec AS. Immunophenotyping of hematologic neoplasms in paraffin-embedded tissue sections. Am J Clin Pathol 1990; 93(4 Suppl 1):S17–26.
17. _____, Olson S, Kurec AS, Eastman-Abaya K, Gottlieb AJ, Mason DY. The immunophenotyping of extramedullary myeloid cell tumors in paraffin-embedded tissue sections. Am J Surg Pathol 1988;12:699–707.
18. Doshi HM, Schochet SS Jr, Gold M, Nugent GR. Granulocytic sarcoma presenting as an epidural mass with acute paraparesis in an aleukemic patient. Am J Clin Pathol 1991;95:228–32.
19. Falini B, Flenghi L, Pileri S, et al. PG-M1: a new monoclonal antibody directed against a fixative-resistant epitope on the macrophage-restricted form of the CD68 molecule. Am J Pathol 1993;142:1359–72.
20. Fellbaum C, Hansmann ML. Immunohistochemical differential diagnosis of granulocytic sarcomas and malignant lymphomas on formalin-fixed materials. Virchows Arch [A] 1990;416:351–5.
21. Foucar K, Foucar E, Willman C, Horrath A, Gerety RL. Nonleukemic granulocytic sarcoma of the heart: a report of a fatal case. Am J Hematol 1987;25:325–32.
22. Frame R, Head D, Lee R, Craven C, Ward JH. Granulocytic sarcoma of the prostate. Two cases causing urinary obstruction. Cancer 1987;59:142–6.
23. Furebring-Freden M, Martinsson U, Sundstrom C. Myelosarcoma without acute leukaemia: immunohistochemical and clinicopathologic characterization of 8 cases. Histopathology 1990;16:243–50.
24. Hanson CA, Ross CW, Schnitzer B. Anti-CD34 immunoperoxidase staining in paraffin sections of acute leukemia: comparison with flow cytometric immunophenotyping. Hum Pathol 1992;23:26–32.
25. Hurwitz BS, Sutherland JC, Walker MD. Central nervous system chloromas preceding acute leukemia by one year. Neurology 1970;20:771–5.
26. Hutchison RE, Kurec AS, Davey FR. Granulocytic sarcoma. Clin Lab Med 1990;10:889–901.
27. Kanavaros P, Lavergne A, Galian A, et al. A primary immunoblastic T-malignant lymphoma of the small bowel with azurophilic intracytoplasmic granules. A histologic, immunologic, and electron microscopy study. Am J Surg Pathol 1988;12:641–7.
28. Keifer J, Zaino R, Ballard JO. Erythroleukemic infiltration of a lymph node: use of hemoglobin immunohistochemical technique in diagnosis. Hum Pathol 1984;15:1090–3.
29. Krause JR. Granulocytic sarcoma preceding acute leukemia: a report of six cases. Cancer 1979;44:1017–21.
30. Kubonishi I, Ohtsuki Y, Machida K, et al. Granulocytic sarcoma presenting as a mediastinal mass tumor. Report of a case and cytological and cytochemical studies of tumor cells in vivo and in vitro. Am J Clin Pathol 1984;82:730–4.
31. Long JC, Mihm MC. Multiple granulocytic tumors of the skin, report of six cases of myelogenous leukemia with initial manifestations in the skin. Cancer 1977;39:2004–16.
32. Lusher JM. Chloroma as a presenting feature of acute leukemia. Am J Dis Child 1984;108:62–6.
33. Mason DY, Taylor CR. The distribution of muramidase (lysozyme) in human tissues. J Clin Pathol 1975;28:124–32.
34. Mason TE, Demaree RS Jr, Margolis CI. Granulocytic sarcoma (chloroma) two years preceding myelogenous leukemia. Cancer 1973;31:423–32.

35. McCarty KS Jr, Wortman J, Daly J, Rundles RW, Hanker JS. Chloroma (granulocytic sarcoma) without evidence of leukemia: facilitated light microscopic diagnosis. Blood 1980;56:104–8.

36. Meis JM, Butler JJ, Osborne BM, Manning JT. Granulocytic sarcoma in nonleukemic patients. Cancer 1986;58:2697–709.

37. Muller S, Sangster G, Crocker J, et al. An immunohistochemical and clinicopathological study of granulocytic sarcoma (chloroma). Hematol Oncol 1986;4:101–12.

38. Muss HB, Moloney WC. Chloroma and other myeloblastic tumors. Blood 1973;42:721–8.

39. Neiman RS, Barcos M, Berard C, et al. Granulocytic sarcoma: a clinicopathologic study of 61 biopsied cases. Cancer 1981;48:1426–37.

40. Pinkus GS, Pinkus JL. Myeloperoxidase: a specific marker for myeloid cells in paraffin sections. Mod Pathol 1991;6:733–41.

41. Pulford KA, Erber WN, Crick JA, et al. Use of monoclonal antibodies against human neutrophil elastase in normal and leukaemic myeloid cells. J Clin Pathol 1988;41:853–60.

42. Ralfkiaer E, Pulford KA, Lauritzen AF, Avnstrom S, Guldhammer B, Mason DY. Diagnosis of acute myeloid leukaemia with the use of monoclonal anti-neutrophil elastase (NP57) reactive with routinely processed biopsy samples. Histopathology 1989;14:637–43.

43. Rappaport H. Tumors of the hematopoietic system. Atlas of Tumor Pathology, 1st Series, Section 3, Fascicle 8. Washington D.C.: Armed Forces Institute of Pathology, 1966:239–63.

44. Sears HF, Reid J. Granulocytic sarcoma, local presentation of a systemic disease. Cancer 1976;37:1808–13.

45. van Veen S, Kluin PM, de Keizer RJW, Kluin-Nelemans HC. Granulocytic sarcoma (chloroma). Presentation of an unusual case. Am J Clin Pathol 1991;95:567–71.

46. Whitcomb CC, Sternheim WL, Borowitz MJ, Davila E, Byrne GE Jr. T-cell lymphoma mimicking granulocytic sarcoma. Am J Clin Pathol 1985;84:760–3.

47. Wiernick PH, Serpick AA. Granulocytic sarcoma (chloroma). Blood 1970;35:361–9.

48. Wong KF, Chan JK. Anti-myeloperoxidase: antibody of choice for labeling of myeloid cells including diagnosis of granulocytic sarcoma. Adv Anat Pathol 1995;2:65–8.

49. _____, Yuen RW, Lok AS, Chan TK. Granulocytic sarcoma presenting as bleeding gastric polyp. Pathology 1989;21:63–4.

Hairy Cell Leukemia

50. Abbondanzo SL, Sulak LE. Ki-1 positive lymphoma developing ten years after the diagnosis of hairy cell leukemia. Cancer 1991;67:3117–22.

51. Anderson KC, Boyd AW, Fisher DC, Leslie D, Schlossman SF, Nadler LM. Hairy cell leukemia: a tumor of pre-plasma cells. Blood 1985;65:620–9.

52. Bartl R, Frisch B, Hill W, Burkhardt R, Sommerfeld W, Sund M. Bone marrow histology in hairy cell leukemia. Identification of subtypes and their prognostic significance. Am J Clin Pathol 1983;79:531–45.

53. Bouroncle BA, Wiseman BK, Doan CA. Leukemic reticuloendotheliosis. Blood 1958;13:609–30.

54. Brunning RD, McKenna RW. Tumors of the bone marrow. Atlas of Tumor Pathology. 3rd Series, Fascicle 8. Washington D.C.: Armed Forces Institute of Pathology, 1994:276–87.

55. Burke JS. The value of the bone-marrow biopsy in the diagnosis of hairy cell leukemia. Am J Clin Pathol 1978;70:876–84.

56. _____, Byrne GE Jr, Rappaport H. Hairy cell leukemia (leukemic reticuloendotheliosis). I. A clinical pathologic study of 21 patients. Cancer 1974;33:1399–410.

57. _____, Rappaport H. The diagnosis and differential diagnosis of hairy cell leukemia in bone marrow and spleen. Semin Oncol 1984;11:334–46.

58. _____, Sheibani K, Winberg CD, Rappaport H. Recognition of hairy cell leukemia in a spleen of normal weight. Am J Clin Pathol 1987;87:276–81.

59. Catovsky D, Foa R. The lymphoid leukaemias. London: Butterworths, 1990:156–81

60. _____, O'Brien M, Melo JV, Wardle J, Brozovic M. Hairy cell leukemia (HCL) variant: an intermediate disease between HCL and B prolymphocytic leukemia. Semin Oncol 1984;11:362–9.

61. _____, Pettit JE, Galton DA, Spiers AS, Harrison CV. Leukaemia reticuloendotheliosis ("Hairy" cell leukemia): a distinct clinico-pathological entity. Br J Haematol 1974:26:9–27.

62. Chadburn A, Inghirami G, Knowles DM. Hairy cell leukemia-associated antigen LeuM5 (CD11c) is preferentially expressed by benign activated and neoplastic CD8 T cells. Am J Pathol 1990;136:29–37.

63. Chang KL, Stroup R, Weiss LM. Hairy cell leukemia. Current status. Am J Clin Pathol 1992;97:719–38.

64. Chilosi M, Pizzolo G. Immunophenotypical diagnosis and monitoring of hairy cell leukemia [Editorial]. Leukemia 1990;4:168–9.

65. Cleary ML, Wood GS, Warnke R, Chao J, Sklar J. Immunoglobulin gene rearrangements in hairy cell leukemia. Blood 1984;64:99–104.

66. Daniel MT, Flandrin G. Fine structure of abnormal cells in hairy cell (tricholeukocytic) leukemia, with special reference to their in vitro phagocytic capacity. Lab Invest 1974;30:1–8.

67. Diez Martin JL, Li CY, Banks PM. Blastic variant of hairy cell leukemia. Am J Clin Pathol 1987;87:576–83.

68. Elkon KB, Hughes GR, Catovsky D, et al. Hairy-cell leukaemia with polyarteritis nodosa. Lancet 1979;2:280–2.

69. Falini B, Pulford K, Erber WN, et al. Use of a panel of monoclonal antibodies for the diagnosis of hairy cell leukaemia, an immunocytochemical study of 36 cases. Histopathology 1986;10:671–87.

70. _____, Schwarting R, Erber W, et al. The differential diagnosis of hairy cell leukemia with a panel of monoclonal antibodies. Am J Clin Pathol 1985;83:289–300.

71. Farcet JP, Weschsler J, Wirquin V, Divine M, Reyes F. Vasculitis in hairy-cell leukemia. Arch Intern Med 1987;147:660–4.

72. Foroni L, Catovsky D, Luzzatto L. Immunoglobulin gene rearrangements in hairy cell leukemia and other chronic B cell lymphoproliferative disorders. Leukemia 1987;1:389–92.

73. Golomb HM. Hairy cell leukemia: an unusual lymphoproliferative disease, a study of 24 patients. Cancer 1978;42:946–56.

74. Hanson CA, Ward PC, Schnitzer B. A multilobular variant of hairy cell leukemia with morphologic similarities to T-cell lymphoma. Am J Surg Pathol 1989;13:671–9.

75. Hassan IB, Hagberg H, Sundstrom C. Immunophenotype of hairy-cell leukemia. Eur J Haematol 1990;45:172–6.

76. Hogan SF, Osborne BM, Butler JJ. Unexpected splenic nodules in leukemic patients. Hum Pathol 1989;20:62–8.

77. Hsu SM, Yang K, Jaffe ES. Hairy cell leukemia: a B cell neoplasm with a unique antigenic phenotype. Am J Clin Pathol 1983;80:421–8.

78. Kalyanaraman VS, Sarngadharan MG, Robert-Guroff M, Miyoshi I, Golde D, Gallo RC. A new subtype of human T-cell leukemia virus (HTLV-II) associated with a T-cell variant of hairy cell leukemia. Science 1982;218:571–3.

79. Kantarjian HM, Schachner J, Keating MJ. Fludarabine therapy in hairy cell leukemia. Cancer 1991;67:1291–3.

80. Klima M, Waddell CC. Hairy cell leukemia associated with focal vascular damage. Hum Pathol 1984;15:657–9.

81. Krol T, Robinson J, Bekeris L, Messmore H. Hairy cell leukemia and a fatal periarteritis nodosa-like syndrome. Arch Pathol Lab Med 1983;107:583–5.

82. Lazzaro B, Munger R, Flick J, Moriber-Katz S. Visualization of the ribosome-lamella complex in plastic-embedded biopsy specimen as an aid to diagnosis of hairy cell leukemia. Arch Pathol Lab Med 1991;115:1259–62.

83. Lennert K, Mohri N. Histopathology and diagnosis of non-Hodgkin's lymphomas. In: Lennert K, ed. Malignant lymphomas other than Hodgkin's disease: histology, cytology, ultrastructure, immunology. Berlin: Springer Verlag, 1978:111–469.

84. Meijer CJ, van der Valk P, Jansen J. Hairy cell leukemia: an immunohistochemical and morphometric study. Semin Oncol 1984;11:347–52.

85. Melo JV, Robinson DS, Gregory C, Catovsky D. Splenic B cell lymphoma with villous lymphocytes in the peripheral blood: a disorder distinct from hairy cell leukemia. Leukemia 1987;1:294–8.

86. Mulligan SP, Travade P, Matutes E, et al. B-ly-7, a monoclonal antibody reactive with hairy cell leukemia, also defines an activation antigen on normal CD8+ T cells. Blood 1990;76:959–64.

87. Naeim F. Hairy cell leukemia: characteristics of the neoplastic cells. Hum Pathol 1988;19:375–88.

88. _____, Hoon DS, Cheng L, Herschman H, Cochran A Jr. Reactivity of neoplastic cells of hairy cell leukemia with antisera to S-100 protein. Am J Clin Pathol 1987;88:86–91.

89. Paoletti M, Bitter MA, Vardiman JW. Hairy-cell leukemia. Morphologic, cytochemical, and immunologic features. Clin Lab Med 1988;8:179–95.

90. Piro LD, Carrera CJ, Carson DA, Beutler E. Lasting remissions in hairy-cell leukemia induced by a single infusion of 2-chlorodeoxyadenosine. N Engl J Med 1990;332:1117–21.

91. Rosenblatt JD, Chen IS, Golde DW. HTLV-II and human lymphoproliferative disorders. Clin Lab Med 1988;8:85–95.

92. _____, Giorgi JV, Golde DW, et al. Integrated human T-cell leukemia virus II genome in CD8+ T cells from a patient with "atypical" hairy cell leukemia: evidence for distinct T and B cell lymphoproliferative disorders. Blood 1988;71:363–9.

93. Sansoni P, Rowden G, Manara GC, Ferrari C, Tonesani C, De Panfilis G. Immunoelectronmicroscopic demonstration of S-100 protein in hairy cell leukemia cells. Am J Clin Pathol 1988;89:374–7.

94. Saxon A, Stevens RH, Golde DW. T-lymphocyte variant of hairy cell leukemia. Ann Intern Med 1978;88:323–6.

95. Schwarting R, Dienemann D, Kruschwitz M, Fritsche G, Stein H. Specificities of monoclonal antibodies B-ly7 and HML-1 are identical [Letter]. Blood 1990;75:320–1.

96. Strickler JG, Schmidt CM, Wick MR. Methods in pathology. Immunophenotype of hairy cell leukemia in paraffin sections. Mod Pathol 1990;3:518–23.

97. Thaler J, Dietze O, Faber V, et al. Monoclonal antibody B-ly7: a sensitive marker for detection of minimal residual disease in hairy cell leukemia. Leukemia 1990;4:170–6.

98. Vardiman JW, Gilewski TA, Ratain MJ, Bitter MA, Bradlow BA, Golomb HM. Evaluation of Leu-M5 (CD11c) in hairy cell leukemia by the alkaline phosphatase anti-alkaline phosphatase technique. Am J Clin Pathol 1988;90:250–6.

99. _____, Variakojis D, Golomb HM. Hairy cell leukemia, an autopsy study. Cancer 1979;43:1339–49.

100. Yam LT, Janckila AJ, Chan CH, Li CY. Hepatic involvement in hairy cell leukemia. Cancer 1983;51:1497–504.

101. _____, Phyliky RL, Li CY. Benign and neoplastic disorders simulating hairy cell leukemia. Semin Oncol 1984;11:353–61.

Systemic Mastocytosis

102. Austen KF. Systemic mastocytosis [Editorial]. N Engl J Med 1992;326:637–40.

103. Brunning RD, Rosai J, McKenna RW, Parkin JL, Risdall R. Systemic mastocytosis. Extracutaneous manifestations. Am J Surg Pathol 1983;7:425–38.

104. Chariot P, Monnet I, Gaulard P, Abd-Alsamad I, Ruffie P, De Cremoux H. Systemic mastocytosis following mediastinal germ cell tumor: an association confirmed. Hum Pathol 1993;24:111–2.

105. Horny HP, Kaiserling E. Lymphoid cells and tissue mast cells of bone marrow lesions in systemic mastocytosis: a histological and immunohistological study. Br J Haematol 1988;69:449–55.

106. _____, Kaiserling E, Campbell M, Parwaresch MR, Lennert K. Liver findings in generalized mastocytosis. A clinicopathologic study. Cancer 1989;63:532–8.

107. _____, Kaiserling E, Parwaresch MR, Lennert K. Lymph node findings in generalized mastocytosis. Histopathology 1992;21:439–46.

108. _____, Parwaresch MR, Kaiserling E, et al. Mast cell sarcoma of the larynx. J Clin Pathol 1986;39:596–602.

109. _____, Parwaresch MR, Lennert K. Bone marrow findings in systemic mastocytosis. Hum Pathol 1985;16:808–14.

110. _____, Ruck MT, Kaiserling E. Spleen findings in generalized mastocytosis. A clinicopathologic study. Cancer 1992;70:459–68.

111. _____, Ruck M, Wehrmann M, Kaiserling E. Blood findings in generalized mastocytosis: evidence of frequent simultaneous occurrence of myeloproliferative disorders. Br J Haematol 1990;76:186–93.

112. _____, Ruck P, Xiao JC, Kaiserling E. Immunore-activity of normal and neoplastic human tissue mast cells with macrophage-associated antibodies, with special reference to the recently developed monoclonal antibody PG-M1. Hum Pathol 1993;24:355–8.

113. Klatt EC, Lukes RJ, Meyer PR. Benign and malignant mast cell proliferations. Diagnosis and separation using a pH-dependent toluidine blue stain in tissue section. Cancer 1983;51:1119–24.

114. Kluin-Nelemans HC, Jansen JH, Breukelman H, et al. Response to interferon alfa-2b in a patient with systemic mastocytosis. N Engl J Med 1992;326:619–23.

115. Leder LD. Subtle clues to diagnosis by histochemistry. Mast cell disease. Am J Dermatopathol 1979;1:261–6.

116. Lennert K, Parwaresch MR. Mast cells and mast-cell neoplasia: a review. Histopathology 1979;3:349–65.

117. Longley BJ, Morganroth GS, Tyrrell L, et al. Altered metabolism of mast-cell growth factor (c-kit ligand) in cutaneous mastocytosis. N Engl J Med 1993;328:1302–7.

118. Metcalfe DD. Classification and diagnosis of mastocytosis: current status. J Invest Dermatol 1991;96:2–4S.

119. _____. The treatment of mastocytosis: an overview. J Invest Dermatol 1991;96:56–59S.

120. Murphy GF, Elder DE. Non-melanocytic tumors of the skin. Atlas of Tumor Pathology. 3rd Series, Fascicle 1. Washington D.C.: Armed Forces Institute of Pathology, 1991:187–9.

121. Parwaresch RM, Horny HP, Bodewadt-Radzun S. Mast cell disease. In: Knowles DM, ed. Neoplastic hematopathology, Baltimore: Williams & Wilkins, 1992:1485–515.

122. Rywlin AM. Mastocytic eosinophilic fibrohistiocytic lesion of the bone marrow. Hematology 1982;H:82–5.

123. _____, Hoffman EP, Ortega RS. Eosinophilic fibrohistiocytic lesion of bone marrow: a distinctive new morphologic finding, probably related to drug hypersensitivity. Blood 1972;40:464–72.

124. te Velde J, Vismans FJ, Leenheers-Binnendijk L, Vos CJ, Smeenk D, Bijvoet OL. The eosinophilic fibrohistiocytic lesion of the bone marrow. A mastocellular lesion in bone disease. Virchows Arch [A] 1978;377:277–85.

125. Torrey E, Simpson K, Wilbur S, Munoz P, Skikne B. Malignant mastocytosis with circulating mast cells. Am J Hematol 1990;34:283–6.

126. Travis WD, Li CY. Pathology of the lymph node and spleen in systemic mast cell disease. Mod Pathol 1988;1:4–14.

127. _____, Li CY, Bergstralh EJ. Solid and hematologic malignancies in 60 patients with systemic mast cell disease. Arch Pathol Lab Med 1989;113:365–8.

128. _____, Li CY, Bergstralh EJ, Yam LT, Swee RG. Systemic mast cell disease. Analysis of 58 cases and literature review. Medicine (Baltimore) 1988;67:345–68.

129. _____, Li CY, Hoagland HC, Travis LB, Banks PM. Mast cell leukemia: report of a case and review of the literature. Mayo Clin Proc 1986;61:957–66.

130. _____, Li CY, Yam LT, Bergstralh EJ, Swee RG. Significance of systemic mast cell disease with associated hematologic disorders. Cancer 1988;62:965–72.

131. Webb TA, Li CY, Yam LT. Systemic mast cell disease: a clinical and hematopathologic study of 26 cases. Cancer 1982;49:927–38.

132. Wong KF, Chan JK, Chan JC, Kwong YL, Ma SK, Chow TC. Concurrent acute myeloid leukemia and systemic mastocytosis. Am J Hematol 1991;38:243–4.

❖❖❖

20

LYMPHOMAS OF THE SPLEEN

Although the spleen is often involved by Hodgkin's disease or non-Hodgkin's lymphoma as part of generalized disease, primary splenic lymphoma is rare. Careful gross examination of the spleen is extremely important for proper histologic sampling and diagnosis (Table 20-1). In this chapter, primary splenic lymphoma and patterns of splenic involvement by various types of lymphoma are discussed.

PRIMARY SPLENIC LYMPHOMA

Definition. There are no precise criteria for making a diagnosis of primary splenic lymphoma, and many cases reported as such in the literature are disseminated lymphomas with prominent splenic involvement. Some authors adopt the stringent criteria that the lymphoma should be confined to the spleen or splenic hilar lymph nodes, without evidence of involvement of other sites (3,7); others have relaxed these criteria to include cases with minimal liver or bone marrow involvement (9). However, to conform with the definition of extranodal lymphoma in general, and to keep the entity pure, use of the more stringent criteria appears advisable, although some cases of primary splenic lymphoma presenting with high-stage disease are inevitably excluded by this definition.

Ahmann et al. (1) proposed a staging system for splenic lymphoma: stage I, tumor limited to

Table 20-1

CORRELATION OF GROSS APPEARANCE OF THE SPLEEN WITH THE UNDERLYING PATHOLOGY

Gross Appearance	Common Causes
Miliary small white nodules involving the entire parenchyma	Follicular lymphoma Small cell lymphomas* (small lymphocytic, lymphoplasmacytoid, mantle cell) B-cell chronic lymphocytic leukemia* Hodgkin's disease (rare) Other (miliary tuberculosis, amyloidosis ["sago" spleen])
Solitary large fleshy nodule or multiple large nodules with or without coalescence	Diffuse large cell lymphoma Follicular large cell lymphoma Hodgkin's disease Other (inflammatory pseudotumor, malignant fibrous histiocytoma, metastasis)
Multiple haphazardly distributed tumor nodules of variable sizes	Hodgkin's disease Large cell lymphoma Bacillary angiomatosis Mycobacterial spindle cell pseudotumor Metastasis
Solitary small nodule or several clustered small nodules	Hodgkin's disease Localized lymphoid hyperplasia
Homogeneous beefy red appearance, with or without blood lakes, with or without recognizable atrophic white pulp	Acute and chronic leukemias, including hairy cell leukemia Some cases of large cell lymphoma ("malignant histiocytosis" pattern) Infectious mononucleosis and other immunologic reactions Congestive splenomegaly Agnogenic myeloid metaplasia Congenital and hemolytic anemia Storage disease Systemic mastocytosis**

*The nodules are often less discrete than those seen in follicular lymphoma.
** Often with thick fibrous trabeculae; some small nodules may be seen in addition.

the spleen; stage II, tumor limited to the spleen and hilar lymph nodes; and stage III, involvement of the liver and nodes beyond splenic hilum. We only accept cases fulfilling the criteria of stages I and II as primary splenic lymphoma.

Incidence. Primary splenic lymphoma is uncommon, accounting for less than 1 percent of all lymphomas. Among 5,100 cases of lymphoma seen at the Mayo Clinic from 1946 through 1963, only 17 fulfilled the strict diagnostic criteria for primary splenic lymphoma (1). Similarly, only 9 cases of primary splenic lymphoma were found among 1,584 cases of non-Hodgkin's lymphoma accessioned at the McGill Cancer Center (3).

Clinical Features. Because of the differences in diagnostic criteria, it is difficult to generalize on the clinicopathologic features of primary splenic lymphoma. Interpretation of the older literature is hampered by the use of old terminology (1). Furthermore, it is not possible to extract information on relevant individual cases from some large series (1,9,17). Most primary splenic lymphomas are non-Hodgkin's lymphomas; Hodgkin's disease confined to the spleen is rare (19,26).

The following clinical features are based on analysis of 47 cases of non-Hodgkin's lymphoma fulfilling the strict diagnostic criteria for primary splenic lymphoma (2–4,7,8,10,13,15,16,18, 21,24,25); biases are inevitable due to erratic reporting in the literature. The patients are adults, with a mean age of 57 years; there is a slight male predominance (1.3 to 1). The most common presentation is upper abdominal pain or discomfort. Systemic symptoms such as fever, malaise, and weight loss are also common. Peripheral blood cytopenia, if present, is generally insignificant. Two cases were diagnosed in human immunodeficiency virus–seropositive patients (2,10). Examination usually reveals splenomegaly only, with no other positive signs. Splenic lymphoma should be considered a likely diagnosis in patients who present with left upper quadrant pain, fever, and radiologic evidence of a splenic mass (15).

An example of primary splenic true histiocytic lymphoma has been reported (11). The tumor was initially localized to the spleen in the form of multiple discrete nodules. The neoplastic cells were malignant-appearing erythrophagocytic histiocytic cells expressing a monocyte/histiocyte immunophenotype in the absence of clonal immunoglobulin and T-cell receptor gene rearrange-

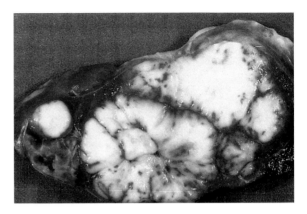

Figure 20-1
PRIMARY LARGE CELL LYMPHOMA OF SPLEEN
Characteristically, coalescent large fleshy nodules are seen on the cut surface.

ments. Since the patient subsequently died from disseminated disease, this may have been an unusual variant of malignant histiocytosis (12).

Gross Findings. The enlarged spleen usually weighs over 500 g, but can weigh up to several kilograms. In general, a "miliary" pattern, characterized by small white nodules evenly distributed over the cut surface, is seen predominantly in small cell lymphomas (Table 20-1). Tumors composed of a single or multiple large fleshy nodules, with or without hemorrhage and necrosis, usually result from involvement by large cell lymphomas (fig. 20-1); these tumor masses can breach the splenic capsule to invade the surrounding structures such as the diaphragm, stomach, and pancreas.

Microscopic Findings. Although small cell lymphomas are reported to greatly outnumber the large cell type in some studies (17,19,20,22,24), these series are not reliable since many cases of disseminated lymphoma are included. Analysis of the 47 reported cases of primary splenic lymphoma shows the following distribution of histologic types: large cell (including anaplastic large cell), 30 cases; small cell, 15 cases; mixed cell lymphoma of follicular center cell type (centroblastic-centrocytic), 1 case; and small noncleaved cell, 1 case.

The small cell lymphomas are of small lymphocytic, lymphoplasmacytoid, or mantle cell type. The infiltrate tends to be localized in the white pulp, with variable spill-over into the red pulp (fig. 20-2). In the small lymphocytic and lymphoplasmacytoid types the infiltrate is composed of

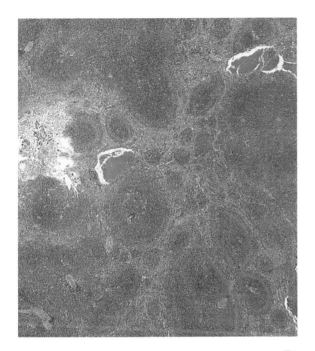
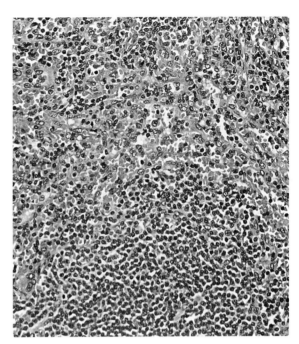

Figure 20-2
PRIMARY B-CELL SMALL LYMPHOCYTIC LYMPHOMA OF THE SPLEEN
Left: The dark-staining nodules of lymphoma in the white pulp do not always appear well delineated because the lymphoma cells merge into the surrounding red pulp.
Right: The lower field shows replacement of the Malpighian corpuscle by a monotonous population of small lymphocytes. Similar lymphoid cells are also seen in the red pulp (upper field).

small lymphoid cells with round nuclei and condensed chromatin; more amphophilic to basophilic cytoplasm can be identified in the lymphoplasmacytoid type (fig. 20-3). For mantle cell lymphoma, the neoplastic cells possess irregular nuclei, fairly condensed chromatin, and scanty cytoplasm.

In the large cell lymphomas, the neoplastic cells often grow in diffuse sheets, totally replacing the splenic architecture in the involved areas (fig. 20-4); they can also show a more permeative growth pattern in the red pulp, with preservation of the sinuses and pulp cords (fig. 20-5) (18). The cytology of the lymphoma cells is highly variable, like their nodal counterpart. The cellular population can be monotonous, pleomorphic, or anaplastic (figs. 20-4, right, 20-6).

Immunophenotypic and Genotypic Findings. Little information is available on the immunophenotypic details of primary splenic lymphoma, although the terminology used in the various studies implies that most cases are of B-cell type. In one series of 10 cases of primary splenic large cell lymphoma, 6 were confirmed to

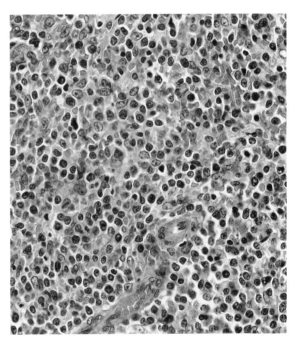

Figure 20-3
PRIMARY LYMPHOPLASMACYTOID
LYMPHOMA OF THE SPLEEN
The small lymphoid cells have a definite rim of amphophilic cytoplasm.

413

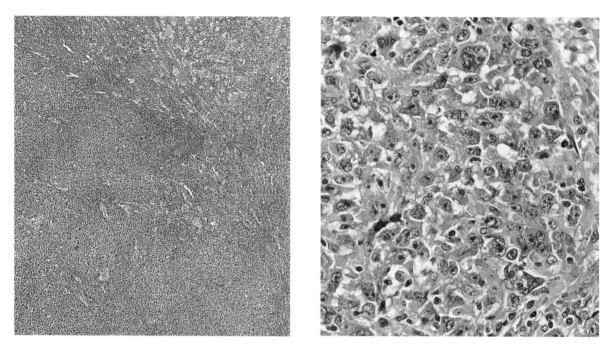

Figure 20-4
PRIMARY SPLENIC LARGE B-CELL LYMPHOMA
Left: The tumor nodule (left and lower field) obliterates the normal splenic architecture.
Right: The large lymphoma cells appear pleomorphic. Residual splenic tissue is not identified among the neoplastic cells.

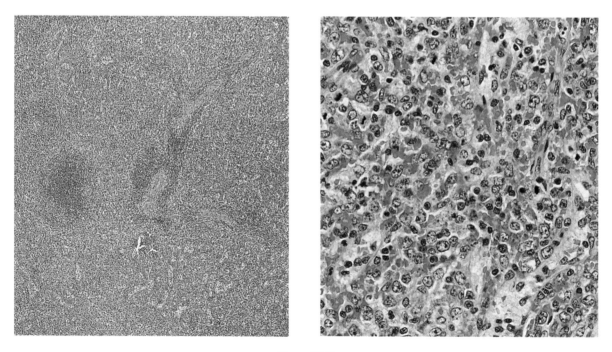

Figure 20-5
PRIMARY SPLENIC LARGE B-CELL LYMPHOMA SHOWING DIFFUSE RED PULP INVOLVEMENT
Left: The red pulp is expanded, but the white pulp is still recognizable.
Right: Despite diffuse infiltration of the red pulp by large lymphoma cells, the sinusoidal and pulp cord structures are still preserved. This pattern of involvement has been considered to be a characteristic of "malignant histiocytosis."

be of B-cell lineage by the demonstration of monotypic immunoglobulin, but the lineage of the other 4 could not be determined because lymphoid markers other than immunoglobulin were not available (15). Of the 17 splenic lymphomas reported by Falk and Stutte (9) (which included cases with minimal involvement of the liver or bone marrow), 14 were of B lineage, and 3 of T lineage. Some cases can express CD30 (2). Two cases showed the *bcl*-6 gene rearrangement typically observed in a subset of diffuse large B-cell lymphomas (23).

Differential Diagnosis. Infectious mononucleosis involving the spleen may mimic malignant lymphoma by virtue of expansion of the red pulp by large numbers of activated lymphoid cells, subendothelial or trabecular infiltration by similar cells, and even occasional Reed-Sternberg–like cells (fig. 20-7). Other viral infections can produce a similar histologic picture (6). The young age of the patient, a positive Monospot test, and the presence of a spectrum of lymphoid cells instead of a monomorphous population should lead to serious consideration of infectious mononucleosis.

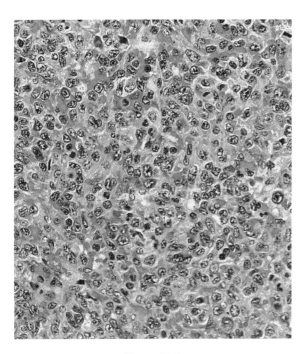

Figure 20-6
PRIMARY SPLENIC POST-THYMIC T-CELL
LYMPHOMA OF LARGE CELL TYPE

The spleen is extensively infiltrated by large lymphoma cells. Distinction from large B-cell lymphoma cannot be made without the help of immunohistochemical studies.

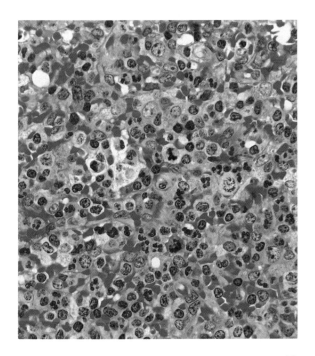

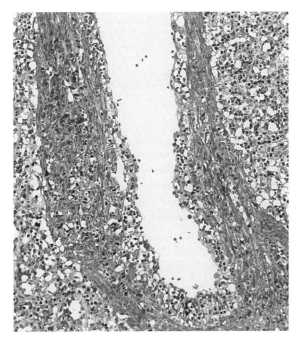

Figure 20-7
INFECTIOUS MONONUCLEOSIS INVOLVING SPLEEN
Left: In the red pulp, there are many interspersed large lymphoid cells.
Right: The lymphoid cells show subendothelial infiltration of the trabecular vessels.

Localized reactive lymphoid hyperplasia of the spleen can be mistaken for malignant lymphoma (5). This is an idiopathic condition characterized by the presence of a solitary fleshy nodule measuring 1 to 10 mm in the parenchyma of the spleen. Histologically, some cases show coalescing reactive lymphoid follicles with prominent germinal centers, while others show a localized proliferation of small lymphocytes, plasma cells, and immunoblasts. Sclerosis may be present. The nodule should be examined at multiple levels to exclude lymphoma, particularly Hodgkin's disease (14).

Treatment and Prognosis. Most of the reported patients with primary splenic lymphoma received postoperative chemotherapy, radiotherapy, or both. The overall survival is slightly over 50 percent, irrespective of histologic type, although the follow-up period is short in some studies (2–4,7,8,10,13,15,16,18,21,24,25). Using strict criteria for diagnosis of primary splenic lymphoma, Brox and Shustik (4) reported a highly favorable outcome in 11 of 12 cases, with many long-term survivors. Most of the reported deaths occurred within 1 year (3,8–10,15,24). However, late recurrences sometimes occurred after many years (7,15); some were successfully treated by chemotherapy or radiotherapy.

SPLENIC INVOLVEMENT BY LYMPHOMA

Hodgkin's Disease

The practice of staging laparotomy, popularized in the 1970s, resulted in greater knowledge of the patterns of spread and splenic involvement by Hodgkin's disease. This surgical procedure is performed more selectively today, because the frequent use of systemic chemotherapy in place of radiotherapy makes knowledge of the exact sites of involvement less important (38,55).

Examination of the Spleen. The recommended method for examination of a spleen removed at staging laparotomy is as follows. The spleen should be received fresh. After removal of the hilar soft tissue and lymph nodes, it is weighed and measured. It should be thinly sliced at intervals of 2 to 3 mm using a long sharp knife, and each slice carefully inspected and lightly palpated for abnormalities (33,38). Representative blocks should be taken from any abnormal areas, in particular whitish nodules, and from normal-looking areas as well. If no abnormality is detected, four random blocks are taken. All splenic hilar lymph nodes should be histologically examined.

Incidence. Splenic involvement is detected in more than one third of patients undergoing staging laparotomy (Table 20-1). However, there is poor correlation between splenic size and likelihood of involvement by Hodgkin's disease. At least one in four patients with Hodgkin's disease have splenic involvement when unsuspected clinically, and as many as half of patients thought to have involvement because of clinical or radiologic enlargement of the spleen do not (55).

Gross Findings. Although the spleen is often enlarged, it can be of normal size. The most common pattern of involvement is in the form of several randomly distributed, white, fleshy nodules that are isolated or confluent (Table 20.1). It can also take the form of a solitary tiny focus as small as 1 mm in diameter (40,45), large fleshy tumor masses, or miliary small white nodules dispersed throughout the parenchyma (fig. 20-8). Microscopic involvement in the absence of a macroscopic lesion is rare (33,36,45).

Microscopic Findings. All types of Hodgkin's disease, with the exception of nodular lymphocyte predominance type, commonly involve the spleen. The earliest site of involvement is the periarterial lymphoid sheath and marginal zone of the white pulp (33,40,62). With time, the entire Malpighian body is replaced, and the lesion coalesces with adjacent involved areas to form larger nodules (figs. 20-9–20-11). Diagnostic Reed-Sternberg cells and their variants are present in a variable inflammatory background which may include small lymphocytes, plasma cells, histiocytes, and eosinophils (figs. 20-12, 20-13). Irrespective of subtype, there can be cellular fibrosis or sclerosis, located within or around the involved nodules (fig. 20-11). In lymphocyte predominance Hodgkin's disease, splenic involvement may be evidenced only by small clusters of epithelioid histiocytes and lymphocytic and histiocytic (L&H) cells within or at the margin of the Malpighian bodies (62). Subtyping of Hodgkin's disease based on the splenic pathology is usually difficult and unnecessary, although the presence of prominent sclerosis and lacunar cells favors a diagnosis of the nodular sclerosis subtype (32).

For patients with well-documented Hodgkin's disease, it is not necessary to adhere to stringent

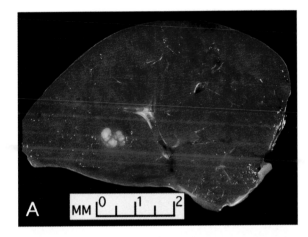

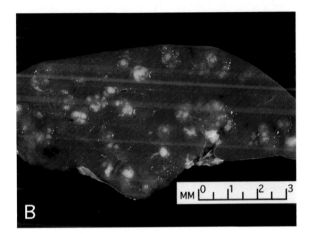

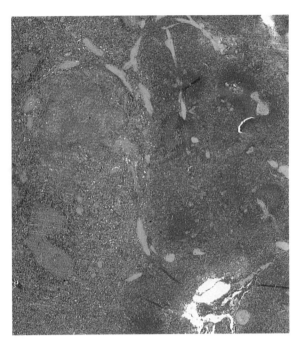

Figure 20-9
SPLENIC INVOLVEMENT BY HODGKIN'S DISEASE
A solitary focus of involvement is present in this spleen, appearing on low magnification as a large pale nodule (left middle field).

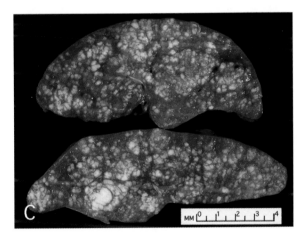

Figure 20-8
SPLENIC INVOLVEMENT BY HODGKIN'S DISEASE
A: A single focus composed of several contiguous small nodules.
B: More extensive involvement, with many variable-sized white nodules haphazardly scattered in the splenic parenchyma.
C: Massive involvement in the form of multiple nodules, some of which coalesce.

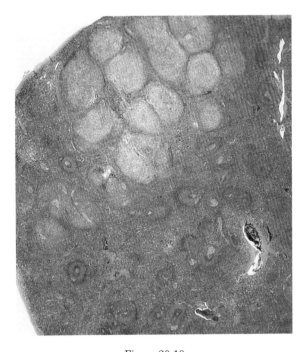

Figure 20-10
SPLENIC INVOLVEMENT BY HODGKIN'S DISEASE
Coalescent pale-staining nodules representing Malpighian corpuscles expanded by Hodgkin's disease are seen in the upper field. Another focus of early involvement is seen in the left middle field, in the form of slightly enlarged Malpighian corpuscles.

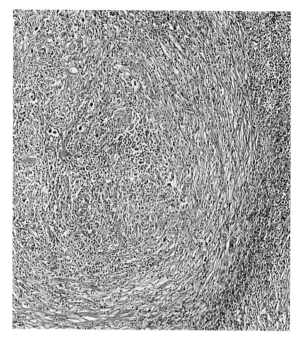

Figure 20-11
SPLENIC INVOLVEMENT BY HODGKIN'S DISEASE
The Malpighian corpuscle is expanded by a mixed cellular infiltrate, and is surrounded by sclerotic stroma.

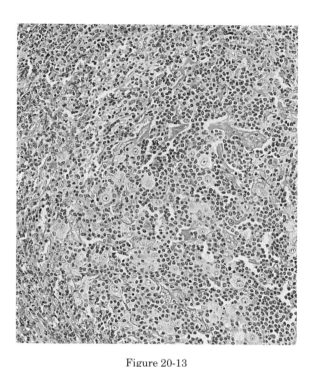

Figure 20-13
SPLENIC INVOLVEMENT BY HODGKIN'S DISEASE
Large cells with prominent nucleoli (consistent with mononuclear Hodgkin cells or lacunar cells) are scattered among small lymphocytes and occasional eosinophils, consistent with involvement by Hodgkin's disease.

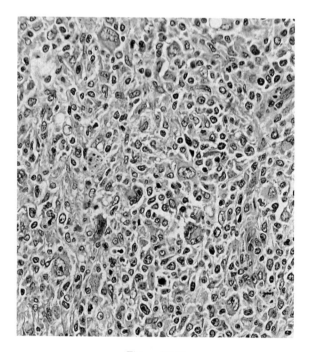

Figure 20-12
SPLENIC INVOLVEMENT BY HODGKIN'S DISEASE
Diagnostic Reed-Sternberg cells and mononuclear Reed-Sternberg cell variants are present in a mixed inflammatory background.

diagnostic criteria to determine whether the spleen is involved. Provided that there are Reed-Sternberg cell variants in an appropriate background, the spleen is considered involved even in the absence of diagnostic Reed-Sternberg cells (fig. 20-13) (36,51); even if only occasional large atypical cells with cytologic features falling short of those of Reed-Sternberg cell variants (so-called atypical reticulum cells) are found in an appropriate background, such features are also considered suggestive of involvement by Hodgkin's disease. Noncaseating epithelioid granulomas may be seen in the spleens of approximately 10 percent of patients with Hodgkin's disease (56), and they can even form macroscopic nodules. However, the presence of these granulomas should not be equated with splenic involvement by Hodgkin's disease, because they can occur in the absence of such involvement (44). After treatment with radiotherapy or chemotherapy, the eradicated disease in the spleen may appear as sclerotic nodules, with or without accumulation of foamy histiocytes (35).

Prognostic Factors. The presence of splenic involvement signifies more advanced disease, and treatment strategy has to be tailored accordingly. There is evidence suggesting that the spleen is a critical station in the hematogenous dissemination of Hodgkin's disease; involvement of the liver or bone marrow is rare in the absence of splenic disease. One study has shown that the presence of more than five grossly visible tumor nodules in the sectioned spleen is associated with a worse prognosis (43). Epithelioid granulomas in the spleen or liver of patients with Hodgkin's disease have been reported to be associated with a better 5-year overall survival as well as 5-year relapse-free survival (54,56); however, on extended follow-up, a significant survival advantage can no longer be demonstrated (27).

Non-Hodgkin's Lymphoma

The spleen is commonly involved in non-Hodgkin's lymphoma, particularly the low-grade type (Table 20-2). There is a propensity to involve the white pulp, with variable degrees of involvement of the red pulp (Table 20-1). The most common patterns of histologic involvement are listed in Table 20-3. Since all types of lymphoma may produce a nodular pattern in the spleen as a result of the normal nodular architecture of the white pulp, it is inappropriate to classify a lymphoma as follicular or diffuse on the basis of the pattern of splenic involvement alone (62).

A different viewpoint, championed by van Krieken (59,60), is that the widely held belief that the white pulp is commonly involved by lymphoma is incorrect, based on the observations that the preexisting white pulp is often atrophic, partially involved follicles are not seen, and the number of tumor nodules greatly exceeds the number of white pulp follicles. The nodules of lymphoma that are observed in the spleen arise instead from the red pulp. Most low-grade B-cell lymphomas involve predominantly the red pulp, with follicular lymphoma and lymphoplasmacytoid lymphoma showing a predilection for nodule formation in the non-filtering areas; sometimes there may be involvement of the T-cell areas. Post-thymic T-cell lymphomas involve predominantly the T-cell areas of the spleen. The large cell lymphomas destroy the splenic architecture and show no preference for certain compartments in the spleen. Inter-

Table 20-2

INCIDENCE OF SPLENIC INVOLVEMENT IN VARIOUS TYPES OF LYMPHOMA

Lymphoma Type	Frequency of Splenic Involvement at Diagnosis* (Percent)
Hodgkin's disease	
Lymphocyte predominance	11–23
Nodular sclerosis	39
Mixed cellularity	63
Lymphocyte depletion	67
Non-Hodgkin's lymphoma	
Small lymphocytic	60–100
Lymphoplasmacytoid	57
Mantle cell	57
Monocytoid B-cell and low-grade B-cell lymphoma of mucosa-associated lymphoid tissue	Rare
Follicular	49-61
Diffuse large cell	6-38
Post-thymic T-cell	?
Mycosis fungoides	25
Small noncleaved cell	?
Lymphoblastic	?

*From references 30,34,37,39,41,42,45-48,50,58,61.
? = Reliable information not available.

ested readers may refer to van Krieken's review on this subject (59,60).

Splenectomy is rarely performed in patients with a confirmed diagnosis of malignant lymphoma, except when complicated by significant hypersplenism. However, splenectomy is sometimes performed for diagnostic purposes in patients presenting with lymphoma confined to intra-abdominal sites.

Follicular Lymphoma

Splenic involvement by follicular lymphoma is common, and the involved spleen can be of normal weight. Grossly, the cut surface reveals miliary, discrete, small white nodules uniformly distributed throughout the entire parenchyma (fig. 20-14); the nodules can appear crowded. Haphazardly distributed large tumor nodules can occur

Table 20-3

COMMON PATTERNS OF SPLENIC INVOLVEMENT BY LYMPHOMA*

Multicentric involvement of white pulp
Follicular lymphoma

Irregular expansion of white pulp with spill-over into red pulp
Small lymphocytic lymphoma
Lymphoplasmacytoid lymphoma
Mantle cell lymphoma
Monocytoid B-cell lymphoma
Marginal zone B-cell lymphoma/splenic lymphoma with circulating villous lymphocytes
Follicular lymphoma
Diffuse large cell lymphoma
Mycosis fungoides
Small noncleaved (Burkitt's) lymphoma
Lymphoblastic lymphoma
Hodgkin's disease

Early localization to periarteriolar lymphoid sheath and/or marginal zone**
Hodgkin's disease
Post-thymic T-cell lymphoma, including Lennert's lymphoma and mycosis fungoides
Lymphoblastic lymphoma
Monocytoid B-cell lymphoma
Marginal zone B-cell lymphoma

Diffuse infiltration of red pulp[†]
Small lymphocytic lymphoma
Mycosis fungoides
Diffuse large cell lymphoma of B- or T-lineage, including so-called malignant histiocytosis

*Adapted from references 31,32.
**Systemic mastocytosis can also exhibit this pattern.
[†]Leukemic infiltration, with the exception of chronic lymphocytic leukemia, typically shows this pattern of splenic infiltration.

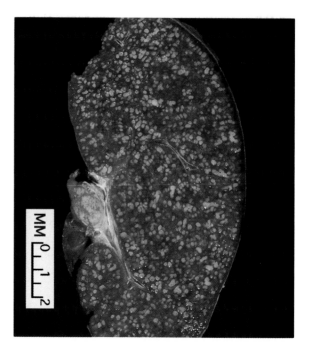

Figure 20-14
SPLENIC INVOLVEMENT BY FOLLICULAR LYMPHOMA
This illustration depicts the classic appearance of spleen involved by follicular lymphoma, namely the presence of discrete, miliary, small, white "pearly" nodules throughout the whole parenchyma.

in follicular lymphoma of large cell type (fig. 20-15) (48). Histologically, the white pulp is uniformly involved, although the replaced Malpighian bodies may vary in size and may coalesce (fig. 20-16). The neoplastic nodules in the white pulp can be surrounded by a residual mantle zone and marginal zone cells. There are often smaller nodules which appear to have "sprouted out" in the red pulp (fig. 20-16, left). Cases composed predominantly of small cleaved cells (centrocytes) are easily recognized by the cytologic monotony, predominance of small cells, and lack of tingible body macrophages (fig. 20-17). Recognition of follicular lymphoma composed of a mixed cell population is more difficult, because the

cytologic composition resembles that of reactive follicles. The best clues are the absence of tingible body macrophages and the identification of smaller nodules composed of similar cells in the red pulp (fig. 20-18). In difficult cases, immunohistochemical studies (light chain restriction and *bcl*-2 protein expression) are required to confirm involvement.

Small Lymphocytic, Lymphoplasmacytoid, and Mantle Cell Lymphomas

Small lymphocytic, lymphoplasmacytoid, and mantle cell lymphomas frequently involve the spleen. The beefy red splenic parenchyma is uniformly studded with miliary small white nodules that are often less well defined than those seen in follicular lymphoma. Some nodules can become confluent. Histologically, the white pulp is irregularly expanded by small lymphoid cells, with concomitant involvement of the red pulp in the form of irregular small clusters and a diffuse

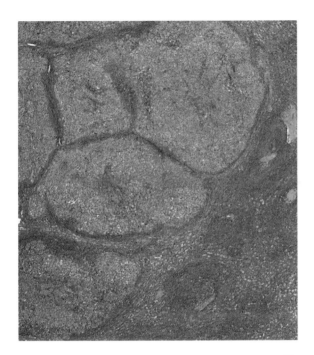
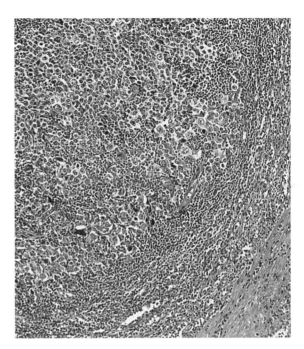

Figure 20-15
SPLENIC INVOLVEMENT BY FOLLICULAR LARGE CELL LYMPHOMA
Left: In this example, the involvement takes the form of several large coalescent nodules with sparing of other parts of the spleen.
Right: The nodules are composed of large noncleaved cells (centroblasts). Normal red pulp tissue is seen in the lower field.

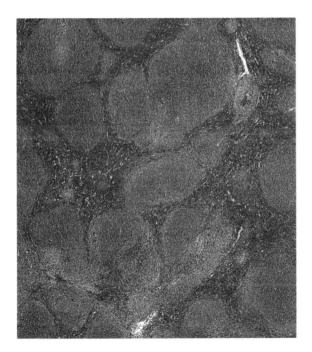
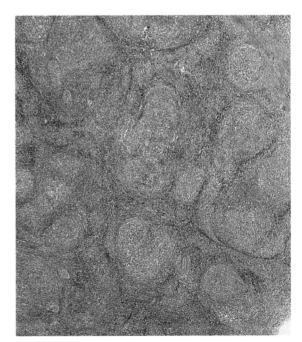

Figure 20-16
SPLENIC INVOLVEMENT BY FOLLICULAR LYMPHOMA
Left: Note the characteristic generalized involvement of the Malpighian bodies, which are variably expanded. Smaller nodules composed of similar cells can also be identified in the red pulp.
Right: Another example showing more extensive involvement. The Malpighian corpuscles are markedly expanded, with little red pulp tissue in between.

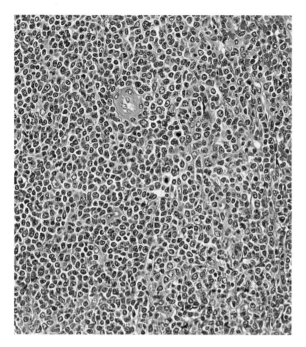

Figure 20-17
SPLENIC INVOLVEMENT BY
FOLLICULAR LYMPHOMA
The Malpighian body is replaced by a fairly monotonous population of small cleaved cells (centrocytes) mixed with small numbers of large noncleaved cells (centroblasts). In this nodule, there is no identifiable mantle zone or marginal zone.

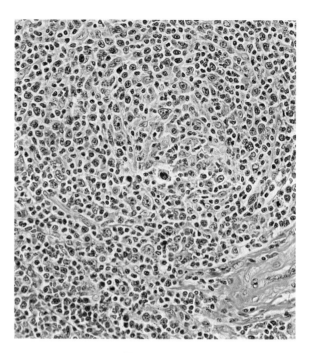

Figure 20-18
SPLENIC INVOLVEMENT BY
FOLLICULAR LYMPHOMA
This example of follicular mixed cell lymphoma comprises a mixture of small cleaved cells (centrocytes) and large noncleaved cells (centroblasts) in the absence of tingible body macrophages. The mantle zone is poorly defined.

infiltrate (figs. 20-19, 20-20, left). The white pulp nodules can also coalesce. The neoplastic nature of the process can be recognized by the monotony of the small lymphoid cells (fig. 20-20, right), involvement of the red pulp, and subendothelial infiltration of the trabecular veins (49); confirmation of diagnosis can be obtained by immunohistochemical studies.

In small lymphocytic lymphoma, the intermingled larger cells (prolymphocytes and paraimmunoblasts) may lead to confusion with mixed cell lymphoma. Some cases are accompanied by numerous clusters of epithelioid histiocytes, which may mask the neoplastic process (32,49).

In lymphoplasmacytoid lymphoma, the neoplastic infiltrate can sometimes be localized predominantly in the mantle zone of the white pulp. There is also a variant form of lymphoplasmacytoid lymphoma displaying a peculiar zonal distribution instead of the usual intermixing of the cell types (28). In these cases, the small lymphocytes occupy the Malpighian bodies, while the lymphoplasmacytoid cells and plasma

cells are seen in the mantle and marginal zones, with spill into the red pulp.

In mantle cell lymphoma, the neoplastic cells grow as broad rims around the residual atrophic germinal centers of the Malpighian bodies, and are surrounded by residual marginal zone cells (53). Sometimes the neoplastic cells invade and replace the germinal centers. Their neoplastic nature is evidenced by the coalescence of the lymphoid mantles of adjacent Malpighian bodies and the presence of large numbers of similar cells in the red pulp. In difficult cases, immunohistochemical studies can be done to demonstrate light chain restriction.

Monocytoid B-Cell Lymphoma

Monocytoid B-cell lymphoma rarely involves the spleen. Although the monocytoid B cells are cytologically very similar to the neoplastic cells of hairy cell leukemia, the two diseases show different patterns of splenic infiltration. The former shows predominant involvement of the white pulp, while the latter predominant involvement of the red pulp (32). The lymphoma cells are often confined to the marginal zones, surrounding the residual germinal centers and their mantles. They can also surround primary follicles. There is variable extension of the neoplastic cells into the red pulp.

Diffuse Large Cell Lymphoma

Splenic involvement by large cell lymphoma can result in a number of patterns: a large solitary fleshy nodule; multiple large coalescent fleshy nodules; or diffuse expansion of the splenic parenchyma, with a beefy red appearance. Necrosis and hemorrhage can occur within the tumor nodules, which histologically are composed of diffuse compact sheets of large lymphoma cells, with total obliteration of the normal splenic architecture (see figs. 20-4, 20-6). Sclerosis is prominent in some cases (49). In those cases showing a diffuse pattern of involvement, there is haphazard permeation of the pulp cords and sinusoids of the red pulp by isolated lymphoma cells (see fig. 20-5), sometimes accompanied by an increase in reactive erythrophagocytic histiocytes. This is also the pattern traditionally considered to be characteristic of so-called malignant histiocytosis (57).

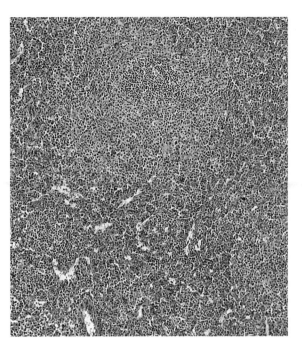

Figure 20-19
SPLENIC INVOLVEMENT BY
LYMPHOPLASMACYTOID LYMPHOMA
In contrast to follicular lymphoma (compare with figure 20-16), the expanded Malpighian corpuscles do not have discrete outlines; smaller lymphoid nodules are also seen in the red pulp.

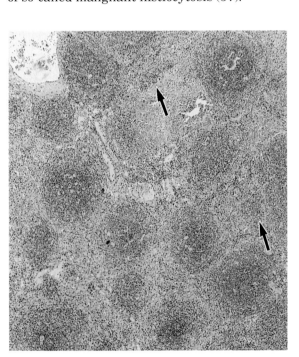

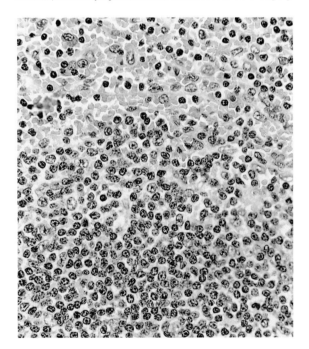

Figure 20-20
SPLENIC INVOLVEMENT BY SMALL LYMPHOCYTIC LYMPHOMA/CHRONIC LYMPHOCYTIC LEUKEMIA
Left: The Malpighian bodies are replaced by dense infiltrates of dark-staining small lymphocytes. Note that the red pulp is also involved by similar infiltrates (arrow).
Right: The white pulp is replaced by a monotonous infiltrate of small lymphocytes mixed with rare larger cells having nuclei with prominent nucleoli (prolymphocytes). The red pulp (upper field) is similarly infiltrated.

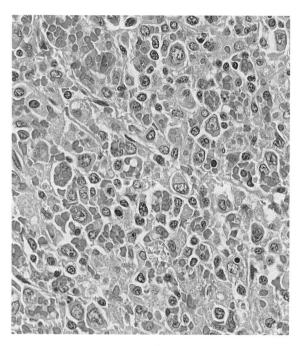

Figure 20-21
SPLENIC INVOLVEMENT BY LARGE T-CELL
LYMPHOMA ASSOCIATED WITH REACTIVE
HEMOPHAGOCYTOSIS
The red pulp of the spleen is diffusely permeated by large lymphoma cells (T lineage) and histiocytes showing erythrophagocytosis. The histiocytes have smaller, bland-looking nuclei with delicate chromatin.

Post-Thymic T-Cell Lymphoma

The patterns of splenic involvement by post-thymic T-cell lymphoma can be indistinguishable from those of large cell lymphoma. However, in some cases, the tumor may be confined to the periarteriolar lymphoid sheaths and marginal zones (32,57,61). Sometimes, epithelioid histiocytes form wreaths around the white pulp nodules. There can be an increase in reactive histiocytes showing erythrophagocytosis (fig. 20-21).

The pattern of splenic involvement in mycosis fungoides is varied (61). It can take the form of a diffuse infiltrate in the red pulp, irregular nodules in the red and white pulp, or localization in the periarteriolar lymphoid sheath.

Other Lymphoma Types

Since splenectomy is rarely performed for patients with small noncleaved cell (Burkitt's) lymphoma and lymphoblastic lymphoma, information on their patterns of splenic involvement is limited. In small noncleaved cell lymphoma, the neoplastic cells usually infiltrate both the white and red pulp, but the white pulp may be selectively involved in occasional cases (29,52,62). In T-lymphoblastic lymphoma, the neoplastic cells are localized to the periarteriolar lymphoid sheath in the early phase, and diffusely infiltrate the red pulp with obliteration of the white pulp in more advanced disease (32).

LYMPHOMA PRESENTING WITH PROMINENT SPLENOMEGALY

Almost any histologic type of non-Hodgkin's lymphoma can present initially with splenomegaly (69). There are, however, several types of lymphoma that present with prominent splenomegaly and distinctive clinicopathologic features, such as *hepatosplenic T-cell lymphoma, lymphoplasmacytoid lymphoma, splenic lymphoma with circulating villous lymphocytes,* and *marginal zone cell lymphoma.* Hollema et al. (68) found that small lymphocytic lymphoma with predominant splenomegaly differs from conventional small lymphocytic lymphoma in that proliferation centers are absent; CD5, CD23, and CD43 are often not expressed; but CD45RO (UCHL1) is sometimes expressed. It is likely that these cases represent marginal zone B-cell lymphoma rather than B-cell small lymphocytic lymphoma/chronic lymphocytic leukemia as strictly defined. Most cases reported in the literature as "nontropical idiopathic splenomegaly" (65) probably represent low-grade small cell lymphoma (69), because half of the patients develop systemic lymphoma on extended follow-up (66).

In 1977, Braylan et al. (63) reported three cases of small cell lymphoma involving the spleen, in which the diagnosis of lymphoma was obscured by extensive epithelioid granulomas (fig. 20-22). A prominent epithelioid histiocytic reaction can in fact be observed in a wide variety of B-cell and T-cell lymphomas, and does not necessarily indicate a specific lymphoma type. It is helpful to assess the lymphoid cells in between the histiocytic components for nuclear atypia (fig. 20-22). Examination of additional histologic materials, such as lymph node biopsy, may help clarify the diagnosis; immunohistochemical and genotypic studies are useful for difficult cases. It should be noted, however, that benign diseases can also be associated with prominent epithelioid granulomas in the spleen (64,67,70).

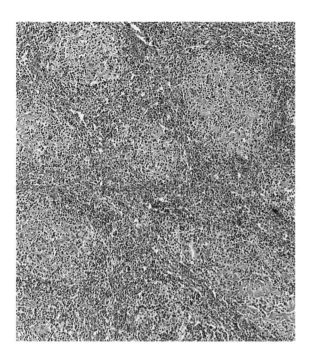 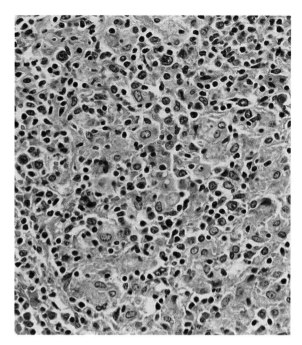

Figure 20-22
SPLENIC LYMPHOMA WITH PROMINENT EPITHELIOID CELL REACTION

Left: The white pulp is irregularly expanded.
Right: In the white pulp, small clusters of epithelioid histiocytes are admixed with lymphoid cells. The diagnosis of lymphoma is suggested by the atypia of the small and large lymphoid cells.

Hepatosplenic T-Cell Lymphoma

Clinical Features. Hepatosplenic T-cell lymphoma is a rare but distinctive form of lymphoma preferentially involving the sinusoids of the spleen, liver, and bone marrow. It typically occurs in young adults (predominantly male), who present with fever, hepatosplenomegaly, and cytopenia. The clinical evolution is highly variable, but most patients die within a few years despite treatment (72,73,75–77). The tumor reported as erythrophagocytic Tγ lymphoma may represent the same entity but with erythrophagocytic activity by the lymphoma cells (74).

Microscopic Findings. The red pulp of the spleen, including the sinuses and pulp cords, is infiltrated by a monotonous population of medium-sized neoplastic lymphoid cells (fig. 20-23). The nuclei of these cells are round or irregularly folded, and nucleoli are usually not prominent. The cells possess an appreciable amount of pale cytoplasm. They do not show erythrophagocytosis. Similar lymphoid cells infiltrate the hepatic and bone marrow sinusoids (fig. 20-24). A deceptive feature of this lymphoma is that the neoplastic cells may appear cohesive, mimicking carcinoma

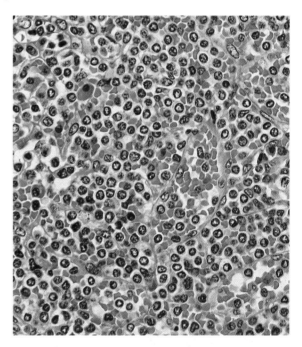

Figure 20-23
HEPATOSPLENIC GAMMA/DELTA T-CELL
LYMPHOMA INVOLVING THE SPLEEN

The splenic sinusoids and pulp cords are infiltrated by medium-sized lymphoid cells. Note the striking resemblance to hairy cell leukemia. (Courtesy of Dr. Philippe Gaulard, Creteil, France.)

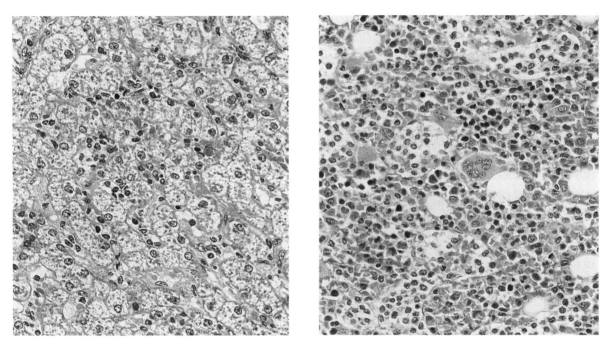

Figure 20-24
HEPATOSPLENIC GAMMA/DELTA T-CELL LYMPHOMA
Left: Medium-sized lymphoid cells are scattered in the sinusoids of the liver.
Right: In the bone marrow, similar cells are confined to the sinusoids.

(76). The histologic appearance of the spleen may strongly mimic hairy cell leukemia (77).

Immunologic Findings. The neoplastic cells stain with various T-lineage markers. They are often CD3 and CD 56 positive. Most cases characteristically express the gamma/delta T-cell receptor (72,73,77), although occasional cases express the alpha/beta receptor (75). A significant percentage of T cells occurring in the normal splenic red pulp also express the gamma/delta T-cell receptor (71), raising the possibility of preferential homing to a distinct histologic microenvironment in hepatosplenic T-cell lymphoma.

Genotypic Findings. On genotypic analysis, tumors expressing the gamma/delta T-cell receptor show clonal rearrangements of the gamma-chain or delta-chain T-cell receptor gene, while the beta-chain T-cell receptor gene is either in germline or rearranged configuration (73,76).

Lymphoplasmacytoid Lymphoma (Immunocytoma) of the Spleen

Clinical Features. Lymphoplasmacytoid lymphoma (immunocytoma) sometimes has prominent splenic involvement, which presents as splenomegaly (the so-called splenomegalic type) (81). Although such cases are often reported in the literature as "primary splenic lymphoma," they do not satisfy the strict criteria required for this diagnosis because of the frequent concomitant involvement of bone marrow and liver (78). Some cases reported in the literature as small lymphocytic lymphoma or well-differentiated lymphocytic lymphoma of the spleen may also represent lymphoplasmacytoid lymphoma (80,82). This type of lymphoma usually occurs in patients over the age of 50 years, who present with systemic symptoms and splenomegaly. Serum M-protein is often detected. The prognosis appears to be favorable, at least in the short term (78,79). Among 11 cases in one study, 9 were alive and well after 1 to 14 years, and 2 died from infection within 1 year. Most of these patients had been treated by splenectomy and chemotherapy (single agent or multiagent chemotherapy including cyclophosphamide, vincristine, and prednisone) (78).

Pathologic Findings. The enlarged spleen usually weighs more than 500 g, and exhibits numerous small whitish nodules on the cut surface. Histologically, the white pulp is replaced by a

 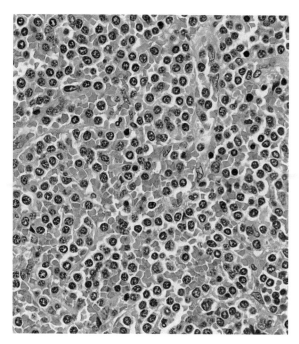

Figure 20-25
SPLENIC INVOLVEMENT BY LYMPHOPLASMACYTOID LYMPHOMA
Left: The red pulp (ill-defined small nodules) is involved in addition to the white pulp (larger nodules with ill-defined outlines).
Right: The small lymphoid cells have an eccentric rim of basophilic cytoplasm.

mixture of small lymphocytes, lymphoplasma-cytoid cells, plasma cells, and immunoblasts (fig. 20-25). A similar infiltrate is often present in the red pulp, sometimes associated with formation of small poorly defined nodules. Light chain restriction can often be demonstrated in the lymphoma cells.

Splenic B-Cell Lymphoma with Circulating Villous Lymphocytes

Clinical Features. In 1987, Melo et al. (87,88) described a form of B-cell lymphoma showing preferential splenic involvement and circulating villous lymphocytes that was distinct from hairy cell leukemia (83,91). This entity had been previously reported in 1979 by Neiman et al. (90) as "malignant lymphoma simulating leukemic reticuloendotheliosis." The lymphoma occurs predominantly in elderly men (median age 68.4 years), who present with gross splenomegaly but little or no lymphadenopathy. Monoclonal gammopathy, usually IgM type, is identified in the serum of two thirds of patients. The disease is indolent, with 5-year survival of 78 percent (89). Most deaths are due to unrelated diseases rather than the underlying lymphoma. Large cell trans-

formation can occur in a minority of cases (92). There may be a higher incidence of splenic lymphoma with villous lymphocytes in tropical West Africa than in the western world (83).

Pathologic Findings. The circulating lymphoma cells have round nuclei slightly larger than those of small lymphocytes, clumped chromatin, and a single small nucleolus. The nuclei are sometimes eccentrically placed. The cytoplasm is relatively abundant and basophilic, with unevenly distributed short thin villi frequently concentrated in one pole of the cell (fig. 20-26). Some cells are obviously plasmacytoid. In contrast to hairy cell leukemia, the neoplastic cells are smaller, the nuclear chromatin is more clumped, the nucleoli are more obvious, the cytoplasm is more basophilic, and the villi are fewer and clustered. They usually lack tartrate-resistant acid phosphatase activity.

The bone marrow is involved in 75 percent of cases. There is patchy infiltration of lymphoma cells, often in a nodular pattern, but the involvement can be minimal and subtle.

The spleen usually weighs over 1 kg. There is predominant involvement of the white pulp, with variable involvement of the red pulp (fig. 20-27);

427

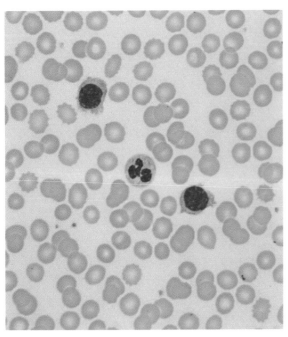

Figure 20-26
SPLENIC B-CELL LYMPHOMA WITH
CIRCULATING VILLOUS LYMPHOCYTES
In the peripheral blood, the small lymphoid cells have
dark round nuclei, lightly basophilic cytoplasm, and bipolar
surface villous processes.

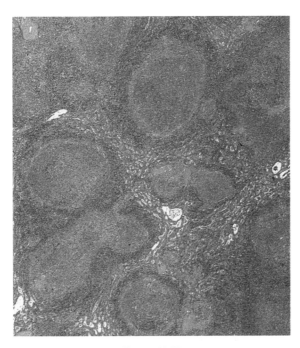

Figure 20-27
SPLENIC B-CELL LYMPHOMA WITH
CIRCULATING VILLOUS LYMPHOCYTES
The spleen shows a "lymphomatous" rather than "leuke-
mic" pattern of involvement, with predominant infiltration
of the white pulp.

Table 20-4

**REPORTED IMMUNOPHENOTYPIC
PROFILE OF SPLENIC LYMPHOMA
WITH VILLOUS LYMPHOCYTES,
BASED ON ANALYSIS OF 100 CASES***

Antibody		Percent Positive Cases
Surface immunoglobulin light chain	Kappa:	60
	Lambda:	40
CD22		95
FMC7		89
CD11c		47
CD10		30
CD23		31
CD25		25
CD5		19
CD103		15
HC2		9

*From reference 86.

there is never exclusive involvement of the red
pulp as usually observed in hairy cell leukemia.
The infiltrate comprises nodular aggregates of
small to medium-sized lymphoid cells with
clumped chromatin; the larger cells are often concentrated in the periphery, producing a zonation
phenomenon. Lymphoplasmacytic differentiation
may be evident (fig. 20-28). The bone marrow
shows variable and patchy infiltration by lymphoma cells, often in a nodular pattern.

**Immunophenotypic and Genotypic Find-
ings.** The immunophenotypic profile of splenic
lymphoma with villous lymphocytes is shown in
Table 20-4 (86,89). The lymphoma cells stain with
various B-cell markers and surface immunoglobulins. No case shows the combined immunophenotype characteristic of hairy cell leukemia:
anti-HC2+, CD25+, CD103 (B-ly7)+, CD11c+; or
the combined phenotype of B-cell chronic lymphocytic leukemia/small lymphocytic lymphoma:
CD5+, CD23+, FMC7-.

Of 22 cases studied, none shows *bcl*-2 gene
rearrangement (84); approximately 15 percent
show the translocation t(11;14)(q13;q32) with
implication of the *bcl*-1 (*CCND*1) gene (85).

Nosologic Considerations. Splenic B-cell
lymphoma with villous lymphocytes appears to be
a heterogeneous entity, encompassing marginal
zone B-cell lymphoma, lymphoplasmacytic/

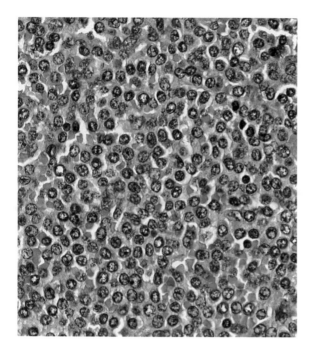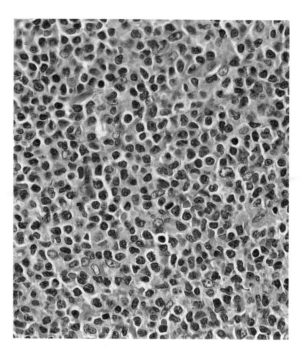

FIGURE 20-28
SPLENIC B-CELL LYMPHOMA WITH CIRCULATING VILLOUS LYMPHOCYTES
Left: In this example, the lymphoma cells have a lymphoplasmacytoid appearance.
Right: In this example, the lymphoma cells have a moderate amount of pale cytoplasm. Note similarity with splenic marginal
zone B-cell lymphoma (figure 20-30).

lymphoplasmacytoid lymphoma (as evidenced by the plasmacytoid appearance of the neoplastic cells and frequent association with monoclonal gammopathy), and mantle cell lymphoma (92). It has also been suggested that this is a single clinicopathologic entity that is identical to splenic marginal zone B-cell lymphoma (84a).

Malignant Lymphoma of Marginal Zone Cells

Clinical Features. In the white pulp of the spleen, a well-defined pale-staining marginal zone normally surrounds the lymphoid follicles in the white pulp. A small number of cases of splenic marginal zone cell lymphoma have now been reported (93,95,96). The patients present with splenomegaly, anemia, and weight loss. Besides the spleen, the bone marrow and other sites such as the liver are commonly involved. There are too few cases and the follow-up is too short for any conclusion to be drawn regarding the behavior of this lymphoma, but the disease appears indolent (96). Palutke et al. (94) reported two cases of splenic large cell lymphoma of alleged marginal

zone cell origin, but the evidence in support of the marginal zone nature is not conclusive.

Pathologic, Immunologic, and Genotypic Findings. The cut surface of the enlarged spleen reveals multiple, small, grey-white nodules. Histologically, broad rims of medium-sized lymphoid cells surround the follicle centers of the white pulp and may coalesce (fig. 20-29). The nuclei of the lymphoid cells are round or indented, the chromatin is moderately condensed, and there is a moderate rim of pale cytoplasm (fig. 20-30). These cells may invade the mantle zones and even replace the germinal centers. Red pulp involvement is common. The bone marrow infiltration is often paratrabecular (96).

The lymphoma cells express various B-cell markers, but not CD5, CD10, CD23, or CD25. There is also light chain restriction. Genotypic studies show rearrangements of the immunoglobulin, but not the *bcl*-1 and *bcl*-2 genes (95,96).

Differential Diagnosis. Cytologically and immunophenotypically, marginal zone cell lymphoma cannot be distinguished from low-grade B-cell lymphoma of mucosa-associated lymphoid

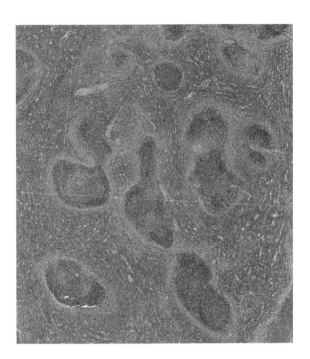
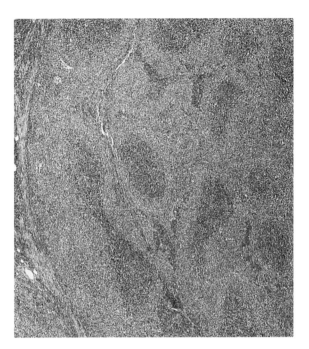

Figure 20-29
MARGINAL ZONE CELL LYMPHOMA

Left: In the spleen, the marginal zone is expanded, with areas of coalescence.
Right: The splenic hilar lymph node also displays a marginal zone pattern (pale-staining areas) of involvement. (Courtesy of Professor Peter Isaacson, London, UK.)

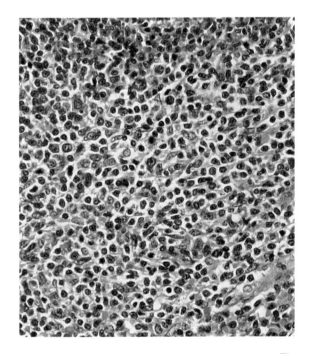
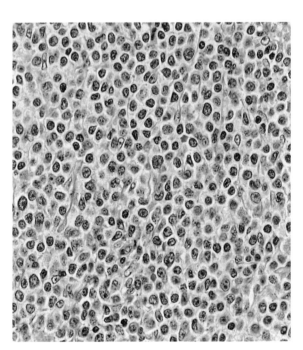

Figure 20-30
MARGINAL ZONE CELL LYMPHOMA INVOLVING SPLEEN

Morphologic spectrum of the neoplastic marginal zone cells.
Left: Relatively small cells with slightly irregular and dark nuclei. There is a thin rim of pale cytoplasm.
Right: Medium-sized cells with slightly irregular nuclei and an appreciable amount of cytoplasm. (Courtesy of Professor Peter Isaacson, London, UK.)

tissue and monocytoid B-cell lymphoma. In fact, the proposed cell of origin of all these lymphoma types is the marginal zone cell. However, based on currently available evidence, it appears justified to keep splenic marginal zone cell lymphoma separate, because it differs clinically from these other lymphoma types by virtue of the disseminated disease process. It has recently been suggested that splenic marginal zone B-cell lymphoma overlaps greatly with splenic lymphoma with villous lymphocytes or may in fact represent the same entity (84a).

REFERENCES

Primary Splenic Lymphoma

1. Ahmann DL, Kiely JM, Harrison EG Jr, Payne WS. Primary lymphoma of the spleen. A review of 49 cases in which the diagnosis was made at splenectomy. Cancer 1966;19:461–9.

2. Bellany CO, Krajewski AJ. Primary splenic large cell anaplastic lymphoma associated with HIV infection. Histopathology 1994;24:481–3.

3. Brox A, Bishinsky JI, Berry G. Primary non-Hodgkin lymphoma of the spleen. Am J Hematol 1991;38:95–100.

4. _____, Shustik C. Non-Hodgkin's lymphoma of the spleen. Leuk Lymphoma 1993;11:165–71.

5. Burke JS, Osborne BM. Localized reactive lymphoid hyperplasia of the spleen simulating malignant lymphoma. A report of seven cases. Am J Surg Pathol 1983;7:373–80.

6. Butler JJ. Pathology of the spleen in benign and malignant conditions. Histopathology 1983;7:453–74.

7. Das Gupta T, Coombes B, Brasfeld RD. Primary malignant neoplasms of the spleen. Surg Gynecol Obstet 1965;120:947–60.

8. Falk S, Karhoff M, Takeshita M, Stutte HJ. Primary pleomorphic T-cell lymphoma of the spleen. Histopathology 1990;16:191–2.

9. _____, Stutte HJ. Primary malignant lymphomas of the spleen, a morphologic and immunohistochemical analysis of 17 cases. Cancer 1990;66:2612–9.

10. Fausel R, Sun NC, Klein S. Splenic rupture in HIV-infected patient with primary splenic lymphoma. Cancer 1990;66:2414–6.

11. Franchino C, Reich C, Distenfeld A, Ubriaco A, Knowles DM. A clinicopathologically distinctive primary splenic histiocytic neoplasm. Demonstration of its histiocytic derivation by immunophenotypic and molecular genetic analysis. Am J Surg Pathol 1988;12:398–404.

12. Gastineau DA, Banks PM, Knowles DM. Primary splenic neoplasm [Letter]. Am J Surg Pathol 1989;13:989.

13. Hara K, Ito M, Shimizu K, Matsumoto T, Suchi T, Iijima S. Three cases of primary splenic lymphoma. Case report and review of the Japanese literature. Acta Pathol Jpn 1985;35:419–35.

14. Harris NL. Localized lymphoid hyperplasia of the spleen [Letter]. Am J Surg Pathol 1984;8:557–8.

15. _____, Aisenberg AC, Meyer JE, Ellman L, Elman A. Diffuse large cell (histiocytic) lymphoma of the spleen. Clinical and pathological characteristics of ten cases. Cancer 1984;54:2460–7.

16. Ishihara T, Takahashi M, Uchino F, Matsumoto N. A filiform large cell lymphoma of the spleen: a case report with immunohistochemical and electron microscopic study. Ultrastruct Pathol 1990;14:193–9.

17. Kehoe J, Straus DJ. Primary lymphoma of the spleen. Clinical features and outcome after splenectomy. Cancer 1988;62:1433–8.

18. Kobrich U, Falk S, Karhoff M, Middeke B, Anselstetter V, Stutte HJ. Primary large cell lymphoma of the splenic sinuses: a variant of angiotropic B-cell lymphoma (neoplastic angioendotheliomatosis)? Hum Pathol 1992;23:1184–7.

19. Kraemer BB, Osborne BM, Butler JJ. Primary splenic presentation of malignant lymphoma and related disorders. A study of 49 cases. Cancer 1984;54:1606–19.

20. Long JC, Aisenberg AC. Malignant lymphoma diagnosed at splenectomy and idiopathic splenomegaly. A clinicopathologic comparison. Cancer 1974;33:1054–61.

21. Montanaro A, Patton R. Primary splenic malignant lymphoma, histiocytic type, with sclerosis: report of a case with long-term survival. Cancer 1976;38:1625–8.

22. Narang S, Wolf BC, Neiman RS. Malignant lymphoma presenting with prominent splenomegaly. A clinicopathologic study with special reference to intermediate cell lymphoma. Cancer 1985;55:1948–57.

23. Offit K, Lo Coco F, Louie DC, et al. Rearrangement of the bcl-6 gene as a prognostic marker in diffuse large-cell lymphoma. N Engl J Med 1994;331:74–80.

24. Spier CM, Kjeldsberg CR, Eyre HJ, Behm FG. Malignant lymphoma with primary presentation in the spleen. A study of 20 patients. Arch Pathol Lab Med 1985;109:1076–80.

25. Weide R, Gorg C, Pfluger KH, et al. Concomitant primary low grade non-Hodgkin's lymphoma of the spleen and breast carcinoma. Leuk Lymphoma 1992;7:337–9.

26. Zellers RA, Thibodeau SN, Banks PM. Primary splenic lymphocyte depletion Hodgkin's disease. Am J Clin Pathol 1990;94:453–7.

Splenic Involvement by Lymphoma

27. Abrams J, Pearl P, Moody M, Schimpff SC. Epithelioid granulomas revisited: long-term follow-up in Hodgkin's disease. Am J Clin Oncol 1988;11:456–60.

28. Alberti VN, Neiman RS. Lymphoplasmacytic lymphoma. A clinicopathologic study of a previously unrecognized composite variant. Cancer 1984;53:1103–8.

29. Banks PM, Arseneau JC, Gralnick HR, Cannelos GP, DeVita VT Jr, Berard CW. American Burkitt's lymphoma: a clinicopathologic study of 30 cases. II. Pathologic correlations. Am J Med 1975;58:322–9.

30. Brittinger G, Bartels H, Common H, et al. Clinical and prognostic relevance of the Kiel classification of non-Hodgkin lymphomas, results of a prospective multicenter study by the Kiel Lymphoma Study Group. Hematol Oncol 1984;2:269–306.

31. Burke JS. The diagnosis of lymphoma and lymphoid proliferations in the spleen. In: Jaffe ES, ed. Surgical pathology of the lymph nodes and related organs. Major problems in pathology, Vol. 16. Philadelphia: WB Saunders, 1985:249–81.

32. _____. The spleen. In: Sternberg SS, Antonioli DA, Carter D, Mills SE, Oberman HA, eds. Diagnostic surgical pathology. 2nd ed. New York: Raven Press, 1994:735–57.

33. Butler JJ. Pathology of the spleen in benign and malignant conditions. Histopathology 1983;7:453–74.

34. Castellani R, Bonadonna G, Spinelli P, Bajetta E, Galante E, Rilke F. Sequential pathologic staging of untreated non-Hodgkin's lymphomas by laparoscopy and laparotomy combined with bone marrow biopsy. Cancer 1977;40:2322–8.

35. Colby TV, Hoppe RT, Warnke RA. Hodgkin's disease at autopsy: 1972-1977. Cancer 1981;47:1852–62.

36. Dorfman RF. Formal discussion of Robert J. Lukes' paper, "Criteria for involvement of lymph node, spleen, and liver in Hodgkin's disease." Cancer Res 1971;31:1768–9.

37. _____. Relationship of histology to site in Hodgkin's disease. Cancer Res 1971;31:1786–93.

38. _____, Colby TV. The pathologist's role in management of patients with Hodgkin's disease. Cancer Treat Rep 1982;66:675–80.

39. Falk S, Stutte HJ. Morphologic manifestations of malignant lymphomas in the spleen; a histologic and immunohistochemical study of 500 biopsy cases. In: Fenoglio-Preiser CM, Wolff M, Rilke F, eds. Field & Wood, 1992:49–95. (Progress in Surgical Pathology, Vol. 12).

40. Farrer-Brown G, Bennett MH, Harrison CV, Millett Y, Jelliffe AM. The diagnosis of Hodgkin's disease in surgically excised spleens. J Clin Pathol 1972;25:294–300.

41. Glatstein E, Trueblood HW, Enright LP, Rosenberg SA, Kaplan HS. Surgical staging of abdominal involvement in unselected patients with Hodgkin's disease. Radiology 1970;97:425–32.

42. Goffinet DR, Warnke R, Dunnick NR, et al. Clinical and surgical (laparotomy) evaluation of patients with non-Hodgkin's lymphomas. Cancer Treat Rep 1977;61:981–92.

43. Hoppe RT, Rosenberg SA, Kaplan HS, Cox RS. Prognostic factors in pathological stage IIIA Hodgkin's disease. Cancer 1980;46:1240–6.

44. Kadin ME, Donaldson SS, Dorfman RF. Isolated granulomas in Hodgkin's disease. N Engl J Med 1970;283:859–61.

45. _____, Glatstein E, Dorfman RF. Clinicopathologic studies of 117 untreated patients subjected to laparotomy for staging of Hodgkin's disease. Cancer 1971; 27:1277–94.

46. Kaplan HS. Hodgkin's disease. 2nd ed. Cambridge: Harvard University Press, 1980:52–115.

47. _____, Dorfman RF, Nelson TS, Rosenberg SA. Staging laparotomy and splenectomy in Hodgkin's disease: analysis of indications and patterns of involvement in 285 consecutive, unselected patients. Natl Cancer Inst Monogr 1973;36:291–301.

48. Kim H, Dorfman RF. Morphological studies of 84 untreated patients subjected to laparotomy for the staging of non-Hodgkin's lymphomas. Cancer 1974;33:657–74.

49. Kraemer BB, Osborne BM, Butler JJ. Primary splenic presentation of malignant lymphoma and related disorders. A study of 49 cases. Cancer 1984;54:1606–19.

50. Lotz MJ, Chabner B, DeVita VT Jr, Johnson RE, Berard CW. Pathological staging of 100 consecutive untreated patients with non-Hodgkin's lymphomas: extramedullary sites of disease. Cancer 1976;37:266–70.

51. Lukes RJ. Criteria for involvement of lymph node, bone marrow, spleen, and liver in Hodgkin's disease. Cancer Res 1971;31:1755–67.

52. Mann RB, Jaffe ES, Braylan RC, Nanba K, Frank MM, Ziegler JL, Berard CW. Non-endemic Burkitt's lymphoma. A B-cell tumor related to germinal centers. N Engl J Med 1976;295:685–91.

53. Narang S, Wolf BC, Neiman RS. Malignant lymphoma presenting with prominent splenomegaly. A clinicopathologic study with special reference to intermediate cell lymphoma. Cancer 1985;55:1948–57.

54. O'Connell MJ, Schimpff SC, Kirschner RH, Abt AB, Wiernik PH. Epithelioid granulomas in Hodgkin's disease. A favorable prognostic sign? JAMA 1975;233:886–9.

55. Rosenberg SA. Exploratory laparotomy and splenectomy for Hodgkin's disease: a commentary [Editorial]. J Clin Oncol 1988;6:574–5.

56. Sacks EL, Donaldson SS, Gordon J, Dorfman RF. Epithelioid granulomas associated with Hodgkin's disease: clinical correlations in 55 previously untreated patients. Cancer 1978;41:562–7.

57. Stroup RM, Burke JS, Sheibani K, Ben-Ezra J, Brownwell M, Winberg CD. Splenic involvement by aggressive malignant lymphomas of B-cell and T-cell types. A morphologic and immunophenotypic study. Cancer 1992;69:413–20.

58. Trudel MA, Krikorian JG, Neiman RS. Lymphocyte predominance Hodgkin's disease. A clinicopatholoic reassessment. Cancer 1987;59:99–106.

59. van Krieken JH. Histopathology of the spleen in non-Hodgkin's lymphoma. Histol Histopathol 1990;5:113–22.

60. _____, Feller AC, te Velde J. The distribution of non-Hodgkin's lymphoma in the lymphoid compartments of the human spleen. Am J Surg Pathol 1989;13:757–65.

61. Variakojis D, Rosas-Uribe A, Rappaport H. Mycosis fungoides: pathologic findings in staging laparotomies. Cancer 1974;33:1589–600.

62. Wolf BC, Neiman RS. Disorders of the spleen. Philadelphia: WB Saunders, 1989:75–98. (Major problems in pathology, vol. 20).

Lymphoma Presenting with Prominent Splenomegaly

63. Braylan RC, Long JC, Jaffe ES, Greco FA, Orr SL, Berard CW. Malignant lymphoma obscured by concomitant extensive epithelioid granulomas: report of three cases with similar clinicopathologic features. Cancer 1977;39:1146–55.

64. Collins RD, Neiman RS. Granulomatous diseases of the spleen. In: Ioachim HL, ed. Pathology of granulomas. New York: Raven Press, 1983:189–207.

65. Dacie JV, Brian MC, Harrison CV, Lewis SM, Worlledge SM. Nontropical idiopathic splenomegaly (primary hypersplenism): a review of 10 cases and their relationship to malignant lymphomas. Br J Hematol 1969;17:317–33.

66. _____, Galton DA, Gordon-Smith EC, Harrison CV. Non-tropical "idiopathic splenomegaly": a follow-up study of 10 patients described in 1969. Br J Hematol 1978;38:185–93.

67. Falk S, Takeshita M, Stutte HJ. Epithelioid granulomatosis with initial and predominant manifestation in the spleen. Morphological and immunohistochemical analysis of six cases. Virchows Arch [A] 1988;414:69–76.

68. Hollema H, Visser L, Poppema S. Small lymphocytic lymphomas with predominant splenomegaly: a comparison of immunophenotype with cases of predominant lymphadenopathy. Mod Pathol 1991;4:712–7.

69. Kraemer BB, Osborne BM, Butler JJ. Primary splenic presentation of malignant lymphoma and related disorders. A study of 49 cases. Cancer 1984;54:1606–19.

70. Wolf BC, Neiman RS. Disorders of the spleen. Philadelphia: W.B. Saunders, 1989:75–98. (Major problems in pathology, vol. 20).

Hepatosplenic T-Cell Lymphoma

71. Bordessoule D, Gaulard P, Mason DY. Preferential localisation of human lymphocytes bearing T cell receptors to the red pulp of the spleen. J Clin Pathol 1990;43:461–4.

72. Cooke CB, Greiner T, Raffeld M, Kingma D, Steller-Stevenson M, Jaffe E. γδ T-cell lymphoma, a distinct clinicopathologic entity [Abstract]. Mod Pathol 1994; 7:106A.

73. Farcet JP, Gaulard P, Marolleau JP, et al. Hepatosplenic T-cell lymphoma: sinusal/sinusoidal localization of malignant cells expressing the T-cell receptor gd. Blood 1990;75:2213–9.

74. Kadin ME, Kamoun M, Lamberg J. Erythrophagocytic T-gamma lymphoma: a clinicopathologic entity resembling malignant histiocytosis. N Engl J Med 1981;304:648–53.

75. Krishnan J, Goodman Z, Frizzera G. Primary hepatic sinusoidal presentation of malignant T-cell lymphoma [Abstract]. Mod Pathol 1992;5:81A.

76. Sun T, Brody J, Susin M, Lichtman S, Boss E, Moskowitz L. Extranodal T-cell lymphoma mimicking malignant histiocytosis. Am J Hematol 1990;35:269–74.

77. Wong KF, Chan JK, Matutes E, et al. Hepatosplenic γδ T-cell lymphoma: a distinctive aggressive lymphoma type. Am J Surg Pathol 1995;6:718–26.

Lymphoplasmacytoid Lymphoma

78. Audouin J, Diebold J, Schvartz H, Le Tourneau A, Bernadou A, Zittoun R. Malignant lymphoplasmacytic lymphoma with prominent splenomegaly (primary lymphoma of the spleen). J Pathol 1988;155:17–33.

79. Juliusson G, Ost A, Biberfeld P, Robert KH. Hematological remission of leukaemic polymorphic immunocytoma following splenectomy. Case report with longitudinal immunological and cytogenic studies. Acta Pathol Microbiol Immunol Scand [A] 1986;94:133–9.

80. Kraemer BB, Osborne BM, Butler JJ. Primary splenic presentation of malignant lymphoma and related disorders. A study of 49 cases. Cancer 1984;54:1606–19.

81. Lennert K, Feller AC. Histopathology of non-Hodgkin's lymphomas (based on the updated Kiel classification). 2nd ed. Berlin: Springer-Verlag, 1992:67.

82. Narang S, Wolf BC, Neiman RS. Malignant lymphoma presenting with prominent splenomegaly. A clinicopathologic study with special reference to intermediate cell lymphoma. Cancer 1985;55:1948–57.

Splenic B-Cell Lymphoma with Circulating Villous Lymphocytes

83. Bates I, Bedu-Addo G, Rutherford T, Bevan DH. Splenic lymphoma with villous lymphocytes in tropical West Africa. Lancet 1992;340:575–7.

84. Dyer MJ, Zani VJ, Lu WZ, et al. BCL2 translocations in leukemias of mature B-cells. Blood 1994;83:3682–8.

84a. Isaacson PG, Matutes E, Burke M, Catovsky D. The histopathology of splenic lymphoma with villous lymphocytes. Blood 1994;84:3828–34.

85. Jadayel D, Matutes E, Dyer MJ, et al. Splenic lymphoma with villous lymphocytes: analysis of BCL-1 rearrangements and expression of the cyclin D1 gene. Blood 1994;83:3664–71.

86. Matutes E, Morilla R, Owusu-Ankomah K, Houlihan A, Catovsky D. The immunophenotype of splenic lymphoma with villous lymphocytes and its relevance to the differential diagnosis with other B-cell disorders. Blood 1994;83:1558–62.

87. Melo JV, Hegde U, Parreira A, Thompson I, Lampert IA, Catovsky D. Splenic B cell lymphoma with circulating villous lymphocytes: differential diagnosis of B cell leukaemias with large spleens. J Clin Pathol 1987;40:642–51.

88. _____, Robinson DS, Gregory C, Catovsky D. Splenic B cell lymphoma with "villous" lymphocytes in the peripheral blood: a disorder distinct from hairy cell leukemia. Leukemia 1987;1:294–8.

89. Mulligan SP, Catovsky D. Splenic lymphoma with villous lymphocytes. Leuk Lymphoma 1992;6:97–105.

90. Neiman RS, Sullivan AL, Jaffe R. Malignant lymphoma simulating leukemic reticuloendotheliosis: a clinicopathologic study of ten cases. Cancer 1979;43:329–42.

91. Spriano P, Barosi G, Invernizzi R, et al. Splenomegalic immunocytoma with circulating hairy cells. Report of eight cases and review of the literature. Haematologica 1986;71:25–33.

92. Sun T, Susin M, Brody J. Splenic lymphoma with circulating villous lymphocytes: report of 7 cases and review of the literature. Am J Hematol 1994;45:39–50.

Splenic Marginal Zone Cell Lymphoma

93. Cousar JB, McKee LC, Greco FA, Glick AD, Collins RD. Report of an unusual B-cell lymphoma, probably arising from the perifollicular cells (marginal zone) of the spleen [Abstract]. Lab Invest 1980;42:109A.
94. Palutke M, Eisenberg L, Narang S, et al. B lymphocytic lymphoma (large cell) of possible splenic marginal zone origin presenting with prominent splenomegaly and unusual cordal red pulp distribution. Cancer 1988;62:593–600.
95. Schmid C, Kirkham N, Diss T, Isaacson PG. Splenic marginal zone cell lymphoma. Am J Surg Pathol 1992;16:455–66.
96. Sendelbach KM, Pugh WC, Rodriguez J, et al. Splenic marginal zone lymphoma (MGZL): clinical and pathologic characteristics of 11 cases [Abstract]. Mod Pathol 1994;7:120A.

21

NONHEMATOLYMPHOID TUMORS AND TUMOR-LIKE LESIONS OF LYMPH NODE AND SPLEEN

CLASSIFICATION

In addition to metastatic deposits, a variety of primary nonhematolymphoid tumors and tumor-like lesions occur in lymph node. These include:

I. Stromal Lesions, including Smooth Muscle and Myofibroblastic
    A. Hemorrhagic spindle cell tumor with amianthoid fibers (palisaded myofibro-blastoma)
    B. Smooth muscle proliferations
        1. Smooth muscle proliferation in nodal hilum
        2. Angiomyolipoma
        3. Lymphangiomyomatosis/Lymphangiomyoma
        4. Leiomyomatosis
        5. Angiomyomatous hamartoma
        6. Intranodal leiomyoma
    C. Inflammatory pseudotumor
    D. Mycobacterial spindle cell pseudotumor
    E. Deciduosis
    F. Lipomatosis
    G. Others, e.g., myelolipoma, plexiform fibrohistiocytic tumor
II. Vascular Lesions
    A. Kaposi's sarcoma
    B. Hemangioma, including epithelioid hemangioma
    C. Lymphangioma
    D. Hemangioendothelioma
        1. Epithelioid hemangioendothelioma
        2. Spindle and epithelioid (histiocytoid) hemangioendotheliomas
        3. Polymorphous hemangioendothelioma
    E. Angiosarcoma
    F. Vascular neoplasm arising in Castleman's disease
    G. Vascular transformation of sinuses
    H. Angiolipomatous hamartoma in association with Castleman's disease
    I. Bacillary angiomatosis
    J. Venolymphatic angiodysplasia
III. Epithelial and Nevus Inclusions in Lymph Node

A. Glandular inclusions
B. Nevus cell aggregates
C. Blue nevus

Nonhematolymphoid tumors and tumor-like conditions of the spleen include:

I. Vascular Lesions
    A. Hemangioma
    B. Littoral cell angioma
    C. Lymphangioma
    D. Peliosis of spleen
    E. Hemangioendothelioma
    F. Angiosarcoma
    G. Kaposi's sarcoma
    H. Angiomyolipoma
    I. Bacillary angiomatosis
    J. Hemangiopericytoma
II. Others
    A. Sarcomas of other types, e.g., malignant fibrous histiocytoma
    B. Inflammatory pseudotumor
    C. Mycobacterial spindle cell pseudotumor
    D. Splenic hamartoma
    E. Cysts
        1. True cysts
            a. Epithelial cyst
            b. Parasitic cyst
        2. False cyst
    F. Lipoma

In this chapter, the various primary non-hematolymphoid lesions of lymph node and spleen are discussed, followed by metastatic tumors in these organs.

HEMORRHAGIC SPINDLE CELL TUMOR WITH AMIANTHOID FIBERS (PALISADED MYOFIBROBLASTOMA)

Definition. Hemorrhagic spindle cell tumor with amianthoid fibers (palisaded myofibroblastoma) is a rare benign mesenchymal tumor of lymph node with myofibroblastic/smooth muscle differentiation, often accompanied by a hemorrhagic rim and formation of amianthoid fibers (7,10).

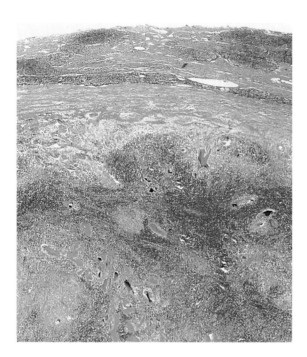 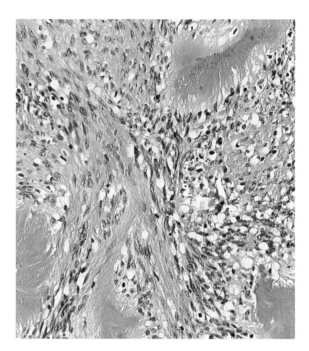

Figure 21-1

HEMORRHAGIC SPINDLE CELL TUMOR WITH AMIANTHOID FIBERS (PALISADED MYOFIBROBLASTOMA)

Left: Low-power view showing an attenuated rim of nodal tissue on top. Note the prominent hemorrhagic rim.

Right: Spindle cells and amianthoid fibers are evident. Note the extravasated red blood cells. (Courtesy of Dr. Saul Suster, Miami, FL.)

Clinical Features. This tumor occurs over a wide age range, with a slight male predominance (1–8,10). The patients present with a solitary mass that may be tender. Although initially reported to involve exclusively inguinal lymph nodes (7,10), it has since been recognized to involve other nodes such as those of the neck and mediastinum (1,3,5). This is a benign lesion which does not recur or metastasize after local excision.

Gross Findings. The tumor is well circumscribed, and measures from 0.6 to 5.0 cm in greatest dimension. The cut surface is grey-white to tan, with hemorrhagic areas, particularly in the rim.

Microscopic Findings. The residual lymph node tissue is compressed to form an attenuated rim on the outermost aspect, on the inner side of which is a hemorrhagic zone with hemosiderin deposits, variable degrees of granulation tissue, and sclerosis (fig. 21-1, left). Sometimes a fibrous pseudocapsule is formed. The core is composed of fascicles of spindle cells which often intersect at right angles, and there may be vague nuclear palisading in areas.

The spindle cells are bland-looking, with elongated nuclei, fine chromatin, and scanty to moderate eosinophilic cytoplasm that may show perinuclear vacuolation (fig. 21-1, right). Mitoses are infrequent. Intracytoplasmic and extracellular fuchsinophilic globules (actin positive) can also be detected in some cases. Interstitial hemorrhage, fresh and old, is commonly present throughout the lesion.

A distinctive feature is the presence of amianthoid fibers, which are abundant to barely developed (2,7). Amianthoid fibers are stellate areas of collagen deposition that may be calcified (fig. 21-1, right). They have been postulated to arise through obliteration of preexisting vascular structures (7) or coalescence of the actin globules extruded from the spindle cells (8,10).

Immunohistochemical and Ultrastructural Findings. The spindle cells are immunoreactive for vimentin, muscle-specific actin, and myosin, but not desmin, S-100 protein, or factor VIII–related antigen (7,10). The amianthoid fibers are immunoreactive for type I collagen; their peripheral portions are also immunoreactive for type III collagen and actin (6). Ultrastructurally, the spindle cells have discontinuous basal laminae. They possess abundant microfilaments with focal densities, pinocytotic vesicles, rough endo-plasmic reticulum, and occasional intercellular junctions, lending support to smooth muscle or myofibroblastic differentiation (3,4,7,8). The amianthoid fibers, in contrast to those occurring in other tumors, are composed of normal native collagen, and giant collagen fibrils are lacking (6).

Differential Diagnosis. The presence of spindle cells and interstitial hemorrhage in a lymph node may raise concern for Kaposi's sarcoma. However, unlike Kaposi's sarcoma, the red blood cells are entirely interstitial rather than in vascular slits, the spindle cell fascicles are straight rather than curved, amianthoid fibers are frequently present, and eosinophilic periodic acid–Schiff (PAS)-positive hyaline globules are absent. Furthermore, well-developed Kaposi's sarcoma frequently shows some degree of nuclear pleomorphism and a higher mitotic rate.

Sarcomas, particularly leiomyosarcoma, can simulate this benign neoplasm, but the former always exhibit some degree of nuclear pleomorphism and readily identifiable mitoses.

The vague nuclear palisading and amianthoid fibers in hemorrhagic spindle cell tumors may suggest intranodal schwannoma. However, in the former tumor, the distinct Antoni A and Antoni B areas are lacking, nuclear palisading is never well developed, and there is no staining for S-100 protein.

Another spindle cell tumor primary in lymph node to consider in the differential diagnosis is true dendritic cell sarcoma (follicular dendritic or inter-digitating dendritic cell sarcoma). In dendritic cell sarcoma, the neoplastic cells are generally plumper and often form nests or whorls, scattered lymphocytes are more commonly seen, and the distinctive interstitial hemorrhage and amian-thoid fibers are lacking (9). A diagnosis of true dendritic cell sarcoma should always be confirmed by extensive immunohistochemical studies.

Benign metastasizing leiomyoma (leiomyomatosis) in lymph node is histologically similar to hemorrhagic spindle cell tumor; it is distin-guished by the more conventional appearance of the smooth muscle cells (oval to elongated cigar-shaped nuclei and more fibrillary eosinophilic cytoplasm) and absence of interstitial hemor-rhage or amianthoid fibers.

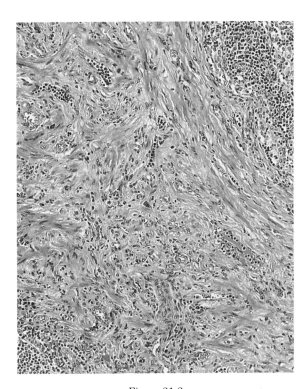

Figure 21-2
SMOOTH MUSCLE PROLIFERATION
IN LYMPH NODE HILUM
The smooth muscle cells are disposed in a collagenous stroma.

SMOOTH MUSCLE PROLIFERATIONS IN LYMPH NODE

Smooth muscle cells are normally found in lymph nodes, either associated with the blood vessels or lymphatics, or in the capsule and trabeculae (29,40). A variety of uncommon pro-liferative lesions involving smooth muscle occur in lymph nodes, and these entities have recently been reviewed in detail (46).

Smooth Muscle Proliferation in Nodal Hilum

A haphazard proliferation of smooth muscle cells, often accompanied by fibrosis and prominent vascularity, may distort the lymph node hilum (fig. 21-2). The nodal parenchyma is spared. This reactive lesion is an uncommon incidental finding in lymph nodes, most notably those of the inguinal region. The smooth muscle proliferation is postu-lated to be of vascular origin, possibly reflecting a previous inflammatory reaction (21).

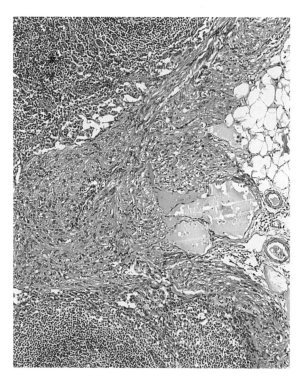

Figure 21-3
ANGIOMYOLIPOMA INVOLVING LYMPH NODE
The lesion is composed of smooth muscle, vascular channels, and adipose cells. This lesion is located predominantly in the subcapsular sinus.

Angiomyolipoma

Angiomyolipoma, a hamartomatous lesion of the kidney that can occur as a component of the tuberous sclerosis complex, is characterized by a haphazard proliferation of adipose cells, thick-walled blood vessels, and smooth muscle; these are present in highly variable proportions (13). The smooth muscle cells often radiate out from the vessel walls, and can appear alarming as a result of epithelioid morphology and nuclear pleomorphism. They typically stain with the melanoma-specific antibody HMB-45 in addition to the usual myoid markers (20). The tumor is invariably benign.

There is a tendency for angiomyolipoma to show multifocal growth. Involvement of retroperitoneal lymph nodes (fig. 21-3), which takes the form of sinusoidal growth or more massive replacement of the nodal parenchyma, is similarly interpreted as a manifestation of multicentricity (15,17,18,26,33,36,42,43). Such cases do not exhibit aneuploidy, and the benign behavior has been confirmed by long-term follow-up (17,42).

Lymphangiomyomatosis

Lymphangiomyomatosis (lymphangioleiomyomatosis) is a malformative or hamartomatous proliferation of lymphatic channels and smooth muscle, occurring exclusively in women, usually during their reproductive years (22,23, 28). Since a small proportion of patients also have angiomyolipoma of the kidney, and changes similar to lymphangiomyomatosis occasionally occur in the lungs of patients with tuberous sclerosis, the possibility of lymphangiomyomatosis representing forme fruste tuberous sclerosis has been raised (23,28,35).

Lymphangiomyomatosis characteristically shows progressive involvement of the lungs, often resulting in death from pulmonary insufficiency within 10 years (23). The thoracic duct, mediastinum, retroperitoneum, and lymph nodes (thoracic, axillary, cervical, or intraabdominal) can also be involved. Occasionally, the disease is confined to the retroperitoneum, forming large masses; this form of disease is associated with a more favorable outcome (14,22,47).

Rarely, lymphangiomyomatosis is an incidental, isolated finding in intra-abdominal lymph nodes (22,37). Because of the solitary nature of the process, the term "lymphangiomyoma" can be applied. Two cases reported as "leiomyomatosis" in a pelvic lymph node, and postulated to arise from vascular smooth muscle, are probably lymphangiomyomatosis, in view of the prominence of interspersed vascular channels (38,41,45).

Grossly, the lymph nodes are spongy, resilient, and pale tan or white. They are involved in a sinusoidal or more extensive fashion (fig. 21-4, left). The smooth muscle cells form short fascicles around an anastomosing network of endothelium-lined spaces, resulting in a pericytomatous pattern (fig. 21-4, right). They are morphologically distinctive, with a plump spindly appearance and regular oval nuclei with no atypia or mitoses. The cytoplasm is lightly eosinophilic to clear (fig. 21-5, left). Besides staining for various myogenic markers such as muscle-specific actin and desmin, the smooth muscle cells stain consistently with HMB-45 (fig. 21-5, right) (20).

Lymphangiomyomatosis must be distinguished from metastatic well-differentiated leiomyosarcoma. The latter has no consistent relationship with the vascular channels; often shows

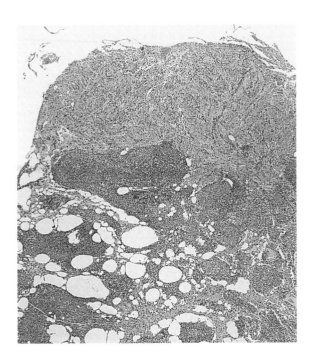
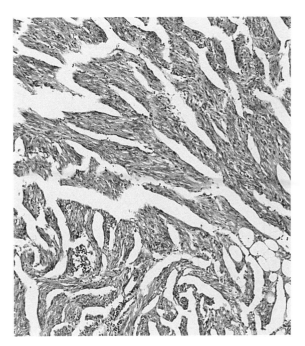

Figure 21-4
LYMPHANGIOMYOMATOSIS INVOLVING LYMPH NODE
Left: The lesion expands the subcapsular sinus focally.
Right: Anastomosing branching lymphatic spaces are surrounded by plump smooth muscle cells with pale to clear cytoplasm.

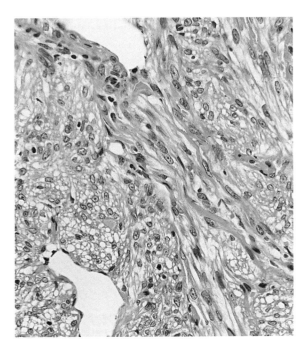
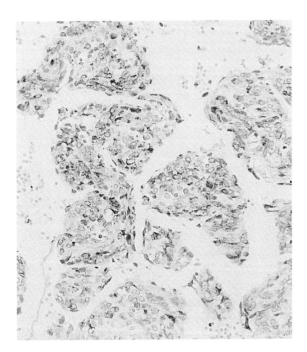

Figure 21-5
LYMPHANGIOMYOMATOSIS INVOLVING PELVIC LYMPH NODE
Left: The smooth muscle cells are plump and possess pale to clear cytoplasm. There are interspersed vascular spaces.
Right: The smooth muscle cells show granular cytoplasmic immunostaining with HMB-45.

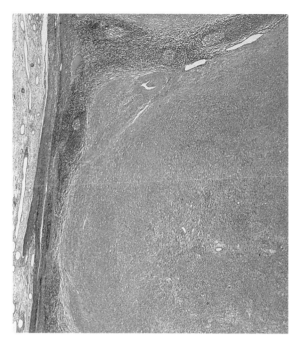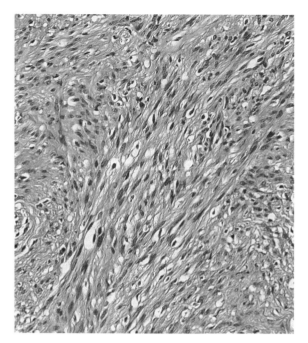

Figure 21-6
LEIOMYOMATOSIS OF PELVIC LYMPH NODE (METASTASIZING UTERINE LEIOMYOMA)
Left: Extensive replacement of lymph node by smooth muscle proliferation.
Right: The smooth muscle cells are bland looking and lack mitoses. (Courtesy of Dr. Akio Horie, Kitakyushu, Japan.)

greater cellularity, atypia, some mitotic figures, and more eosinophilic-staining cytoplasm; and lacks HMB-45 immunoreactivity (28).

Leiomyomatosis of Lymph Node

Proliferation of compact bundles of bland-looking and mitotically inactive smooth muscle cells can occur, although rarely, in lymph nodes; the nodes are usually intra-abdominal. The smooth muscle proliferation causes partial (such as subcapsular) or complete replacement of the nodal parenchyma (fig. 21-6). The reported outcome is benign except for one patient with benign metastasizing leiomyoma who died of complications of the disease (11,16,24,31,34).

Leiomyomatosis of lymph node is believed to arise in the following circumstances. 1) Metastasizing uterine leiomyoma can involve lymph node, and is believed to result from uterine tumor gaining access to lymphatic channels spontaneously or during manipulations at uterine curetting (fig. 21-6) (11,16,24,31,34). However, since uterine leiomyomas are so common (25), it is difficult to prove that the uterine tumor is indeed

the source of the nodal lesion. Alternatively, the nodal smooth muscle can be derived directly from the subcoelomic mesenchyme (32). 2) Leiomyomatosis peritonealis disseminata can show lymph node involvement (30,32). 3) Leiomyomatosis of lymph node may rise through organization of intranodal decidua or endometriosis (27,32) by myofibroblasts or smooth muscle cells, reflecting the multipotentiality of the pelvic subcoelomic mesenchyme that can be found in the peripheral sinus of lymph nodes (39). 4) So-called primary nodal leiomyomatosis (vascular leiomyomatosis) (38,41) is morphologically indistinguishable from nodal involvement by lymphangiomyomatosis, and may in fact represent the same entity with lymph node involvement alone (fig. 21-5) (45).

Angiomyomatous Hamartoma

Angiomyomatous hamartoma is a distinctive form of smooth muscle proliferation involving the inguinal lymph nodes almost exclusively (19). It affects patients of a wide age range, with a male predominance. The patients present with enlarged lymph nodes, which can be matted; the enlargement is often of long duration. Edema of the ipsilateral limb sometimes accompanies the lymphadenopathy. This lesion is innocuous.

Grossly, the lymph node is extensively replaced by firm white tissue (fig. 21-7). Histologically, there is proliferation of thick-walled blood vessels in the hilum, often accompanied by an increase in fibrous tissue. The process extends into and replaces the nodal parenchyma in the form of more haphazardly and sparsely disposed bland-looking smooth muscle cells in a sclerotic stroma (figs. 21-8, 21-9). The smooth muscle appears to be vascular in origin since it is closely related to narrow or ectatic vascular spaces (fig. 21-9). In some cases, the process appears more angiomatous, with many congested, proliferated, thin-walled blood vessels interspersed within the lesion (fig. 21-10). Occasionally, there can be interspersed adipocytes (12). Angiomyomatous hamartoma differs from hilar smooth muscle proliferation by the extensive intranodal involvement. The features that distinguish it from nodal vascular leiomyomatosis or lymphangiomyomatosis are listed in Table 21-1.

Intranodal Leiomyoma

Smooth muscle tumors with histologic features identical to those of somatic soft tissue have rarely been reported to occur as primary tumors of lymph node (44). One of the two reported cases

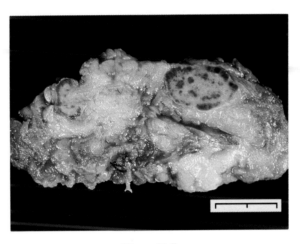

Figure 21-7
ANGIOMYOMATOUS HAMARTOMA OF INGUINAL LYMPH NODES
In this groin dissection, abnormal lymph nodes are embedded in the fat. The nodes show extensive replacement by tan, firm tissue.

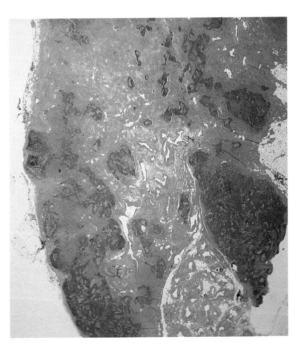
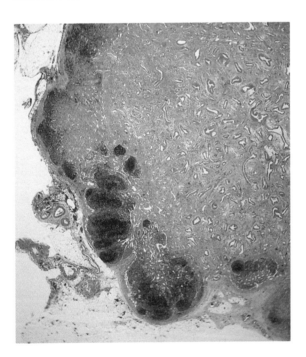

Figure 21-8
ANGIOMYOMATOUS HAMARTOMA OF LYMPH NODE
There is extensive and multifocal involvement of the nodal parenchyma. Note better-formed blood vessels in the hilum; they are more prominent in the right figure than in the left.

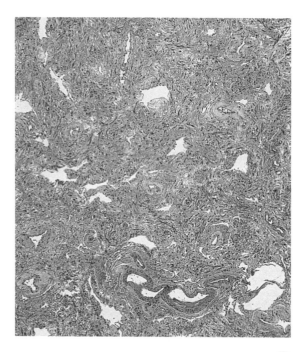 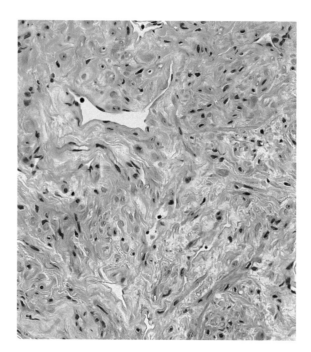

Figure 21-9
ANGIOMYOMATOUS HAMARTOMA OF LYMPH NODE
Left: In the hilar and medullary regions (lower field), proliferated thick-walled vessels merge into a fibromuscular stroma in the cortex (upper field).
Right: In the cortical regions, smooth muscle cells are haphazardly disposed in a sclerotic stroma.

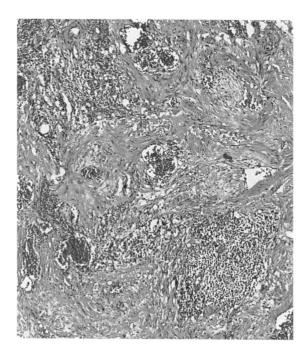

Figure 21-10
ANGIOMYOMATOUS HAMARTOMA OF LYMPH NODE
This example shows a more angiomatous component.

occurred in a patient with acquired immunodeficiency syndrome (AIDS).

One case showing overlapping features of leiomyoma and myofibroblastoma has also been recently reported (46a).

INFLAMMATORY PSEUDOTUMOR OF LYMPH NODE

Definition. A distinct nodal reaction resembling inflammatory pseudotumor of other organs is a rare cause of lymphadenopathy. The pathogenesis is unknown, but the lesion probably is the end result of an inflammatory process in response to diverse etiologies (49,52). A case reported as benign vascular proliferation in lymph node following acute toxoplasmosis probably represents the same entity (53). In occasional cases of Kikuchi's necrotizing lymphadenitis, foci of fibrovascular tissue indistinguishable from inflammatory pseudotumor are present (54).

Clinical Features. Inflammatory pseudotumor of lymph node affects predominantly young adults, who present with prominent lymphadenopathy involving a single or multiple

442

Table 21-1

COMPARISON BETWEEN ANGIOMYOMATOUS HAMARTOMA AND VASCULAR LEIOMYOMATOSIS/LYMPHANGIOMYOMATOSIS OF LYMPH NODE

	Angiomyomatous Hamartoma	Vascular Leiomyomatosis or Lymphangiomyomatosis
Sex	Male predominance	Exclusively female
Presentation	Inguinal lymph node enlargement	Incidental finding in abdominal lymph nodes or part of more widespread disease
Distribution	Hilum, medulla, and portions of the cortex	Subcapsular sinuses or more extensive involvement
Smooth muscle	Spindly cells with eosinophilic cytoplasm haphazardly arranged; proliferation of thick-walled vessels in continuity with lesion	Plump cells with pale to clear cytoplasm in compact bundles; interspersed endothelium-lined anastomosing vascular channels
Lesional sclerosis	Prominent	Minimal
HMB-45 immuno-staining	Negative	Positive

sites, often accompanied by constitutional symptoms (such as fever, anorexia, night sweats). Some patients present with fever of unknown origin (49,50–52). The lymph node involved may be superficial or deep (retroperitoneal, mediastinal). Laboratory abnormalities such as raised erythrocyte sedimentation rate, anemia, and hypergammaglobulinemia are common. Surgical excision of the mass lesion is often curative, and can be accompanied by dramatic resolution of symptoms. The disease is benign, although some cases may relapse. Indomethacin or steroid treatment can result in symptomatic relief in some patients with systemic lymphadenopathy and prominent symptoms (52).

Microscopic Findings. The lymph nodes often exceed 3 cm in diameter, and may be matted. The disease process mainly involves the connective tissue framework of the lymph node (hilum, trabecula, capsule) with variable involvement of the nodal parenchyma and perinodal tissue (fig. 21-11). There is a proliferation of spindle cells, blood vessels lined by flat endothelium, and acute and chronic inflammatory cells, associated with sclerosis (fig. 21-12). The spindle cells, which possess oval nuclei with fine chromatin, can assume a storiform pattern in areas. There is frequent involvement of medium-sized and large veins by the inflammatory or fibro-obliterative reaction (fig. 21-13) (50,52). Uncommon findings include parenchymal infarction,

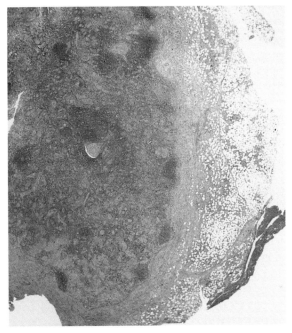

Figure 21-11
INFLAMMATORY PSEUDOTUMOR OF LYMPH NODE
There is predominant involvement of the connective tissue framework of the node.

fibrinoid vascular necrosis, and karyorrhexis (49). Immunohistochemical studies have shown that the spindle cells are composed mostly of activated histiocytes and fibroblasts, with a minor population of myofibroblasts (49,50). The uninvolved nodal parenchyma shows nonspecific

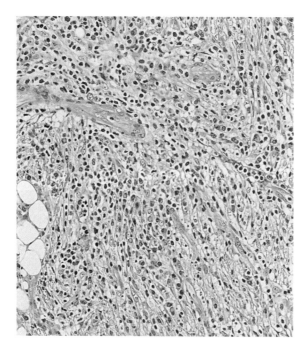

Figure 21-12
INFLAMMATORY PSEUDOTUMOR
OF LYMPH NODE
Blood vessels, spindle cells, lymphocytes, and plasma cells are the main constituents of the lesion.

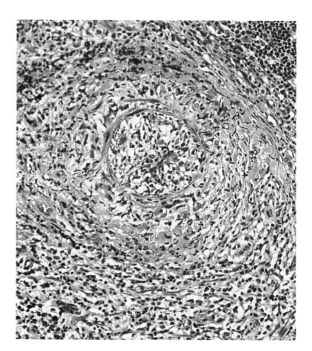

Figure 21-13
INFLAMMATORY PSEUDOTUMOR
OF LYMPH NODE
Venulitis is a common finding in the perinodal tissue.

reactive changes; cytologically atypical cells are absent and mitoses are infrequent.

The differential diagnoses include Kaposi's sarcoma, mycobacterial spindle cell pseudotumor, Castleman's disease, Hodgkin's disease, and postthymic T-cell lymphoma (48). In contrast to Kaposi's sarcoma, inflammatory pseudotumor of lymph node shows more prominent sclerosis, the spindle cells are not associated with vascular slits, and eosinophilic hyaline globules are absent.

MYCOBACTERIAL SPINDLE CELL PSEUDOTUMOR OF LYMPH NODE AND SPLEEN

In patients with *Mycobacterium avium intracellulare* infection, particularly in a setting of AIDS, the lymph nodes and spleen may exhibit an unusual spindle cell growth imparted by the sheets of histiocytes that are engorged with mycobacteria (55–57). The descriptive term, mycobacterial spindle cell pseudotumor, has been applied (55). This pattern is similar to the "histoid" pattern that has previously been observed in some cases of leprosy (58).

Histologically, the lesion is multinodular or diffuse, and is characterized by spindly cells admixed with capillaries, lymphocytes, and plasma cells. A storiform pattern is commonly observed. The spindly cells have eosinophilic granular cytoplasm and oval nuclei; occasional cells may exhibit nuclear enlargement and distinct nucleoli (figs. 21-14–21-16). Numerous acid-fast bacilli can be demonstrated in the spindly cells (fig. 21-14C), which can be shown by immunohistochemical and ultrastructural studies to represent histiocytes.

This pseudotumor may be mistaken for inflammatory pseudotumor or smooth muscle tumor. The latter mistake is particularly likely to be made because of the frequent (but unexplained) immunoreactivity of the spindly histiocytes for desmin (57). Distinction from inflammatory pseudotumor is important because of the need for antimicrobial therapy. Mycobacterial spindle cell pseudotumor usually occurs in a setting of AIDS and lacks the vasculitis and extracapsular extension characteristic of inflammatory pseudotumor. A firm diagnosis can be made by the Ziehl-Neelsen stain (fig. 21-14C) (55).

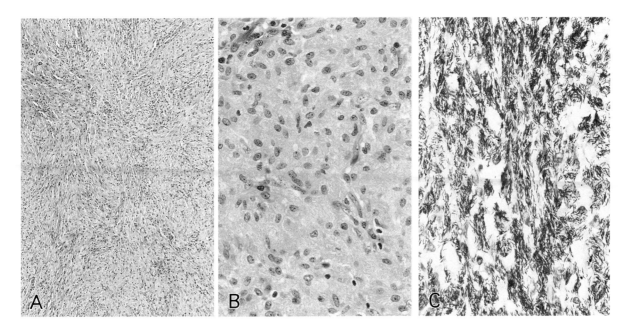

Figure 21-14
MYCOBACTERIAL SPINDLE CELL PSEUDOTUMOR OF LYMPH NODE
A: Spindly cells (histiocytes) with a vague storiform arrangement.
B: The plump spindly cells have ovoid nuclei with fine chromatin and abundant finely granular cytoplasm.
C: Myriads of acid-fast bacilli can be demonstrated in the spindly cells by Ziehl-Neelsen stain.

DECIDUOSIS OF LYMPH NODE

Decidual cells may occur as compact masses in the abdominal lymph nodes of pregnant women, mimicking metastatic carcinoma, particularly if the lymph nodes are removed as part of cancer surgery (59–61). Deciduosis can arise in endometriosis of lymph node during pregnancy (62,64); under such circumstances, narrow endometrial glands lined by attenuated epithelium may be found on further search. Alternatively, deciduosis of lymph node may arise in the absence of endometriosis and is probably derived from the multipotential subcoelomic mesenchymal cells under the influence of pregnancy (59–61,63,64,65,67).

The decidual cells are found mainly in the subcapsular areas and sometimes the superficial cortex. They are polygonal or plump and spindled, and possess distinct cell membranes, abundant amphophilic (sometimes vacuolated) cytoplasm, and round to oval nuclei (fig. 21-17). A mild degree of nuclear pleomorphism can occur.

Decidual cells can be distinguished from metastatic squamous cell carcinoma by the lack of desmoplastic reaction, mitotic figures, and keratinization (63). Furthermore, similar decidual cell clusters

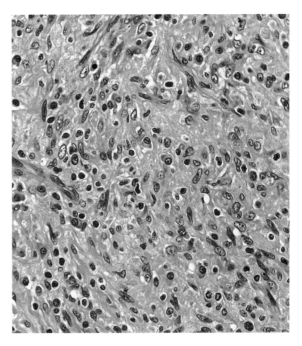

Figure 21-15
MYCOBACTERIAL SPINDLE CELL
PSEUDOTUMOR OF LYMPH NODE
In this example, the spindly cells are elongated and resemble myofibroblasts or fibroblasts. There are intermixed blood vessels and plasma cells, resembling inflammatory pseudotumor.

445

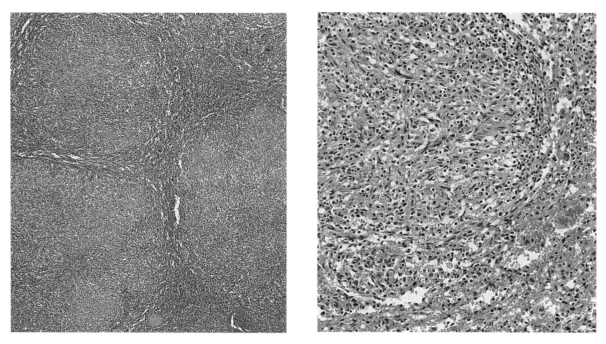

Figure 21-16
MYCOBACTERIAL SPINDLE CELL PSEUDOTUMOR OF SPLEEN
Left: Multiple spindle cell nodules are found in the splenic parenchyma.
Right: The expansile nodule comprises spindly cells and mononuclear cells.

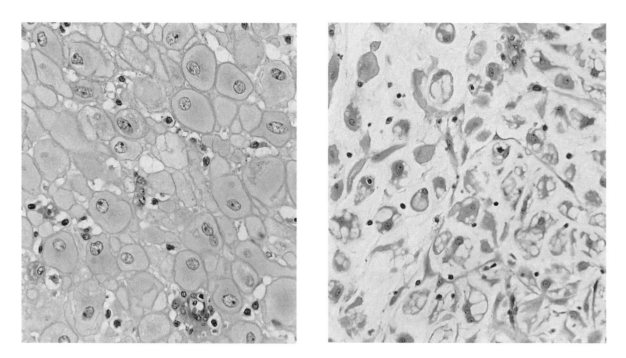

Figure 21-17
DECIDUOSIS OF LYMPH NODE
Left: The cells are polygonal and have sharp cell borders.
Right: The cells can appear vacuolated.

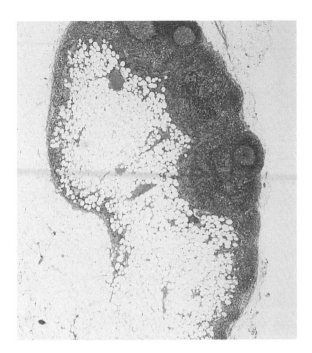

Figure 21-18
LIPOMATOSIS OF LYMPH NODE
In this axillary lymph node, the hilum is expanded by adipose cells. There is some extension of the process into the nodal parenchyma.

can often be found in the submesothelial tissue elsewhere in the pelvis. Immunohistochemical studies can help in difficult cases because decidual cells are not immunoreactive for cytokeratin (66).

"LIPOMATOSIS" OF LYMPH NODE

"Lipomatosis" or fatty infiltration is a fairly common occurrence in lymph nodes, particularly the axillary nodes. The nodal parenchyma is almost totally replaced by adipose tissue, with only a thin rim of residual lymphoid tissue (fig. 21-18). This lesion is of no importance except that it may cause palpable enlargement of lymph node.

KAPOSI'S SARCOMA OF LYMPH NODE

Definition. Kaposi's sarcoma (KS) is a distinctive tumor of probable vascular nature, characterized histologically by an admixture of spindle cells and narrow vascular spaces, and frequently showing multicentric growth (162). There is controversy as to whether KS is a hyperplastic lesion or a true neoplasm (85,132). The multifocal growth, which does not conform to a metastatic pattern; the heterogeneous cellular

composition; and the lack of DNA aneuploidy have been cited to support the probable hyperplastic nature of KS (69,85). On the other hand, in vitro studies have demonstrated transforming genes in KS (127). DNA obtained from KS transforms the fibroblast cell line NIH/3T3; when the transfected cells are injected into nude mice, tumors histologically similar to KS are formed. It is possible that early KS is a hyperplastic state that may progress into a true neoplasm when secondary genetic changes occur (102,169).

Clinical Features and Epidemiology. KS occurs in a variety of clinical settings, but it was rare in non-Africans until the recent epidemic of AIDS (109,123). In the following discussion, the emphasis will be on the lymph node manifestations of KS.

Classic Kaposi's Sarcoma. The classic form of KS occurs mostly in elderly men of Jewish and Mediterranean descent, in the form of skin lesions usually confined to the lower extremities. Lymph node involvement is uncommon. The disease typically pursues an indolent course for 10 to 15 years; systemic lesions may eventually develop in the gastrointestinal tract, lymph nodes, and other organs in long-term cases (86, 99,123,169). One third of patients have or subsequently develop second primary cancers, especially lymphoreticular malignancies (152).

African (Endemic) Kaposi's Sarcoma. KS is endemic in the native population of equatorial Africa, accounting for 9 percent of all cancers in Ugandan males. Cutaneous KS occurs in young adults (aged 15 to 40 years), with a marked male predominance. Regional lymph node involvement sometimes occurs, and there may be clinically quiescent visceral lesions (76,93,114,123,156,160,169). Patients with localized nodular skin lesions have indolent disease, while those with large exophytic or deeply invasive tumors have a slowly progressive disease that results in death within 5 to 8 years.

There is a lymphadenopathic form occurring mainly in children (aged 2 to 13 years); the male to female ratio is 3 to 1. The patients present with localized or generalized lymphadenopathy, and skin lesions are uncommon. A similar lymphadenopathic form sometimes occurs in young adults, but is almost always accompanied by widespread skin lesions. There is no association with human immunodeficiency virus (HIV) infection. This form is rapidly progressive, resulting in death within 1 to 3 years.

In recent years, there has been a marked increase in aggressive, AIDS-related KS in Africa as well (143).

Epidemic Kaposi's Sarcoma. KS occurs in approximately 30 percent of patients with AIDS, primarily in homosexual men; it is uncommon in patients contracting HIV infection through the parenteral route (74,117,123,151,169). The risk of developing KS is fairly constant after HIV seroconversion, unlike the risk of infections or lymphoma which increases as the immunodeficiency worsens. The disorder is often disseminated, involving mucocutaneous sites, lymph nodes, and visceral organs (especially the gastrointestinal tract and lungs). AIDS-related KS has a fulminant course, with less than 20 percent survival at 2 years if associated with opportunistic infection. Rarely, KS has been documented in homosexual males in the absence of HIV infection (123).

Organ Transplant–Associated Kaposi's Sarcoma. Organ transplant recipients on immunosuppressive therapy are at increased risk for developing KS. Approximately 0.4 percent of patients with renal transplant develop KS, and the risk is higher in patients of Jewish or Mediterranean extraction. KS may be localized to the skin and oral/pharyngeal mucosa, or may be widespread with systemic involvement (115,119, 123,143,145). In contrast to epidemic KS, lymph node involvement is rare, visceral disease is less common, and fatalities from KS are less frequent. The behavior varies from indolent (localized skin lesions) to rapidly progressive. Some cases may regress with reduction or discontinuation of immunosuppressive therapy.

Kaposi's Sarcoma Associated with Other Forms of Immunosuppression. There appears to be a slightly increased risk of developing KS in patients on deliberate or unintentional immunosuppressive therapy for malignancies (mostly lymphoma) and autoimmune diseases (such as rheumatoid arthritis, systemic lupus erythematosus). Skin lesions are always present, and about one third of patients have concomitant visceral or lymph node involvement (111,122,143,144,166).

Other Associations. KS is a rare complication of multicentric Castleman's disease (fig. 21-19) (83,91,106,125,150). The "lymphoma-like lymph node changes" reported in KS (130) have been reinterpreted as multicentric Castleman's disease (89,106,150). It is unclear whether KS is a

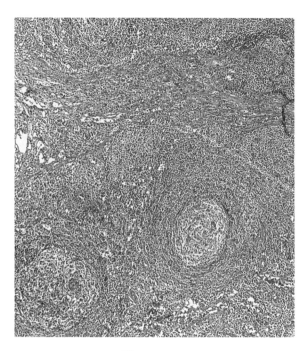

Figure 21-19
KAPOSI'S SARCOMA ASSOCIATED WITH
MULTICENTRIC CASTLEMAN'S DISEASE
In the center field, a focus of Kaposi's sarcoma is present among hyaline-vascular follicles.

consequence of immunologic alterations associated with multicentric Castleman's disease or whether both processes are due to a primary disorder in immune regulation. Of interest, hypervascular follicular hyperplasia similar to that seen in Castleman's disease is commonly observed in the residual lymphoid tissue adjacent to AIDS-related KS (81,114,147), epitomizing the dynamic interaction between the lymphoreticular and vascular systems.

Nodal KS may coexist with malignant lymphoma or leukemia (141,152,162,164,167). Rarely, primary lymphadenopathic KS can occur in apparently healthy subjects with no evidence of immunodeficiency or HIV infection (75,78,126). KS has also been reported as an incidental finding in regional lymph nodes draining carcinomas (126).

Microscopic Findings. The histologic features of KS involving lymph node are the same regardless of the clinical context (94,95), except that early nodal involvement is more commonly encountered as an incidental finding in patients with HIV infection (105).

The histologic patterns of KS in lymph node are varied. There may be a single nodule or

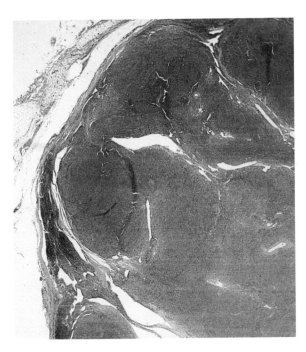

Figure 21-20
KAPOSI'S SARCOMA OF LYMPH NODE
Extensive replacement of lymph node in a multinodular pattern.

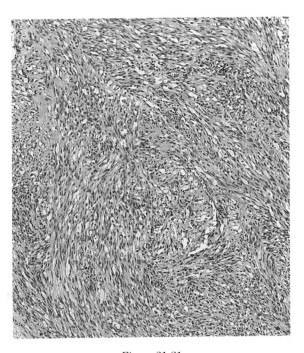

Figure 21-21
KAPOSI'S SARCOMA OF LYMPH NODE
Intersecting curved fascicles of spindle cells, among which are many vascular slits.

multiple confluent nodules scattered throughout the node (fig. 21-20), or almost total replacement of the parenchyma by KS (141). Small, peripherally located tumor nodules are found in regional lymph nodes of patients with cutaneous KS, a pattern similar to that observed in metastatic carcinoma (76,162). Some cases show a predominantly sinusoidal infiltration (141), with irregular extension into the interfollicular zones like fibrous septa (113). However, a mixture of these patterns is not uncommon in a single case.

The well-developed lesion is characterized by curved fascicles of spindle cells with intertwined short slits containing extravasated erythrocytes (figs. 21-21, 21-22). There can be interspersed better-formed capillary spaces congested with blood (100,141). The proportion of these elements varies greatly from case to case (figs. 21-22, 21-23). The spindle cell fascicles interweave in such a way that longitudinally sectioned bundles are often juxtaposed with transversely sectioned bundles. In cross-section, the fascicles show a characteristic sieve-like pattern in which the erythrocyte-containing intercellular slits are easier to appreciate (fig. 21-22) (103). In some cases,

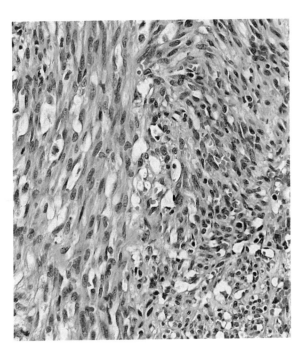

Figure 21-22
KAPOSI'S SARCOMA OF LYMPH NODE
Typical criss-crossing pattern, with longitudinally sectioned fascicles alternating with transversely sectioned fascicles. Note the sieve-like pattern in the latter. Nuclear pleomorphism is minimal, and red blood cells are seen in the vascular slits.

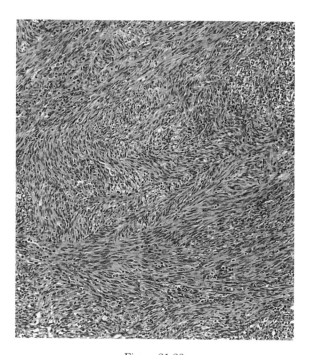

Figure 21-23
KAPOSI'S SARCOMA OF LYMPH NODE
This example resembles fibrosarcoma; its vascular nature is not immediately apparent.

the fascicular growth pattern is poorly developed, with poorly canalized vascular channels haphazardly mixed with spindly cells (fig. 21-24).

The spindle cells possess elongated nuclei with pale to dark chromatin, inconspicuous nucleoli, and lightly stained cytoplasm (fig. 21-22). Individual cell necrosis is common. Nuclear pleomorphism is minimal to mild, and the mitotic count is typically low, although some cases have more mitoses (103). However, a rare anaplastic variant characterized by significant nuclear atypia, with or without anastomosing vascular channels, is also recognized (140,160). This angiosarcoma-like anaplastic variant is recognized by the identification of foci with histologic features of typical KS.

Within the lesion, hemosiderin deposits, lymphoplasmacytic aggregates, and histiocytes are frequently present. A highly distinctive, although not pathognomonic (107), feature found in practically all cases of KS is the eosinophilic hyaline globules, which are variable in size (2 to 10 mm) and stain a lighter color than red blood cells (fig. 21-25) (97,113,140). These globules are

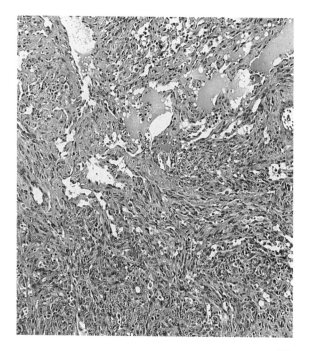

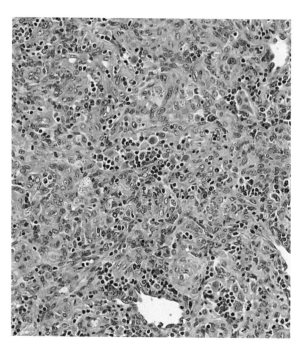

Figure 21-24
KAPOSI'S SARCOMA OF LYMPH NODE
Left: Solid growth of spindle cells mixed with narrow vascular channels, some of which anastomose, resembling the pattern seen in angiosarcoma (upper field).
Right: Barely canalized small blood vessels are haphazardly mixed with spindly cells, without formation of well-defined fascicles. Plasma cells are typically interspersed. Eosinophilic hyaline globules are seen in some plump cells.

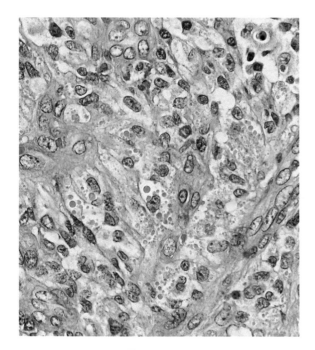

Figure 21-25
KAPOSI'S SARCOMA OF LYMPH NODE
Distinctive cytoplasmic eosinophilic hyaline globules are abundant in this field.

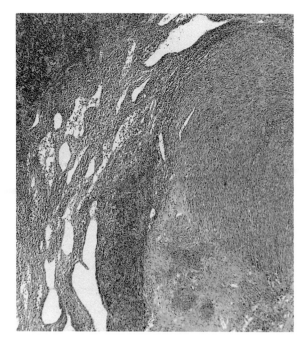

Figure 21-26
KAPOSI'S SARCOMA OF LYMPH NODE
Lymphangiectasia around the tumor nodule.

PAS-positive, diastase-resistant (94), and stain with phosphotungstic acid hematoxylin (PTAH) and phloxine tartrazine (113). Most are located within the cytoplasm of spindle cells or histiocytes, and are often surrounded by clear halos (95,98). Occasionally, the globules are extracellular. Ultrastructurally, they are osmiophilic bodies, some of which may be membrane bound (130). They are believed to be products of lysosomal degeneration or effete red blood cells (71,94,107,121,131).

Ectatic blood vessels and lymphatics are sometimes identified at the periphery of the lesion (fig. 21-26) (94), but it is unclear whether they are part of the disease process or are merely reactive. A variety of changes occur in the residual lymphoid parenchyma, such as reactive follicular hyperplasia, diffuse lymphoid hyperplasia with plasmacytosis, simple plasmacytosis, sinus hyperplasia, hypervascular follicular hyperplasia resembling Castleman's disease, lymphocyte depletion, and dermatopathic lymphadenopathy (81,100,114,141,147,148,153).

The earliest lesion of KS usually involves the capsule of the lymph node; variable extension into the node is along the fibrous trabeculae (fig. 21-27)

(95,105,109,113). There is an increase in irregularly shaped miniature vascular channels, which are ectatic or narrow. Rudimentary fascicles of spindle cells, plasma cells, and hemosiderin are often present (fig. 21-28).

Involvement of the spleen by KS is uncommon and manifests as irregular vascular spaces and spindle cells in the fibrous trabeculae and around the blood vessels (fig. 21-29). Discrete nodules are rarely formed (162).

Moskowitz et al. (134) described an *inflammatory variant* of KS, characterized by arborizing hyalinized thickened blood vessels, a dense lymphoplasmacytic infiltrate, and frequently, hemosiderin deposits. However, these features have not been universally accepted as diagnostic of KS; they can also be interpreted as a nonspecific reactive change preceding the development of KS rather than a morphologically distinct phase of KS (162).

Immunohistochemical Findings. The spindle cells of KS show inconsistent and variable staining for factor VIII–related antigen and *Ulex europaeus,* but usually stain strongly with CD31 and CD34 (73,110,112,124,128,135). There is no staining for muscle-specific actin.

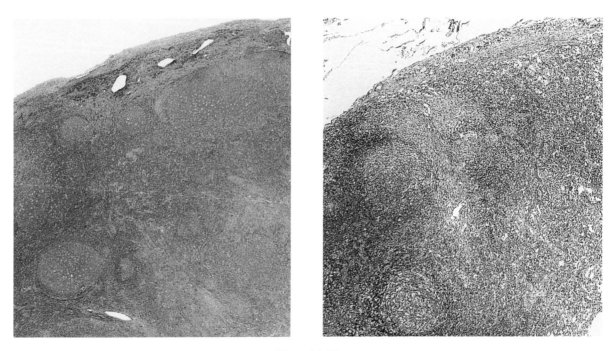

Figure 21-27
EARLY KAPOSI'S SARCOMA OF LYMPH NODE

Left: This lesion takes the form of thickening of the nodal capsule. The patient has AIDS, as evidenced by the explosive follicles that lack well-defined mantles.

Right: A different case, showing that the lesion extends from the nodal capsule into the node along the fibrous trabeculae.

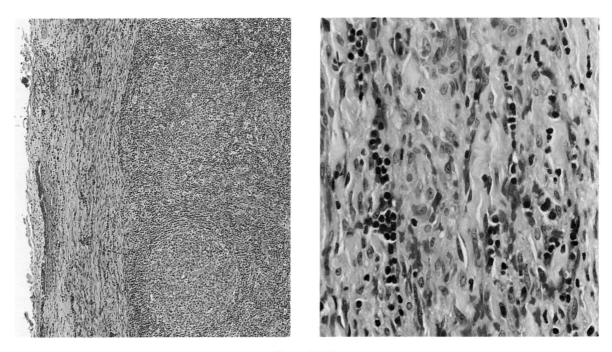

Figure 21-28
EARLY KAPOSI'S SARCOMA OF LYMPH NODE

Left: The nodal capsule shows fibrous thickening with increased cellularity.

Right: Typically, narrow vascular channels and isolated spindly cells are mixed with plasma cells. The finding of hyaline globules (upper field) provides strong support for the diagnosis of Kaposi's sarcoma.

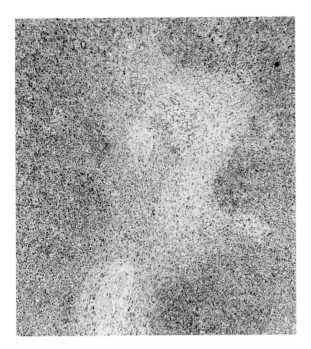

Figure 21-29
KAPOSI'S SARCOMA OF SPLEEN
The involvement is mainly in the fibrous trabeculae.

Histogenesis. There is much controversy on the nature of the cellular proliferation in KS (108). Suggestions of cell origin include reticuloendothelial cell (87,93), primitive mesenchymal cell (134,161), Schwann cell (72,146), fibroblast (159), smooth muscle cell (158), dermal dendrocyte (138), neuromyoarterial apparatus (142), lymphatic endothelium (73,96,138), blood vascular endothelium (80,107,116,135,155,157), vascular related elements including pericytes (69,129), or a combination of vascular and lymphatic endothelia (70,92). Recent studies have favored an endothelial origin for the tumor cells, which have been reported to display overlapping histochemical and immunophenotypic profiles of lymphatic and vascular endothelial cells (73,92,110,120,155). Staining for 5'-nucleotidase, lack of staining for HLA-DR and alkaline phosphatase, and the selective expression of various basement membrane components favor a lymphatic nature for KS (73,96,137). The predominant localization of lesions corresponding to the normal distribution of lymphatics and the absence of lesions in organs devoid of lymphatics (brain, eyeball) also favor a lymphatic origin (98). On the other hand, staining with several monoclonal antibodies that

react with capillary but not lymphatic endothelium favors a vascular endothelial origin (149). Furthermore, the spindle cells of KS exhibit the immunophenotypic profile of activated endothelial cells (168), and often simultaneously coexpress some macrophage antigens (such as CD68, CD14, PAM-1) (163).

Pathogenesis. The pathogenesis of KS remains speculative, but epidemiologic and molecular genetic studies have provided clues about the possible pathogenesis of AIDS-associated KS.

AIDS-associated KS is much more common among the homosexual population than any other AIDS risk group. The proportion of homosexual or bisexual male AIDS patients developing KS has declined, from more than 40 percent in 1983 to around 15 percent in 1988 (74,90,123). The data strongly implicate a sexually transmitted agent/virus as a cofactor in the development of KS (74, 77,79). The agent probably acts rapidly, has no persistent effect, and is now much less common in the homosexual lifestyle (probably resulting from a decrease in high-risk sexual practices and the use of condoms in response to rigorous education campaigns). Some recent studies implicate human papillomavirus type 16 in the genesis of some cases of KS (118,139), but the findings are inconclusive.

HIV itself has also been suggested to have a role in the development of KS, even though the virus genome is not incorporated into the tumor cells (88,104). Implantation of the *tat* gene of HIV into the germline of mice results in skin tumors histologically similar to human KS (165). The *tat* protein is believed to induce vascular growth by enhancing response to basic fibroblast growth factor. *Tat* has been postulated to be the factor responsible for the higher frequency and aggressiveness of KS in HIV-seropositive subjects as compared to the classic form of KS in which basic fibroblastic growth factor is not enhanced (100a).

In vitro studies have provided evidence that a cascade of autocrine- and paracrine-mediated events contributes to the development of KS (101, 112,136,154). Cells derived from AIDS-associated KS can be successfully propagated in culture only if the medium contains growth factors released by cultured T lymphocytes infected with human retroviruses. The cultured KS cells induce their own growth and the growth of normal endothelial cells, fibroblasts, and other cell types; they also induce angiogenesis and KS-like lesions when injected into nude mice.

The exact role played by immunosuppression remains to be defined. There is no satisfactory explanation for why KS develops in patients with AIDS or patients on immunosuppressive therapy, but not in those with congenital immune deficiencies (119). Furthermore, there is no evidence of humoral or cell-mediated immune deficiency in patients with endemic KS (143). Thus, immunosuppression probably plays only a permissive role in the development of KS, through the decrease in immune surveillance or activation of oncogenic viruses.

The suggestion that cytomegalovirus (CMV) infection plays an etiologic role in KS (84) has not been substantiated by recent studies (68,77,82, 123). CMV-DNA sequences have not been identified in KS except when associated with generalized CMV infection (88,104) Recent studies strongly implicate a new herpes virus as the etiologic agent of KS of both the AIDS-associated and non-AIDS–associated types (82a,83a).

Differential Diagnosis. The major differential diagnoses of KS include vascular transformation of sinuses, intranodal hemorrhagic spindle cell tumor with amianthoid fibers, nodal vascular tumors such as cellular hemangioma and spindle/ histiocytoid hemangioendothelioma, bacillary angiomatosis, and inflammatory pseudotumor.

Diagnosing early nodal involvement by KS may be extremely difficult. The subtle thickening and vascular proliferation in the capsule may resemble granulation tissue (105). It is helpful to examine deeper cuts from the tissue block in order to search for more diagnostic, although often rudimentary, spindle cell fascicles (fig. 21-28). Identification of PAS-positive hyaline globules in PAS-diastase preparations strongly favors the diagnosis of KS.

VASCULAR TUMORS OF LYMPH NODE

Primary vascular tumors of lymph node, other than Kaposi's sarcoma, are rare, with only a limited number of cases recorded in the literature (170,171,179,181,182,184,186). These tumors have a range of histologic appearances, but most are benign. Interested readers may refer to a recent review article detailing a pattern recognition approach for the diagnosis of vasoproliferative le-

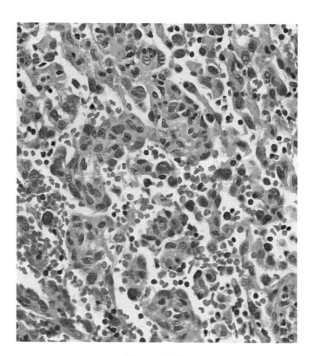

Figure 21-30
METASTATIC ANGIOSARCOMA IN LYMPH NODE
Note the papillary tufts and anastomosing vascular channels, as well as the cytologic atypia.

sions of lymph node (192). If an angiosarcoma is found within a lymph node, it probably represents a metastatic deposit (fig. 21-30). Angiomyomatous hamartoma is discussed under the section, Smooth Muscle Proliferations.

Nodal Hemangioma

Nodal hemangioma presents either as solitary lymphadenopathy or as an incidental finding in lymph nodes (170,171,179,181,182,184). The association with malignancy in some cases is probably fortuitous, because these small lesions would not have been discovered had the lymph nodes not been removed as part of the cancer surgery (171). Occasional cases have shown an association with vascular lesions elsewhere, such as intestinal angiodysplasia (170), oral hemangiopericytoma (170), and vascular esophageal polyp (174). The case reported by Goldstein and Bartal (179) as "hemangioendothelioma" appears to be a cellular hemangioma rather than a vascular tumor of borderline/low-grade malignancy, while a case considered to be "nodal hemangioendothelioma" (186) has been reinterpreted as angiomatoid malignant fibrous histiocytoma

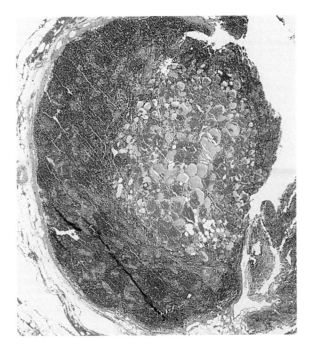 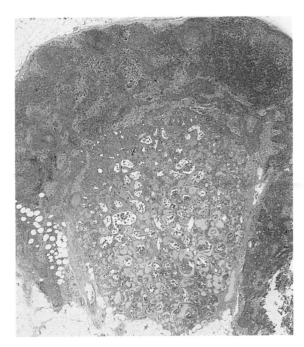

Figure 21-31
HEMANGIOMA OF LYMPH NODE
Left: This capillary/cavernous hemangioma is characterized by a localized collection of vascular channels.
Right: This capillary/cavernous hemangioma mainly involves the medulla and hilum of the lymph node.

(177). The lesion termed "hemangiomatoid" is probably a form of hemangioma (185), but the entity reported as "nodal angiomatosis" (178) appears to be more related to vascular transformation of sinuses (173).

Histologically, hemangioma forms a discrete circumscribed or ill-defined mass of variable size within the lymph node. The lesion is often centered on the nodal hilum or medulla (fig. 21-31), but can almost totally replace the nodal parenchyma.

The hemangiomas are composed of closely packed capillaries, veins, or cavernous vessels, or a combination of these elements (fig. 21-32). The vascular channels can be congested with blood or empty. Variable amounts of fibrous tissue and even fat may be interposed between the proliferated blood vessels (182,184,191). Sometimes, a loose fibromyxoid stroma separates the lobules of capillaries, a pattern reminiscent of granuloma pyogenicum (lobular capillary hemangioma) (fig. 21-33). Some hemangiomas are highly cellular, being formed by closely packed, poorly canalized, pericyte-rich blood vessels (fig. 21-34); the cellular atypia and maze-like anastomosing channels typical of angiosarcoma are lacking. In contrast to

vascular transformation of sinuses, hemangioma forms a discrete mass lesion rather than having a pure sinusoidal distribution, and there is no association with lymphatic/venous obstruction.

Epithelioid Vascular Tumors

Epithelioid vascular tumors, characterized histologically by plump (histiocytoid) endothelial cells with abundant eosinophilic hyaline and often vacuolated cytoplasm, can occur primarily in lymph nodes. There is a continuous spectrum of differentiation, with epithelioid hemangioma on the benign end, epithelioid hemangioendothelioma in the middle (borderline or low-grade malignancy), and epithelioid angiosarcoma on the malignant end (172,187,189,191,193). Some cases may show overlapping features (191).

Epithelioid Hemangioma. Epithelioid hemangioma, also known as *angiolymphoid hyperplasia with eosinophilia,* can occur primarily in lymph node (171,189,191). It is benign. The epithelioid endothelium–lined vascular channels are generally well formed (fig. 21-35), and the stroma is often, but not invariably, rich in lymphocytes and eosinophils. The disease process

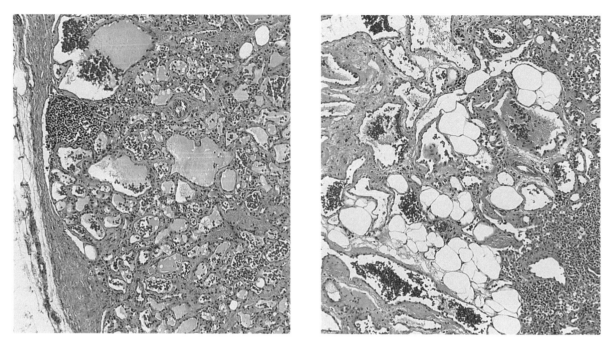

Figure 21-32
HEMANGIOMA OF LYMPH NODE
Left: This hemangioma is formed by congested capillaries.
Right: This nodal hemangioma is composed of thin-walled veins. There are interspersed fat cells.

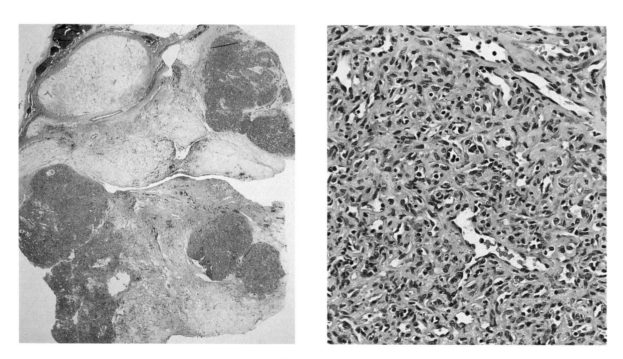

Figure 21-33
LOBULAR CAPILLARY HEMANGIOMA OF LYMPH NODE
Left: There is extensive replacement by capillary lobules that are separated by edematous stroma. Residual nodal tissue is seen in the left upper field.
Right: The lobules are composed of closely packed narrow capillaries.

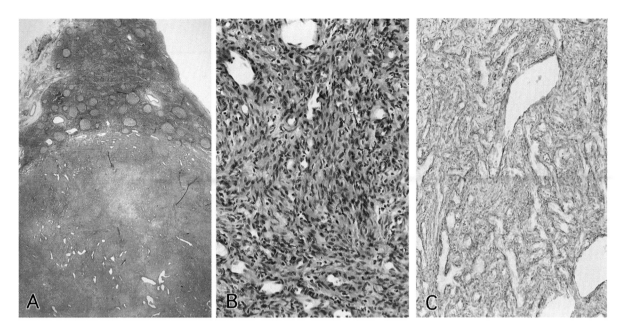

Figure 21-34
CELLULAR HEMANGIOMA OF LYMPH NODE

A: Most of the lymph node is replaced by an expansile tumor.

B: Note the closely packed blood vessels with barely visible lumina. A spindle cell pattern is created.

C: The individual blood vessels are best highlighted by immunostaining for muscle-specific actin, which outlines the pericytes around the vessels.

frequently involves the endothelial lining and muscle coat of the larger hilar blood vessels. Although epithelioid hemangioma was often considered synonymous to Kimura's disease in the past, these are now recognized as two distinct entities (172,183). Kimura's disease is basically an inflammatory/allergic process, and lacks the distinctive endothelial proliferation of epithelioid hemangioma.

Epithelioid Hemangioendothelioma. Primary epithelioid hemangioendothelioma of lymph node is very rare, but has been well documented (171,176,193). Local excision is usually curative, but the lesion may recur; metastasis is a potential complication. The possibility that the nodal lesion is a metastasis from a primary tumor elsewhere (such as lung, liver, bone, or soft tissue) should be excluded before accepting the lesion as a lymph node primary. Epithelioid hemangioendothelioma is characterized by short cords of polygonal, stellate, or plump spindle cells disposed in an abundant hyaline or myxochondroid matrix (fig. 21-36). Necrosis and hyalinization are common in the central portion of the tumor (fig. 21-37). The tumor cells have abundant eosinophilic hyaline

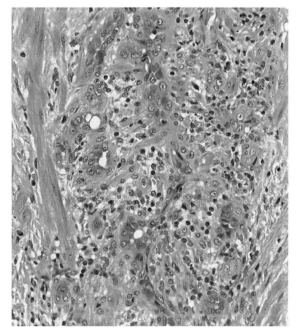

Figure 21-35
EPITHELIOID HEMANGIOMA OF LYMPH NODE

The vessels are lined by plump cells which sometimes show vacuolation. The stroma is infiltrated by eosinophils.

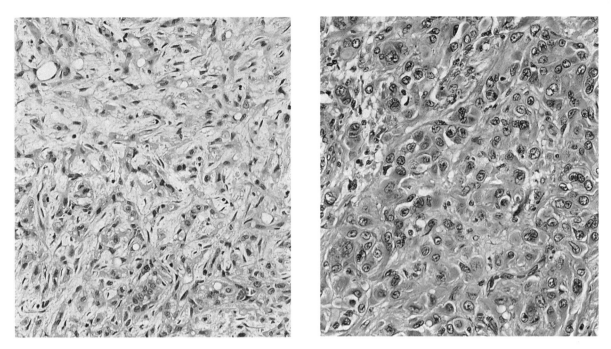

Figure 21-36
EPITHELIOID HEMANGIOENDOTHELIOMA OF LYMPH NODE
Left: Cords of tumor cells lie in a myxoid matrix. Note the cytoplasmic vacuoles.
Right: Predominantly solid growth of polygonal cells with abundant eosinophilic hyaline cytoplasm.

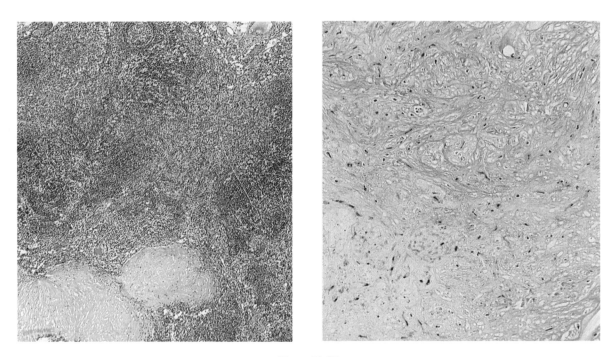

Figure 21-37
EPITHELIOID HEMANGIOENDOTHELIOMA OF LYMPH NODE WITH REGRESSIVE CHANGES
Left: There is extensive hyalinization and focal calcification.
Right: A diagnosis can hardly be made from the hyalinized areas, but the few residual "strangulated" tumor cords should provide a clue to the correct diagnosis.

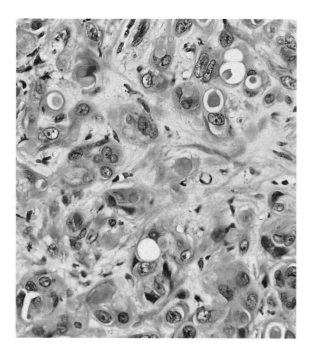

Figure 21-38
EPITHELIOID HEMANGIOENDOTHELIOMA
OF LYMPH NODE

Polygonal cells with abundant hyaline cytoplasm are seen. The vacuoles and primitive vascular channels contain red blood cells or lysed blood. Nuclear pleomorphism is mild to moderate.

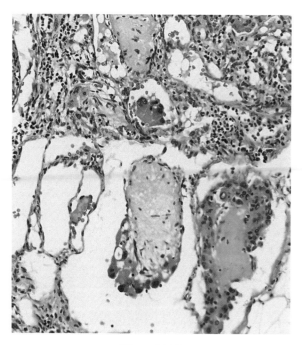

Figure 21-39
EPITHELIOID HEMANGIOENDOTHELIOMA
OF LYMPH NODE

In the peripheral portion of the tumor, papillary tufts of epithelioid cells are often found projecting into lymphovascular spaces. These papillary tufts often have hyalinized cores.

cytoplasm, which is frequently vacuolated. The nuclei show mild to moderate pleomorphism, and nuclear pseudoinclusions are common (fig. 21-38). Mitotic figures are infrequent. There are usually no or few well-formed vascular channels, but red blood cells can often be identified in some of the cytoplasmic vacuoles. In some areas, the tumor cells are more compact and form nondescript sheets (fig. 21-36, right). Nodal epithelioid hemangioendothelioma can be mistaken for metastatic carcinoma because of its growth pattern and cytology. Whenever the following features are present in combination, the diagnosis of epithelioid hemangioendothelioma should be suspected (191): tumor cells growing in cords; an abundant myxoid, hyaline, or cartilage-like stroma; and prominent cytoplasmic vacuoles (mucin negative). Search should then be made for primitive vascular channels and red blood cells in the cytoplasmic vacuoles. It is usually helpful to examine the peripheral portions of the tumor, where intravascular or intralymphatic growth in the form of character-

istic papillary tufts is often found (fig. 21-39). The diagnosis can be further confirmed by immunostaining for CD34, CD31, and factor VIII–related antigen; labeling with *Ulex europaeus* (fig. 21-40); or finding Weibel-Palade bodies on ultrastructural examination. It should be noted, however, that cytokeratin can be positive in this tumor (180). Another important differential diagnosis is bacillary angiomatosis.

Spindle and Epithelioid Hemangioendothelioma. Spindle and epithelioid (histiocytoid) hemangioendothelioma, reported as a primary tumor of lymph node by Silva et al. (188), appears to be a variant of epithelioid hemangioendothelioma. It differs from typical epithelioid hemangioendothelioma by the presence of a more prominent spindle cell component and a much less abundant hyaline matrix (fig. 21-41). In contrast to Kaposi's sarcoma, the spindle cells are plumper, a significant number of polygonal "histiocytoid" endothelial cells are present, and eosinophilic hyaline globules are absent.

459

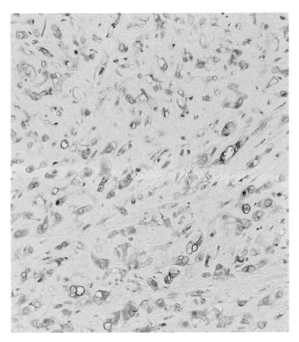

Figure 21-40
EPITHELIOID HEMANGIOENDOTHELIOMA
OF LYMPH NODE
Positive immunostaining of the tumor cells for factor VIII–related antigen is seen. The reactivity is strongest in the vacuoles (early vascular lumen formation).

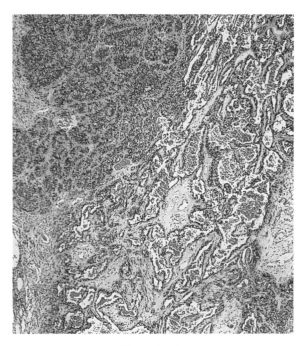

Figure 21-42
POLYMORPHOUS HEMANGIOENDOTHELIOMA
OF LYMPH NODE
This tumor is characterized by a variegated pattern: solid areas, narrow anastomosing vascular spaces, and cavernous vascular spaces.

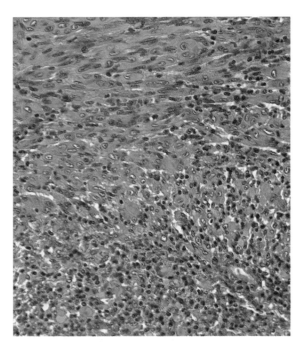

Figure 21-41
SPINDLE AND EPITHELIOID
(HISTIOCYTOID) HEMANGIOENDOTHELIOMA
There is a mixture of spindle cells and plump epithelioid cells. In this example, many eosinophils are admixed.

Polymorphous Hemangioendothelioma

Polymorphous hemangioendothelioma is an uncommon low-grade malignant vascular tumor occurring in lymph nodes (171). The histologic patterns vary in different portions of the same tumor. Of two patients with follow-up information, one remained well at 6 years and one died with metastatic disease at 3.3 years (190).

Polymorphous hemangioendothelioma is characterized by an intimate blend of solid, primitive vascular and angiomatous components (fig. 21-42). The solid component consists of sheets, packets, cords, and complex trabeculae of polygonal cells with uniform nuclei, fine chromatin, and scanty cytoplasm (fig. 21-43). In areas, vascular differentiation is evident in the form of occasional cytoplasmic vacuoles, narrow clefts, irregular branching channels, and papillary formations. The angiomatous component is formed by ectatic or congested vascular spaces lined by plump cells. The tumor cells stain for *Ulex europaeus,* but not factor VIII–related antigen.

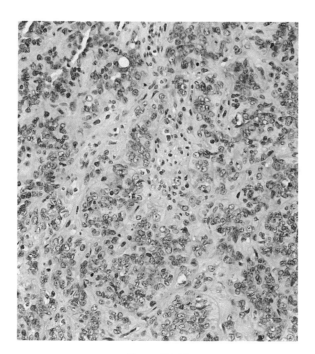

Figure 21-43
POLYMORPHOUS HEMANGIOENDOTHELIOMA
OF LYMPH NODE

The solid area is formed by islands and broad trabeculae of cells with mild nuclear pleomorphism. Occasional cells are vacuolated, indicating early vascular differentiation at the cellular level. Some early vascular slits are seen in the upper field.

Lymphangioma

Lymphangioma of lymph node is almost always accompanied by involvement of the surrounding soft tissues or other sites (such as the spleen) (171,186). It is noncircumscribed, and partially or completely replaces the nodal parenchyma. It is composed of variably sized, endothelium-lined lymphatic spaces filled with proteinaceous fluid which may contain collections of small lymphocytes (fig. 21-44). Lymphoid aggregates are also frequently found in the fibrous septa between the lymphatic spaces. Rarely, the lesion is composed of large cystic spaces, justifying the designation "cystic hygroma" (175).

VASCULAR NEOPLASM ARISING IN LOCALIZED FORM OF CASTLEMAN'S DISEASE

Kaposi's sarcoma can complicate some cases of multicentric Castleman's disease (195,197), but an unusual vascular neoplasm distinct from Kaposi's sarcoma has also been recognized to

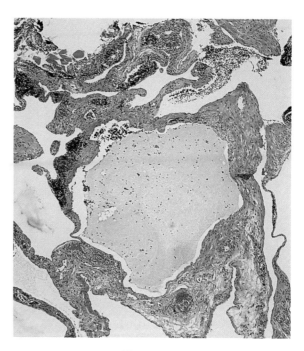

Figure 21-44
LYMPHANGIOMA OF LYMPH NODE
Large lymph-filled cystic spaces replace the nodal parenchyma.

arise in the solitary form of hyaline-vascular Castleman's disease (198). Earlier descriptions of this uncommon association include a case alluded to by Symmers (200) and a case of "Kaposi's sarcoma" complicating Castleman's disease reported by Nagai et al. (199).

The vascular tumor is located in the retroperitoneum, mediastinum, or axilla, and measures 4 to 20 cm (198,201). The cut surface is solid and tan, and sometimes shows areas of hemorrhage. Histologically, in addition to the component of hyaline-vascular Castleman's disease, there is a mesenchymal neoplasm which forms discrete nodules or blends with the interfollicular proliferation of high endothelial venules that are typical of Castleman's disease (figs. 21-45, 21-46). This tumor differentiates into vascular and vascular-related elements, and is composed of swirling fascicles of spindle or plump cells that occasionally form vascular lumina. The tumor cells show mild to marked nuclear pleomorphism, and the mitotic count is highly variable. Hyaline globules typical of Kaposi's sarcoma are absent. There are often foci of fibrosis and necrosis. Neutrophils, lymphocytes, and macrophages are

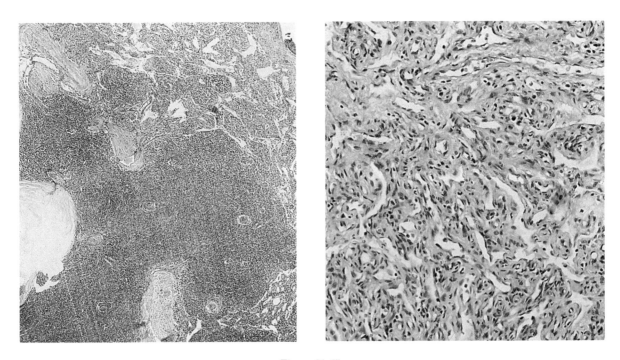

Figure 21-45
VASCULAR NEOPLASM COMPLICATING HYALINE-VASCULAR CASTLEMAN'S DISEASE

Left: The vascular neoplasm is evident in the upper field. In the lower field, hyaline-vascular follicles that characterize Castleman's disease are seen.

Right: This case of vascular neoplasm is formed by irregular narrow vascular channels with no cellular atypia.

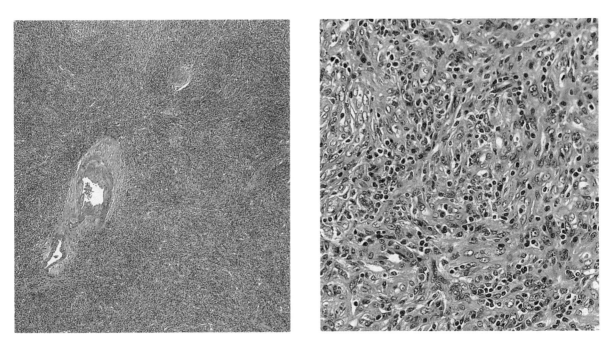

Figure 21-46
HYALINE-VASCULAR CASTLEMAN'S DISEASE WITH VASCULAR HYPERPLASIA:
A POSSIBLE PRECURSOR OF VASCULAR NEOPLASM

Left: There is marked expansion of the interfollicular tissue by vascular proliferation, to the extent that only one hyaline-vascular follicle is evident in this field.

Right: Note the proliferation of vessels resembling high endothelial venules.

often interspersed throughout the tumor. Immunostaining for factor VIII–related antigen is often negative, while a variable proportion of the tumor cells stain for vimentin and muscle-specific actin (198). While some cases appear to be genuine vascular tumors (with factor VIII–related antigen reactivity) (194,201), the endothelial nature of many reported cases has not been proven, and some may even represent hyperplasia or neoplasm of stromal cells or follicular dendritic cells (196).

The behavior of this uncommon tumor awaits clarification by further long-term studies, but at least two cases exhibiting significant nuclear atypia and frequent mitoses metastasized and were fatal. Five patients have remained disease-free 1 to 3 years after surgery (198). The occurrence of a vascular neoplasm in association with Castleman's disease suggests that the former develops from the background of vascular hyperplasia (fig. 21-46), possibly mediated by angiogenic factors released by the lymphoid component.

VASCULAR TRANSFORMATION OF LYMPH NODE SINUSES

Definition. Vascular transformation of sinuses refers to the conversion of lymph node sinuses into complex, anastomosing, endothelium-lined channels, frequently accompanied by fibrosis (210). This is a fairly common nodal reaction which may be mistaken for Kaposi's sarcoma. The lesion termed "nodal angiomatosis" probably refers to the same entity (203,205, 209); an alternative designation, *stasis lymphadenopathy,* has also been proposed (212).

Clinical Features. Vascular transformation of sinuses occurs in any age group of either sex. Lymph nodes of any location can be involved. In most instances, it is an incidental finding in lymph nodes obtained in a variety of surgical procedures, such as dissections of regional lymph nodes draining cancer, but it can also present as lymphadenopathy alone (205). The lesion is innocuous.

Pathogenesis. In the initial description of vascular transformation of sinuses, venous obstruction was considered to be the major underlying etiology (210). Subsequent studies on rabbits have shown that occlusion of the efferent lymphatics, with or without venous obstruction,

can produce the changes of vascular transformation of sinuses (215). In most cases, factors contributing to lymphovascular obstruction can often be identified (such as tumor in the vicinity, vascular thrombosis, severe heart failure, previous surgery) (205,208,210,212–214,216); however, the occasional occurrence of vascular sinus transformation in the regional lymph nodes draining cancer or hemangioma in the absence of lymphovascular obstruction suggests that angiogenic factors may contribute to the development of the vasoproliferation in some cases (205).

Microscopic Findings. Vascular sinus transformation can involve some or all of the lymph node sinuses; the capsule is spared (fig. 21-47). The expanded sinuses often exhibit sclerosis, and the intervening lymphoid parenchyma shows variable degrees of atrophy (fig. 21-47, right). The proliferated vessels within the sinuses are in the form of irregular sinuous vascular slits or rounded vascular spaces lined by flat endothelium (fig. 21-48). Commonly, there are solid foci formed by bland-looking spindle or plump oval cells, among which irregular anastomosing vascular clefts can be identified (fig. 21-48). Extravasation of red blood cells is common, and there can be interstitial fibrin deposits (fig. 21-49). Furthermore, the solid areas often show gradual "maturation" into well-formed vascular spaces towards the capsular aspect (fig. 21-50). A less common variant is characterized by complex maze-like vascular channels, morphologically identical to the plexiform vascularization of lymph node described in cats (fig. 21-51); this pattern has so far been observed only in intra-abdominal nodes in humans (205,211).

The perinodal blood vessels often appear prominent by virtue of their thickened walls. Thrombosis is only infrequently identified.

Nodular Spindle Cell Variant. The nodular spindle cell variant of vascular transformation of sinuses, which is particularly liable to be mistaken histologically for Kaposi's sarcoma, is characterized by spindle cell nodules superimposed on the sinusoidal vascular proliferation (fig. 21-52) (206). The nodules comprise interlacing fascicles of spindle cells with interspersed vascular clefts. The cuffing of spindle cells around the vascular spaces is often easier to appreciate in areas cut in cross section. Most of the spindle cells are pericytes or smooth muscle

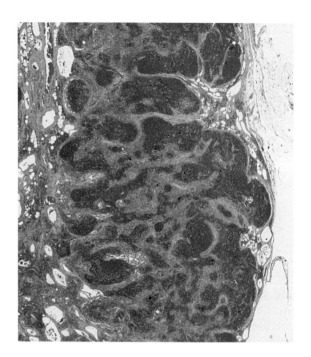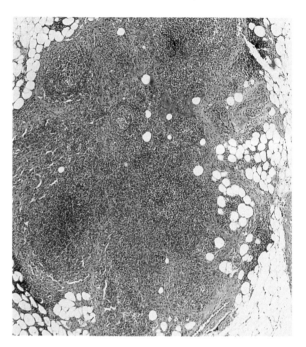

Figure 21-47
VASCULAR TRANSFORMATION OF SINUSES
Left: Expansion and fibrosis of the sinuses is evident.
Right: The striking vascular transformation of the sinuses in this example is associated with lymphoid atrophy.

cells. This variant occurs most frequently in retroperitoneal lymph nodes removed because of renal cell carcinoma, and is presumably caused by angiogenic factors that drain into the regional lymph nodes from the highly vascularized renal cell carcinoma, although it can also occur in superficial lymph nodes in patients without a history of malignant neoplasm.

Differential Diagnosis. The most important differential diagnosis is Kaposi's sarcoma (207, 217). Vascular transformation of sinuses occurs in diverse clinical circumstances, whereas, with the exception of its recognized incidence in African children, nodal involvement by Kaposi's sarcoma occurs most frequently in immunocompromised hosts; however, vascular sinus transformation has also been recorded in patients with AIDS (218). The histologic features that help distinguish the two are listed in Table 21-2. The vascular slits in vascular transformation of sinuses, which are complex and branching, are accompanied by a significant component of pericytes as demonstrated by immunostaining; this contrasts with the short vascular slits of Kaposi's sarcoma, which lack a pericytic component.

Nodal hemangioma forms a more discrete mass lesion, and is basically identical to analogous tumors in the soft tissues (202,204,205).

ANGIOLIPOMATOUS HAMARTOMA IN ASSOCIATION WITH CASTLEMAN'S DISEASE

Angiolipomatous hamartoma is occasionally associated with hyaline-vascular Castleman's disease (219-221,223). The lesions occur in the posterior mediastinum or retroperitoneum, forming large masses measuring 12 to 15 cm. All patients have remained well after surgical excision.

Grossly, within the noncircumscribed, yellow, fatty mass, a single firm tan nodule or multiple scattered nodules are present. The component of Castleman's disease corresponds to the tan nodules, and consists of hyaline-vascular follicles separated by a lymphocyte-rich stroma with plentiful high endothelial venules (fig. 21-53, left). The angiolipomatous hamartoma is composed predominantly of fibroadipose tissue and haphazardly scattered thick-walled blood vessels (fig. 21-53, right).

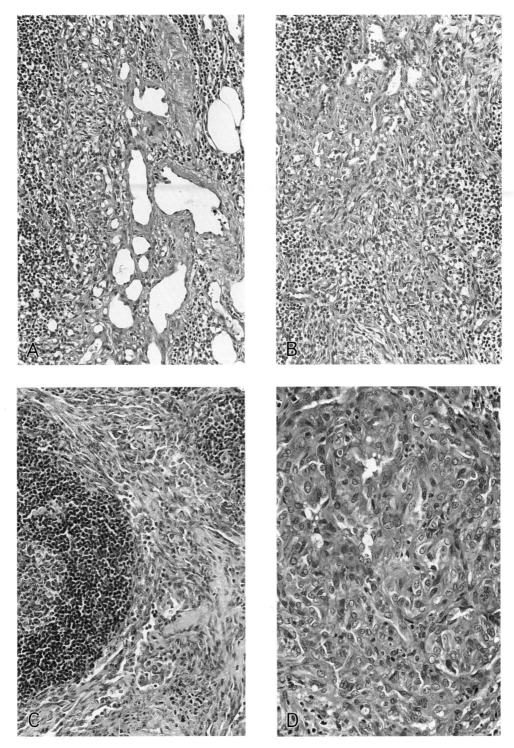

Figure 21-48
VASCULAR TRANSFORMATION OF SINUSES: THE MORPHOLOGIC SPECTRUM

A: Well-formed capillary-sized vessels occur in the fibrosed sinus.

B: Spindly cells and narrow vascular clefts in a fibrous stroma.

C: Irregular branching vascular clefts in a fibrous stroma, which differ from the short nonbranching vascular slits seen in Kaposi's sarcoma.

D: Plump cells with a solid pattern and some poorly formed vascular channels.

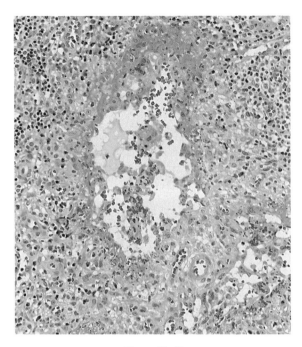

Figure 21-49
VASCULAR TRANSFORMATION OF SINUSES
This example is associated with fibrin deposits.

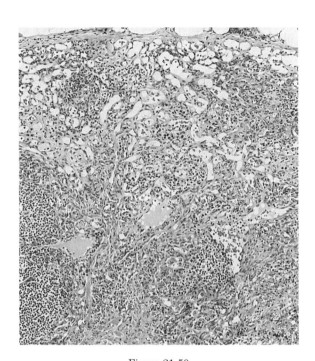

Figure 21-50
VASCULAR TRANSFORMATION OF SINUSES
The solid spindle cell foci (lower field) merge and "mature"
into better-formed vessels towards the capsule (upper field).

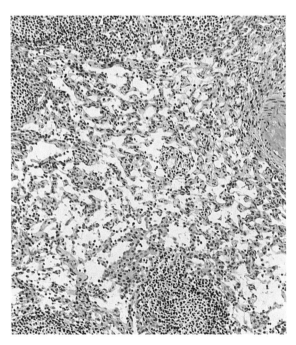

Figure 21-51
VASCULAR TRANSFORMATION OF SINUSES IN
AN INTRA-ABDOMINAL LYMPH NODE
This example exhibits a plexiform pattern.

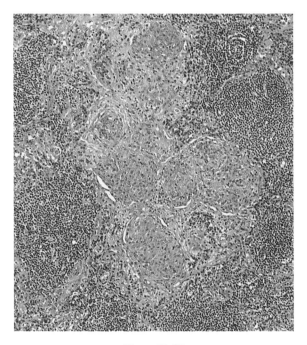

Figure 21-52
NODULAR SPINDLE CELL VASCULAR
TRANSFORMATION OF LYMPH NODE
(NODULAR VARIANT OF
VASCULAR TRANSFORMATION OF SINUSES)
Nodular aggregates of spindly cells and blood vessels are
formed in the expanded sinuses.

Table 21-2

COMPARISON BETWEEN VASCULAR TRANSFORMATION OF SINUSES AND NODAL KAPOSI'S SARCOMA

	Vascular Transformation of Sinuses	Nodal Kaposi's Sarcoma
Pattern of nodal involvement	Confined to sinuses; does not involve capsule	Capsule, parenchyma, or sinuses; capsular involvement common
Spindle cells	Narrow short fascicles sometimes formed; when present, accompanied by irregular branching vascular slits and showing maturation into well-formed vascular channels towards capsular aspect	Broad, curved fascicles common in well-developed lesions; vascular slits short and nonbranching
Cellular atypia	Absent	Sometimes present
Sclerosis	Common and often prominent	Usually insignificant in well-developed lesions
PAS+ hyaline globules	Only found in exceptional cases	Almost always present, particularly in well-developed lesions

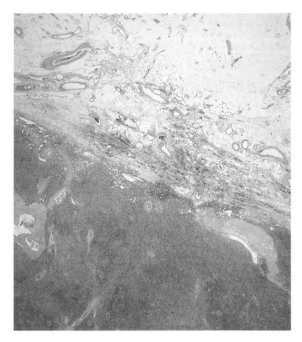 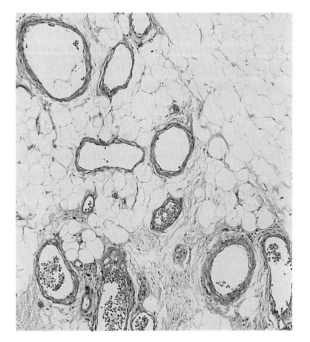

Figure 21-53

ANGIOLIPOMATOUS HAMARTOMA IN ASSOCIATION WITH CASTLEMAN'S DISEASE

Left: The angiolipomatous hamartoma (upper field) is associated with the hyaline-vascular type of Castleman's disease (lower field).
Right: Prominent blood vessels are found among mature fat cells in the angiolipomatous hamartoma.

The association of Castleman's disease of hyaline-vascular type with an obviously hamartomatous component has been invoked to support a possible hamartomatous origin for Castleman's disease. Alternatively, the vasoproliferation in both the Castleman's lesion and the angiolipomatous component may result from the action of angiogenic factors secreted by the stimulated lymphocytes within the lymphoid component (220). Also, hamartomatous thick-walled vessels (in the absence of an adipose component) can also be rarely observed within a Castleman's lesion (222).

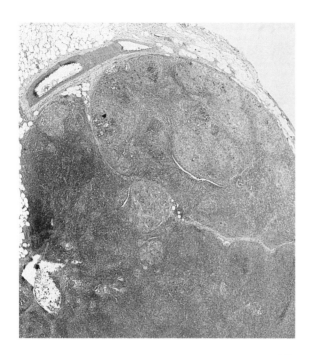 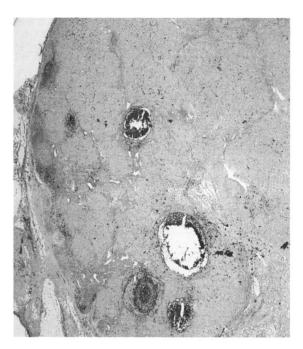

Figure 21-54
BACILLARY ANGIOMATOSIS OF LYMPH NODE
Left: Lymph node showing a multinodular pattern of involvement.
Right: Another example showing extensive replacement of nodal parenchyma by confluent nodules. There are also peliotic spaces.

BACILLARY ANGIOMATOSIS

Definition. Bacillary angiomatosis, originally known as epithelioid angiomatosis, is an unusual but distinctive reactive tumor-like vascular proliferation in response to infection by a bacterium morphologically similar to the cat-scratch disease bacillus *Afipia felis* (224,227,233,241,243). Although the bacilli exhibit many properties of *A. felis*, they differ by producing a completely different histologic reaction, showing dramatic response to antibiotics, and having a different whole-cell fatty acid chromatographic profile (231,237). Molecular analysis further suggests that the bacillary angiomatosis agent is a previously uncharacterized rickettsia closely related to *Rochalimaea quintana* (240), named *Rochalimaea henselae*, or by the new nomenclature, *Bartonella henselae* (239,244); however, *R. quintana* may also be responsible for some cases of bacillary angiomatosis (230). Of interest, *R. henselae* has recently been shown to be a more common etiologic agent of cat scratch disease than *A. felis* (223a).

Clinical Features. Bacillary angiomatosis occurs almost exclusively in the setting of immu-nodeficiency, especially in patients with AIDS (226,227,231–233,241). It commonly presents as multiple skin nodules, but many other sites including lymph node and spleen can be involved. Lymphadenopathy may be the sole manifestation or may occur in association with other sites of disease (225,231,235). The disease can disseminate and is potentially lethal, but it shows an excellent response to antibiotics such as erythromycin (226,231).

Microscopic Findings. Scattered throughout the lymph node or spleen are multiple coalescent nodules of proliferated vessels (figs. 21-54, 21-55) (225,229). The vessels, which range from being barely canalized to ectatic, are lined by plump endothelial cells with pale or finely vacuolated cytoplasm (figs. 21-56–21-58). There may be mild to moderate nuclear pleomorphism in the endothelial cells (fig. 21-57) (225,235). A distinctive feature is an abundant eosinophilic to amphophilic, amorphous or granular interstitial material which, on Warthin-Starry stain, proves to be aggregated bacilli (figs. 21-59, 21-60). The bacilli are short and morphologically indistinguishable from those seen in cat-scratch disease.

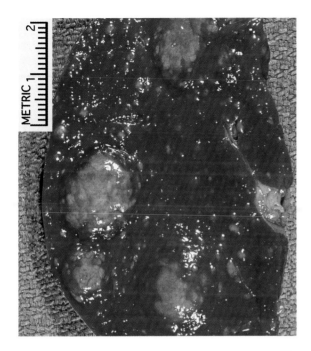 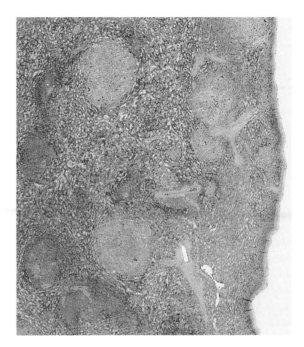

Figure 21-55
BACILLARY ANGIOMATOSIS OF THE SPLEEN
Left: The cut surface of the spleen is studded with small and large fleshy nodules of bacillary angiomatosis.
Right: Histologically, these nodules are haphazardly distributed in the splenic parenchyma.

Neutrophils are frequently but not invariably found in the interstitium. Extravasation of erythrocytes is common. Less common findings include foamy histiocytes, loculated edema, granuloma, and peliosis (figs. 21-54, left; 21-61) (225,228,234, 236). In the spleen, there may be peliotic spaces rimmed by myxoid stroma harboring bacilli (236).

The bacilli occur in clumps extracellularly, and are best demonstrated by the Warthin-Starry stain (fig. 21-59), or in semi-thin Epon sections. The bacilli can also be demonstrated by the Giemsa stain (242), and by immunohistochemical techniques using *R. quintana* antibodies (238) or cultured cat-scratch disease bacilli antisera (233). Trilaminar cell walls are seen on electron microscopy.

Differential Diagnosis. Bacillary angiomatosis should not be mistaken for vascular tumors because of the potential for systemic involvement if not treated with appropriate antibiotics. Unlike epithelioid hemangioma or hemangioendothelioma, the endothelial cells in bacillary angiomatosis have pale rather than eosinophilic hyaline cytoplasm, there is no prominent cytoplasmic vacuolation, and there is a distinctive interstitial

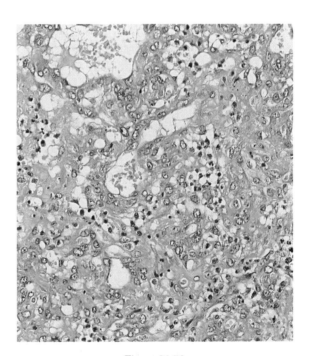

Figure 21-56
BACILLARY ANGIOMATOSIS OF LYMPH NODE
Ectatic vessels are lined by plump endothelium. Note the eosinophilic to amphophilic interstitial material and neutrophils in the stroma.

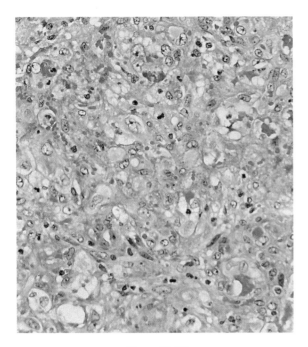

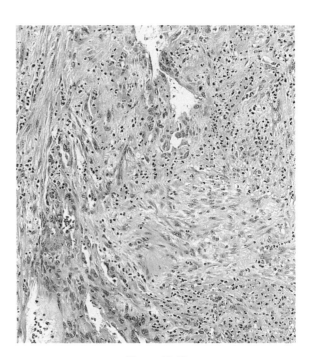

Figure 21-57
BACILLARY ANGIOMATOSIS OF LYMPH NODE

Barely canalized proliferated blood vessels are lined by plump cells with atypical nuclei. In this example, neutrophils are sparse, but amphophilic interstitial materials are evident.

Figure 21-58
BACILLARY ANGIOMATOSIS OF SPLEEN

Irregular, branching narrow vascular channels are separated by a fibrous stroma containing amphophilic interstitial deposits and neutrophils.

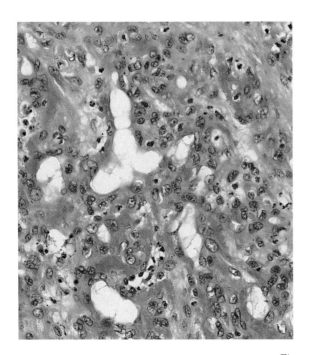

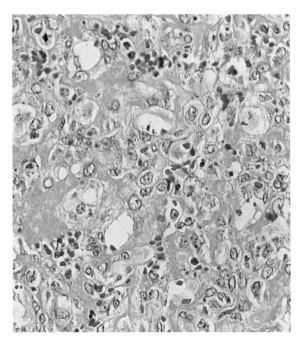

Figure 21-59
BACILLARY ANGIOMATOSIS

Left: Proliferated blood vessels are separated by abundant eosinophilic, vaguely fibrillary material. Some neutrophils are also seen.
Right: Barely canalized blood vessels separated by eosinophilic interstitial materials in the absence of neutrophils.

470

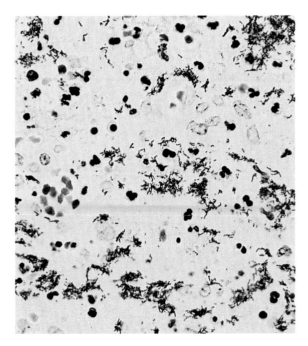

Figure 21-60
BACILLARY ANGIOMATOSIS
The Warthin-Starry stain demonstrates numerous bacilli, corresponding to the deep-staining eosinophilic or amphophilic interstitial material.

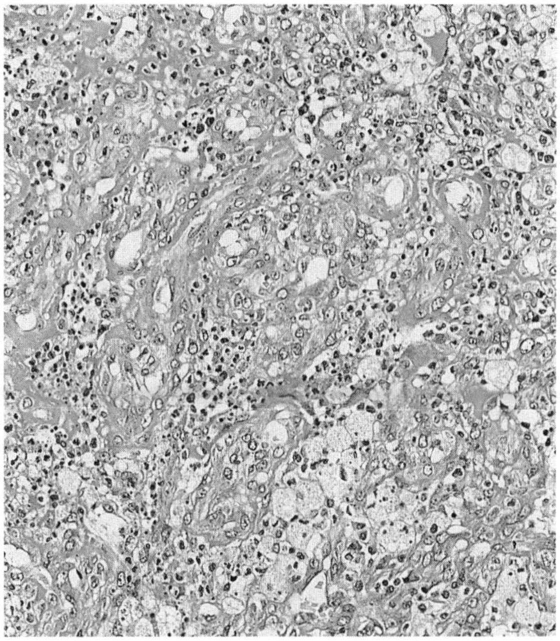

Figure 21-61
BACILLARY ANGIOMATOSIS OF LYMPH NODE
Foamy histiocytes are found between the proliferated blood vessels.

material formed by myriads of bacilli. Bacillary angiomatosis differs from Kaposi's sarcoma by the presence of plump cells, better-formed blood vessels, and a lack of well-defined spindle cell fascicles. Although nuclear pleomorphism can occur, bacillary angiomatosis is distinguished from angiosarcoma (metastatic or primary in lymph node) by the well-formed vascular channels, the distinctive interstitial material, and the frequent neutrophilic infiltrate. In case of doubt, the diagnosis can be readily clarified by a Warthin-Starry stain.

GLANDULAR INCLUSIONS IN LYMPH NODE

Müllerian Inclusions

Clinical Features. Benign Müllerian inclusions can occur in intra-abdominal (249,266,268, 270,285,286) and occasionally, inguinal and femoral (287) lymph nodes of females, and more rarely of males (264,290). They have been documented in 5 to 41 percent of intra-abdominal lymph nodes obtained from surgical excisions or autopsy in women (255,262,266,268,285). They

are generally believed to result from metaplastic proliferation of the peritoneal mesothelium (264, 266,267,290), but the possibility of "benign metastasis" cannot be completely discounted (246). These inclusions are usually incidental findings with no clinical manifestations, but on occasion may cause lymph node enlargement, false-positive lymphangiogram results, or ureteric obstruction (267,295).

Microscopic Findings. The Müllerian inclusions are usually located in the capsule or superficial cortex of the lymph node (266,282), but more extensive involvement sometimes occurs (267, 268). Rarely, they are found within the subcapsular sinuses (268,286). They may be surrounded by a thin rim of sclerotic stroma, or appear "naked" within the lymphoid tissue (282). Psammoma bodies can be present. The glands are round, irregular-contoured, or cystic, sometimes with papillary projections. They are usually lined by columnar ciliated cells and secretory cells with regular basal nuclei which may be pseudostratified, morphologically identical to endosalpingiosis (fig. 21-62). However, the epithelium can be of endometrial

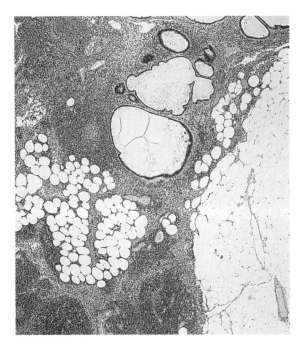 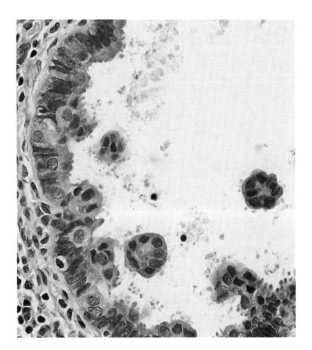

Figure 21-62
MÜLLERIAN INCLUSION IN PELVIC LYMPH NODE
Left: Several cystic epithelial inclusions are seen in this node.
Right: Note the cilia in some of the lining cells.

(255,282), endocervical (256,282), or metaplastic squamous (276,284) type. Nuclear pleomorphism and mitoses are lacking. Rarely, the glandular epithelium shows mild atypia and proliferates to form cribriform or solid patterns (249,253,267). A unique case of miniature adenoacanthoma arising in a nodal Müllerian inclusion has been reported (269).

Differential Diagnosis. It is most important to distinguish benign Müllerian inclusions from metastatic adenocarcinoma (although the two elements may coexist in the same node) (266, 282,285). The distinction is usually not difficult except when the patient has an ovarian borderline serous tumor; in this case the distinction may be extremely difficult and even arbitrary (253). The following features favor a diagnosis of benign inclusion over metastasis: capsular or interfollicular location within the node; presence of ciliated cells; lack of significant cellular atypia and mitotic activity; and absence of a desmoplastic reaction.

Squamous metaplasia of the Müllerian inclusions can also lead to a mistaken diagnosis of metastatic squamous cell carcinoma (276,295). However, in contrast to the latter, the cells are cytologically bland and mitotically inactive, a prominent basal cell layer is present, desmoplastic reaction is absent, and serial sectioning of the tissue may reveal the metaplastic origin from benign glands.

Endometriosis

Endometriosis involving lymph nodes can cause enlargement of the lymph node or may be an incidental microscopic finding (250,265). In contrast to Müllerian inclusions, endometriosis is located more centrally within the node, an endometrial stromal component is present, and frequently there are siderophages and pseudoxanthoma cells. A unique example accompanied by a prominent smooth muscle component has been reported, appropriately termed "endomyometriosis" (280).

Salivary Gland Inclusions

Heterotopic salivary gland ducts and acini are commonly found within intraparotid lymph nodes, since the parotid epithelium invaginates and lymphoid tissue condenses during the same

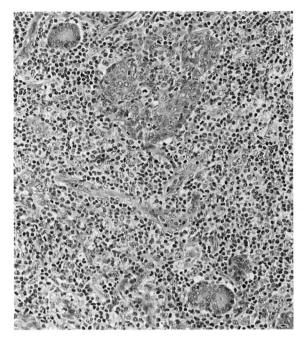

Figure 21-63
SALIVARY GLAND INCLUSION IN LYMPH NODE
In this patient with AIDS, the salivary gland inclusions show epithelial proliferation, resembling the epimyoepithelial islands seen in Sjögren's syndrome.

Thyroid Inclusions

Heterotopic thyroid follicles occur rarely in cervical lymph nodes (258,275). They have been identified in up to 3 percent of autopsies after thorough search (275), but others have reported a less than 1 percent incidence (258) based on examination of surgical materials. Thyroid inclusions appear as aggregates of 20 to 30 normal-appearing colloid-filled follicles in the subcapsular or intracapsular regions (or occasionally deeper parenchyma) of the lymph node (258). There can be a thin sclerotic rim around the follicles.

The distinction from metastatic papillary thyroid carcinoma can be very difficult, because papillary carcinoma can appear deceptively bland. Thyroid follicles identified in lymph nodes should be considered metastatic thyroid carcinoma unless the following strict criteria are satisfied (275): microscopic size; round or oval follicles, loosely arranged and without papillae; nuclei not enlarged and not crowded, with fine chromatin; nucleoli not enlarged; lack of stromal reaction; and absence of psammoma bodies.

If a large portion of the lymph node is replaced by thyroid follicles or multiple nodes are involved, the diagnosis of metastatic thyroid carcinoma is more likely (281).

Mammary Inclusions

Epithelial inclusions occurring within axillary lymph nodes are rare (252,257,260,261,274,277, 292). They appear as groups of ducts or small cysts lined by a double-layered epithelium, often devoid of stroma. Larger cysts lined by apocrine or keratinizing stratified squamous epithelium can occur. These inclusions are often interpreted as heterotopic mammary tissue, although it is also possible that they have a sweat gland origin (257,274). Exceptionally, florid hyperplasia (292), papilloma (274), or carcinoma (277,293) can arise primarily in ectopic breast inclusions in axillary lymph nodes (fig. 21-64).

Other Epithelial Inclusions

Rarely, glandular inclusions have been reported in unusual sites such as mediastinal lymph node and celiac lymph node; the latter can be caused by pancreatic heterotopia with and without cystic or proliferative change in the ductal component (248,270). Exceptionally, simple

embryonic period (247,288,291). Similar inclusions are sometimes found in extraparotid cervical lymph nodes. The ducts are lined by a double layer of epithelium and myoepithelium, and the acinic cells contain abundant zymogen granules. They are believed to be the source of the lymphoepithelial lesions (Sjögren's syndrome–like changes) and cysts occurring in patients with AIDS (fig. 21-63) (283).

A variety of tumors can arise from the salivary inclusions within lymph nodes. The most common are Warthin tumors, which are believed to arise within intraparotid lymph nodes (245,251, 254). Other tumors include sebaceous lymphadenoma (259,272), sebaceous lymphadenocarcinoma (259), pleomorphic adenoma (263,272), dermal analogue type of basal cell adenoma (272, 273), monomorphic adenoma (272), mucoepidermoid carcinoma (272,289), acinic cell carcinoma (272,279), and adenocarcinoma (271). Thus the finding of salivary gland carcinoma within a lymph node does not always indicate that the lesion is a metastasis from some other site (289).

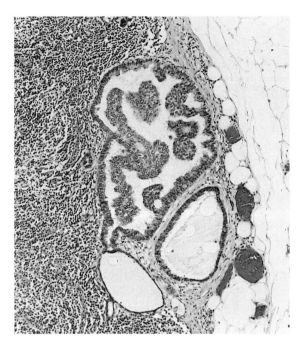

Figure 21-64
MAMMARY EPITHELIAL INCLUSION
IN AXILLARY LYMPH NODE

This mammary inclusion shows changes of intraductal carcinoma.

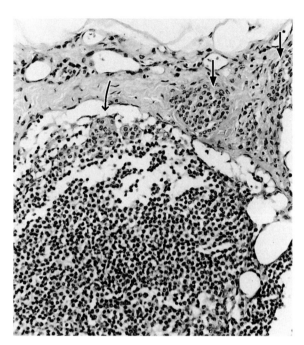

Figure 21-65
NEVUS CELLS IN LYMPH NODE

In this example, aggregates of nevus cells are present both within the capsule (straight arrows) and in the subcapsular sinus (curved arrows).

tubular colonic type glands occur in nodal sinuses, presumably resulting from embolization following surgical manipulation or biopsy (278). Epithelial Tamm-Horsfall inclusions have recently been described in the renal hilar or periaortic lymph nodes in children with renal neoplasms; they are cytologically benign glandular structures embedded in protein matrix within the marginal sinuses. They are believed to arise through rupture of renal tubules (due to tumor obstruction) and inspissation of protein into the renal interstitium, which is carried to the lymph nodes through the lymphatics (294). Mesothelial inclusions in the form of small tubules can occur in the connective tissue of the nodal capsule in abdominal lymph nodes (294).

NEVUS CELLS IN LYMPH NODE

Nevus Cell Aggregates

Clinical Features. Nevus cell aggregates are uncommon incidental findings in lymph nodes. On examination of regional lymph nodes from patients with malignant melanoma or breast cancer, 0.33 to 7.30 percent of cases have nevus cell aggre-

gates (296,298,306,308). Lymph nodes of various locations can be involved, including axillary, inguinal, and cervical (302,303,306,308,311).

A case of malignant melanoma arising from nevus cell inclusions in a lymph node, with features in transition between the two elements, has been documented (312). Some cases of malignant melanoma in a lymph node without an identifiable primary may have arisen in a similar manner.

Microscopic Findings. The nevus cells form bands, nodules, or cords in the nodal fibrous capsule, with variable extension into the fibrous trabeculae and perinodal soft tissues (fig. 21-65). Rarely, they occur within the nodal parenchyma (306,308) or lymphatics (306,311,314). They are morphologically identical to benign melanocytic nevi, and are round to ovoid cells with round nuclei, fine chromatin, and a moderate amount of pale to clear cytoplasm. They lack nuclear pleomorphism or mitosis. Melanin pigment is absent or present only focally.

Histogenesis. The histogenesis of nevus cell aggregates in lymph node has been much debated. Some authors favor the migration-arrest hypothesis (299,301,303,308,311), but Azzopardi and associates (297) question this by pointing out that melanocytes arrested in the dermis before completion of their journey to the epidermis become bipolar pigmented melanocytes and not ordinary nevus cells. Other authors propose that nodal nevus inclusions represent benign metastasis, because pigmented nevi can be identified in the skin drained by the affected lymph node in most cases, nevus cell aggregates have occasionally been found within lymphatics, and nevus inclusions are not found in visceral or deep lymph nodes (298,306, 314). However, the predominant location of the nevus cells in the nodal capsule rather than subcapsular sinus argues against the "benign metastasis" theory.

Differential Diagnosis. Nevus cell aggregates must not be confused with metastatic carcinoma or melanoma. Awareness of their existence reduces this risk. In contrast to metastases, nevus cells are often localized in the fibrous capsule and trabeculae instead of the sinuses, and they lack cytologic atypia. With immunohistochemical studies, nevus cells are cytokeratin negative and S-100 protein positive (315), while carcinoma cells are cytokeratin positive and S-100 protein variable.

A variant of Spitz's nevus (so-called malignant Spitz's nevus) can occasionally metastasize to regional lymph nodes, but this phenomenon apparently does not alter the benign evolution of this tumor, with all patients remaining disease-free on follow-up (313). Spitz's nevus cells differ from nodal nevus cells in being larger, and having vesicular nuclei, prominent nucleoli, and abundant eosinophilic hyaline cytoplasm.

Nevus cell aggregates differ from blue nevi of lymph node by the absence of spindle/dendritic cells and absence of heavy pigmentation. Rarely, the two elements may coexist in the same node (312).

Blue Nevi of Lymph Node

Clinical Features. Blue nevi are rare incidental findings in axillary lymph nodes (297–300, 305,310), and sometimes in lymph nodes at other sites (296,307). In some patients, blue nevi are also present in the skin of the drainage areas (297,307). The favored theory of histogenesis is that of arrest of melanocytes on their migration towards their final destination (297,305), but Nodl favors the hypothesis of benign metastasis (307).

Microscopic Findings. Histologically, heavily pigmented slender spindle and dendritic cells form a band of variable thickness within the nodal capsule, but the fibrous trabeculae and surrounding fibroadipose tissue can also be affected (297–300). The abundant melanin pigment often obscures the nuclear details (fig. 21-66). Therefore, examination of sections stained with hematoxylin and eosin after bleaching may help confirm the lack of nuclear atypia and absence of mitosis.

Cellular blue nevus sometimes develops benign metastases in regional lymph nodes, but the cells often occur in the sinuses and parenchyma, and are not heavily pigmented (304,306,309). Long-term follow-up has documented the benign nature of these lesions despite metastasis (304,309).

RARE LESIONS OF LYMPH NODE

Rare nonhematolymphoid lesions occurring in lymph nodes include *myelolipoma* (320), *plexiform fibrohistiocytic tumor* (fig. 21-67) (317), *neurilemmoma* (318), and *veno-lymphatic angiodysplasia* (319). The latter is a penetration of one or several inguinal lymph nodes by the long saphenous vein or one of its major branches. *Plexiform neurofibroma* can involve the hilum of lymph node as part of the diffuse process of neurofibromatosis (316). Symmers (321) has described but not illustrated an example of *fibroma*, but this may represent the end-stage of a variety of disease processes including metastatic sclerosing carcinoma.

LYMPH NODE METASTASIS

Lymph nodes, which are interposed along the course of lymphatic channels, are commonly involved by metastatic cancer. The role of the surgical pathologist in assessment of lymph node metastasis includes: 1) identification of metastatic tumor in the regional or distant lymph nodes of cancer, for staging purposes or for documentation of recurrence; 2) distinction of metastatic cancer from malignant lymphoma; and 3) prediction of the primary site for metastatic tumor of unknown primary, if possible. Increasingly, fine needle aspiration is used for the documentation of malignancy in lymph nodes, either in patients with known malignancy or in patients presenting with lymphadenopathy (402,405,436).

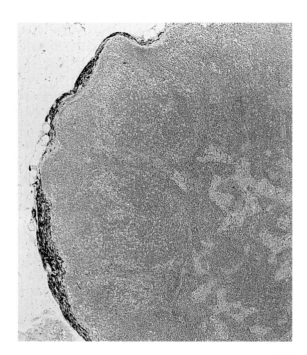
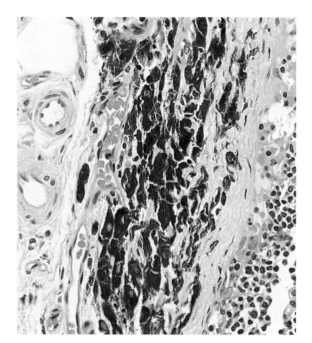

Figure 21-66
BLUE NEVUS OF LYMPH NODE
Left: A pigmented band is present in the capsule on one pole.
Right: Higher magnification shows the deeply pigmented blue nevus cells.

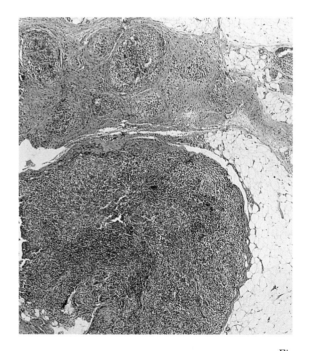
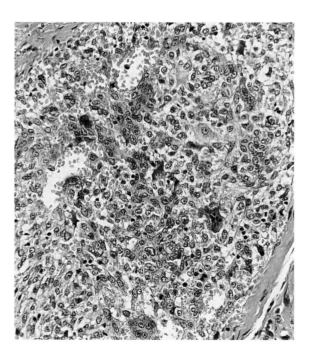

Figure 21-67
PLEXIFORM FIBROHISTIOCYTIC TUMOR IN LYMPH NODE
This occurred in the axillary lymph node of a 9-year-old boy.
Left: Multiple plexiform nodules are found both within and outside the nodal parenchyma.
Right: The nodules are composed of plump cells mixed with multinucleated giant cells.

Staging of Cancer or Documentation of Recurrence

Malignant melanomas and most carcinomas show a propensity to metastasize to lymph nodes. Although sarcomas more commonly disseminate through the blood stream, some, such as malignant fibrous histiocytoma and clear cell sarcoma of tendons and aponeurosis, also tend to involve lymph nodes (363).

Metastatic cancer usually poses no problem in diagnosis if the patient is known to have cancer. Isolated clusters of tumor in the subcapsular sinuses represent the earliest phase of involvement. With time, the nodal parenchyma is involved in a patchy or diffuse pattern; this may be accompanied by desmoplasia, necrosis, inflammatory reaction, or epithelioid granulomas. Involvement can sometimes be so extensive that it is practically impossible to recognize that the specimen is a lymph node. The metastatic tumor deposits are generally morphologically identical to the primary tumor, but they can appear better or less differentiated. Involvement of perinodal tissue confers a worse prognosis in some cancers (368,417).

Sometimes, lymph node involvement may be extremely subtle, with isolated or small groups of tumor cells lying in the sinuses. Such lymph nodes may be falsely interpreted as being free of tumor. Immunohistochemical studies can improve the detection of these microscopic metastases. In axillary lymph nodes draining breast cancer, about 25 percent of those cases reported to be "negative" are shown to contain cytokeratin- or epithelial membrane antigen–positive tumor cells (335,442,477), and such cases are found in some studies to fare worse than the truly negative cases (374,452,464). In regional lymph nodes draining malignant melanoma, 14 percent of cases previously reported as "negative" are shown to have S-100 protein–positive melanoma cells; a higher mortality is observed in this group of patients compared with the truly node-negative patients (351). In patients with stage A or B colorectal carcinoma, immunohistochemical staining of the regional lymph nodes for cytokeratin shows micrometastases in approximately 25 percent of cases; the prognostic implication of this finding has been conflicting (no effect or worsened prognosis) (388,394). Whether immunohistochemical detection of micrometastases in regional lymph nodes of cancer should be carried out routinely remains unresolved, pending further studies to document whether microscopic metastasis is a significant independent prognostic factor, especially since isolated tumor cells found in lymph nodes may not always survive. A potential pitfall in interpreting immunohistochemical preparations is mistaking positively stained indigenous cells in the lymph node for metastatic cancer. Interfollicular dendritic cells can stain for cytokeratin (372,392); rarely, cytokeratin-positive reactive mesothelial cells can occur in mediastinal lymph nodes (333). The S-100 protein–positive interdigitating dendritic/Langerhans cells and nodal nevus cells should not be mistaken for occult metastatic melanoma.

Differential Diagnosis. Benign nodal inclusions such as Müllerian inclusions, nevus cell inclusions, and deciduosis should not be mistaken for metastatic cancer. An unusual sinus reaction featuring signet ring histiocytes may mimic metastatic lobular carcinoma of breast or signet ring carcinoma (382). A variety of spindle cell lesions can potentially be mistaken for metastatic sarcoma, for example, nodal smooth muscle proliferations, hemorrhagic spindle cell tumor with amianthoid fibers, mycobacterial spindle cell pseudotumor, and follicular dendritic cell sarcoma.

On the other hand, metastatic carcinoma in lymph node can appear so deceptively bland that it may be mistaken for developmental lesions. This poses a greater problem in diagnosis if lymphadenopathy is the initial manifestation of the occult malignancy. Lymph node metastasis from squamous cell carcinoma of the head and neck region (particularly the palatine tonsil) may be cystic and composed of bland-looking squamous cells, raising the possibility of a branchial cyst (fig. 21-68) (352, 423). However, a careful search often reveals cytologic atypia in at least some squamous islands. In practical terms, any squamous cyst occurring within a cervical lymph node should be presumed to be metastatic carcinoma until proven otherwise. Metastatic papillary thyroid carcinoma can sometimes manifest as a unilocular or multi-nodular cyst in lymph node, with the lining cells being attenuated and the typical nuclear features of papillary carcinoma obscured (fig. 21-69). In this circumstance, immunostaining for thyroglobulin can confirm the thyroid origin of the lesion. Alternatively, metastatic thyroid carcinoma may be composed of groups of follicles lined

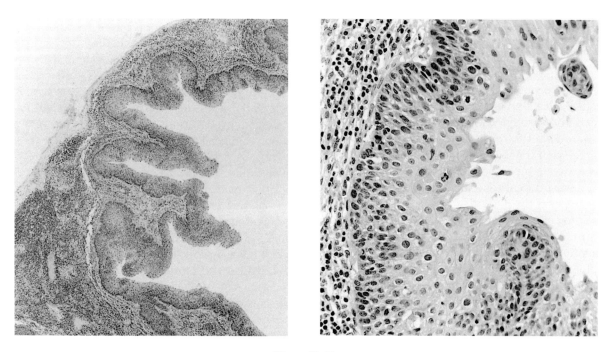

Figure 21-68
CYSTIC METASTATIC SQUAMOUS CARCINOMA IN LYMPH NODE
Cystic metastatic squamous carcinoma in lymph node, from a tonsillar primary.
Left: The tumor is predominantly cystic.
Right: The tumor cells show only mild nuclear atypia, and may lead to an erroneous diagnosis of branchial cyst.

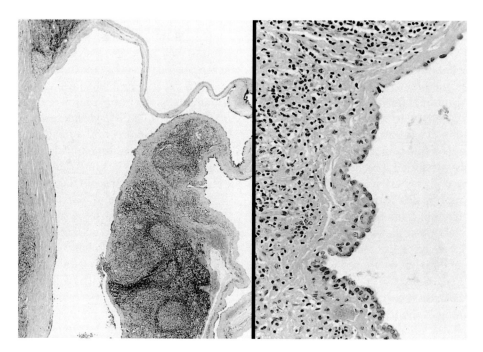

Figure 21-69
CYSTIC METASTATIC PAPILLARY THYROID CARCINOMA IN LYMPH NODE
Left: The tumor deposit is entirely cystic.
Right: The cystic spaces are lined by attenuated cells that are barely recognizable as being characteristic of papillary thyroid carcinoma. The cells are immunoreactive for thyroglobulin.

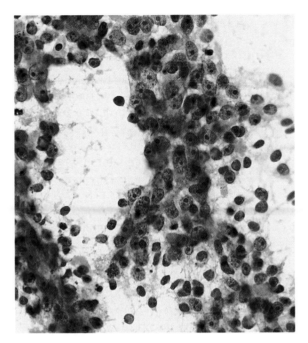

Figure 21-70
CYTOLOGY OF METASTATIC UNDIFFERENTIATED
CARCINOMA FROM NASOPHARYNX
Fine needle aspiration of lymph node harboring metastatic nasopharyngeal carcinoma. The cells often occur in "syncytial" clusters with ill-defined cytoplasm. Note the characteristic prominent nucleoli.

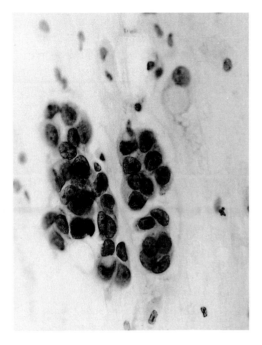

Figure 21-71
CYTOLOGY OF METASTATIC
ADENOCARCINOMA IN LYMPH NODE
Metastatic adenocarcinoma, with small glandular clusters and mucin vacuoles.

by bland-looking cells, mimicking benign thyroid inclusions in lymph node (377).

Fine Needle Aspiration. Fine needle aspiration is a helpful and safe procedure for detection of metastatic cancer in lymph node, provided that the potential pitfalls are recognized (391,402,405,436). A negative result does not exclude the presence of metastasis, which may be focal. The yield may be poor for sclerotic lesions, e.g., after radiation therapy. The presence of epithelial elements in a lymph node aspirate is not conclusive evidence of metastatic carcinoma either, because benign epithelial inclusions and skin adnexal structures may have been included in the aspirate material (436). Close attention to cytologic details is important.

Metastatic cancer can often be easily recognized in aspirate smears by the presence of sheets and clusters of cohesive cells with nuclear pleomorphism (figs. 21-70–21-72), although some tumors, such as malignant melanoma and lobular carcinoma of the breast, may appear noncohesive (441). Epithelioid granulomas, which manifest as cohesive aggregates of plump to spindle cells,

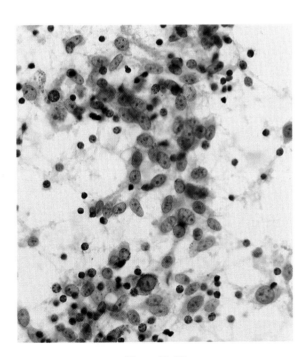

Figure 21-72
CYTOLOGY OF METASTATIC
MELANOMA IN LYMPH NODE
Brown pigment (melanin) is evident in some of the malignant cells.

may be mistaken for metastatic carcinoma; cyto-logic atypia, however, is lacking (345,391). Fol-licular lymphomas can also yield cohesive cellu-lar clusters in smears (441), but the lymphoid nature of the lesion can be recognized from the tumor cells that lie singly.

Table 21-3

METASTATIC CANCERS THAT MAY BE MISTAKEN FOR LYMPHOMA HISTOLOGICALLY

Nasopharyngeal undifferentiated (lymphoepithe-lial) carcinoma

Undifferentiated carcinoma from a variety of sites

Malignant melanoma

Lobular carcinoma of breast

Small cell carcinoma of lung and other sites

Merkel cell carcinoma

Alveolar rhabdomyosarcoma

Ewing's sarcoma and peripheral neuroepithelioma

Neuroblastoma

Germinoma

Metastatic Cancer Versus Malignant Lymphoma ("Undifferentiated Malignant Tumor")

Metastatic cancers that lack obvious differenti-ation may resemble malignant lymphoma (Table 21-3). There can be significant problems in diagno-sis; an accurate diagnosis is important because the treatment of these various tumors is substan-tially different from that of malignant lymphoma.

In most cases, a definitive diagnosis can be reached after morphologic assessment and special studies, but some cases still remain unclassifiable. In this circumstance, the only designation one can give is "undifferentiated malignant tumor." Fur-ther biopsies and observation of the clinical course sometimes clarify the diagnostic dilemma.

Histologic Assessment. Careful morpho-logic assessment is most important. However, should there be any uncertainty, ancillary tests must be performed to clarify the diagnosis.

In general, carcinoma is characterized by cohe-sive growth in the form of sheets and clusters which show a sharp interface with the lymphoid or fibrous stroma (fig. 21-73). In some carcinomas

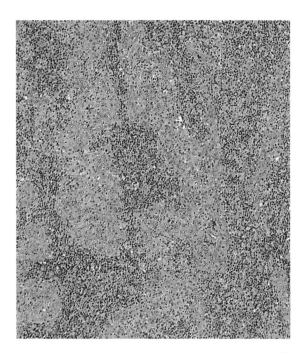 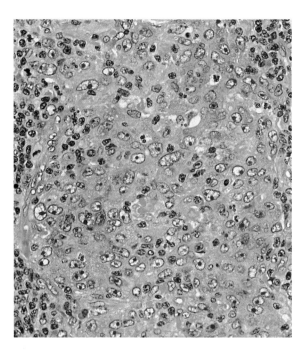

Figure 21-73
METASTATIC NASOPHARYNGEAL CARCINOMA IN LYMPH NODE
Left: Metastatic undifferentiated carcinoma from nasopharynx typically shows cohesive growth pattern, with the islands of tumor sharply demarcated from the surrounding stroma.
Right: The tumor cells typically have an indistinct cellular outline and distinct nucleoli.

(such as undifferentiated carcinoma from the nasopharynx), intermingling of the tumor cells with lymphocytes may obscure the cohesive quality of the tumor (fig. 21-74); however, the tumor clusters can often be appreciated under low to medium magnification examination (fig. 21-75). Furthermore, the tumor cells of nasopharyngeal carcinoma often have a syncytial quality, contrasting with the well-defined cytoplasmic outline of large lymphoma cells. Lack of cellular cohesiveness, however, does not exclude carcinoma. Arrangement of the tumor cells in trabeculae favors a diagnosis of carcinoma, but this must be distinguished from the cords formed passively by lymphoma or leukemic cells insinuating between collagen fibers.

Rarely, metastatic carcinoma can simulate Hodgkin's disease as a result of intermingling of the large tumor cells exhibiting prominent nucleoli with lymphocytes and neutrophils (fig. 21-76) (326,485); marked nuclear pleomorphism, presence of spindly cells, focal cohesive tumor clusters, and emperipolesis of neutrophils in tumor cells should favor a diagnosis of metastatic carcinoma (fig. 21-76, left). Metastatic lobular carcinoma of

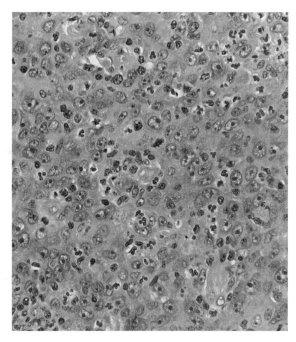

Figure 21-74
METASTATIC NASOPHARYNGEAL CARCINOMA
IN LYMPH NODE

The large neoplastic cells are intermingled with the lymphoid cells and neutrophils, and may be mistaken for immunoblasts. In contrast to the latter, the cellular outline is poorly defined.

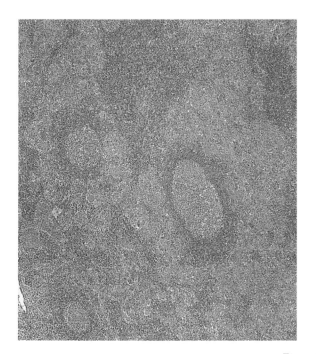

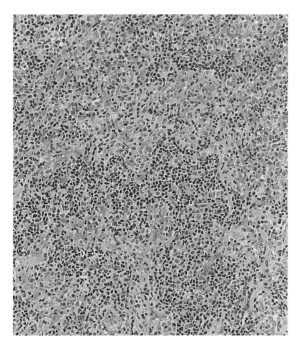

Figure 21-75
METASTATIC UNDIFFERENTIATED NASOPHARYNGEAL CARCINOMA IN LYMPH NODE
Examination of the lymph node at medium magnification helps appreciate the cohesive growth pattern.
Left: In this example, the growth (pink staining) occurs predominantly between lymphoid follicles.
Right: The cohesive quality of the tumor can be appreciated as irregular discrete trabeculae.

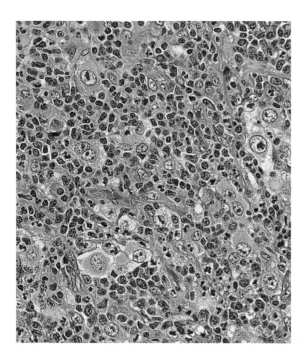 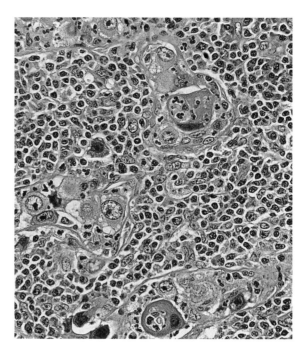

Figure 21-76
METASTATIC CARCINOMA SIMULATING HODGKIN'S DISEASE
Left: Dispersed in the inflammatory background are isolated large cells (carcinoma cells) with big nucleoli, mimicking Reed-Sternberg cells.
Right: The definite cohesive epithelial growth pattern found focally identifies it as a carcinoma (diagnosis further confirmed by cytokeratin immunoreactivity).

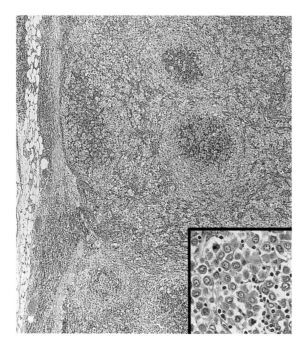

Figure 21-77
METASTATIC LOBULAR CARCINOMA OF BREAST
The tumor frequently appears noncohesive. Inset: The individual tumor cells may resemble lymphoma cells.

the breast is known to mimic lymphoma (fig. 21-77) and metastatic small cell or Merkel cell carcinoma can simulate lymphoblastic lymphoma by virtue of the medium-sized cells, fine chromatin pattern, and frequent mitoses (figs. 21-78–21-80). The pattern of growth of melanoma is best described as being "cohesively noncohesive," because the tumor cells often fall apart from one another within the clusters and sheets (figs. 21-81, 21-82). Rarely, lymphoma can appear deceptively cohesive and even "squamoid" (342,467).

The presence of nuclear molding favors the diagnosis of carcinoma, and this feature is most noticeable in small cell carcinoma (fig. 21-78, left). However, some lymphomas, particularly Burkitt's lymphoma, can exhibit a similar phenomenon. Streaming of nuclei is another feature favoring a diagnosis of carcinoma over lymphoma.

If the neoplastic cells diffusely permeate the blood vessel walls, lymphoma is the more likely diagnosis (fig. 21-83), although rare carcinomas, such as anaplastic carcinoma of the thyroid (337)

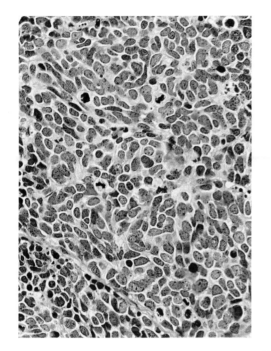 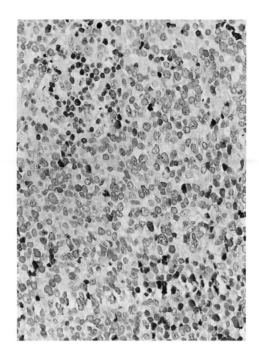

Figure 21-78
METASTATIC SMALL CELL CARCINOMA FROM LUNG

Left: This example shows the typical spindling of the hyperchromatic nuclei ("oat cells"). The nuclear streaming favors the diagnosis of carcinoma over lymphoma.

Right: Another example shows a striking resemblance to lymphoblastic lymphoma. Immunohistochemical studies are required to clarify the diagnosis.

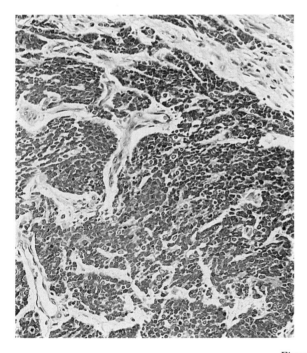 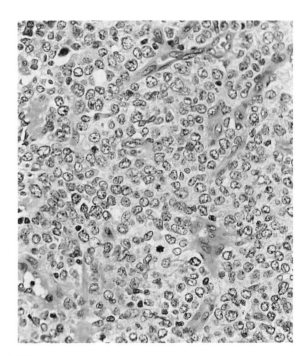

Figure 21-79
METASTATIC MERKEL CELL CARCINOMA FROM SKIN

Left: Growth is in the form of irregular islands and trabeculae.

Right: This example shows a diffuse pattern, and the tumor mimics lymphoma. Note the characteristic vascular hyperplasia.

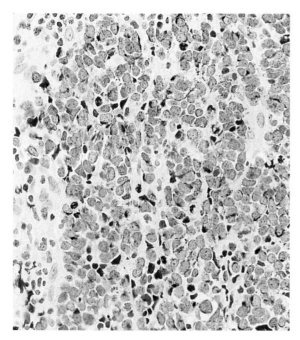

Figure 21-80
METASTATIC MERKEL CELL CARCINOMA
The tumor cells typically show a dot-like pattern of cytokeratin immunoreactivity, a pattern of staining that can be observed in small cell carcinomas of various sites.

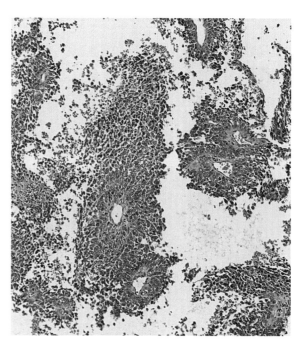

Figure 21-81
METASTATIC MELANOMA IN LYMPH NODE
A pseudopapillary pattern is created by the dehiscence of the tumor cells.

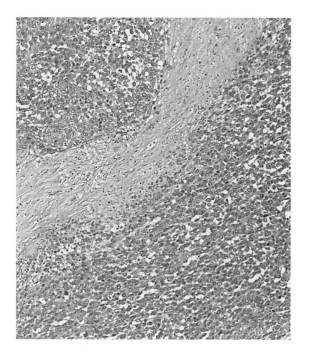

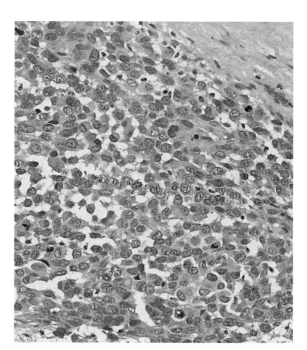

Figure 21-82
METASTATIC MELANOMA IN LYMPH NODE
Left: The tumor cells often appear "cohesively noncohesive," with the tumor cells "falling apart" from one another within the discrete large islands.
Right: The tumor cells often have an appreciable amount of eosinophilic cytoplasm.

and desmoplastic malignant melanoma (393), can permeate vascular walls in a similar fashion.

The presence of cytoplasmic mucin-like vacuoles should raise the possibility of carcinoma, and fine brown pigment the possibility of malignant melanoma. If the cytoplasm is basophilic or plasmacytoid, malignant lymphoma is the more likely diagnosis.

Since lymphoma and melanoma can assume histologic appearances traditionally associated with carcinoma, it is important not to exclude them from consideration. A sinusoidal distribution of tumor within a lymph node can be seen not only in metastatic cancer, but also in lymphoma (342). A prominent myxoid stroma or signet ring cells can occur in melanoma, lymphoma, as well as myeloma (figs. 21-84, 21-85) (330,340,346,365,373,401,433,454,468). Lymphoma and melanoma can also, though rarely, have a spindled configuration (329).

Small round cell tumors of childhood pose a different problem. The major differential diagnoses are neuroblastoma, rhabdomyosarcoma, Ewing's

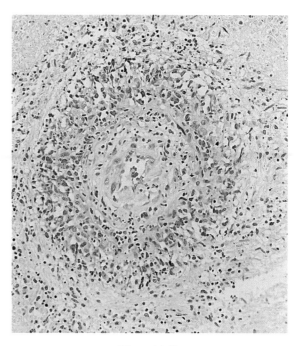

Figure 21-83
VASCULAR PERMEATION BY LYMPHOMA
Malignant lymphoma showing permeation of blood vessel wall and subintima. This pattern is rarely seen in carcinoma.

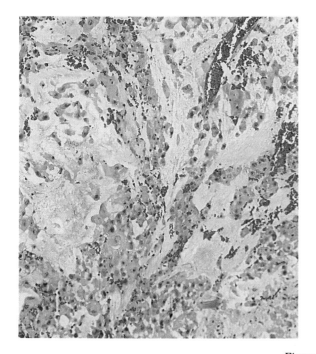

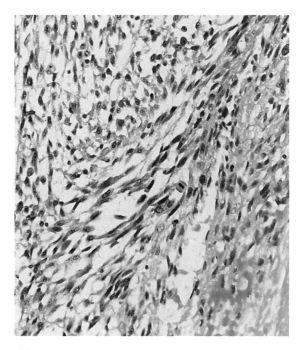

Figure 21-84
METASTATIC MELANOMA IN LYMPH NODE
Left: Metastatic melanoma showing a prominent myxoid pattern.
Right: The melanoma shows spindling of the tumor cells and myxoid change, mimicking sarcoma.

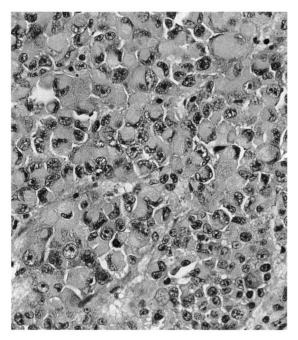

Figure 21-85
METASTATIC MELANOMA IN LYMPH NODE

This case is composed of signet ring cells, in which the nuclei are displaced by the cytoplasmic eosinophilic globules (aggregates of intermediate filaments).

sarcoma, primitive neuroectodermal tumor, and lymphoblastic lymphoma/leukemia. Frequently, a definitive diagnosis cannot be reached without the aid of special investigations. The presence of large packets of cells in which the central cells appear dehiscent favors the diagnosis of alveolar rhabdomyosarcoma, especially if cells with an appreciable amount of eosinophilic cytoplasm are identified (fig. 21-86). Multinucleated giant cells are rarely ever seen in Ewing's sarcoma or lymphoblastic lymphoma. A fibrillary matrix or ganglion cell differentiation suggests neuroblastoma (fig. 21-87), and marked nuclear convolution suggests lymphoblastic lymphoma/leukemia.

Histochemistry. When there is striking paucity of reticulin fibers, a diagnosis of lymphoma is unlikely. Successful demonstration of cytoplasmic mucosubstance confirms a diagnosis of carcinoma or mesothelioma. If the differential diagnosis is between germinoma and malignant lymphoma, abundance of glycogen strongly favors the former, because glycogen is usually (but not always) absent in the latter (fig. 21-88) (325). Abundance of glycogen in a small round cell tumor of childhood

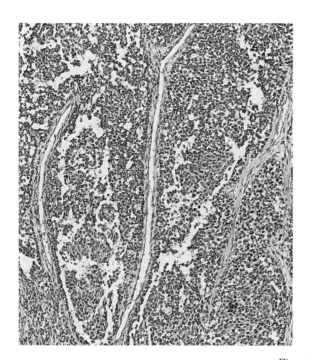

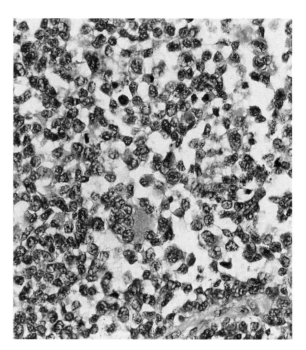

Figure 21-86
METASTATIC ALVEOLAR RHABDOMYOSARCOMA IN LYMPH NODE
Left: Alveolar packets of tumor, with central cellular dehiscence.
Right: Among the small tumor cells, there are larger cells with more cytoplasm (recognizable rhabdomyoblasts).

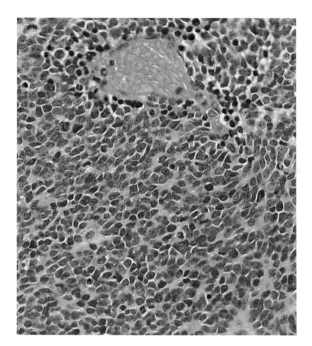

Figure 21-87

METASTATIC NEUROBLASTOMA IN LYMPH NODE

The scanty fibrillary matrix among the tumor cells provides a clue to the neural nature of this neoplasm.

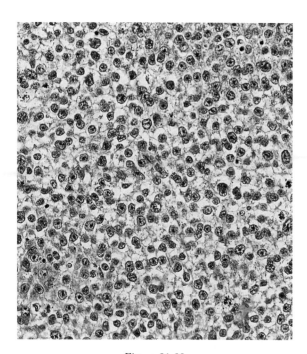

Figure 21-88

METASTATIC SEMINOMA IN LYMPH NODE

The tumor cells are polygonal and possess clear cytoplasm. The nuclei are typically round, with prominent nucleoli.

favors the diagnosis of Ewing's sarcoma or rhabdomyosarcoma, although neuroblastoma can sometimes be glycogen-rich (463). Positive staining for melanin (with Masson-Fontana, Schmorl's, or Warthin-Starry at pH 3.2) in an undifferentiated tumor favors a diagnosis of melanoma, but other substances with reducing properties (such as lipofuscin and argentaffin granules) react similarly.

Enzyme studies, which usually require fresh or frozen tissues, are rarely used nowadays. A positive 3,4-dihydroxyphenylalanine (DOPA) reaction (which detects tyrosinase) suggests that a tumor is melanocytic (448). Among the small round cell tumors of childhood, acetylcholinesterase is positive in neuroblastoma and focally positive in rhabdomyosarcoma, but not in Ewing's sarcoma or lymphoma (443). The chloroacetate esterase stain can confirm the granulocytic nature of a malignant tumor, provided that mast cells are excluded (409); this stain works well on paraffin sections.

Immunohistochemistry. A panel of antibodies should always be used, because unexpected cross reactions are not uncommon. The panel chosen depends on the differential diagnoses being

considered, but should at least include antibodies to cytokeratin, leukocyte common antigen (CD45RB), and S-100 protein. The immunohistochemical findings must be interpreted in light of the histologic and clinical findings, and in most instances a positive result is much more significant than a negative one (which can be due to technical factors, overfixation, etc.).

Cytokeratin. The cytokeratins are a complex family of intermediate-filament polypeptides with a wide range of molecular weights (40 to 67 kD). Since most cytokeratin antibodies do not react with all cytokeratin types, it is important to use a mixture of cytokeratin antibodies or a pan-keratin antibody (such as MNF-116) (329). Neuroendocrine, hepatocellular, and renal cell carcinomas often express only low molecular weight cytokeratins (such as cytokeratin 18) (329,356,395,480).

Positive staining for cytokeratin in an "undifferentiated" malignant tumor, in the proper context, strongly favors a diagnosis of carcinoma (fig. 21-89) (329). However, malignant mesothelioma, some sarcomas (such as synovial sarcoma, epithelioid sarcoma, malignant rhabdoid tumor), and chordoma are also consistently positive

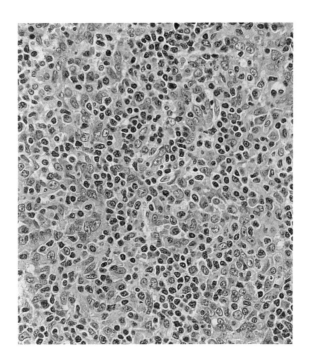
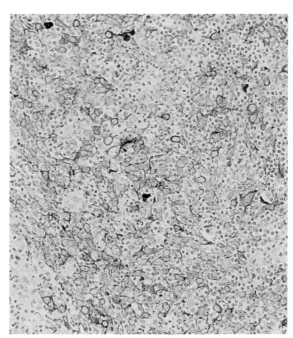

Figure 21-89
METASTATIC UNDIFFERENTIATED CARCINOMA FROM NASOPHARYNX
Left: The carcinoma cells are so intimately intermingled with the lymphoid cells that they may be missed or misinterpreted as lymphoma cells.
Right: Immunostaining for cytokeratin highlights the carcinoma cells.

(329,470). In addition, a growing list of tumors have been recognized as showing occasional unexpected (aberrant) staining for cytokeratin, such as malignant melanoma (376,426), myogenic tumor (334), glioma (353,434), malignant fibrous histiocytoma (427), vascular tumor (385), nerve sheath tumor (386), Ewing's sarcoma (429), plasmacytoma (483), and lymphoma (358,389).

Leukocyte Common Antigen (CD45RB). Leukocyte common antigen is a highly sensitive and specific marker for the hematolymphoid lineage in neoplasms (407,424,476); false positives are extremely rare if only membrane or Golgi staining is regarded as characteristic (422,475). In the immunohistochemical evaluation of an undifferentiated tumor, antibody against leukocyte common antigen should not be omitted from the antibody panel even if the histologic features appear to favor carcinoma or sarcoma, because lymphomas occasionally assume unusual appearances (340, 342,373,401,437,467,468). Lack of staining for leukocyte common antigen, however, does not completely exclude the possibility of lymphoma,

because negativity may result from overfixation and antigen loss, an insensitive detection technique, or true lack of expression (such as some cases of lymphoblastic lymphoma, anaplastic large cell CD30-positive lymphoma, plasmacytoma, and large cell lymphoma) (342,366, 389,407,471a). Therefore, if malignant lymphoma is strongly suspected, this possibility should be further pursued with B-cell markers, T-cell markers, anti-immunoglobulin antibodies, and CD30 antibody (341,342,366,389).

S-100 Protein. S-100 protein is a highly sensitive marker for malignant melanoma. The staining pattern is characteristically both nuclear and cytoplasmic; cytoplasmic staining alone should not be accepted. However, S-100 protein lacks specificity, and is demonstrable in many other types of tumor including breast carcinoma (361,398, 432,457). Should there be any uncertainty, staining with additional melanoma-specific antibodies such as HMB-45 and NK1/C3 (357,384,412,426) (which, however, are not entirely specific either; 331,412) and electron microscopy are helpful.

488

Table 21-4

IMMUNOHISTOCHEMICAL PROFILE OF SMALL ROUND CELL TUMORS OF CHILDHOOD

Tumor	LCA	Neural Markers	Muscle Markers	Vimentin	MIC2 (CD99)
Lymphoma/leukemia	+	–	–	–/+	+
Neuroblastoma	–	+	–	–/+	–
Rhabdomyosarcoma	–	–*	+	+	–
Ewing's sarcoma and peripheral primitive neuroectodermal tumor	–	–/+	–	+	+

LCA: leukocyte common antigen (CD45RB); neural markers: neuron-specific enolase, synaptophysin, neurofilament, CD57 (Leu-7), CD56 (NKH1) (the antibody NB-84, which is applicable in paraffin sections, is useful for staining neuroblastoma); muscle markers: desmin, myoglobin, creatine kinase MM, myosin, MyOD1; MIC2: recognized by antibodies such as HBA-71, 013, 12E7.
+ = positive; – = negative; –/+ = highly variable staining.
*Commonly positive for neuron-specific enolase.

For small round cell tumors of childhood, the panel of antibodies used should reflect the diagnostic possibilities (Table 21-4) (383,400,411, 426,439,440,445,451,461,462,465,469). Desmin immunoreactivity in this setting provides strong support for the diagnosis of rhabdomyosarcoma because leiomyosarcoma is not among the differential diagnoses. The MIC2 antibody (CD99) is a useful marker for Ewing's sarcoma and peripheral neuroepithelioma, although it also stains lymphoblastic lymphoma (440,445). The recently available antibody MyoD1 holds promise of being the most sensitive and specific marker for skeletal muscle neoplasms (466).

Electron Microscopy. Although the role of electron microscopy in elucidating the nature of undifferentiated malignant tumors has diminished with the availability of a wide range of antibodies reactive in formalin-fixed materials, useful information can still be obtained in some cases (378,415).

There are no ultrastructural features that are pathognomonic of lymphoma, but the presence of nuclear pockets and abundance of rough endoplasmic reticulum should raise this possibility. The finding of well-formed desmosomes supports a diagnosis of carcinoma or mesothelioma, although desmosomal attachments are occasionally seen in lymphomas (404,408,413). The presence of premelanosomes is indicative of malignant melanoma.

Electron microscopy plays an important role in the diagnosis of small round cell tumors of childhood (425,461,462,473). The presence of neurites and dense core granules supports the diagnosis of neuroblastoma or primitive neuroectodermal tumor. A diagnosis of rhabdomyosarcoma is supported by finding alternating arrays of thick and thin filaments, Z-band materials, or single-file deposits of ribosomes along thin filaments. There are generally no distinctive features in Ewing's sarcoma except an abundance of glycogen and occasional cell junctions.

Cytogenetic Studies. Cytogenetic studies are very informative if specific chromosomal abnormalities are identified (368,451), for example, t(2;5) in CD30-positive (Ki-1) large cell lymphoma (418); t(11;22)(q23;q11-12) in Ewing's sarcoma and peripheral primitive neuroectodermal tumor (324,369,416,450,478,479); double minutes, homogeneous staining regions, and deletion of the short arm of chromosome 1 in neuroblastoma (380,471,478); and t(2;13) in alveolar rhabdomyosarcoma (369,435,473).

Chromosomal translocations can also be detected by the fluorescence in situ hybridization (FISH) technique on interphase nuclei of the tumor cells (339).

Molecular Analysis. Molecular studies are useful for diagnosing an undifferentiated neoplasm. Immunoglobulin or T-cell receptor gene rearrangement strongly suggests a diagnosis of lymphoid neoplasia and its possible lineage (323,

350,354,370,399,406,443). Although the presence of such gene rearrangements is fairly specific, the results have to be interpreted in conjunction with other findings, because false negative results are possible, and clonal T-cell receptor or immunoglobulin gene rearrangements have occasionally been observed in nonlymphoid neoplasms such as myeloid leukemia (354,406,443,455).

Detection of the specific genes that are known to be rearranged in certain tumor types (such as *EWS/FLI1* in Ewing's sarcoma and peripheral neuroepithelioma, *NPM/ALK* in anaplastic large cell lymphoma, *PAX3/FKHR* in alveolar rhabdomyosarcoma, and *bcl*-2/IgH in some large B-cell lymphomas) by Southern blot analysis or polymerase chain reaction provides strong support for these diagnoses (338,339). Detection of the mRNA transcripts of the skeletal muscle regulator gene *MyOD1* in a malignant neoplasm strongly favors a diagnosis of rhabdomyosarcoma or alveolar soft part sarcoma (466).

Other Specialized Techniques. Formaldehyde- or glycoxylic acid–induced fluorescence may help in detection of catecholamines and their precursors in suspected neuroblastoma (461,473).

Tissue culture studies occasionally prove helpful, because tumor cells may show better differentiation in vitro, either spontaneously or upon stimulation by exogenous agents (355,381, 430). Development of neurites on culture favors the diagnosis of neuroblastoma or related tumors (430). Amelanotic melanoma can become pigmented on culture (355,381), providing a clue to its melanocytic nature.

Prediction of Origin of a Metastatic Carcinoma

Between 3 and 4 percent of all cancers present with metastases from an occult primary neoplasm (328). By far, carcinoma and melanoma account for most cases. Prediction of the probable primary site by the pathologist is important for patient work-up. In addition to pathologic assessment, knowledge of the sex, age, and exact location of the lymph node is of prime importance. It is important to identify tumors for which effective treatment or palliation is available, such as germ cell tumors, prostatic carcinoma, breast carcinoma, thyroid carcinoma, and ovarian carcinoma (447). Rare examples of neuroendocrine carcinoma (Merkel cell carcinoma) of lymph node in the absence of primary elsewhere have also been reported (364).

Location of Involved Lymph Node. *Cervical Lymph Node.* Cervical lymph nodes are most commonly involved by metastatic cancers of unknown origin. A thorough examination of the upper aerodigestive tract with multiple-site biopsies is necessary (328), although the primary site is ultimately detected in only one third of cases. In the study by Molinari et al. (428), there was a correlation between the primary site and the location of the lymph node containing the metastatic deposits, e.g., floor of mouth and anterior third of tongue with submental node metastases, and nasopharynx with metastatic deposits in posterior cervical triangle nodes.

Supraclavicular Lymph Node. For metastatic tumors presenting in supraclavicular lymph nodes, most primary tumors are discovered in organs below the level of the clavicle (lung, gastrointestinal tract, genitourinary tract including the testis and prostate); others are identified in the thyroid or upper aerodigestive tract (397,428,444).

Axillary Lymph Node. Most patients presenting with cancer of unknown origin in axillary lymph nodes are women. Successful localization of the primary can be achieved in 50 to 75 percent of cases (444,449). Most primary tumors are identified in the breast; others are found in the lung, gastrointestinal tract, or pancreas (444).

The prognosis for occult breast carcinoma presenting with axillary node metastasis is still favorable, being comparable to patients with equivalent extent of disease who present with palpable breast tumors (449). Histologic features favoring the diagnosis of metastatic breast carcinoma include sheets of large apocrine-like pleomorphic cells with pale to granular pink cytoplasm, large nuclei, and prominent nucleoli (fig. 21-90) (390). Cytoplasmic mucin, although often focal, can usually be detected (390,449). Only a small proportion of cases exhibit the more widely recognized trabecular, cribriform, or comedo patterns (fig. 21-91) (390).

Inguinal Lymph Node. Inguinal lymph node metastases represent an uncommon presentation of cancer of unknown origin; most primary tumors are melanoma or squamous carcinoma from the trunk, lower extremities, lower genital tract, and rectum (444).

Histopathology and Histochemistry. If preliminary assessment fails to identity the primary site of a metastatic carcinoma, the next important step is to review all histologic materials to ascertain that this is indeed a carcinoma and not a lymphoma misinterpreted as carcinoma, so as not to waste efforts in searching for a nonexistent primary.

It is generally difficult to predict the primary site of a metastatic carcinoma from histologic assessment alone, because carcinomas of a certain histologic type look similar regardless of the location. In the uncommon circumstance of finding bile production by tumor cells, hepatocellular carcinoma is most likely. Histologic features favoring mammary origin have already been discussed in a previous section. Clear cell tumors should prompt serious consideration of renal cell adenocarcinoma, hepatocellular carcinoma, and germ cell tumor, although carcinoma from other sites can also have clear cells.

Undifferentiated carcinoma of the nasopharynx, which occurs with a particularly high frequency in Orientals and often presents as cervical lymphadenopathy, can often be suspected on

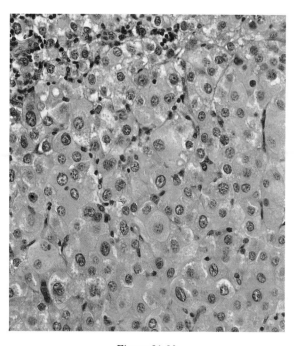

Figure 21-90
METASTATIC MAMMARY CARCINOMA
IN AXILLARY LYMPH NODE
The large polygonal tumor cells possess finely granular ("apocrine") cytoplasm.

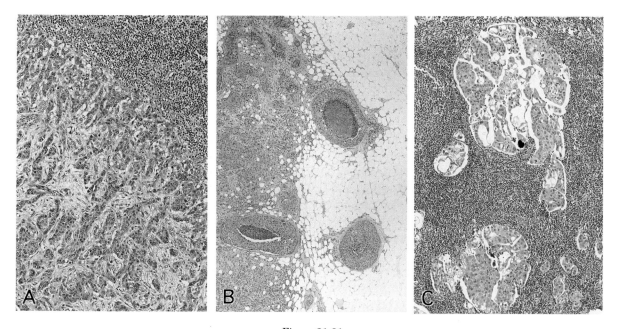

Figure 21-91
METASTATIC MAMMARY CARCINOMA IN LYMPH NODE
A: Typical growth pattern in the form of cords.
B: Typical comedo pattern of growth.
C: Papillary growth with occasional psammoma bodies.

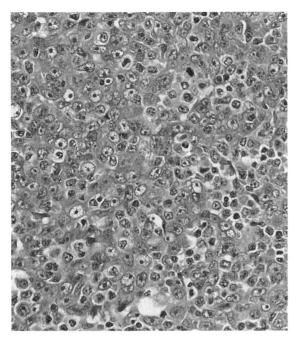

Figure 21-92
METASTATIC NASOPHARYNGEAL CARCINOMA
IN LYMPH NODE
Typical syncytial appearance, vesicular nuclei, and prominent nucleoli.

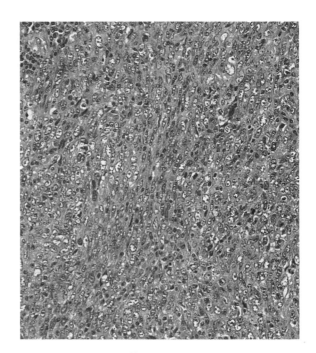

Figure 21-93
METASTATIC NASOPHARYNGEAL CARCINOMA
IN LYMPH NODE
Spindle cell growth can sometimes be seen.

histologic grounds (379). The tumor is composed of sheets of cells with crowded vesicular nuclei and prominent nucleoli (figs. 21-73, 21-74, 21-92). The cell borders are poorly defined, giving a syncytial-like appearance. Occasionally, fascicles of plump spindle cells can be present (fig. 21-93).

Among adenocarcinomas, demonstration of cytoplasmic mucin renders the diagnosis of renal cell adenocarcinoma unlikely (371). The previous belief that mucin positivity excludes a thyroid primary has not been substantiated by recent studies (343). Failure to demonstrate mucin in a signet ring carcinoma should raise the possibility of prostatic primary (446).

Immunohistochemistry. Immunohistochemical studies can occasionally help in suggesting the origin of a metastatic cancer. There are few organ-specific markers; some of the more useful ones are listed in Table 21-5. The value of immunostaining for alpha-fetoprotein to suggest a liver primary is limited, because the sensitivity is low, and alpha-fetoprotein positivity can occur in other tumors, such as germ cell tumor, gastric carcinoma, and pancreatic carcinoma (375). A

tumor staining only for low molecular weight cytokeratins (CAM5.2+, AE1/AE3-) in a cell membrane pattern strongly suggests a diagnosis of hepatocellular carcinoma, although such staining may be seen in some renal cell carcinomas (395). A canalicular pattern of staining for carcinoembryonic antigen strongly supports a diagnosis of hepatocellular carcinoma (fig. 21-94). A small cell tumor showing dot-like staining for cytokeratin may raise the possibility of Merkel cell carcinoma (fig. 21-80) (329), but this pattern is by no means pathognomonic.

For men over the age of 45 years, it is imperative to immunostain for prostatic-specific antigen or prostatic acid phosphatase on encountering metastatic adenocarcinoma or undifferentiated carcinoma of unknown origin, because this may represent the initial presentation of prostatic cancer (fig. 21-95) (336,337,397). For young patients presenting with carcinoma of unknown primary, it is important to immunostain for beta-human chorionic gonadotropin, alpha-fetoprotein, and placental alkaline phosphatase. Positive staining suggests a diagnosis of germ cell tumor, as either a metastasis from an

Table 21-5

**COMMERCIALLY AVAILABLE ANTIBODIES HELPFUL FOR
DETERMINING THE POSSIBLE PRIMARY SITE OF A METASTATIC CARCINOMA**

Antibody	Organ	Cautionary Note
Thyroglobulin (322,337)	Thyroid	Anaplastic and mucoepidermoid carcinomas of the thyroid are usually thyroglobulin negative
Calcitonin (337,359,414,482)	Thyroid (medullary carcinoma)	Some other neuroendocrine carcinomas such as those of the larynx can be immunoreactive for calcitonin; some antibody preparations contain "impurities," resulting in nonspecific staining
Prostatic acid phosphatase (PAP) (347,367,456, 458,472,484)	Prostate	PAP is a sensitive marker for prostatic cancer, including undifferentiated type; however, PAP immunoreactivity has also been demonstrated in rectal carcinoids, carcinoids of other sites, islet tumors, breast carcinomas (rare), and salivary gland tumors (rare)
Prostatic-specific antigen (PSA) (347,367,431, 459,472)	Prostate	PSA is a specific marker for prostatic carcinoma (except that occasionally salivary gland tumors can be PSA positive), although it may not be as sensitive as PAP for undifferentiated prostatic carcinomas; use of both PAP and PSA antibodies is therefore advised
Alpha-lactalbumin (327,349,362, 410,474,481)	Breast	The reported results of staining for alpha-lactalbumin in breast carcinoma is highly variable (0 to 67 percent); this marker is not very sensitive, and staining can be very focal; positive results have also been noted in skin adnexal, salivary gland, ovarian, colonic, and pancreatic cancers, and mesotheliomas
GCDFP-15 (BRST-2) (362,419–421,481)	Breast	Gross cystic disease fluid protein-15 (GCDFP-15) stains about 50 to 74 percent of breast carcinomas, but some authors have not found it to be a sensitive marker; extramammary Paget's disease, some sweat gland neoplasms, and salivary gland tumors can stain with GCDFP-15; rarely, prostatic carcinoma and carcinomas of other sites also stain
"Ovarian markers": OC125 (CA-125, celomic antigen); OV632 (403)	Ovary	OC125 stains a high proportion of ovarian carcinomas (especially serous type) and adenocarcinomas of the uterine corpus and cervix, but it can also stain some carcinomas occurring outside the genital tract and reactive mesothelium; OV632 shows much higher but not absolute specificity for female genital tract carcinomas, but it works only on frozen sections
Carcinoembryonic antigen (CEA) with canalicular pattern of staining (348,453)	Liver	The distinctive canalicular pattern of staining for CEA is pathognomonic of hepatocellular carcinoma; positivity rate tends to be lower for the less-differentiated tumors; polyclonal unabsorbed antiserum or monoclonal antibody that cross reacts with canalicular biliary glycoprotein 1 has to be used

occult testicular primary or the so-called extragonadal germ cell cancer syndrome, which is potentially curable with cisplatinum-based chemotherapy (387,396,447).

Electron Microscopy. Electron microscopy plays a limited role in elucidating the probable primary site of a metastatic carcinoma (357,360, 415). The presence of numerous microvilli with prominent cores of microfilaments that extend down into an apical zone of cytoplasm relatively free of organelles strongly suggests gastrointestinal carcinoma, especially if glycocalyx, glycocaly-

ceal bodies, and apical cytoplasmic electron-dense granules are also present. An abundant smooth endoplasmic reticulum and mitochondria with tubulovesicular cristae suggests adrenal cortical carcinoma or steroid-producing tumors of the gonads. The following features suggest a renal origin for an adenocarcinoma: brush border-like microvilli, lipid droplets, glycogen lakes, complexly infolded basal plasma membrane, and frequent vesicles and vacuoles in the apical cytoplasm. The presence of laminated, osmiophilic, myelin-like inclusions similar to surfactant-containing inclusions

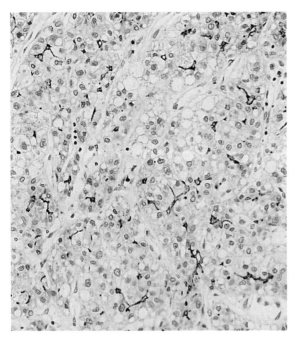

Figure 21-94
METASTATIC HEPATOCELLULAR CARCINOMA
IN LYMPH NODE

Carcinoembryonic antigen gives a typical canalicular pattern of staining, highlighting the bile canaliculi.

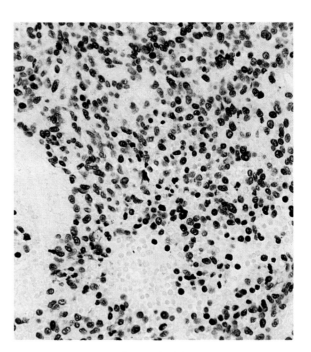

Figure 21-96
METASTATIC NASOPHARYNGEAL CARCINOMA
IN LYMPH NODE PRESENTING AS METASTATIC
CARCINOMA OF UNKNOWN PRIMARY

Nuclear labeling of the carcinoma cells for Epstein-Barr virus–encoded RNA strongly suggests that the primary is nasopharyngeal.

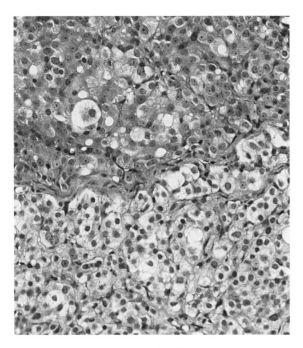

Figure 21-95
METASTATIC PROSTATIC ADENOCARCINOMA
IN A SUPRACLAVICULAR LYMPH NODE

Despite the relatively solid growth, the nuclei do not show great variation in size. Note the typical prominent nucleoli. Some cells have eosinophilic cytoplasm, while others have pale cytoplasm.

favors a pulmonary origin. The presence of numerous long slender branching microvilli, specialized desmosomes, and perinuclear intermediate filaments suggests malignant mesothelioma, which may rarely present as lymph node metastasis (460).

Molecular and Cytogenetic Studies. Positive in situ hybridization for albumin mRNA provides good evidence for the hepatocellular origin of a carcinoma; immunohistochemical detection of albumin cannot serve the same purpose because passive diffusion of albumin into tumor is common (438). In situ demonstration of Epstein-Barr virus (EBV) DNA or RNA in the neoplastic cells of an undifferentiated carcinoma strongly suggests a nasopharyngeal primary, although carcinomas of other sites can also occasionally harbor EBV (fig. 21-96) (344,437).

Detection of i(12p) either by conventional cytogenetic study or by fluorescence in situ hybridization in a malignant tumor strongly supports a diagnosis of germ cell tumor (332).

SPLENIC HEMANGIOMA, LYMPHANGIOMA, HEMANGIOENDOTHELIOMA, AND HEMANGIOPERICYTOMA

Splenic Hemangioma

Clinical Features. Hemangioma of the spleen, although rare, is the most common benign primary neoplasm in this organ (493,496). It occurs mostly in young or middle-aged adults (average age, 30 to 40 years); some studies show no sex predilection (487), but others, a male predominance (493,496). Most splenic hemangiomas are small incidental findings at laparotomy or autopsy (493,501), but they can occasionally cause considerable splenomegaly. Complications include rupture, consumption coagulopathy, microangiopathic anemia, and thrombocytopenia (493, 496,499,505). In symptomatic patients, splenectomy is curative (496).

When splenic hemangioma is a component of a more widespread vascular proliferation in the viscera (such as liver, skin), the term *angiomatosis* is appropriate (493,500,502). Symmers (507) described a case associated with hereditary telangiectasia. Rarely, angiomatosis is limited to the spleen (503).

Pathologic Findings. Splenic hemangioma forms a solitary nodule or multiple blue-red, spongy nodules in the spleen. They are either well demarcated from the surrounding parenchyma or are ill-defined. Most splenic hemangiomas are cavernous hemangiomas, similar to those occurring in soft tissues (501). They are composed of large blood-filled spaces lined by flat endothelium, and separated by thin fibrous septa or splenic pulp tissue (fig. 21-97). Infarction, thrombosis, or fibrosis can occur (493,496). Less commonly, they are of the capillary type.

In diffuse angiomatosis of the spleen, the whole spleen is replaced by neoplastic vascular channels (503,505). In at least one case, the endothelial cells showed immunohistochemical features of splenic sinus endothelium, and the term "diffuse sinusoidal hemangiomatosis" was applied (503).

Differential Diagnosis. The differential diagnosis of splenic hemangioma includes angiosarcoma, lymphangioma, and peliosis of spleen. The latter is an idiopathic condition characterized by widespread blood-filled spaces in the spleen. It usually, but not invariably, occurs in conjunction

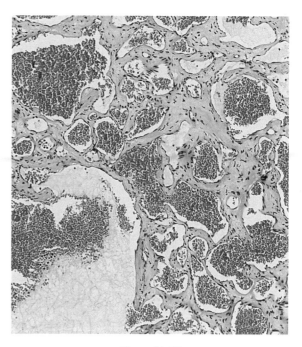

Figure 21-97
SPLENIC HEMANGIOMA
Cavernous hemangioma of spleen, characterized by large blood-filled spaces.

with peliosis hepatis (508,509), and is discovered incidentally or presents with rupture (489,492, 498,508,509). Most cases show an association with use of anabolic steroids or wasting diseases (such as tuberculosis or malignancies). Peliosis of spleen differs from hemangioma in that the blood spaces are haphazardly scattered in the red pulp instead of forming a more discrete tumor. Histologically, the blood lakes are not necessarily completely lined by endothelium, and there is preferential involvement of the parafollicular areas.

Littoral Cell Angioma

Clinical Features. Littoral cell angioma is a very rare but distinctive benign tumor of the spleen composed of splenic sinus elements; there is no counterpart of this tumor in other organs or somatic soft tissues (490). It occurs over a wide age range, with a mean of 49 years. There is no sex predilection. Most patients present with splenomegaly of unknown origin, with or without features of hypersplenism. Some patients also have fever, which abates after splenectomy. Although the tumor is benign in most cases, a malignant variant may exist.

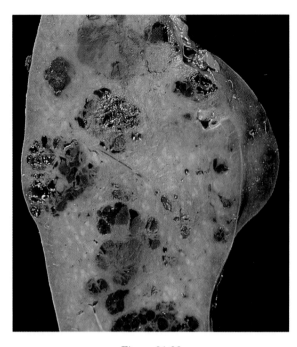

Figure 21-98
LITTORAL CELL ANGIOMA OF SPLEEN
Multiple blood-filled nodules are scattered throughout the spleen.

Pathologic Findings. Littoral cell angioma appears grossly as a solitary nodule or multiple circumscribed blood-filled spongy nodules (fig. 21-98). It is characterized histologically by anastomosing vascular channels, which attain a pseudopapillary pattern in some areas (fig. 21-99). These vascular channels often anastomose with the normal splenic sinuses at the periphery. There can also be markedly dilated cavernous vascular spaces. The channels are lined by tall or flat cells with regular indented nuclei and infrequent mitoses (fig. 21-100). Exfoliated cells are often found within the lumina. Rarely, an extensive intraluminal sheet-like proliferation of lining cells is observed. PAS-positive cytoplasmic globules may be present, and annular reticulin fibers can be demonstrated in areas (fig. 21-101). Immunohistochemical studies show that the lining cells stain for endothelial markers (such as factor VIII–related antigen) and histiocytic markers (such as CD68 and lysozyme).

Differential Diagnosis. Littoral cell angioma must not be mistaken for the highly malignant splenic angiosarcoma. It differs from angiosarcoma

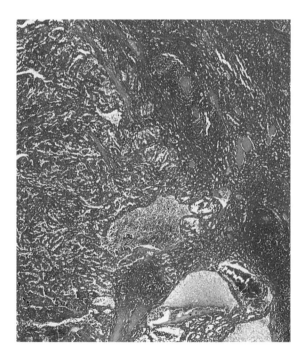
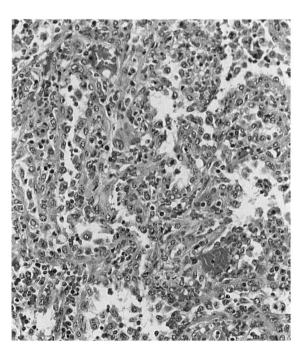

Figure 21-99
LITTORAL CELL ANGIOMA OF SPLEEN
Left: In addition to large blood-filled vascular channels, there are complex narrow vascular channels which appear papillary focally. Normal splenic tissue is seen in right upper field.
Right: Anastomosing vascular channels with a pseudopapillary pattern. Exfoliated cells are present in the lumina.

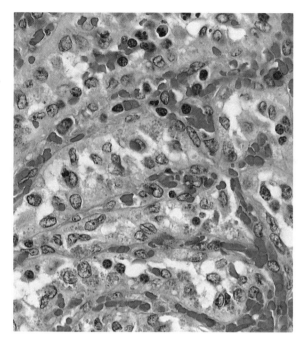

Figure 21-100
LITTORAL CELL ANGIOMA OF SPLEEN
The vascular channels are lined by bland-looking plump cells, some of which contain cytoplasmic eosinophilic globules.

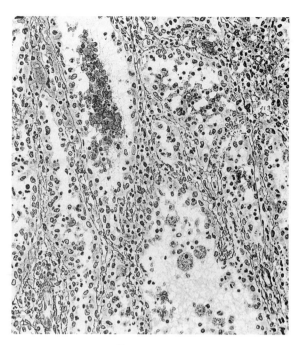

Figure 21-101
LITTORAL CELL ANGIOMA OF SPLEEN
Reticulin stain demonstrates incomplete ring fibers around the vascular spaces, typical of splenic sinuses. (Gordon and Sweets reticulin impregnation)

in exhibiting architectural features of splenic sinuses; absence of irregular, anastomosing maze-like vascular channels; and absence of cellular atypia or mitoses.

Splenic Lymphangioma

Splenic lymphangioma, which is probably a hamartomatous rather than neoplastic lesion, is even less common than splenic hemangioma. It can be a small incidental finding, or can be large and multicentric (488,493). There is often concurrent involvement of other viscera (486,495,504).

Lymphangioma involves the spleen in the form of a solitary nodule, multiple nodules, or diffuse growth (fig. 21-102). It is microcystic or solid, and may show central scarring (486,488). As in other sites, distinction of lymphangioma from hemangioma is not always easy (493). Unlike the random localization of hemangioma, lymphangioma often involves the capsule and trabeculae, where lymphatics are normally concentrated (fig. 21-103). The endothelium-lined spaces are filled with eosinophilic proteinaceous material instead of blood. The endothelium is typically flat (fig. 21-103); however, in several reported cases,

it is focally plump and vacuolated, and forms papillary projections into the vascular lumen (fig. 21-104) (488,491,494), reminiscent of epithelioid hemangioma. Two of these cases were interpreted as probable malignant change in a lymphangioma (491,494), but neither tumor has metastasized on short-term follow-up. Only long-term follow-up will clarify whether such histologic features are indicative of malignancy or merely represent an unusual morphologic expression of the endothelial cells.

Hemangioendothelioma

Hemangioendothelioma, a vascular tumor occupying an intermediate position both in terms of histology and behavior between a hemangioma and conventional angiosarcoma, can occur as a primary tumor of the spleen (497,506). It should be noted, however, that most cases reported in the literature as "splenic hemangioendothelioma" are in fact angiosarcomas.

Kaw et al. (497) described a hemangioendothelioma composed of blood vessels with moderate cellular atypia and rare mitoses in a 48-year-old man. Suster (506) reported a case composed

497

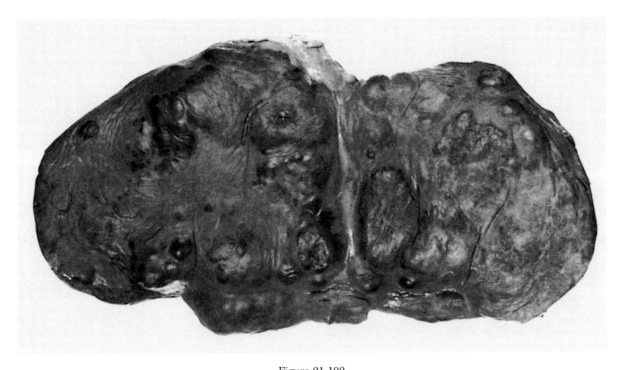

Figure 21-102
CYSTIC LYMPHANGIOMA OF SPLEEN
This spleen weighs 3360 g. Multiple nodules are evident in the spleen. (Fig. 336 from Fascicle 8, 1st Series.)

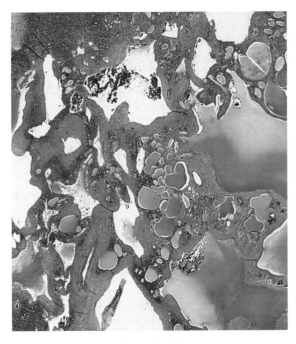

Figure 21-103
SPLENIC LYMPHANGIOMA
Many of the vascular spaces are closely associated with the fibrous trabeculae. The vascular spaces are filled with proteinaceous fluid.

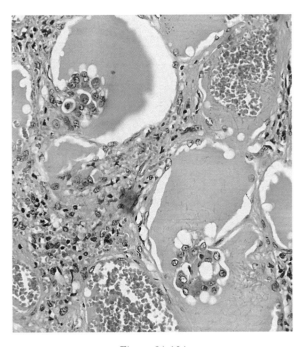

Figure 21-104
SPLENIC LYMPHANGIOMA
Papillary tufts of endothelial cells are sometimes seen.

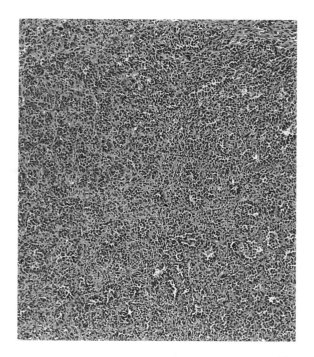 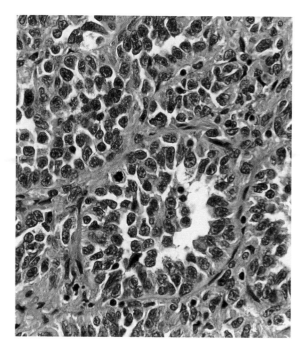

Figure 21-105
HEMANGIOENDOTHELIOMA OF SPLEEN
Left: The spleen is largely overrun by narrow vascular channels, but necrosis is not seen.
Right: The vascular channels are lined by plump cells with mild to moderate atypia and occasional mitoses. The resemblance to splenic sinuses suggests that this might represent the malignant counterpart of littoral cell angioma.

of epithelioid and spindly cells, occurring in a 3-year-old boy. Both patients have remained well after surgery. These tumors can be distinguished from the highly aggressive angiosarcoma by the absence of dissecting growth and lack of striking cellular atypia (fig. 21-105).

Hemangiopericytoma

Rarely, hemangiopericytoma occurs in the spleen as a primary tumor (510,511). It is either asymptomatic or results in palpable splenomegaly. Histologically, it is identical to the same tumor occurring in the soft tissues.

ANGIOSARCOMA OF SPLEEN

Clinical Features. Primary angiosarcoma of the spleen is rare: slightly over 100 cases have been reported in the literature (513,516,522). It has been reported under a variety of designations, such as hemangiosarcoma, malignant hemangioendothelioma, and endothelial sarcoma (512,513,522). It occurs mostly in older individuals, with a mean age of 53 years (516,517,522). Few patients are

under 40 years of age (525). There is no predilection for either sex (516,520).

The patients usually present with an abdominal mass or pain. Some present with hemoperitoneum as a result of rupture of the tumor (512, 517). Some develop hematologic complications such as normochromic normocytic anemia, microangiopathic anemia, thrombocytopenia, leukocytosis, and consumption coagulopathy (516,517, 523). Systemic symptoms of fever, fatigue, and weight loss can also be present (516,520). Distant blood-borne metastasis is common, mostly to liver, lung, bone, bone marrow, and lymph node (514). The prognosis is grave: most patients die within 1 year of diagnosis (517,524), and according to a study of 38 cases, 79 percent died by 6 months (516). Splenectomy is the usual treatment; chemotherapy has not been proven to be beneficial (520).

Unlike angiosarcoma of the liver, no definite etiologic association has been identified (525). Only sporadic cases are associated with previous chemotherapy (for lymphoma) (516,525) and radiotherapy (for breast cancer) (523).

Gross Findings. Angiosarcoma often causes massive enlargement of the spleen, which often weighs 0.5 to 1 kg. The cut surface reveals multiple ill-defined, purple-red nodules of tumor or diffuse replacement of the entire spleen by tumor (fig. 21-106). There are typically large areas of hemorrhage and necrosis, with occasional blood-filled cavities (519,522).

Microscopic Findings. Angiosarcoma of spleen is histologically identical to angiosarcoma of soft tissues (515). The degree of differentiation may differ significantly from area to area within the same tumor, but significant nuclear pleomorphism is at least focally present. There are often anastomosing vascular channels, spindle cell fascicles, papillary formations, and solid areas (fig. 21-107). The better differentiated areas often have a honeycomb or sponge-like pattern, cavernous vessels, or splenic sinus-like structures (fig. 21-108). The poorly differentiated areas of the tumor may resemble malignant fibrous histiocytoma or fibrosarcoma (fig. 21-107A).

Based on the in situ cytologic atypia of sinus lining cells in some splenic angiosarcomas, Wolf and Neiman (524) postulated that these tumors arise from the sinus endothelium. Recently, a splenic angiosarcoma showing histochemical and immunohistochemical features of splenic sinus endothelial cells was reported (521); since areas of the tumor appear to be indistinguishable from littoral cell angioma, this case could represent the malignant variant of that lesion.

Differential Diagnosis. Angiosarcoma is distinguished from hemangioma by nuclear pleomorphism, mitoses, and frequent presence of solid growth. Since angiosarcoma may appear deceptively bland in foci, extensive sampling may be required to reveal the true nature of the tumor. The diagnosis of splenic hemangioma should be based on strict morphologic criteria, namely, bland cytology and absence of anastomosing vascular channels (522).

It is important not to mistake bacillary angiomatosis, a reactive vasoproliferative process which may exhibit mild to moderate nuclear pleomorphism, for angiosarcoma. In the gross specimen, the tumor-like nodules of bacillary angiomatosis appear fleshy, lacking the hemorrhagic/ necrotic quality of angiosarcoma (see fig. 21-55, left). Histologic clues for diagnosis of bacillary angiomatosis include abundant interstitial material

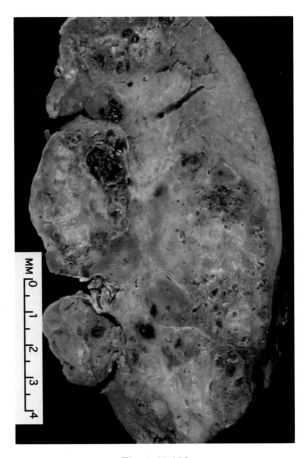

Figure 21-106
ANGIOSARCOMA OF SPLEEN
Most of the spleen is replaced by tumor, which is hemorrhagic and necrotic. (Courtesy of Dr. Louis T.C. Chow, Hong Kong.)

(bacillary clumps), many neutrophils, and absence of irregular anastomosing vascular clefts.

In spleens involved by hairy cell leukemia, the irregular blood lakes ("pseudosinuses") may mimic vascular tumors (518). This disorder can be recognized by the monomorphous population of mitotically inactive and bland-looking medium-sized cells with abundant pale to clear cytoplasm replacing the splenic parenchyma, and absence of true endothelial cells lining the blood-filled spaces.

Poorly differentiated angiosarcoma may exhibit solid areas indistinguishable morphologically from malignant fibrous histiocytoma. Vasoformative areas should be carefully searched for in all sarcomas of the spleen. Immunostaining for endothelial markers is particularly helpful (516,524).

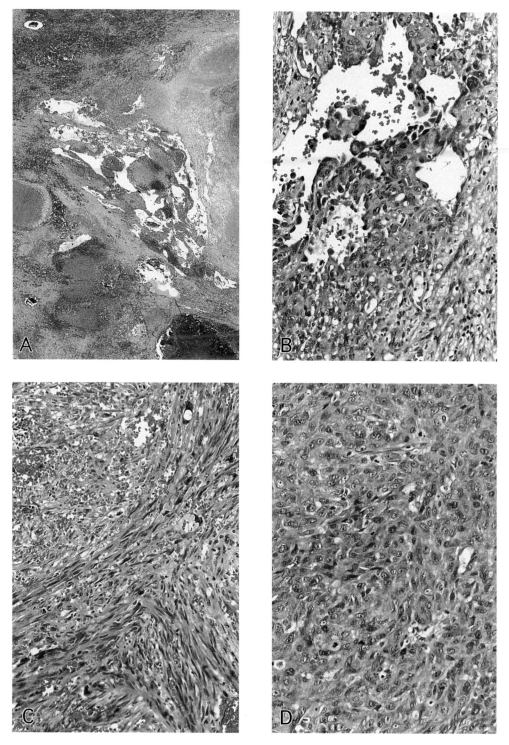

Figure 21-107
ANGIOSARCOMA OF SPLEEN

A: Irregular vascular channels, hemorrhage, and necrosis are evident.

B: Complex vascular channels are lined by highly atypical endothelial cells.

C: Solid spindle cell growth with interspersed vascular slits, reminiscent of Kaposi's sarcoma.

D: Solid growth, in which the vascular nature of the tumor is not evident. Elsewhere in the tumor, some neoplastic vessels are identified.

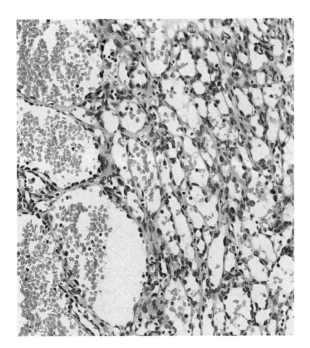

Figure 21-108
ANGIOSARCOMA OF SPLEEN WITH
DECEPTIVELY "BENIGN" APPEARANCE

This focus looks like a hemangioma, but the plump and dark nuclei of the endothelial cells should be suspicious for malignancy. Elsewhere in the tumor, a more definite malignant pattern is seen.

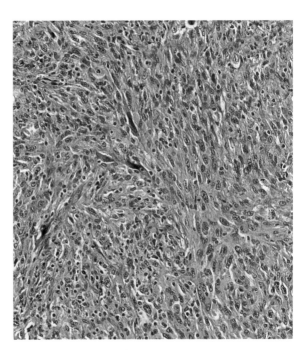

Figure 21-109
MALIGNANT FIBROUS
HISTIOCYTOMA OF SPLEEN

Note the prominent storiform pattern of growth. (Courtesy of Dr. Steven C. Siber, Danbury, CT.)

NONVASCULAR SARCOMAS OF SPLEEN

Primary sarcomas other than angiosarcoma are rare in the spleen. Several cases of malignant fibrous histiocytoma have been reported (528, 535,536), and examples of fibrosarcoma reported in the older literature may represent the same tumor (527,529,530,532,534). The occurrence of leiomyosarcoma in the human spleen has also been suggested but not well documented (527,531).

Patients with *splenic malignant fibrous histiocytoma* are usually middle-aged, and present with splenomegaly, abdominal pain, and constitutional symptoms. These tumors are highly aggressive. At least two of the four cases reported in the literature developed distant metastases (535,536).

Malignant fibrous histiocytomas cause massive enlargement of the spleen. They are histologically identical to those occurring in the soft tissues, being composed of pleomorphic spindle cells and plump cells disposed in a storiform pattern (fig. 21-109). Interspersed inflammatory cells and foamy histiocytes may be abundant in some

cases. Angiosarcoma must be excluded in all cases, since a malignant fibrous histiocytoma–like pattern may be present in this tumor.

Although most studies of malignant fibrous histiocytoma of soft tissues show that the neoplastic cells are phenotypically mesenchymal rather than histiocytic (533,537), one report demonstrated a histiocytic phenotype (535). This supports the current view that malignant fibrous histiocytoma represents a heterogeneous entity, encompassing tumors of different histogenesis (526).

INFLAMMATORY PSEUDOTUMOR OF SPLEEN

Definition. Inflammatory pseudotumor, which is well recognized in other sites such as the lung, gastrointestinal tract, and liver, is rare in the spleen (538–546). It is a reactive mass lesion showing a spectrum of nonspecific inflammatory and reparative changes (539). In the spleen, it can mimic malignant lymphoma clinically, radiologically, and macroscopically. The etiology is not known, but some cases show an association with prior systemic bacterial infection (546). Other

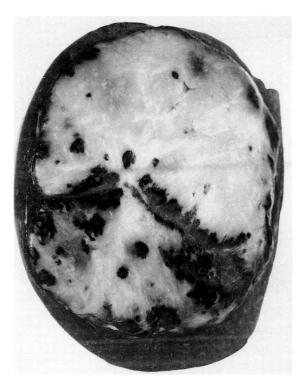

Figure 21-110
INFLAMMATORY PSEUDOTUMOR OF SPLEEN
The lesion is circumscribed and firm, with hemorrhagic foci. (Courtesy of Dr. K.H. Fu, Hong Kong.)

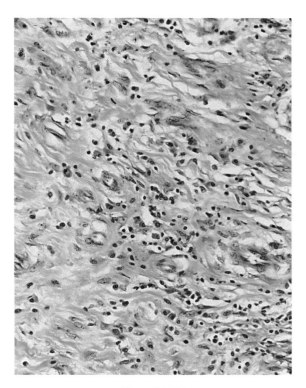

Figure 21-111
INFLAMMATORY PSEUDOTUMOR OF SPLEEN
Bland-looking spindle cells are mixed with blood vessels, lymphocytes, and plasma cells. Sclerosis is often prominent in inflammatory pseudotumor of spleen. (Courtesy of Dr. K.H. Fu, Hong Kong.)

suggested causes are vascular obstruction and autoimmune disorders (545).

Clinical Features. Inflammatory pseudotumor of the spleen occurs mostly in adults (especially middle-aged and older individuals), with no sex predilection (543,545). Some splenic lesions are incidentally found (especially small ones), while others manifest with fever or symptoms referable to the mass lesion such as upper abdominal pain. All patients have remained well after splenectomy.

Gross Findings. The lesion is usually solitary, firm, white, vaguely lobulated, and bulging, and may be punctuated by areas of hemorrhage or necrosis (fig. 21-110). It is well circumscribed or partly infiltrative, adhering to the surrounding structures. Its size ranges from 0.5 to 12.7 cm in greatest dimension. Rarely, it manifests in the form of multiple nodules (542,545).

Microscopic Findings. Inflammatory pseudotumor of the spleen is characterized by myofibroblastic cells with bland-looking oval nu-clei, chronic inflammatory cells, and variable numbers of neutrophils, and is often accompanied by sclerosis which may be extensive (fig. 21-111). In areas, the spindly myofibroblasts may be so prominent that fibrous histiocytoma is mimicked. In other areas, plasma cells may be so prominent ("plasma cell granuloma") that plasmacytoma is mimicked, necessitating immunostaining for immunoglobulin to prove its polytypic nature. There may be a "zoning" phenomenon, with central coagulative necrosis surrounded by a zone of inflammatory cells, which is further surrounded by the spindle cell proliferation. Less common findings include foamy histiocytes, multinucleated giant cells, hematoidin or hemosiderin pigment, eosinophils, and noncaseating granulomas (538–541,543–545).

Immunohistochemical studies have shown the inflammatory infiltrate to comprise predominantly T-lineage small lymphocytes, polytypic plasma cells, and histiocytes (545).

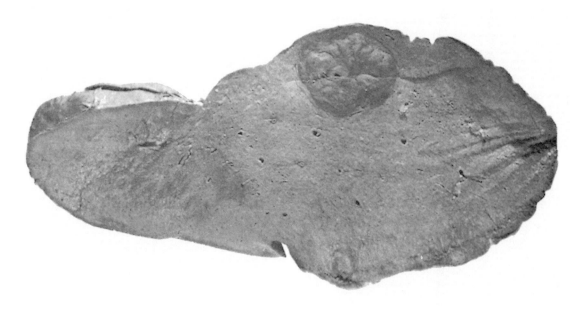

Figure 21-112
SPLENIC HAMARTOMA
The hamartoma appears as a single, spherical, subcapsular nodule. (Fig. 357 from Fascicle 8, 1st Series.)

SPLENIC HAMARTOMA

Definition. Splenic hamartoma, also known as *splenoma,* is a tumor-like malformation composed of normal splenic red pulp elements in an abnormal quantitative relationship and a faulty structural arrangement (551,559). It is postulated to represent a focal developmental disturbance in the spleen, but some authors consider it to be a neoplasm (a special form of hemangioma/lymphangioma) or a post-traumatic lesion (548,563).

Clinical Features. Splenic hamartomas are uncommon, with only slightly over 100 cases reported in the literature. They occur in any age group, with no apparent sex predilection. Most are incidental findings in splenectomy specimens or at autopsy (563), but some cause upper abdominal discomfort as a result of splenomegaly (557,567) or even rupture (549,556). Some patients present with hematologic complications such as thrombocytopenia or anemia, presumably resulting from sequestration of hemopoietic cells in the hamartoma (547,551,558, 560,564,566). This is a benign lesion, and splenectomy is curative for symptomatic patients. Some cases have been reported in association with tuberous sclerosis (550,565), thus providing

further support to the proposed hamartomatous nature of this distinctive splenic lesion.

Gross Findings. Splenic hamartomas are spherical, circumscribed, bulging nodules which compress the surrounding parenchyma (fig. 21-112). Most are solitary, but some form multiple nodules (551,553,554,556,562,566). They appear dark red to grayish white, and range in size from less than 1 cm to over 15 cm. They often lack the fibrous trabeculae and white pulp of the normal splenic parenchyma. Some lesions may show hyalinization or calcification (551,561).

Microscopic Findings. Despite the sharp demarcation grossly, splenic hamartoma paradoxically does not appear as well-defined microscopically (fig. 21-113). The expansile nodule compresses the surrounding red pulp (fig. 21-113), a phenomenon best highlighted by a reticulin stain. It is composed of irregularly arranged, tortuous vascular channels of variable caliber, lined by endothelium similar to splenic sinus lining cells (which can be plump) (551). The vascular channels are surrounded by loose aggregates of lymphocytes and macrophages that resemble the pulp cords (fig. 21-114). The reticulin fiber architecture is disorganized, and the annular fibers typical of normal splenic sinuses may be absent.

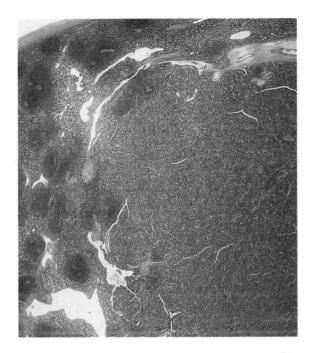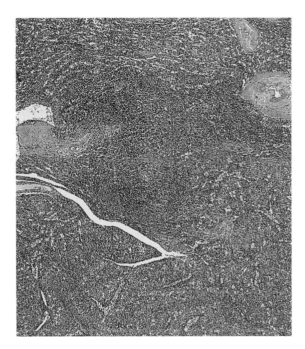

Figure 21-113
SPLENIC HAMARTOMA
Left: The expansile nodule is devoid of a white pulp component.
Right: The haphazard and disorganized sinuses of splenic hamartoma (lower field) contrast with the orderly sinuses in the normal splenic parenchyma (upper field).

There are no organized lymphoid follicles (Malpighian corpuscles). Additional features found in some cases include focal sclerosis; plasmacytosis; extramedullary hemopoiesis; and accumulation of macrophages, lipid-laden macrophages, eosinophils, and mast cells (551,563).

Differential Diagnosis. Distinction of splenic hamartoma from hemangioma may be difficult; in fact, some authors have postulated that hamartomas are sclerosed angiomas (552). However, splenic hamartomas can be recognized by the presence of both sinus-like structures and pulp cord–like elements. Immunohistochemically, the endothelial cells of splenic hamartoma are CD8 positive, which is typical of sinus-type endothelium, whereas those of hemangioma are not (568). Hemangiomas often encompass well-organized lymphoid tissue, whereas splenic hamartomas do not. Although sclerosis may occur in splenic hamartoma, prominent sclerosis would favor the alternative diagnosis of sclerosed hemangioma.

Using antibodies to factor VIII–related antigen (F8) and CD34, Krishnan et al. (555) have reinterpreted some splenic hamartomas as cord capillary

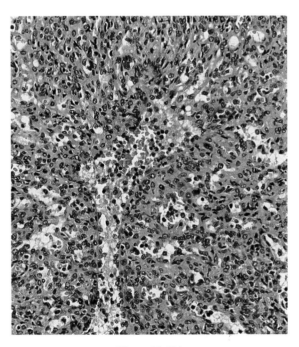

Figure 21-114
SPLENIC HAMARTOMA
Irregular sinuses mixed with pulp cord-like elements.

hemangiomas because of an immunophenotype of F8-, CD34+ rather than F8+, CD34-.

In patients with Hodgkin's disease undergoing staging laparotomy, the presence of a hamartoma (with scattered lymphocytes and eosinophils) may raise concern for involvement by Hodgkin's disease (563). However, the hamartomatous nature of the lesion can be recognized by the disordered vasculature and absence of Reed-Sternberg cells or their variants.

SPLENIC CYSTS

Several types of cysts can occur in the spleen (575): true cysts, which can be epithelial or parasitic, and false cysts. Excluding parasitic cysts, epithelial cysts account for about 20 percent of all splenic cysts, whereas false cysts make up about 80 percent (576).

Epithelial Cysts

Definition. Epithelial cysts, often termed *epidermoid cysts,* are benign unilocular cysts of the spleen (583). The former designation is preferred because the lining is not always epidermoid. The term "congenital cyst" is not entirely appropriate either because it is often impossible to prove that these cysts are indeed congenital (584).

General Features. The origin of epithelial cysts of the spleen is controversial. Their development has been attributed to embryonic inclusion of epithelial tissue (ectoderm, mesoderm, or endoderm) from adjacent structures or to inclusion of mesothelial lining with subsequent squamous metaplasia (571,572,582,583). Indeed, some patients do give a history of previous trauma, raising the possibility that a subclinical tear in the spleen with mesothelial entrapment was etiologic in the formation of the cyst (571). A recent study using scanning and transmission electron microscopy has shown ultrastructural features of mesothelial cells in some of the lining cells (571). On the other hand, study of the cytokeratin profile of one case suggests that the epithelium is either of teratomatous derivation or originates from inclusions of fetal squamous epithelium (577).

Clinical Features. Epithelial cysts occur in children and young adults, with male predominance (576) or no sex predilection (569,571,

580,585,590). They can be asymptomatic or may cause symptoms referable to the mass lesion. Rarely, the cysts rupture or are complicated by secondary bacterial infection (578). Splenectomy is curative. Two unusual examples lined by mucinous epithelium, with one complicated by pseudomyxoma peritonei after rupture, have been recorded (579,587). Malignant transformation (squamous cell carcinoma) has also been reported (573). A few epithelial cysts have occurred in intrapancreatic accessory spleens (589).

Pathologic Findings. Grossly, the luminal surface of an epithelial cyst of the spleen is typically coarsely trabeculated and glistening, reminiscent of the endocardium of the right ventricle (fig. 21-115) (576). The average size is 10 cm. The cyst may adhere to surrounding structures, and is filled with clear fluid or turbid fluid that contains cholesterol crystals (583). Although most are solitary, some may be multiple (570).

Histologically, the cyst wall is variably fibrous, and is usually lined by stratified squamous epithelium which may show keratinization (576, 588). Rete ridges and skin appendages are absent. It may be lined partly or wholly by transitional cell epithelium (574,585), or by a single layer of flattened, cuboidal or hobnail cells (figs. 21-116, 21-117) (571). The latter is often interpreted as being mesothelial in nature. Less commonly, isolated mucinous cells are scattered in the stratified squamous or transitional epithelium, and smaller cysts reminiscent of cystitis cystica may be found in the fibrous wall (fig. 21-117) (571). The epithelium can also be partly or largely denuded. True dermoid cysts with hair follicles and sebaceous glands are exceptional (570,575, 587). An example of low-grade mucinous cystadenocarcinoma of the spleen, morphologically identical to the ovarian counterpart, has also been reported (581).

Parasitic Cysts

The histologic details of parasitic cysts, which are identical to those occurring in other sites, will not be further expanded (586). Hydatid (echinococcal) cysts account for a highly variable percentage of splenic cysts, but are common only in endemic areas (576); other parasitic cysts are caused by *Cysticercus* and *Pentastoma* larvae (587).

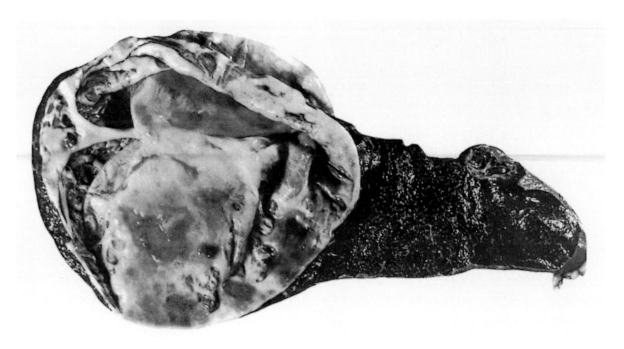

Figure 21-115
EPIDERMOID CYST OF SPLEEN
Note the typical trabeculation, resembling the endocardial surface. (Fig. 366 from Fascicle 8, 1st Series.)

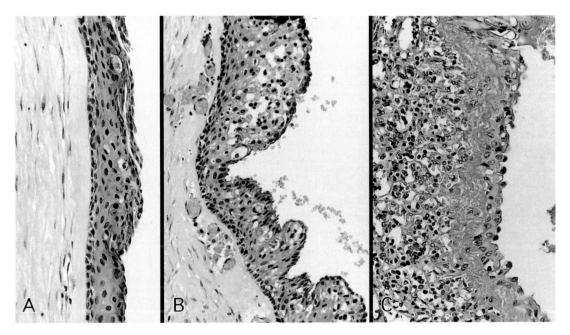

Figure 21-116
EPITHELIAL CYSTS OF SPLEEN
The variable cytologic composition of epithelial cyst of spleen.
A: Nonkeratinizing stratified squamous epithelium.
B: Stratified squamous epithelium with interspersed mucinous cells (upper field).
C: Hobnail cells.

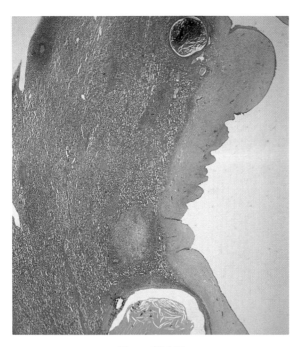

Figure 21-117
EPIDERMOID CYST OF SPLEEN
The luminal surface is rugged. A few cystic inclusions are seen in the fibrous wall.

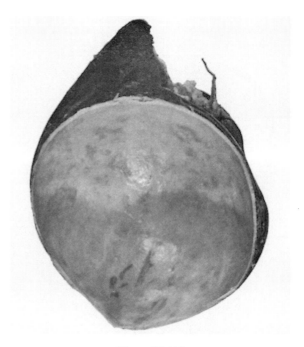

Figure 21-118
FALSE CYST OF SPLEEN
The cut surface reveals a thick cyst wall with a smooth internal surface. (Fig. 371 from Fascicle 8, 1st Series.)

False Cysts

Clinical Features. False cysts (pseudocysts or secondary cysts) are so named because they lack a cellular lining. They occur mostly in children and young adults (576). Most are incidental findings, but some are large (over 20 cm) (587) and cause symptoms. Rarely, they rupture and cause hemoperitoneum. Since many patients give a history of previous trauma, it is postulated that these cysts arise from liquefaction of hematomas. Even so, it is very difficult to prove conclusively that the trauma was etiologic (583). It is also conceivable that some false cysts arise through cystic degeneration of hamartoma, infarct, or angioma, or from denudation of epithelial cysts (583).

Pathologic Findings. Grossly, false cysts differ from epithelial cysts in that the luminal surface of the unilocular or multilocular cyst is often smooth or shaggy rather than trabeculated (figs. 21-118, 21-119). They are often filled with opaque or cloudy fluid (587). The wall is formed by fibrous tissue which may be focally or exten-

sively calcified; the calcific rim may sometimes be visible on radiographs. Cholesterol crystals and hemosiderin are often present in the fibrous wall (576). An epithelial lining, by definition, is absent (fig. 21-119).

RARE LESIONS OF SPLEEN

Rare nonlymphoid lesions of the spleen include lipoma (593), fibroma (which may merely be a sclerosed hemangioma or hamartoma) (591,595), Dabska's endovascular papillary angioendothelioma (594), carcinosarcoma (which is postulated to be of mesothelial origin) (596), and malignant teratoma (592).

SPLENIC METASTASES

The spleen is involved by nonhematolymphoid solid tumors either through direct invasion by tumors in the vicinity (such as the stomach, pancreas, kidney, and adrenal gland), or through metastasis. The latter usually results from hematogenous spread, and is almost always accompanied by metastasis in other organs (598,599,616).

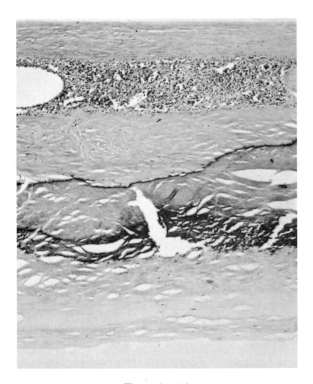

Figure 21-119
FALSE CYST OF SPLEEN
The cyst wall shows five zones from above downward: 1) splenic fibrous capsule; 2) splenic pulp; 3) outer fibrous zone composed of dense collagenous tissue; 4) calcified zone with cholesterol crystals; and 5) inner fibrous zone with many cholesterol clefts but no cellular lining. (Fig. 372 from Fascicle 8, 1st Series.)

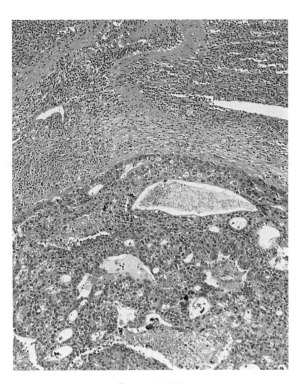

Figure 21-120
METASTATIC ADENOCARCINOMA IN SPLEEN
Neoplastic glands replace portions of the splenic parenchyma.

The reported frequency of splenic metastasis varies greatly from series to series (1.6 to 30 percent) (597,598,601,606,608,612,613), depending on the thoroughness of examination and selection of cases. The suggestion that the spleen exhibits antineoplastic properties prohibiting the development of metastasis (607) has not been fully substantiated, since the frequency of splenic metastasis as detected at autopsy in patients with cancer is comparable to that of the kidney and brain, all of which are sites involved mostly as a result of blood-borne metastasis (598).

Splenic metastasis is usually detected only at autopsy, and rarely poses problems in diagnosis. Among the various tumors, malignant melanoma, breast cancer, and lung cancer account for most cases (598,600). The pattern of metastatic deposit in the spleen varies from being macroscopic (solitary nodule, multiple nodules, mili-ary, or diffuse replacement) to microscopic (598,609,612,616). In the latter, the tumor cells are confined to the venous sinuses, red pulp, white pulp, or trabecular vessels, or are found in several compartments of the spleen (fig. 21-120) (600,612). Rarely, the metastatic tumor is confined to the trabecular lymphatics in the spleen (fig. 21-121), a phenomenon often interpreted as retrograde permeation of splenic lymphatics, usually from tumor deposits in the hilum (606,615). Exceptionally, metastatic carcinoma in the spleen is accompanied by nodular transformation of the red pulp (603).

On rare occasions, splenomegaly resulting from splenic metastasis may be the first manifestation of recurrent solid cancer, a phenomenon observed with a disproportionally high frequency with gynecologic malignancies (597, 605,610,611,614). Exceptionally, splenic metastasis is detected simultaneously with the primary cancer (602,604).

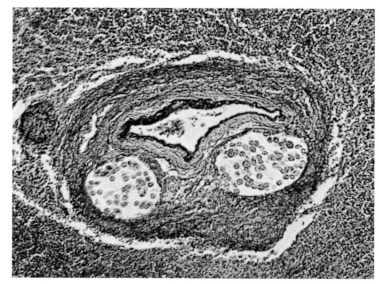

Figure 21-121
METASTATIC UNDIFFERENTIATED
CARCINOMA IN SPLEEN
In this example, tumor cells are found in the lymphatics in the adventitia of a trabecular artery. This unusual occurrence is caused by retrograde permeation of the splenic lymphatics by neoplastic cells, usually from tumor deposits in the splenic hilum. (Van Gieson and Weigert elastica stains)(Fig. 405 from Fascicle 8, 1st Series.)

REFERENCES

Hemorrhagic Spindle Cell Tumor with Amianthoid Fibers

1. Alguacil-Garcia A. Intranodal myofibroblastoma in a submandibular lymph node. A case report. Am J Clin Pathol 1992;97:69–72.
2. Barbareschi M, Mariscotti C, Ferrero S, Pignatiello U. Intranodal haemorrhagic spindle cell tumor: a benign Kaposi-like nodal tumor. Histopathology 1990;17:93–6.
3. Fletcher CD, Stirling RW. Intranodal myofibroblastoma presenting in the submandibular region: evidence of a broader clinical and histological spectrum. Histopathology 1990;16:287–93.
4. Lee JY, Abell E, Shevechik GJ. Solitary spindle cell tumor with myoid differentiation of the lymph node. Arch Pathol Lab Med 1989;113:547–50.
5. Michal M, Chlumska A, Povysilova V. Intranodal "amianthoid" myofibroblastoma. Report of six cases: immunohistochemical and electron microscopical study. Pathol Res Pract 1992;188:199–204.
6. Skalova A, Michal M, Chlumska A, Leivo I. Collagen composition and ultrastructure of the so-called amianthoid fibers in palisaded myofibroblastoma. Ultrastructural and immunohistochemical study. J Pathol 1992;167:335–40.
7. Suster S, Rosai J. Intranodal hemorrhagic spindle-cell tumor with "amianthoid" fibers. Report of six cases of a distinctive mesenchymal neoplasm of the inguinal region that simulates Kaposi's sarcoma. Am J Surg Pathol 1989;13:347–57.
8. Tanda F, Massarelli G, Cossu A, Bosincu L, Cossu S, Ibba M. Primary spindle cell tumor of lymph node with amianthoid fibers: a histological, immunohistochemical and ultrastructural study. Ultrastruct Pathol 1993;17:195–205.
9. Weiss LM, Berry GJ, Dorfman RF, et al. Spindle cell neoplasms of lymph nodes of probable reticulum cell lineage. True reticulum cell sarcoma? Am J Surg Pathol 1990;14:405–14.
10. Weiss SW, Gnepp DR, Bratthauer GL. Palisaded myofibroblastoma. A benign mesenchymal tumor of lymph node. Am J Surg Pathol 1989;13:341–6.

Smooth Muscle Proliferations in Lymph Node

11. Abell MR, Littler ER. Benign metastasizing uterine leiomyoma, multiple lymph nodal metastasis. Cancer 1975;36:2206–13.
12. Allen PW, Hoffman GJ. Fat in angiomyomatous hamartoma of lymph node [Letter]. Am J Surg Pathol 1993;17:748–9.
13. Bennington JL, Beckwith JB. Tumors of the kidney, renal pelvis and ureter. Altas of Tumor Pathology, 2nd Series, Fascicle 12. Washington DC: Armed Forces Institute of Pathology, 1975:204–12.
14. Bhattacharyya AK, Balogh K. Retroperitoneal lymphangioleiomyomatosis. A 36-year benign course in a postmenopausal woman. Cancer 1985;56:1144–6.
15. Bloom DA, Scardino PT, Ehrlich RM, Waisman J. The significance of lymph nodal involvement in renal angiomyolipoma. J Urol 1982;128:1292–5.
16. Boyce CR, Buddhdev HN. Pregnancy complicated by metastasizing leiomyoma of the uterus. Obstet Gynecol 1973;42:252–8.
17. Brecher ME, Gill WB, Straus FH II. Angiomyolipoma with regional lymph node involvement and long-term follow-up study. Hum Pathol 1986;17:962–3.
18. Busch FM, Bark CJ, Clydine HR. Benign renal angiomyolipoma with regional lymph node involvement. J Urol 1976;116:715–7.

19. Chan JK, Frizzera G, Fletcher CD, Rosai J. Primary vascular tumors of lymph nodes other than Kaposi's sarcoma: analysis of 39 cases and delineation of two new entities. Am J Surg Pathol 1992;16:335–50.
20. _____, Tsang WY, Pau MY, Tang MC, Pang SW, Fletcher CD. Lymphangiomyomatosis and angiomyolipoma: closely related entities characterized by hamartomatous proliferation of HMB-45-positive smooth muscle. Histopathology 1993;22:445–55.
21. Channer JL, Davies JD. Smooth muscle proliferation in the hilum of superficial lymph nodes. Virchows Arch [A] 1985;406:261–70.
22. Cornog JL, Enterline HT. Lymphangiomyoma, a benign lesion of chyliferous lymphatics synonymous with lymphangiopericytoma. Cancer 1966;19:1909–30.
23. Corrin B, Liebow AA, Friedman PJ. Pulmonary lymphangiomyomatosis. Am J Pathol 1975;79:348–82.
24. Cramer SF, Meyer JS, Kraner JF Camel M, Mazur MT, Tenenbaum MS. Metastasizing leiomyoma of the uterus. S-phase fraction, estrogen receptor, and ultrastructure. Cancer 1980;45:932–7.
25. _____, Patel A. The frequency of uterine leiomyomas. Am J Clin Pathol 1990;94:435–8.
26. Dao AH, Pinto AC, Kirchner FK, Halter SA. Massive nodal involvement in a case of renal angiomyolipoma [Letter]. Arch Pathol Lab Med 1984;108:612–3.
27. Davies JD. Gut-associated lymph nodes. In: Whitehead R, ed. Gastrointestinal and oesophageal pathology. Edinburgh: Churchill Livingstone, 1989:611–6.
28. Enzinger FM, Weiss SW. Soft tissue tumors. 2nd ed. St. Louis: CV Mosby, 1988:627–35.
29. Folse DS, Beathard GA, Granholm NA. Smooth muscle in lymph node capsule and trabeculae. Anat Rec 1975;183:517–21.
30. Fujii S, Okamura H, Nakashima N, Bann C, Aso T, Nishimura T. Leiomyomatosis peritonealis disseminata. Obstet Gynecol 1980;55:79s–83s.
31. Horie A, Ishii N, Matsumoto M, Hashizume Y, Kawakami M, Sato Y. Leiomyomatosis in the pelvic lymph node and peritoneum. Acta Pathol Jpn 1984;34:813–9.
32. Hsu YK, Rosenshein NB, Parmley TH, Woodruff JD, Elberfeld HT. Leiomyomatosis in pelvic lymph nodes. Obstet Gynecol 1981;57:91s–3s.
33. Hulbert JC, Graf R. Involvement of the spleen by renal angiomyolipoma: metastasis or multicentricity? J Urol 1983;130:328–9.
34. Idelson MG, Davids AM. Metastasis of uterine fibroleiomyomata. Obstet Gynecol 1963;21:78–85.
35. Lack EE, Dolan MF, Finisio J, Grover G, Singh M, Triche TJ. Pulmonary and extrapulmonary lymphangioleiomyomatosis: report of a case with bilateral renal angiomyolipomas, multifocal lymphangioleiomyomatosis, and a glial polyp of the endocervix. Am J Surg Pathol 1986;10:650–7.
36. Longo S. Benign lymph node inclusions. Hum Pathol 1976;7:349–54.
37. Magrini U, Rosso R, Paulli M, et al. Solitary nodal lymphangiomyoma: incidental findings in pelvic lymph nodes [Abstract]. Mod Pathol 1992;5:82A.
38. Mazzoleni G, Salerno A, Santini D, Marabini A, Martinelli G. Leiomyomatosis of pelvic lymph nodes. Histopathology 1992;21:588–9.
39. Ober WB, Black MB. Neoplasms of the subcoelomic mesenchyme. Arch Pathol 1955;59:698–705.
40. Pinkus GS, Warhol MJ, O'Connor EM, Etheridge CL, Fujiwara K. Immunohistochemical localization of smooth muscle myosin in human spleen, lymph node, and other lymphoid tissues. Unique staining patterns in splenic white pulp and sinuses, lymphoid follicles, and certain vasculature with ultrastructural correlations. Am J Pathol 1986;123:440–53.
41. Rigaud C, Bogomoletz WV. Leiomyomatosis in pelvic lymph node [Letter]. Arch Pathol Lab Med 1983;107:153–4.
42. Ro JY, Ayala AG, el-Naggar A, Grignon DJ, Hogan SF, Howard DR. Angiomyolipoma of kidney with lymph node involvement. DNA flow cytometric analysis. Arch Pathol Lab Med 1990;114:65–7.
43. Sant GR, Ucci AA Jr, Meares EM Jr. Multicentric angiomyolipoma: renal and lymph node involvement. Urology 1986;28:111–3.
44. Starasoler L, Vuitch F, Albores-Saavedra J. Intranodal leiomyoma. Another distinctive primary spindle cell neoplasm of lymph node. Am J Clin Pathol 1991;95:858–62.
45. Tsang WY, Chan JK. Primary leiomyomatosis of lymph node or nodal lymphangiomyoma? [Letter] Histopathology 1993;23:393–4.
46. _____, Chan JK, Dorfman RF, Rosai J. Vasoproliferative lesions of lymph node. Pathol Annu 1994;29(Pt 1):63–133.
46a. White JE, Chan YF, Miller MV. Intranodal leiomyoma or myofibroblastoma: an identical lesion? Histopathology 1995;26:188–90.
47. Wolff M. Lymphangiomyoma: clinicopathologic study and ultrastructural confirmation of its histogenesis. Cancer 1973;31:988–1007.

Inflammatory Pseudotumor of Lymph Node

48. Chan JK, Tsang WY. Uncommon syndromes of reactive lymphadenopathy. Semin Oncol 1993;20:648–57.
49. Davis RE, Warnke RA, Dorfman RF. Inflammatory pseudotumor of lymph nodes: additional observations and evidence for an inflammatory etiology. Am J Surg Pathol 1991;15:744–56.
50. Facchetti F, De Wolf Peeters C, de Wever I, Frizzera G. Inflammatory pseudotumor of lymph nodes. Immunohistochemical evidence for its fibrohistiocytic nature. Am J Pathol 1990;137:281–9.
51. Kemper CA, Davis RE, Deresinski SC, Dorfman RF. Inflammatory pseudotumor of intra-abdominal lymph nodes manifesting as recurrent fever of unknown origin: a case report. Am J Med 1991;90:519–23.
52. Perrone T, De Wolf Peeters C, Frizzera G. Inflammatory pseudotumor of lymph nodes. A distinctive pattern of nodal reaction. Am J Surg Pathol 1988;12:351–61.
53. Rousselet MC, Saint-Andre JP, Beaufils JM, Diebold J. Benign vascular proliferation in a lymph node following acute toxoplasmosis. A differential diagnosis from Kaposi's sarcoma. Arch Pathol Lab Med 1988;112:1264–6.
54. Tsang WY, Chan JK, Ng CS. Kikuchi's lymphadenitis. A morphologic study of 75 cases with special reference to unusual features. Am J Surg Pathol 1994;18:219–31.

Mycobacterial Spindle Cell Pseudotumor of Lymph Node and Spleen

55. Chen KT. Mycobacterial spindle cell pseudotumor of lymph nodes. Am J Surg Pathol 1992;16:276–81.
56. Suster S, Moran CA, Blanco M. Mycobacterial spindle cell pseudotumor of the spleen. Am J Clin Pathol 1994; 101:539–42.
57. Umlas J, Federman M, Crawford C, O'Hara CJ, Fitzgibbon JS, Modeste A. Spindle cell pseudotumor due to Mycobacterium avium-intracellulare in patients with acquired immunodeficiency syndrome (AIDS). Positive staining of mycobacteria for cytoskeleton filaments. Am J Surg Pathol 1991;15:1181–7.
58. Wade HW. The histoid variety of lepromatous leprosy. Int J Lepr 1963;31:129–42.

Deciduosis of Lymph Node

59. Ashraf M, Boyd CB, Beresford WA. Ectopic decidual cell reaction in para-aortic and pelvic lymph nodes in the presence of cervical squamous cell carcinoma during pregnancy. J Surg Oncol 1984;26:6–8.
60. Burnett RA, Millan D. Decidual change in pelvic lymph nodes: a source of possible diagnostic error. Histopathology 1986;10:1089–92.
61. Covell LM, Disciullo AJ, Knapp RC. Decidual change in pelvic lymph nodes in the presence of cervical squamous cell carcinoma during pregnancy. Am J Obstet Gynecol 1977;127:674–6.
62. Javert CT. The spread of benign and malignant endometrium in the lymphatic system with a note on coexisting vascular involvement. Am J Obstet Gynecol 1952;64:780–806.
63. Mills SE. Decidua and squamous metaplasia in abdominopelvic lymph nodes. Int J Gynecol Pathol 1983;2:209–15.
64. Ober WB, Black MB. Neoplasms of the subcoelomic mesenchyme. Arch Pathol 1955;59:698–705.
65. Russell HB. Decidual reaction of endometrium ectopic in an abdominal lymph node. Surg Gynecol Obstet 1945;81:218–20.
66. Young RH, Kurman RJ, Scully RE. Proliferations and tumors of intermediate trophoblast of the placental site. Semin Diagn Pathol 1988;5:223–37.
67. Zaytsev P, Taxy JB. Pregnancy-associated ectopic decidua. Am J Surg Pathol 1987;11:526–30.

Kaposi's Sarcoma of Lymph Node

68. Armes J. A review of Kaposi's sarcoma. Adv Cancer Res 1989;53:73–87.
69. Auerbach HE, Brooks JJ. Kaposi's sarcoma: neoplasia or hyperplasia? Surg Pathol 1989;2:19–28.
70. Autio-Harmainen H, Karttunen T, Apaja-Sarkkinen M, Dammert K, Risteli L. Laminin and type IV collagen in different histological stages of Kaposi's sarcoma and other vascular lesions of blood vessel or lymphatic vessel origin. Am J Surg Pathol 1988;12:469–76.
71. Aziz DC, Srolovitz HD, Brisson ML, Begin LR. Characterization of eosinophilic hyaline bodies in Kaposi's sarcoma [Abstract]. Lab Invest 1985;52:4A.
72. Becker BJ. The histogenesis of Kaposi's sarcoma. Acta Union Int Contre Cancer 1962;18:477–86.
73. Beckstead JH, Wood GS, Fletcher V. Evidence for the origin of Kaposi's sarcoma from lymphatic endothelium. Am J Pathol 1985;119:294–300.
74. Beral V, Peterman TA, Berkelman RL, Jaffe HW. Kaposi's sarcoma among persons with AIDS: a sexually transmitted infection? Lancet 1990;335:123–8.
75. Berman MA, Nalesnik MA, Kapadia SB, Rinaldo CR Jr, Jensen F. Primary lymphadenopathic Kaposi's sarcoma in an immunocompetent 25-year-old man. Am J Clin Pathol 1986;86:366–9.
76. Bhana D, Templeton AC, Master SP, Kyalwazi SK. Kaposi sarcoma of lymph nodes. Br J Cancer 1970;24:464–70.
77. Biggar RJ. Cancer in acquired immunodeficiency syndrome: an epidemiological assessment. Semin Oncol 1990;17:251–60.
78. Bonzanini M, Togni R, Barabareschi M, Parenti A, Palma PD. Primary Kaposi's sarcoma of intraparotid lymph node. Histopathology 1992;21:489–91.
79. Bowden FJ, McPhee DA, Deacon NJ, et al. Antibodies to gp41 and nef in otherwise HIV-negative homosexual man with Kaposi's sarcoma. Lancet 1991;337:1313–4.
80. Braun-Falco O, Schmoeckel C, Hubner G. The histogenesis of Kaposi's sarcoma, a histochemical and electron microscopic study. Virchows Arch [A] 1976;369:215–27.
81. Burns BF, Wood GS, Dorfman RF. The varied histopathology of lymphadenopathy in the homosexual male. Am J Surg Pathol 1985;9:287–97.
82. Cerimele D, Scappaticci S, Cattaneo E, Cottoni F. Failure to demonstrate early and late antigens of cytomegalovirus in tissue cultures from Kaposi's sarcoma patients. Arch Dermatol Res 1983;275:197–8.
82a. Chang Y, Cesarman E, Pessin MS, et al. Identification of herpes virus-like DNA sequences in AIDS-associated Kaposi's sarcoma. Science 1994;266:1865–9.
83. Chen KT. Multicentric Castleman's disease and Kaposi's sarcoma. Am J Surg Pathol 1984;8:287–93.
83a. Cohen J. AIDS mood upbeat—for a change. Science 1995;267:959–60.
84. Conant MA. Speculations on the viral etiology of acquired immune deficiency syndrome and Kaposi's sarcoma. J Invest Dermatol 1984;83(Suppl):57s–62s.
85. Costa J, Rabson AS. Generalized Kaposi's sarcoma is not a neoplasm [Letter]. Lancet 1983:1:58.
86. Cox FH, Helwig EB. Kaposi's sarcoma. Cancer 1959;12:289–98.
87. Dayan AD, Lewis PD. Origin of Kaposi's sarcoma from the reticulo-endothelial system. Nature 1967;213:889–90.
88. Delli Bovi P, Donti E, Knowles DM, et al. Presence of chromosomal abnormalities and lack of AIDS retrovirus DNA sequences in AIDS-associated Kaposi's sarcoma. Cancer Res 1986;46:6333–8.

89. De Rosa G, Barra E, Guarino M, Gentile R. Multicentric Castleman's disease in association with Kaposi's sarcoma. Appl Pathol 1989;7:105–10.

90. Des Jarlais DC, Stoneburner R, Thomas P, Friedman SR. Declines in proportion of Kaposi's sarcoma among cases of AIDS in multiple risk groups in New York City [Letter]. Lancet 1987;2:1024–5.

91. Dickson D, Ben-Ezra JM, Reed J, Flax H, Janis R. Multicentric giant lymph node hyperplasia, Kaposi's sarcoma, and lymphoma. Arch Pathol Lab Med 1985;109:1013–8.

92. Dictor M, Andersson C. Lymphaticovenous differentiation in Kaposi's sarcoma. Cellular phenotypes by stage. Am J Pathol 1988;130:411–7.

93. Dörffel J. Histogenesis of multiple idiopathic hemorrhagic sarcoma of Kaposi. Arch Dermatol Syphil 1932;26:608–34.

94. Dorfman RF. Cutaneous and lymphadenopathic Kaposi's sarcoma in Africa and the U.S.A. with observations on persistent lymphadenopathy in homosexual men at risk for the acquired immunodeficiency syndrome. Front Radiat Ther Oncol 1985;19:105–16.

95. _____. Kaposi's sarcoma. With special reference to its manifestations in infants and children and to the concepts of Arthur Purdy Stout. Am J Surg Pathol 1986;10(Suppl 1):68–77.

96. _____. Kaposi's sarcoma, the contribution of enzyme histochemistry to the identification of cell types. Acta Union Int Cortre Cancer 1962;18:464–76.

97. _____. Kaposi's sarcoma revisited. Hum Pathol 1984;15:1013–7.

98. _____, Wood GS, Beckstead JH. Histogenesis. In: Ziegler JL, Dorfman RF, eds. Kaposi's sarcoma: pathophysiology and clinical management. New York: Marcel Dekkerm, 1988:71–112.

99. Dutz W, Stout AP. Kaposi's sarcoma in infants and children. Cancer 1960;13:684–93.

100. Ecklund RE, Valaitis J. Kaposi's sarcoma of lymph nodes. A case report. Arch Pathol 1962;74:224–9.

100a. Ensoli B, Gendelman R, Markham P, et al. Synergy between basic fibroblastic growth factor and HIV-1 Tat protein in induction of Kaposi's sarcoma. Nature 1994;371:674–80.

101. _____, Nakamura S, Salahuddin SZ, et al. AIDS-Kaposi's sarcoma-derived cells express cytokines with autocrine and paracrine growth effects. Science 1989;243:223–6.

102. _____, Salahuddin SZ, Gallo RC. AIDS-associated Kaposi's sarcoma: a molecular model for its pathogenesis. Cancer Cells 1989;1:93–6.

103. Enzinger FM, Weiss SW. Soft tissue tumors. 2nd ed. St. Louis: CV Mosby, 1988:489–532.

104. Fauci AS, Masur H, Gelmann EP, Markham PD, Hahn BH, Lane HC. NIH conference; the acquired immunodeficiency syndrome: an update. Ann Intern Med 1985;102:800–13.

105. Finkbeiner WE, Egbert BM, Groundwater JR, Sagebiel RW. Kaposi's sarcoma in young homosexual men: a histopathologic study with particular reference to lymph node involvement. Arch Pathol Lab Med 1982;106:261–4.

106. Frizzera G, Banks PM, Massarelli G, Rosai J. A systemic lymphoproliferative disorder with morphologic features of Castleman's disease. Pathological findings in 15 patients. Am J Surg Pathol 1983;7:211–31.

107. Fukunaga M, Silverberg SG. Hyaline globules in Kaposi's sarcoma: a light microscopic and immunohistochemical study. Mod Pathol 1991;4:187–90.

108. Gokel JM, Kurzl R, Hubner G. Fine structure and origin of Kaposi's sarcoma. Pathol Europ 1976;11:45–7.

109. Gottlieb GJ, Ackerman AB. Kaposi's sarcoma: an extensively disseminated form in young homosexual men. Hum Pathol 1982;13:882–92.

110. Gray M, Smoller B, McNutt N, Hsu A. The histogenesis of spindle cell nodules of Kaposi's sarcoma [Abstract]. Mod Pathol 1990;3:39A.

111. Greenfield DI, Trinh P, Fulenwider WA, Barth WF. Kaposi's sarcoma in a patient with systemic lupus erythematosus. J Rheumatol 1986;13:637–40.

112. Guarda LG, Silva EG, Ordonez NG, Smith TL Jr. Factor VIII in Kaposi's sarcoma. Am J Clin Pathol 1981;76:197–200.

113. Harawi SJ. Kaposi's sarcoma. In: Harawi SJ, O'Hara CJ. Pathology and pathophysiology of AIDS and HIV-related diseases. London: Chapman and Hall, 1989:83–133.

114. Harris NL. Hypervascular follicular hyperplasia and Kaposi's sarcoma in patients at risk for AIDS [Letter]. N Engl J Med 1984;310:462–3.

115. Harwood AR. Kaposi's sarcoma in renal transplant patients. In: Friedman-Kien AE, Laubenstein LJ, eds. AIDS, the epidemic of Kaposi's sarcoma and opportunistic infections. New York: Masson, 1984:41–44.

116. Hashimoto K, Lever WF. Kaposi's sarcoma. Histochemical and electron microscopic studies. J Invest Dermatol 1964;43:539–49.

117. Haverkos HW, Drotman DP. Prevalence of Kaposi's sarcoma among patients with AIDS [Letter]. N Engl J Med 1985;312:1518.

118. Huang YQ, Li JJ, Rush MG, et al. HPV-16-related DNA sequences in Kaposi's sarcoma. Lancet 1992;339:515–8.

119. Ioachim HL. Neoplasms associated with immune deficiencies. Pathol Annu 1987;22(Pt 2):177–222.

120. Jones RR, Spaull J, Spry C, Jones EW. Histogenesis of Kaposi's sarcoma in patients with and without acquired immune deficiency syndrome (AIDS). J Clin Pathol 1986;39:742–9.

121. Kao GF, Johnson FB, Sulica VI. The nature of hyaline (eosinophilic) globules and vascular slits of Kaposi's sarcoma. Am J Dermatopathol 1990;12:256–67.

122. Kapadia SB, Krause JR. Kaposi's sarcoma after long-term alkylating agent therapy for multiple myeloma. South Med J 1977;70:1011–3.

123. Krigel RL, Friedman-Kien AE. Epidemic Kaposi's sarcoma. Semin Oncol 1990;17:350–60.

124. Kuzu I, Bicknell R, Harris AL, Jones M, Gatter K, Mason DY. Heterogeneity of vascular endothelial cells with relevance to diagnosis of vascular tumors. J Clin Pathol 1992;45:143–8.

125. Lachant NA, Sun NC, Leong LA, Oseas RS, Prince HE. Multicentric angiofollicular lymph node hyperplasia (Castleman's disease) followed by Kaposi's sarcoma in two homosexual males with AIDS. Am J Clin Pathol 1985;83:27–33.

126. Lee SC, Moore OS. Kaposi's sarcoma of lymph nodes. Arch Pathol 1965;80:651–4.

127. Lo SC, Liotta LA. Vascular tumors produced by NIH/3T3 cells transfected with human AIDS Kaposi's sarcoma DNA. Am J Pathol 1985;118:7–13.

128. Longacre TA, Rouse RV. CD31: a new marker for vascular neoplasia. Adv Anat Pathol 1994;1:16–20.

129. Loring WE, Wolman SR. Idiopathic multiple hemorrhagic sarcoma of lung (Kaposi's sarcoma). N Y State J Med 1965;65:668–76.

130. Lubin J, Rywlin AM. Lymphoma-like lymph node changes in Kaposi's sarcoma. Two additional cases. Arch Pathol 1971;92:338–41.

131. Massarelli G, Scott CA, Mura A, Tanda F, Cossu A. Hyaline bodies in Kaposi's sarcoma: an immunocytochemical and ultrastructural study. Appl Pathol 1989;7:26–33.

132. Mirra JM. Kaposi's sarcoma—is it a sarcoma at all? International Symposium on Kaposi's sarcoma and AIDS. Am J Trop Med & Hygiene 1986;28(Suppl):47–62.

133. Moskowitz LB, Hensley GT, Gould EW, Weiss SD. Frequency and anatomic distribution of lymphadenopathic Kaposi's sarcoma in the acquired immunodeficiency syndrome: an autopsy series. Hum Pathol 1985;16:447–56.

134. Mustakallio KK, Levonen E, Raekallio J. Histochemistry of Kaposi's sarcoma. I. Hydrolases and phosphorylase. Exp Molec Pathol 1963;2:303–16.

135. Nadji M, Morales AR, Ziegles-Weissman J, Penneys NS. Kaposi's sarcoma: immunohistologic evidence for an endothelial origin. Arch Pathol Lab Med 1981;105:274–5.

136. Nakamura S, Salahuddin SZ, Biberfeld P, et al. Kaposi's sarcoma cells: long-term culture with growth factor from retrovirus-infected CD4+ T cells. Science 1988;242:426–30.

137. Nerlich A, Zietz C, Schleicher E. Distribution of basement membrane-associated heparan sulfate proteoglycan in idiopathic and AIDS-associated Kaposi's sarcoma. Pathol Res Pract 1991;187:444–50.

138. Nickoloff BJ, Griffiths CE. The spindle-shaped cells in cutaneous Kaposi's sarcoma. Histologic simulators include factor XIIIa dermal dendrocytes. Am J Pathol 1989;135:793–800.

139. _____, Huang YQ, Li JJ, Friedman-Kien AE. Immunohistochemical detection of papillomavirus antigens in Kaposi's sarcoma [Letter]. Lancet 1992;339:548–9.

140. O'Connell KM. Kaposi's sarcoma: histopathological study of 159 cases from Malawi. J Clin Pathol 1977;30:687–95.

141. _____. Kaposi's sarcoma in lymph nodes: histological study of lesions from 16 cases in Malawi. J Clin Pathol 1977;30:696–703.

142. Pautrier LM, Diss A. Kaposi's sarcoma is not a genuine sarcoma but a neurovascular dysgenesis. Br J Dermatol 1929;41:93–105.

143. Penn I. Etiology: immunodeficiency. In: Ziegler JL, Dorfman RF, eds. Kaposi's sarcoma, pathophysiology and clinical management. New York: Marcel Dekker, 1988:129–50.

144. _____. Kaposi's sarcoma in immunosuppressed patients. J Clin Lab Immunol 1983;12:1–10.

145. _____. Kaposi's sarcoma in organ transplant recipients, report of 20 cases. Transplantation. 1979;27:8–11.

146. Pepler WJ. The origin of Kaposi's hemangiosarcoma: a histochemical study. J Pathol Bacteriol 1959;78:553–7.

147. Perlow LS, Taff ML, Orsini JM, et al. Kaposi's sarcoma in a young homosexual man. Associated with angiofollicular lymphoid hyperplasia and a malignant lymphoproliferative disorder. Arch Pathol Lab Med 1983;107:510–3.

148. Ramos CV, Taylor HB, Hernandez BA, Tucker ER. Kaposi's sarcoma of lymph nodes. Am J Clin Pathol 1976;66:998–1003.

149. Rutgers JL, Wieczorek R, Bonetti F, et al. The expression of endothelial cell surface antigens by AIDS-associated Kaposi's sarcoma. Evidence for a vascular endothelial cell origin. Am J Pathol 1986;122:493–9.

150. Rywlin AM, Rosen L, Cabello B. Coexistence of Castleman's disease and Kaposi's sarcoma. Report of a case and speculation. Am J Dermatopathol 1983;5:277–81.

151. Safai B, Johnson KG, Myskowski PL, et al. The natural history of Kaposi's sarcoma in the acquired immunodeficiency syndrome. Ann Intern Med 1985;103:744–50.

152. _____, Mike V, Giraldo G, Beth E, Good RA. Association of Kaposi's sarcoma with second primary malignancies: possible etiopathogenic implications. Cancer 1980;45:1472–9.

153. Said JW. AIDS-related lymphadenopathies. Semin Diagn Pathol 1988;5:365–75.

154. Salahuddin SZ, Nakamura S, Biberfeld P, et al. Angiogenic properties of Kaposi's sarcoma-derived cells after long-term culture in vitro. Science 1988;242:430–3.

155. Scully PA, Steinman HK, Kennedy C, Trueblood K, Frisman DM, Voland JR. AIDS-related Kaposi's sarcoma displays differential expression of endothelial surface antigens. Am J Pathol 1988;130:244–51.

156. Slavin G, Cameron HM, Forbes C, Mitchell RM. Kaposi's sarcoma in East African children: a report of 51 cases. J Pathol 1970;100:187–99.

157. Sperry W, Steigleder G, Bodeau E. Kaposi's sarcoma: venous capillary haemangioblastoma. A histochemical and ultrastructural study. Arch Dermatol Res 1979;266:253–67.

158. Sternberg C. Uber das sarcoma multiplex hemorrhagicum (Kaposi). Arch Dermatol Syph 1912;111:331–40.

159. Symmers D. Kaposi's disease. Arch Pathol 1941;32:764–86.

160. Taylor JF, Templeton AC, Vogel CL, Ziegler JL, Kyalwazi SK. Kaposi's sarcoma in Uganda: a clinicopathological study. Int J Cancer 1971;8:122–35.

161. Tedeschi CG. Some considerations concerning the nature of the so-called sarcoma of Kaposi. Arch Pathol 1958;66:656–84.

162. Templeton AC. Pathology of Kaposi's sarcoma. In: Ziegler JL, Dorfman RF, eds. Kaposi's sarcoma, pathophysiology and clinical management. New York: Marcel Dekker, 1988:23–70.

163. Uccini S, Ruco LP, Monardo F, et al. Coexpression of endothelial cell and macrophage antigens in Kaposi's sarcoma cells. J Pathol 1994;173:23–31.

164. Ulbright TM, Santa Cruz DJ. Kaposi's sarcoma: relationship with hematologic, lymphoid, and thymic neoplasia. Cancer 1981;47:963–73.

165. Vogel J, Hinrichs SH, Reynolds RK, Luciw PA, Jay G. The HIV tat gene induces dermal lesions resembling Kaposi's sarcoma in transgenic mice. Nature 1988;335:606–11.

166. Weiss VC, Serushan M. Kaposi's sarcoma in a patient with dermatomyositis receiving immunosuppressive therapy. Arch Dermatol 1982;118:183–5.

167. Weshler Z, Leviatan A, Krasnokuki D, Kopolovitch J. Primary Kaposi's sarcoma in lymph nodes concurrent with chronic lymphatic leukemia. Am J Clin Pathol 1979;71:234–7.

168. Zhang YM, Bachmann S, Hemmer C, et al. Vascular origin of Kaposi's sarcoma. Expression of leukocyte adhesion molecule-1, thrombomodulin, and tissue factor. Am J Pathol 1994;144:51–9.

169. Ziegler JL, Dorfman RF. Overview of Kaposi's sarcoma: history, epidemiology, and biomedical features. In: Ziegler JL, Dorfman RF, eds. Kaposi's sarcoma, pathophysiology and clinical management. New York: Marcel Dekker, 1988:1–22.

Primary Vascular Tumors of Lymph Node Other than Kaposi's Sarcoma

170. Almagro UA, Choi H, Rouse TM. Hemangioma in a lymph node. Arch Pathol Lab Med 1985;109:576–8.
171. Chan JK, Frizzera G, Fletcher CD, Rosai J. Primary vascular tumors of lymph nodes other than Kaposi's sarcoma. Analysis of 39 cases and delineation of two new entities. Am J Surg Pathol 1992;16:335–50.
172. _____, Hui PK, Ng CS, Yuen NW, Kung IT, Gwi E. Epithelioid hemangioma (angiolymphoid hyperplasia with eosinophilia) and Kimura's disease in Chinese. Histopathology 1989;15:557–74.
173. _____, Warnke RA, Dorfman RF. Vascular transformation of sinuses in lymph nodes, a study of its morphological spectrum and distinction from Kaposi's sarcoma. Am J Surg Pathol 1991;15:732–43.
174. Davies JD. Gut-associated lymph node. In: Whitehead R, ed. Gastrointestinal and esophageal pathology. Edinburgh: Churchill Livingstone, 1989:611–6.
175. _____. Vascular disturbances. In: Stansfeld AG, ed. Lymph node biopsy interpretation. Edinburgh: Churchill Livingstone, 1985:142–58.
176. Ellis GL, Kratochvil FJ. Epithelioid hemangioendothelioma of the head and neck: a clinicopathologic report of 12 cases. Oral Surg Oral Med Oral Pathol 1986;61:61–8.
177. Enzinger FM. Angiomatoid malignant fibrous histiocytoma, a distinctive fibrohistiocytic tumor of children and young adults simulating a vascular neoplasm. Cancer 1979;44:2147–57.
178. Fayemi AO, Toker C. Nodal angiomatosis. Arch Pathol 1975;99:170–2.
179. Goldstein J, Bartal N. Hemangioendothelioma of the lymph node: a case report. J Surg Oncol 1985;28:314–7.
180. Gray MH, Rosenberg AE, Dickersin GR, Bhan AK. Cytokeratin expression in epithelioid vascular neoplasms. Hum Pathol 1990;21:212–7.
181. Gupta IM. Hemangioma in a lymph node. Ind J Pathol Microbiol 1964;71:110–1.
182. Har-El G, Heffner D, Ruffy M. Hemangioma in a cervical lymph node. J Laryngol Otol 1990;104:513–5.
183. Hui PK, Chan JK, Ng CS, Kung IT, Gwi E. Lymphadenopathy of Kimura's disease. Am J Surg Pathol 1989;13:177–86.
184. Kasznica J, Sideli RV, Collins MH. Lymph node hemangioma. Arch Pathol Lab Med 1989;113:804–7.
185. Lott MF, Davies JD. Lymph node hypervascularity: hemangiomatoid lesions and pan-nodal vasodilatation. J Pathol 1983;140:209–19.
186. Rappaport H. Tumors of the hematopoietic system. Atlas of Tumor Pathology. 1st Series, Fascicle 8. Washington D.C.: Armed Forces Institute of Pathology, 1966:357–63.
187. Rosai J, Gold J, Landy R. The histiocytoid hemangiomas. A unifying concept embracing several previously described entities of skin, soft tissue, large vessels, bone, and heart. Hum Pathol 1979;10:707–30.
188. Silva EG, Phillips MJ, Langer B, Ordonez NG. Spindle and histiocytoid (epithelioid) hemangioendothelioma. Primary in lymph node. Am J Clin Pathol 1986;85:731–5.
189. Suster S. Nodal angiolymphoid hyperplasia with eosinophilia. Am J Clin Pathol 1987;88:236–9.
190. Tsang WY. Retiform hemangioendothelioma: a new member of the group of hemangioendotheliomas. Adv Anat Pathol 1995;2:33–8.
191. _____, Chan JK. The family of epithelioid vascular tumors [Invited Review]. Histol Histopathol 1993;8:187–211.
192. _____, Chan JK, Dorfman RF, Rosai J. Vasoproliferative lesions of the lymph node. Pathol Annu 1994;29(Pt 1):63–133.
193. Weiss SW, Ishak KG, Dail DH, Sweet DE, Enzinger FM. Epithelioid hemangioendothelioma and related lesions. Semin Diagn Pathol 1986;3:259–87.

Vascular Neoplasm Arising in Castleman's Disease

194. Chan JK, Tsang WY, Ng CS. Follicular dendritic cell tumor and vascular neoplasm complicating hyaline-vascular Castleman's disease. Am J Surg Pathol 1994;18:517–25.
195. Chen KT. Multicentric Castleman's disease and Kaposi's sarcoma. Am J Surg Pathol 1984;8:287–93.
196. Danon AD, Krishnan J, Frizzera G. Morpho-immunophenotypic diversity of Castleman's disease, hyaline-vascular type: with emphasis on a stroma-rich variant and a new pathogenetic hypothesis. Virchows Arch [A] 1993;423:369–82.
197. Frizzera G, Banks PM, Massarelli G, Rosai J. A systemic lymphoproliferative disorder with morphologic features of Castleman's disease. Pathological findings in 15 patients. Am J Surg Pathol 1983;7:211–31.
198. Gerald W, Kostianovsky W, Rosai J. Development of vascular neoplasia in Castleman's disease. Report of seven cases. Am J Surg Pathol 1990;14:603–14.
199. Nagai K, Sato I, Shimoyama N. Pathohistological and immunohistochemical studies on Castleman's disease of the lymph node. Virchows Arch [A] 1986;409:287–97.
200. Symmers WS. The lymphoreticular system. In: Symmers WS, ed. Systemic pathology, 2nd ed, vol. 2. Edinburgh: Churchill Livingstone, 1978:544–8.
201. Tsang WY, Chan JK, Dorfman RF, Rosai J. Vasoproliferative lesions of lymph node. Pathol Annu 1994;29(Pt 1):63–133.

Vascular Transformation of Lymph Node Sinuses

202. Almagro UA, Choi H, Rouse TM. Hemangioma in a lymph node. Arch Pathol Lab Med 1985;109:576–8.
203. Bedrosian SA, Goldman RL. Nodal angiomatosis: relationship to vascular transformation of lymph nodes [Letter]. Arch Pathol Lab Med 1984;108:864–5.
204. Chan JK, Frizzera G, Fletcher CD, Rosai J. Primary vascular tumors of lymph nodes other than Kaposi's sarcoma. Analysis of 39 cases and delineation of two new entities. Am J Surg Pathol 1992;16:335–50.
205. _____, Warnke RA, Dorfman RF. Vascular transformation of sinuses in lymph nodes. A study of its morphological spectrum and distinction from Kaposi's sarcoma. Am J Surg Pathol 1991;15:732–43.

206. Cook PD, Czerniak B, Chan JK, et al. Nodular spindle cell vascular transformation of lymph nodes: a benign process occurring predominantly in retroperitoneal lymph nodes draining carcinomas that can simulate Kaposi's sarcoma and metastatic tumor [Abstract]. Mod Pathol 1995;8:4A.

207. Dorfman RF. Kaposi's sarcoma. With special reference to its manifestations in infants and children and to the concepts of Arthur Purdy Stout. Am J Surg Pathol 1986;10(suppl 1):68–77.

208. _____, Warnke R. Lymphadenopathy simulating the malignant lymphomas. Hum Pathol 1974;5:519–50.

209. Fayemi AO, Toker C. Nodal angiomatosis. Arch Pathol Lab Med 1975;99:170–2.

210. Haferkamp O, Rosenau W, Lennert K. Vascular transformation of lymph node sinuses due to venous obstruction. Arch Pathol 1971;92:81–3.

211. Lucke VM, Davies JD, Wood CM, Whitbread TJ. Plexiform vascularization of lymph nodes: an unusual but distinctive lymphadenopathy in cats. J Comp Pathol 1987;97:109–19.

212. Michal M, Koza V. Vascular transformation of lymph node sinuses—a diagnostic pitfall. Histopathologic and immunohistochemical study. Pathol Res Pract 1989;185:441–4.

213. Ostrowski ML, Siddiqui T, Barnes RE, Howton MJ. Vascular transformation of lymph node sinuses. A process displaying a spectrum of histologic features. Arch Pathol Lab Med 1990;114:656–60.

214. Scherrer C, Maurer R. La transformation vasculaire sinusienne du ganglion lymphatique, analyse morphologique et immunohistochimique de six cas. Ann Pathol 1985;5:231–8.

215. Steinmann G, Foldi E, Foldi M, Racz P, Lennert K. Morphologic findings in lymph nodes after occlusion of their efferent lymphatic vessels and veins. Lab Invest 1982;47:43–50.

216. Symmers WS. The lymphoreticular system. In: Symmers WS, ed. Systemic pathology, 2nd ed., vol. 2. Edinburgh: Churchill Livingstone, 1978:549.

217. Taylor JF, Templeton AC, Vogel CL, Ziegler JL, Kyalwazi SK. Kaposi's sarcoma in Uganda: a clinicopathological study. Int J Cancer 1971;8:122–35.

218. Tenner-Racz K, Kruse R, Schmidt H, Racz P. Vascular sinus transformation in AIDS: a pathologic condition of lymph nodes resembling Kaposi's sarcoma [Abstract]. Lab Invest 1988;58:92A.

Angiolipomatous Hamartoma in Association with Castleman's Disease

219. Al-Jabi M, Tolnai G, McCaughey WT. Angiofollicular lymphoid hyperplasia in an angiolipomatous mass. Arch Pathol Lab Med 1980;104:313–5.

220. Gerald W, Kostianovsky M, Rosai J. Development of vascular neoplasia in Castleman's disease. Report of seven cases. Am J Surg Pathol 1990;14:603–14.

221. Madero S, Onate JM, Garzon A. Giant lymph node hyperplasia in an angiolipomatous mediastinal mass. Arch Pathol Lab Med 1986;110:853–5.

222. Martin C, Pena ML, Angulo F, Garcia F, Vaca D, Serrano R. Castleman's disease in identical twins. Virchows Arch [A] 1982;395:77–85.

223. Muretto P, Lungarotti F, Lemma E. Giant lymph node hyperplasia in angiohamartomatous soft tissues. Tumori 1981;67:383–90.

Bacillary Angiomatosis

223a. Alkan S, Morgan MB, Sandin R, Ross C, Moscinski LC. Cat scratch disease: a dual etiologic role for Afipia felis and Rochalimaea henselae [Abstract]. Mod Pathol 1995;8:125A.

224. Brenner DJ, Hollis DG, Moss CW, et al. Proposal of Afipia gen. nov., with Afipia felis sp. nov. (formerly the cat scratch disease bacillus), Afipia clevelandensis sp. nov. (formerly the Cleveland Clinic Foundation strain), Afipia broomeae sp. nov., and three unnamed genospecies. J Clin Microbiol 1991;29:2450–60.

225. Chan JK, Lewin KJ, Lombard CM, Teitelbaum S, Dorfman RF. The histopathology of bacillary angiomatosis of lymph nodes. Am J Surg Pathol 1991;15:430–7.

226. Cockerell CJ, LeBoit PE. Bacillary angiomatosis: a newly characterized, pseudoneoplastic, infectious, cutaneous vascular disorder. J Am Acad Dermatol 1990;22:501–12.

227. _____, Whitlow MA, Webster GF, Friedman-Kien AE. Epithelioid angiomatosis: a distinct vascular disorder in patients with the acquired immunodeficiency syndrome or AIDS-related complex. Lancet 1987;2:654–6.

228. Humberson CS. The histopathologic spectrum of cat-scratch bacillus infection in patients with human immunodeficiency virus disease [Abstract]. Mod Pathol 1991;4:87A.

229. Kemper CA, Lombard CM, Deresinski SC, Tompkins LS. Visceral bacillary epithelioid angiomatosis: possible manifestations of disseminated cat scratch disease in the immunocompromised host: a report of two cases. Am J Med 1990;89:216–22.

230. Koehler JE, Quinn FD, Berger TG, LeBoit PE, Tappero JW. Isolation of Rochalimaea species from cutaneous and osseous lesions of bacillary angiomatosis. N Engl J Med 1992;327:1625–31.

231. LeBoit PE. The expanding spectrum of a new disease, bacillary angiomatosis [Editorial]. Arch Dermatol 1990;126:808–11.

232. _____, Berger TG, Egbert BM, Beckstead JH, Yen TS, Stoler MH. Bacillary angiomatosis. The histopathology and differential diagnosis of a pseudoneoplastic infection in patients with human immunodeficiency virus disease. Am J Surg Pathol 1989;13:909–20.

233. _____, Berger TG, Egbert BM, et al. Epithelioid hemangioma-like vascular proliferation in AIDS: manifestations of cat-scratch disease bacillus infection? Lancet 1988;2:960–3.

234. Leong SS, Cazen RA, Yu GS, LeFevre L, Carson JW. Abdominal visceral peliosis associated with bacillary angiomatosis. Ultrastructural evidence of endothelial destruction by bacilli. Arch Pathol Lab Med 1992;116:866–71.

235. Macher AM, Angritt P, Tur SM, Robinson JJ. AIDS case for diagnosis series, 1988. Mil Med 1988;153:M26–M32.

236. Perkocha LA, Ferrell L, Yen TS, et al. Extracutaneous manifestations of bacillary angiomatosis [Abstract]. Mod Pathol 1991;4:88A.
237. Perkocha LA, Geaghan SM, Yen TSB, et al. Clinical and pathological features of bacillary peliosis hepatis in association with human immunodeficiency virus infection. N Engl J Med 1990;323:1581–6.
238. Reed JA, Brigati DJ, Flynn SD, et al. Immunocytochemical identification of Rochalimaea henselae in bacillary (epithelioid) angiomatosis, parenchymal bacillary peliosis, and persistent fever with bacteremia. Am J Surg Pathol 1992;16:650–7.
239. Regnery RL, Anderson BE, Clarridge JE, Rodriguez-Barradas MC, Jones DC, Carr JH. Characterization of a novel Rochalimaea species, R. henselae sp. nov., isolated from blood of a febrile, human immunodeficiency virus-positive patient. J Clin Microbiol 1992;30:265–74.
240. Relman DA, Loutit JS, Schmidt TM, Falkow S, Tompkins LS. The agent of bacillary angiomatosis. An approach to the identification of uncultured pathogens. N Engl J Med 1990;323:1573–80.
241. Tsang WY, Chan JK. Bacillary angiomatosis. A new disease with a broadening clinicopathologic spectrum. Histol Histopathol 1992;7:143–52.
242. _____, Chan JK, Wong CS. Giemsa stain for histological diagnosis of bacillary angiomatosis [Letter]. Histopathology 1992;21:299.
243. Wear DJ, Margileth AM, Hadfield TL, Fischer GW, Schlagel CT, King FM. Cat scratch disease: a bacterial infection. Science 1983;221:1403–5.
244. Welch DF, Pickett DA, Slater LN, Steigerwalt AG, Brenner DJ. Rochalimaea henselae sp. nov., a cause of septicemia, bacillary angiomatosis, and parenchymal bacillary peliosis. J Clin Microbiol 1992;30:275–80.

Glandular Inclusions and Endometriosis in Lymph Node

245. Bernier JL, Bhaskar SN. Lymphoepithelial lesions of salivary glands. Histogenesis and classification based on 186 cases. Cancer 1958;11:1156–79.
246. Blackshaw AJ. Metastatic tumors in lymph nodes. In: Stansfeld AG, ed. Lymph node biopsy Interpretation. Edinburgh: Churchill Livingstone, 1985:380–97.
247. Brown RB, Gaillard RA, Turner JA. The significance of aberrant or heterotopic parotid gland tissue in lymph nodes. Ann Surg 1953;138:850–6.
248. Carr RF, Tang CK, Carrozza MJ, Rodriguez FC. Unusual cystic epithelial choristoma in a celiac lymph node. Hum Pathol 1987;18:866–9.
249. Chen KT. Benign glandular inclusions of the peritoneum and paraaortic lymph nodes. Diagn Gynecol Obstet 1981;3:265–8.
250. Clement PB. Pathology of endometriosis. Pathol Annu 1990;25(Pt 1):245–95.
251. Dietert SE. Papillary cystadenoma lymphomatosum (Warthin's tumor) in patients in a general hospital over a 24-year period. Am J Clin Pathol 1975;63:866–75.
252. Edlow DW, Carter D. Heterotopic epithelium in axillary lymph nodes. Am J Clin Pathol 1973;59:666–73.
253. Ehrmann RL, Federschneider JM, Knapp RC. Distinguishing lymph node metastases from benign glandular inclusions in low-grade ovarian carcinoma. Am J Obstet Gynecol 1980;136:737–46.
254. Fantozzi RD, Bone RC, Fox R. Extraglandular Warthin's tumors. Laryngoscope 1985;95:682–8.
255. Farhi DC, Silverberg SG. Pseudometastases in female genital cancer. Pathol Annu 1982;17(Pt 1):47–76.
256. Ferguson BR, Bennington JL, Haber SL. Histochemistry of mucosubstances and histology of mixed mullerian pelvic lymph node glandular inclusions. Evidence for histogenesis by mullerian metaplasia of coelomic epithelium. Obstet Gynecol 1969;33:617–25.
257. Garret R, Adas AE. Epithelial inclusion cysts in an axillary lymph node. Report of a case simulating metastatic adenocarcinoma. Cancer 1957;10:173–8.
258. Gerard-Marchant R, Caillou B. Thyroid inclusions in cervical lymph nodes. Clin Endocrinol Metab 1981;10:337–49.
259. Gnepp DR, Brannon R. Sebaceous neoplasms of salivary gland origin. Report of 21 cases. Cancer 1984;53:2155–70.
260. Haagensen CD. Diseases of the breast. 3rd ed. Philadelphia: WB Saunders, 1986:555–7.
261. Holdsworth PJ, Hopkinson JM, Leveson SH. Benign axillary epithelial lymph node inclusions—a histological pitfall. Histopathology 1988;13:226–8.
262. Huhn FO. Druseneinschlusse in Becken lymphknoten der Frau. Virchows Arch [A] 1962;335:84–100.
263. Hulbert JC. Ectopic mixed salivary tumor in the neck. J Laryngol Otol 1978;92:533–6.
264. Huntrakoon M. Benign glandular inclusions in the abdominal lymph nodes of a man. Hum Pathol 1985;16:644–6.
265. Javert CT. The spread of benign and malignant endometrium in the lymphatic system with a note on coexisting vascular involvement. Am J Obstet Gynecol 1952;64:780–806.
266. Karp LA, Czernobilsky B. Glandular inclusions in pelvic and abdominal para-aortic lymph nodes. A study of autopsy and surgical material in males and females. Am J Clin Pathol 1969;52:212–8.
267. Kempson RL. Consultation case—benign glandular inclusions in iliac lymph nodes. Am J Surg Pathol 1978;2:321–5.
268. Kheir SM, Mann WJ, Wilkerson JA. Glandular inclusions in lymph nodes. The problem of extensive involvement and relationship to salpingitis. Am J Surg Pathol 1981;5:353–9.
269. Koss LG. Miniature adenoacanthoma arising in an endometriotic cyst in an obturator lymph node. Report of a case. Cancer 1963;16:1369–72.
270. Longo S. Benign lymph node inclusions. Hum Pathol 1976;7:349–54.
271. Ludmer B, Joachims HZ, Ben-Arie J, Eliachar I. Adenocarcinoma in heterotopic salivary tissue. Arch Otolaryngol 1981;107:547–8.
272. Luna M, Monheit J. Salivary gland neoplasms arising in lymph nodes: a clinicopathologic analysis of 13 cases [Abstract]. Lab Invest 1988;58:58A.
273. _____, Tortoledo ME, Allen M. Salivary dermal analogue tumors arising in lymph nodes. Cancer 1987;59:1165–9.
274. McDivitt RW, Stewart FW, Berg JW. Tumors of the breast. Atlas of Tumor Pathology. Series 2, Fascicle 2. Washington D.C.: Armed Forces Institute of Pathology, 1968:116.
275. Meyer JS, Steinberg LS. Microscopically benign thyroid follicles in cervical lymph nodes. Serial section study of lymph node inclusions and entire thyroid gland in 5 cases. Cancer 1969;24:302–11.

276. Mills SE. Decidua and squamous metaplasia in abdominopelvic lymph nodes. Int J Gynecol Pathol 1983;2:209–15.

277. Osmond R, Kalinovsky P. Epithelial inclusion cysts in axillary nodes associated with malignant disease. Med J Aust 1972;2:834–6.

278. Perrone T. Embolization of benign colonic glands to mesenteric lymph nodes [Letter]. Am J Surg Pathol 1985;9:538–41.

279. Perzin KH, LiVolsi VA. Acinic cell carcinoma arising in ectopic salivary gland tissue. Cancer 1980;45:967–72.

280. Rohlfing MB, Kao KJ, Woodard BH. Endomyometriosis: possible association with leiomyomatosis disseminata and endometriosis [Letter]. Arch Pathol Lab Med 1981;105:556–7.

281. Rosai J. Ackerman's surgical pathology. 7th ed. St. Louis: CV Mosby, 1989:435–6.

282. Russell P, Laverty CR. Test and teach. Number twenty. Diagnosis: benign Mullerian rests in pelvic lymph nodes. Pathology 1980;12:31:129–30.

283. Ryan JR, Ioachim HL, Marmer J, Loubeau JM. Acquired immune deficiency syndrome-related lymphadenopathies presenting in the salivary gland lymph nodes. Arch Otolaryngol 1985;111:554–6.

284. Schneider V. Benign glandular lymph node inclusions. Diagn Gynecol Obstet 1980;2:313–20.

285. Schnurr RC, Delgado G, Chun B. Benign glandular inclusions in para-aortic lymph nodes in women undergoing lymphadenectomies. Am J Obstet Gynecol 1978;130:813–6.

286. Shen SC, Bansal M, Purrazzella R, Malviya V, Strauss L. Benign glandular inclusions in lymph nodes, endosalpingiosis, and salpingitis isthmicus nodosa in a young girl with clear cell adenocarcinoma of the cervix. Am J Surg Pathol 1983;7:293–300.

287. Silton RM. More glandular inclusions [Letter]. Am J Surg Pathol 1979;3:285–6.

288. Singer MI, Applebaum EL, Ley KD. Heterotopic salivary tissue in the neck. Laryngoscope 1979;89:1772–8.

289. Smith A, Winkler B, Perzin KH, Wazen J, Blitzer A. Mucoepidermoid carcinoma arising in intraparotid lymph node. Cancer 1985;55:400–3.

290. Tazelaar HD, Vareska G. Benign glandular inclusions [Letter]. Hum Pathol 1986;17:100–1.

291. Thackray AC, Lucas RB. Tumors of the major salivary glands. Atlas of Tumor Pathology. 2nd Series, Fascicle 10. Washington D.C.: Armed Forces Institute of Pathology, 1974:1–2.

292. Turner DR, Millis RR. Breast tissue inclusions in axillary lymph nodes. Histopathology 1980;4:631–6.

293. Walker AN, Fechner RE. Papillary carcinoma arising from ectopic breast tissue in an axillary lymph node. Diagn Gynecol Obstet 1982;4:141–5.

294. Weeks DA, Beckwith JB, Mierau GW. Benign nodal lesions mimicking metastases from pediatric renal neoplasms: a report of the National Wilms' Tumor Study Pathology Center. Hum Pathol 1990;21:1239–44.

295. Weir JH, Janovski NA. Paramesonephric lymph node inclusions—a cause of obstructive uropathy. Obstet Gynecol 1963;21:363–7.

Nevus Cells in Lymph Node

296. Andreola S, Clemente C. Nevus cells in axillary lymph nodes from radical mastectomy specimens. Pathol Res Pract 1985;179:616–8.

297. Azzopardi JG, Ross CM, Frizzera G. Blue nevi of lymph node capsule. Histopathology 1977;1:451–61.

298. Bautista NC, Cohen S, Anders KH. Benign melanocytic nevus cells in axillary lymph nodes. A prospective incidence and immunohistochemical study with literature review. Am J Clin Pathol 1994;102:102–8.

299. Epstein JI, Erlandson RA, Rosen PP. Nodal blue nevi. A study of three cases. Am J Surg Pathol 1984;8:907–15.

300. Goldman RL. Blue nevus of lymph node capsule: report of a unique case. Histopathology 1981;5:445–50.

301. Ioannides G. Lymph nodes with aggregates of nevus cells, a thesis. In: Ackerman AB, ed. Pathology of malignant melanoma. New York: Masson Publishing, 1981:297–300.

302. Jensen JL, Correll RW. Nevus cell aggregates in submandibular lymph nodes. Oral Surg Oral Med Oral Pathol 1980;50:552–6.

303. Johnson WT, Helwig EB. Benign nevus cells in the capsule of lymph nodes. Cancer 1969;23:747–53.

304. Lambert WC, Brodkin RH. Nodal and subcutaneous cellular blue nevi. A pseudometastasizing pseudomelanoma. Arch Dermatol 1984;120:367–70.

305. Lamovec J. Blue nevus of the lymph node capsule. Report of a new case with review of the literature. Am J Clin Pathol 1984;81:367–72.

306. McCarthy SW, Palmer AA, Bale PM, Hirst E. Nevus cells in lymph nodes. Pathology 1974;6:351–8.

307. Nodl F. Spindelzelliger blauer naevus mit lymphknoten—"metastasen." Arch Dermatol Res 1979;264:179–84.

308. Ridolfi RL, Rosen PP, Thaler H. Nevus cell aggregates associated with lymph nodes: estimated frequency and clinical significance. Cancer 1977;39:164–71.

309. Rodriguez HA, Ackerman LV. Cellular blue nevus. Clinicopathologic study of 45 cases. Cancer 1968;21:393–405.

310. Roth JA. Ectopic blue nevi in lymph nodes. In: Ackerman AB, ed. Pathology of malignant melanoma. New York: Masson Publishing, 1981:293–6.

311. _____. Nevus cells in lymph nodes in a patient with malignant melanoma arising in a giant congenital nevus. In: Ackerman AB, ed. Pathology of malignant melanoma. New York: Masson Publishing, 1981:285–92.

312. Shenoy BV, Fort L III, Benjamin SP. Malignant melanoma primary in lymph node. The case of a missing link. Am J Surg Pathol 1987;11:140–6.

313. Smith KJ, Barrett TL, Skelton HG III, Lupton GP, Graham JH. Spindle cell and epithelioid nevi with atypia and metastasis (malignant Spitz nevus). Am J Surg Pathol 1989;13:931–9.

314. Subramony C, Lewin JR. Nevus cells within lymph nodes. Possible metastases from a benign intradermal nevus. Am J Clin Pathol 1985;84:220–3.

315. Yazdi HM. Nevus cell aggregates associated with lymph nodes. Immunohistochemical observations. Arch Pathol Lab Med 1985;109:1044–6.

Rare Lesions of Lymph Node

316. Enzinger FM, Weiss SW. Soft tissue tumors. 2nd ed., St. Louis: CV Mosby, 1988:747–51.
317. _____, Zhang R. Plexiform fibrohistiocytic tumor presenting in children and young adults. An analysis of 65 cases. Am J Surg Pathol 1988;11:818–26.
318. Griffiths AP, Ironside JW, Gray C. True neurilemmoma arising in a lymph node in infancy. Histopathology 1991;18:180–3.
319. Leu HJ. A rare case of angiodysplasia: penetration of inguinal lymph nodes by large superficial leg veins. Report of five cases. Virchows Arch [A] 1990;417:185–6.
320. Stengel B, Dunker H. Extraadrenal intralymphonodular myelolipoma. Pathol Res Pract 1989;184:639–41.
321. Symmers WS. The lymphoreticular system. In: Symmers WS, ed. Systemic pathology, 2nd ed, vol. 2. Edinburgh: Churchill Livingstone, 1978:711.

Metastatic Cancer in Lymph Node

322. Albores-Saavedra J, Nadji M, Civantos F, Morales AR. Thyroglobulin in carcinoma of the thyroid: an immunohistochemical study. Hum Pathol 1983;14:62–6.
323. Arnold A, Cossman J, Bakhshi A, Jaffe ES, Waldmann TA, Korsmeyer SJ. Immunoglobulin-gene rearrangements as unique clonal markers in human lymphoid neoplasms. N Engl J Med 1983;309:1593–9.
324. Aurias A, Rimbaut C, Buffe D, Dubousset J, Mazabraud A. Chromosome translocations in Ewing's sarcoma. N Engl J Med 1983;309:496–7.
325. Azar HA, Jaffe ES, Berard CW, et al. Diffuse large cell lymphomas (reticulum cell sarcomas, histiocytic lymphomas). Correlation of morphologic features with functional markers. Cancer 1980;46:1428–41.
326. Bacchi CE, Dorfman RF, Hoppe RT, Chan JK, Warnke RA. Metastatic carcinoma in lymph nodes simulating syncytial variant of nodular sclerosing Hodgkin's disease. Am J Clin Pathol 1991;96:589–93.
327. Bailey AJ, Sloane JP, Trickey BS, Ormerod MG. An immunocytochemical study of alpha-lactalbumin in human breast tissue. J Pathol 1982;137:13–23.
328. Batsakis JG. The pathology of head and neck tumors: the occult primary and metastases to the head and neck. Head Neck Surg 1981;3:409–23.
329. Battifora H. The biology of the keratins and their diagnostic application. In: DeLellis RA, ed. Advances in immunohistochemistry. New York: Raven Press, 1988:191–221.
330. Bhuta S, Mirra JM, Cochran AJ. Myxoid malignant melanoma. A previously undescribed pattern noted in metastatic lesions and a report of four cases. Am J Surg Pathol 1986;10:203–11.
331. Bonetti F, Colombari R, Manfrin E. Breast carcinoma with positive results for melanoma marker (HMB-45). HMB-45 immunoreactivity in normal and neoplastic breast. Am J Clin Pathol 1989;92:491–5.
332. Bosl GJ, Ilson DH, Rodriguez E, Motzer RJ, Reuter VE, Chaganti RSK. Clinical relevance of the i(12p) marker chromosome in germ cell tumors. JNCI 1994;86:349–55.
333. Brooks JJ, LiVolsi VA, Pietra GG. Mesothelial cell inclusions in mediastinal lymph nodes mimicking metastatic carcinoma. Am J Clin Pathol 1990;93:741–8.
334. Brown DC, Theaker JM, Banks PM, Gatter KC, Mason DY. Cytokeratin expression in smooth muscle and smooth muscle tumours. Histopathology 1987;11:477–86.
335. Bussolati G, Gugliotta P, Morra I, Pietribiasi F, Berardengo E. The immunohistochemical detection of lymph node metastases from infiltrating lobular carcinoma of the breast. Br J Cancer 1986;54:631–6.
336. Butler JJ, Howe CD, Johnson DE. Enlargement of the supraclavicular lymph nodes as the initial sign of prostatic carcinoma. Cancer 1971;27:1055–63.
337. Carcangiu ML, Steeper T, Zampi G, Rosai J. Anaplastic thyroid carcinoma. A study of 70 cases. Am J Clin Pathol 1985;83:135–58.
338. Chan JK. CD30+ (Ki-1) lymphoma: t(2;5) translocation, the implicated genes, and more. Adv Anat Pathol 1995;2:99–104.
339. _____. Molecular analysis of primitive neuroectodermal tumors: a new model for the study of solid tumors showing specific chromosomal translocations. Adv Anat Pathol 1994;1:87–91.
340. _____, Buchanan R, Fletcher CD. Sarcomatoid variant of anaplastic large cell Ki-1 lymphoma. Am J Surg Pathol 1990;14:983–8.
341. _____, Ng CS, Hui PK. A simple guide to the terminology and application of leucocyte monoclonal antibodies. Histopathology 1988;12:461–80.
342. _____, Ng CS, Hui PK, et al. Anaplastic large cell Ki-1 lymphoma. Delineation of two morphological types. Histopathology 1989;15:11–34.
343. _____, Tse CC. Mucin production in metastatic papillary carcinoma of thyroid. Hum Pathol 1988;19:195–200.
344. _____, Yip TT, Tsang WY, Poon YF, Wong CS, Ma VW. Specific association of Epstein-Barr virus with lymphoepithelial carcinoma among tumors and tumor like lesions of the salivary gland. Arch Pathol Lab Med 1994;118:994–7.
345. Chan MK, McGuire LJ, Lee JC. Fine needle aspiration cytodiagnosis of nasopharyngeal carcinoma in cervical lymph nodes, a study of 40 cases. Acta Cytol 1989;33:344–50.
346. Chen KT, Ma CK, Nelson JW, Padmanabhan A, Brittin GM. Clear cell myeloma. Am J Surg Pathol 1985;9:149–54.
347. Cho KR, Epstein JI. Metastatic prostatic carcinoma to supradiaphragmatic lymph nodes. A clinicopathologic and immunohistochemical study. Am J Surg Pathol 1987;11:457–63.
348. Christensen WN, Boitnott JK, Kuhajda FP. Immunoperoxidase staining as a diagnostic aid for hepatocellular carcinoma. Mod Pathol 1989;2:8–12.
349. Clayton F, Ordonez NG, Hanssen GM, Hannsen H. Immunoperoxidase localization of lactalbumin in malignant breast neoplasm. Arch Pathol Lab Med 1982;106:268–70.
350. Cleary ML, Chao J, Warnke R, Sklar J. Immunoglobulin gene rearrangement as diagnostic criterion of B-cell lymphoma. Proc Natl Acad Sci USA 1984;81:593–7.

351. Cochran AJ, Wen DR, Morton DL. Occult tumor cells in the lymph nodes of patients with pathological stage I malignant melanoma. An immunohistological study. Am J Surg Pathol 1988;12:612–8.

352. Compagno J, Hyams VJ, Safavian M. Does branchiogenic carcinoma really exist? Arch Pathol Lab Med 1976;100:311–4.

353. Cosgrove M, Fitzgibbons PL, Sherrod A, Chandrasoma PT, Martin SE. Intermediate filament expression in astrocytic neoplasms. Am J Surg Pathol 1989;13:141–5.

354. Cossman J, Uppenkamp M, Sundeen J, Coupland R, Raffeld M. Molecular genetics and the diagnosis of lymphoma. Arch Pathol Lab Med 1988;112:117–27.

355. Costa J, Rosai J, Rhilpott GW. Pigmentation of "amelanotic" melanoma in culture. A finding of diagnostic relevance. Arch Pathol 1973;95:371–3.

356. Cote RJ, Cordon-Cardo C, Reuter VE, Rosen PP. Immunopathology of adrenal and renal cortical tumors. Coordinated change in antigen expression is associated with neoplastic conversion in the adrenal cortex. Am J Pathol 1990;136:1077–84.

357. Dardick I. Diagnostic electron microscopy. In: Gnepp DR, ed. Pathology of the head and neck. Contemporary issues in surgical pathology, Vol. 10. New York: Churchill Livingstone, 1988:101–90.

358. de Mascarel A, Merlio JP, Coindre JM, Goussot JF, Broustet A. Gastric large cell lymphoma expressing cytokeratin but no leukocyte common antigen: a diagnostic dilemma. Am J Clin Pathol 1989;91:478–81.

359. DeLellis RA, Wolfe HJ. Calcitonin immunohistochemistry. In: DeLellis RA, ed. Diagnostic immunohistochemistry. New York: Masson Publishing, 1981:61–74.

360. Dvorak AM, Monahan RA. Metastatic adenocarcinoma of unknown primary site: diagnostic electron microscopy to determine the site of tumor origin. Arch Pathol Lab Med 1982;106:21–4.

361. Egan MJ, Newman J, Crocker J, Collard M. Immunohistochemical localization of S100 protein in benign and malignant conditions of the breast. Arch Pathol Lab Med 1987;111:28–31.

362. Ellis GK, Gown AM. New applications of monoclonal antibodies to the diagnosis and prognosis of breast cancer. Pathol Annu 1990;25(Pt 2):193–235.

363. Enzinger FM, Weiss SW. Soft tissue tumors. 2nd ed. St. Louis: CV Mosby, 1988:1–965.

364. Eusebi V, Capella C, Cossu A, Rosai J. Neuroendocrine carcinoma within lymph nodes in the absence of a primary tumor, with special reference to Merkel cell carcinoma. Am J Surg Pathol 1992;16:658–66.

365. Eyden BP, Banerjee SS. Multiple myeloma showing signet-ring cell change. Histopathology 1990;7:170–2.

366. Falini B, Pileri S, Stein H, et al. Variable expression of leucocyte-common (CD45) antigen in CD30 (Ki-1)-positive anaplastic large cell lymphoma: implications for the differential diagnosis between lymphoid and non-lymphoid malignancies. Hum Pathol 1990;21:624–9.

367. Feiner HD, Gonzalez R. Carcinoma of the prostate with atypical immunohistological features. Clinical and histologic correlates. Am J Surg Pathol 1986;10:765–70.

368. Fisher ER, Gregorio RM, Redmond C, Kim WS, Fisher B. Pathologic findings from the National Surgical Adjuvant Breast Project (Protocol no. 4). III. The significance of extranodal extension of axillary metastases. Am J Clin Pathol 1976;65:439–44.

369. Fletcher JA, Kozakewich HP, Hoffer FA, et al. Diagnostic relevance of clonal cytogenetic aberrations in malignant soft-tissue tumors. N Engl J Med 1991;324:436–42.

370. Flug F, Pelicci PG, Bonetti F, Knowles DM II, Dalla-Favera R. T-cell receptor gene rearrangements as markers of lineage and clonality in T-cell neoplasms. Proc Natl Acad Sci USA 1985;82:3460–4.

371. Foster EA, Levine AJ. Mucin production in metastatic carcinomas. Cancer 1963;16:506–9.

372. Franke WW, Moll R. Cytoskeletal components of lymphoid organs. I. Synthesis of cytokeratins 8 and 18 and desmin in subpopulations of extrafollicular reticulum cells of human lymph nodes, tonsils and spleen. Differentiation 1987;36:145–63.

373. Fung DT, Chan JK, Tse CC, Sze WM. Myxoid change in malignant lymphoma. Pathogenetic considerations. Arch Pathol Lab Med 1992;116:103–5.

374. Galea MH, Athanassiou E, Bell J, et al. Occult regional lymph node metastases from breast carcinoma: immunohistological detection with antibodies CAM5.2 and NCRC-11. J Pathol 1991;165:221–7.

375. Ganjei P, Nadji M, Albores-Saavedra J, Morales AR. Histologic markers in primary and metastatic tumors of the liver. Cancer 1988;62:1994–8.

376. Gatter KC, Ralfkiaer E, Skinner J, et al. An immunocytochemical study of malignant melanoma and its differential diagnosis from other malignant tumors. J Clin Pathol 1985;38:1353–7.

377. Gerard-Marchant R, Caillou B. Thyroid inclusions in cervical lymph nodes. Clin Endocrinol Metab 1981;10:337–49.

378. Ghadially FN. Diagnostic electron microscopy of tumors. London: Butterworth, 1980:3–242.

379. Giffler RF, Gillespie JJ, Ayala AG, Newland JR. Lymphoepithelioma in cervical lymph nodes of children and young adults. Am J Surg Pathol 1977;1:293–302.

380. Gilbert F, Feder M, Balaban G, et al. Human neuroblastomas and abnormalities of chromosome 1 and 17. Cancer Res 1984;44:5444–9.

381. Giuffre L, Schreyer M, Mach JP, Carrel S. Cyclic AMP induces differentiation in vitro of human melanoma cells. Cancer 1988;61:1132–41.

382. Gould E, Perez J, Albores-Saavedra J, Legaspi A. Signet ring cell sinus histiocytosis. A previously unrecognized histologic condition mimicking metastatic adenocarcinoma in lymph nodes. Am J Clin Pathol 1989;92:509–12.

383. Gould VE, Lee I, Wiedenmann B, Moll R, Chejfec G, Franke WW. Synaptophysin: a novel marker for neurons, certain neuroendocrine cells, and their neoplasms. Hum Pathol 1986;17:979–83.

384. Gown AM, Vogel AM, Hoak D, Gough F, McNutt MA. Monoclonal antibodies specific for melanocytic tumors distinguish subpopulations of melanocytes. Am J Pathol 1986;123:195–203.

385. Gray MH, Rosenberg AE, Dickersin GR, Bhan AK. Cytokeratin expression in epithelioid vascular neoplasms. Hum Pathol 1990;21:212–7.

386. _____, Rosenberg AE, Dickersin GR, Bhan AK. Glial fibrillary acidic protein and keratin expression by benign and malignant nerve sheath tumors. Hum Pathol 1989;20:1089–96.

387. Greco FA, Oldham RK, Fer MF. The extragonadal germ cell cancer syndrome. Semin Oncol 1982;9:448–55.

388. Greenson JK, Isenhart CE, Rice R, Mojzisik C, Houchens D, Martin EW. Identification of occult micrometastases in pericolic lymph nodes of Dukes' B colorectal cancer patients using monoclonal antibodies against cytokeratin and CC49, correlation with long-term survival. Cancer 1994;73:563–9.

389. Gustmann C, Altmannsberger M, Osborn M, Griesser H, Feller AC. Cytokeratin expression and vimentin content in large cell anaplastic lymphomas and other non-Hodgkin's lymphomas. Am J Pathol 1991;138:1413–22.

390. Haupt HM, Rosen PP, Kinne DW. Breast carcinoma presenting with axillary lymph node metastases. An analysis of specific histopathologic features. Am J Surg Pathol 1985;9:165–75.

391. Hsu C, Leung BS, Lau SK, Sham JS, Choy D, Engzell U. Efficacy of fine-needle aspiration and sampling of lymph nodes in 1,484 Chinese patients. Diagn Cytopathol 1990;6:154–9.

392. Iuzzolino P, Bontempini L, Doglioni C, Zanetti G. Keratin immunoreactivity in extrafollicular reticular cells of the lymph node [Letter]. Am J Clin Pathol 1989;91:239–40.

393. Jain S, Allen PW. Desmoplastic malignant melanoma and its variants. A study of 45 cases. Am J Surg Pathol 1989;13:358–73.

394. Jeffers MD, O'Dowd GM, Mulcahy H, Stagg M, O'Donoghue DP, Toner M. The prognostic significance of immunohistochemically detected lymph node micrometastases in colorectal carcinoma. J Pathol 1994;172:183–7.

395. Johnson DE, Herndier BG, Medeiros LJ, Warnke RA, Rouse RV. The diagnostic utility of the keratin profiles of hepatocellular carcinoma and cholangiocarcinoma. Am J Surg Pathol 1988;12:187–97.

396. Jones A, Farrow G, Richardson RL. The extragonadal germ cell cancer syndrome: the Mayo Clinic experience. In: Fer MF, Greco FA, Oldham RK, eds. Poorly differentiated neoplasms and tumors of unknown origin. Orlando: Grune & Stratton, 1986:203–15.

397. Jones H, Anthony PP. Metastatic prostatic carcinoma presenting as left-sided cervical lymphadenopathy: a series of 11 cases. Histopathology 1992;21:149–54.

398. Kahn HJ, Marks A, Thom H, Baumal R. Role of antibody to S100 protein in diagnostic pathology. Am J Clin Pathol 1983;79:341–7.

399. Kamat D, Laszewski MJ, Kemp JD, et al. The diagnostic utility of immunophenotyping and immunogenotyping in the pathologic evaluation of lymphoid proliferations. Mod Pathol 1990;3:105–112.

400. Kawaguchi K, Koike M. Neuron-specific enolase and Leu-7 immunoreactive small round-cell neoplasm. The relationship to Ewing's sarcoma in bone and soft tissue. Am J Clin Pathol 1986;86:79–83.

401. Kim H, Dorfman RF, Rappaport H. Signet ring cell lymphoma. A rare morphologic and functional expression of nodular (follicular) lymphoma. Am J Surg Pathol 1978;2:119–32.

402. Kline TS, Kannan V, Kline IK. Lymphadenopathy and aspiration biopsy cytology. Review of 376 superficial nodes. Cancer 1984;54:1076–81.

403. Koelma IA, Nap M, van Steenis GJ, Fleuren GJ. Tumor markers for ovarian cancer. A comparative immunohistochemical and immunocytochemical study of two commercial monoclonal antibodies (OV632 and OC125). Am J Clin Pathol 1988;90:391–6.

404. Kojima M, Imai Y, Mori N. A concept of follicular lymphoma: a proposal for the existence of neoplasm originating from germinal center. In Berard CW, Bennett JM, Ishikawa E, eds. Malignant diseases of the hematopoietic system. Baltimore: University Park Press, 1973:195–202. (Gann Monogr Cancer Res, vol. 15).

405. Koss LG, Woyke S, Olszewski W. Aspiration biopsy: cytologic interpretation and histologic bases. New York: Igaku-Shoin, 1984:105–53.

406. Krolewski JJ, Dalla-Favera R. Molecular genetic approaches in the diagnosis and classification of lymphoid malignancies. Hematol Pathol 1989;3:45–61.

407. Kurtin PJ, Pinkus GS. Leukocyte common antigen—a diagnostic discriminant between hematopoietic and nonhematopoietic neoplasms in paraffin sections using monoclonal antibodies: correlation with immunologic studies and ultrastructural localization. Hum Pathol 1985;16:353–65.

408. Lamoureux D, Daya D, Simon GT. Cell junctions in lymphomas: study of a primary ovarian T-cell lymphoma and review of 56 other cases of lymphoma. Ultrastruct Pathol 1990;14:247–52.

409. Leder LD. The chloroacetate esterase reaction. A useful means of histological diagnosis of hematological disorders from paraffin sections of skin. Am J Dermatopathol 1979;1:39–42.

410. Lee AC, DeLellis RA, Rosen PP, et al. Alpha-lactalbumin as an immunohistochemical marker for metastatic breast carcinomas. Am J Surg Pathol 1984;8:93–100.

411. Leong AS, Kan AE, Milios J. Small round cell tumors in childhood: immunohistochemical studies in rhabdomyosarcoma, neuroblastoma, Ewing's sarcoma, and lymphoblastic lymphoma. Surg Pathol 1989;2:5–17.

412. ———, Milios J. An assessment of a melanoma-specific antibody (HMB-45) and other immunohistochemical markers of malignant melanoma in paraffin-embedded tissues. Surg Pathol 1989;2:137–45.

413. Levine GD, Dorfman RF. Nodular lymphoma: an ultrastructural study of its relationship to germinal centers and a correlation of light and electron microscopic findings. Cancer 1975;35:148–64.

414. Lloyd RV, Sisson JC, Marangos PJ. Calcitonin, carcinoembryonic antigen and neuron-specific enolase in medullary thyroid carcinoma. Cancer 1983;51:2234–9.

415. MacKay B, Ordonez NG. The role of the pathologist in the evaluation of poorly differentiated tumors and metastatic tumors of unknown origin. In: Fer MF, Greco FA, Oldham RK, eds. Poorly differentiated neoplasms and tumors of unknown origin. Orlando: Grune & Stratton, 1986:3–73.

416. Maletz N, McMorrow LE, Greco A, Wolman SR. Ewing's sarcoma. Pathology, tissue culture, and cytogenetics. Cancer 1986;58:252–7.

417. Mambo NC, Gallager HS. Carcinoma of the breast: the prognostic significance of extranodal extension of axillary disease. Cancer 1977;39:2280–5.

418. Mason DY, Bastard C, Rimokh R, et al. CD30 positive large cell lymphomas ("Ki-1 lymphoma") are associated with a chromosomal translocation involving 5q35. Br J Hematol 1990;74:161–8.

419. Mazoujian G. Gross cystic disease fluid protein-15. In: Wick MR, Siegal GP, eds. Monoclonal antibodies in diagnostic immunohistochemistry. New York: Marcel Dekker, 1988:505–20.

420. _____, Pinkus GS, Davis S, Haagensen DE Jr. Immunohistochemistry of a gross cystic disease fluid protein (GCDFP-15) of the breast. A marker of apocrine epithelium and breast carcinomas with apocrine features. Am J Pathol 1983;110:105–12.

421. _____, Pinkus GS, Haagensen DE Jr. Extramammary Paget's disease—evidence for an apocrine origin. Am J Surg Pathol 1984;8:43–50.

422. McDonnell JM, Beschorner WE, Kuhajda FP, deMent SH. Common leukocyte antigen staining of a primitive sarcoma. Cancer 1987;59:1438–41.

423. Micheau C, Cachin Y, Caillon B. Cystic metastasis in the neck revealing occult carcinoma of the tonsil. A report of six cases. Cancer 1974;33:228–33.

424. Michels S, Swanson PE, Frizzera G, Wick MR. Immunostaining for leukocyte common antigen using an amplified avidin-biotin-peroxidase complex method and paraffin sections. A study of 735 hematopoietic and nonhematopoietic human neoplasms. Arch Pathol Lab Med 1987;111:1035–9.

425. Mierau GW, Berry PJ, Orsini EN. Small round cell neoplasms: can electron microscopy and immunohistochemical studies accurately classify them? Ultrastruct Pathol 1985;9:99–111.

426. Miettinen M, Franssila K. Immunohistochemical spectrum of malignant melanoma. The common presence of keratins. Lab Invest 1989;61:623–8.

427. _____, Soini Y. Malignant fibrous histiocytoma. Heterogeneous patterns of intermediate filament proteins by immunohistochemistry. Arch Pathol Lab Med 1989;113:1363–6.

428. Molinari R, Cantu G, Chiesa F, Podrecca S, Milani F, Del Vecthio M. A statistical approach to detection of the primary cancer based on the site of neck lymph node metastasis. Tumori 1977;63:267–82.

429. Moll R, Lee I, Gould VE, Berndt R, Roessner A, Franke WW. Immunocytochemical analysis of Ewing's tumors. Patterns of expression of intermediate filaments and desmosomal proteins indicate cell-type heterogeneity and pluripotential differentiation. Am J Pathol 1987;127:288–304.

430. Murray MR, Stout AP. Distinctive characteristics of the sympathicoblastoma cultivated in vitro. A method for prompt diagnosis. Am J Pathol 1947;23:429–41.

431. Nadji M, Tabei SZ, Castro A, et al. Prostatic specific-antigen: an immunohistologic marker for prostatic neoplasms. Cancer 1981;48:1229–32.

432. Nakajima T, Watanabe S, Sato Y, Kameya T, Hirota T, Shimosato Y. An immunoperoxidase study of S-100 protein distribution in normal and neoplastic tissues. Am J Surg Pathol 1982;6:715–27.

433. Nakhleh RE, Wick MR, Rocamora A, Swanson PE, Dehner LP. Morphologic diversity in malignant melanomas. Am J Clin Pathol 1990;93:731–40.

434. Ng HK, Lo ST. Cytokeratin immunoreactivity in gliomas. Histopathology 1989;14:359–68.

435. Nojima T, Abe S, Yamaguchi H, Matsuno T, Inoue K. A case of alveolar rhabdomyosarcoma with a chromosomal translocation, t(2;13)(q37;q14). Virchows Arch [A] 1990;417:357–9.

436. Orell SR, Sterrett GF, Walters MN, Whitaker D. Manual and atlas of fine needle aspiration cytology. Edinburgh: Churchill Livingstone. 1986:44–64.

437. Pacchinoni D, Negro F, Valente G, Bussolati G. Epstein-Barr virus detection by in situ hybridization in fine-needle aspiration biopsies. Diagn Mol Pathol 1994;3:100–4.

438. Papotti M, Pacchioni D, Negro F, Bonino F, Bussolati G. Albumin gene expression in liver tumors: diagnostic interest in fine needle aspiration biopsies. Mod Pathol 1994;7:271–5.

439. Perentes E, Rubinstein LJ. Recent applications of immunoperoxidase histochemistry in human neuro-oncology. An update. Arch Pathol Lab Med 1987;111:796–812.

440. Perlman EJ, Dickman PS, Askin FB, Grier HE, Miser JS, Link MP. Ewing's sarcoma—routine diagnostic utilization of MIC2 analysis: a Pediatric Oncology Group/Children's Cancer Group Intergroup study. Hum Pathol 1994;25:304–7.

441. Pitts WC, Weiss LM. Fine needle aspiration biopsy of lymph nodes. Pathol Annu 1988;23(Pt 2):329–60.

442. Raymond WA, Leong AS. Immunoperoxidase staining in the detection of lymph node metastasis in stage I breast cancer. Pathology 1989;21:11–5.

443. Reis MD, Griesser H, Mak TW. T cell receptor and immunoglobulin gene rearrangements in lymphoproliferative disorders. Adv Cancer Res 1989;52:45–80.

444. Ringenberg QS, Yarbro JW. Presentation and clinical syndromes of tumor of unknown origin. In: Fer MF, Greco FA, Oldham RK, eds. Poorly differentiated neoplasms and tumors of unknown origin. Orlando: Grune & Stratton, 1986:101–20.

445. Riopel M, Dickman PS, Link MP, Perlman EJ. MIC2 analysis in pediatric lymphoma and leukemias. Hum Pathol 1994;25:396–9.

446. Ro JY, El-Naggar A, Ayala AG, Mody DR, Ordonez NG. Signet-ring-cell carcinoma of the prostate. Electron-microscopic and immunohistochemical studies of eight cases. Am J Surg Pathol 1988;12:453–60.

447. Robert NJ, Garnick MB, Frei E III. Cancers of unknown origin: current approaches and future perspectives. Semin Oncol 1982;9:526–31.

448. Rodriguez HA, McGavran MH. A modified DOPA reaction for the diagnosis and investigation of pigment cells. Am J Clin Pathol 1969;52:219–27.

449. Rosen PP, Kimmel M. Occult breast carcinoma presenting with axillary lymph node metastases: a follow up study of 48 patients. Hum Pathol 1990;21:518–23.

450. Sandberg AA, Turc-Carel C. The cytogenetics of solid tumors. Relation to diagnosis, classification and pathology. Cancer 1987;59:387–95.

451. Scupham R, Gilbert EF, Wilde J, Wiedrich TA. Immunohistochemical studies of rhabdomyosarcoma. Arch Pathol Lab Med 1986;110:818–21.

452. Sedmak DD, Meineke TA, Knechtges DS, Anderson J. Prognostic significance of cytokeratin-positive breast cancer metastases. Mod Pathol 1989;2:516–20.

453. Sheahan K, O'Brien MJ, Burke B, et al. Differential reactivities of carcinoembryonic antigen (CEA) and CEA-related monoclonal and polyclonal antibodies in common epithelial malignancies. Am J Clin Pathol 1990;94:157–64.

454. Sheibani K, Battifora H. Signet ring-cell melanoma. A rare morphologic variant of malignant melanoma. Am J Surg Pathol 1988;12:28–34.

455. _____, Wu A, Ben-Ezra J, Stroup R, Rappaport H, Winberg C. Rearrangement of kappa-chain and T-cell receptor b-chain genes in malignant lymphomas of T-cell phenotype. Am J Pathol 1987;129:201–7.

456. Shevchuk MM, Romas NA, Ng PY, Tannenbaum M, Olsson CA. Acid phosphatase localization in prostatic carcinoma. A comparison of monoclonal antibody to heteroantisera. Cancer 1983;52:1642–6.

457. Shiro BC, Siegal GP. The use of monoclonal antibodies to S100 protein in diagnostic immunohistochemistry. In: Wick MR, Siegal GP, eds. Monoclonal antibodies in diagnostic immunohistochemistry. New York: Marcel Dekker, 1988:455–503.

458. Sobin LH, Hjermstad BM, Sesterhenn IA, Helwig EB. Prostatic acid phosphatase activity in carcinoid tumors. Cancer 1986;58:136–8.

459. Stein BS, Vangore S, Petersen RO, Kendall AR. Immunoperoxidase localization of prostate-specific antigen. Am J Surg Pathol 1982;6:553–7.

460. Sussman J, Rosai J. Lymph node metastasis as the initial manifestation of malignant mesothelioma. Report of six cases. Am J Surg Pathol 1990;14:819–28.

461. Triche TJ, Askin FB. Neuroblastoma and the differential diagnosis of small-, round-, blue-cell tumors. Hum Pathol 1983;14:569–95.

462. _____, Askin FB, Kissane JM. Neuroblastoma, Ewing's sarcoma, and the differential diagnosis of small-, round-, blue-cell tumors. In: Finegold M, ed. Pathology of neoplasia in children and adolescents. Major problems in pathology, vol. 18. Philadelphia: WB Saunders, 1986:145–95.

463. _____, Ross WE. Glycogen-containing neuroblastoma with clinical and histopathologic features of Ewing's sarcoma. Cancer 1978;41:1425–32.

464. Trojani M, de Mascarel I, Bonichon F, et al. Micrometastases to axillary lymph nodes from carcinomas of the breast: detection by immunohistochemistry and prognostic significance. Br J Cancer 1987;55:303–6.

465. Truong LD, Rangdaeng S, Cagle P, Ro JY, Hawkins H, Font RL. The diagnostic utility of desmin. A study of 584 cases and review of the literature. Am J Clin Pathol 1990;93:305–14.

466. Tsang WY. The MyoD1 gene: the skeletal muscle differentiation regulator gene. Adv Anat Pathol 1994;1:173–5.

467. _____, Chan JK, Tang SK, Tse CC, Cheung MM. Large cell lymphoma with fibrillary matrix. Histopathology 1992;20:80–2.

468. Tse CC, Chan JK, Yuen RW, Ng CS. Malignant lymphoma with myxoid stroma: a new pattern in need of recognition. Histopathology 1991;18:31–5.

469. Tsokos M. The role of immunohistochemistry in the diagnosis of rhabdomyosarcoma [Editorial]. Arch Pathol Lab Med 1986;110:776–8.

470. Tsuneyoshi M, Diamaru Y, Hashimoto H, Enjoji M. Malignant soft tissue neoplasms with histologic features of renal rhabdoid tumors: an ultrastructural and immunohistochemical study. Hum Pathol 1985;16:1235–42.

471. Turc-Carel C, Lizard-Nacol S, Justrabo E, Favrot M, Philip T, Tabone E. Consistent chromosomal transloca-

tion in alveolar rhabdomyosarcoma. Cancer Genet Cytogenet 1986;19:361–2.

471a. Van Eyken P, De Wolf-Peeters C, Van den Oord J, Tricot G, Desmet V. Expression of leukocyte common antigen in lymphoblastic lymphoma and small noncleaved undifferentiated non-Burkitt's lymphoma: an immunohistochemical study. J Pathol 1987;151:257–61.

472. van Krieken JH. Prostate marker immunoreactivity in salivary gland neoplasm. A rare pitfall in immunohistochemistry. Am J Surg Pathol 1994;17:410–4.

473. Variend S. Small cell tumors in childhood, a review. J Pathol 1985;145:1–25.

474. Walker RA. The demonstration of alpha-lactalbumin in human breast carcinomas. J Pathol 1979;129:37–42.

475. Warnke RA, Rouse RV. Limitations encountered in the application of tissue section immunodiagnosis to study of lymphomas and related disorders. Hum Pathol 1985;16:326–31.

476. _____, Gatter KC, Falini D, et al. Diagnosis of human lymphoma with monoclonal antileukocyte antibodies. N Engl J Med 1983;309:1275–81.

477. Wells CA, Heryet A, Brochier J, et al. The immunocytochemical detection of axillary micrometastases in breast cancer. Br J Cancer 1984;50:193–7.

478. Whang-Peng J, Triche TJ, Knutsen T, et al. Cytogenetic characterization of selected small round cell tumors of childhood. Cancer Genet Cytogenet 1986;21:185–208.

479. _____, Triche TJ, Knutsen T, Miser J, Douglass EC, Israel MA. Chromosome translocation in peripheral neuroepithelioma. N Engl J Med 1983;311:584–5.

480. Wick MR, Cherwitz DL, McGlennen RC, Dehner LP. Adrenocortical carcinoma. An immunohistochemical comparison with renal cell carcinoma. Am J Pathol 1986;122:343–52.

481. _____, Lillemoe TJ, Copland GT, Swanson PE, Manivel JC, Kiang DT. Gross cystic disease fluid protein-15 as a marker for breast cancer: immunohistochemical analysis of 690 human neoplasms and comparison with alpha-lactalbumin. Hum Pathol 1989;20:281–7.

482. Woodruff JM, Huvos AG, Erlandson RA, Shah JP, Gerold FP. Neuroendocrine carcinomas of the larynx. A study of two types, one of which mimics thyroid medullary carcinoma. Am J Surg Pathol 1985;9:771–90.

483. Wotherspoon AC, Norton AJ, Isaacson PG. Immunoreactive cytokeratin in plasmacytomas. Histopathology 1989;14:141–5.

484. Yam LT, Winkler CF, Janckila AJ, Li CY, Lam KW. Prostatic cancer presenting as metastatic adenocarcinoma of undetermined origin. Immunodiagnosis by prostatic acid phosphate. Cancer 1983;51:283–7.

485. Zarate-Osorno A, Jaffe ES, Medeiros LJ. Metastatic nasopharyngeal carcinoma initially presenting as cervical lymphadenopathy. A report of two cases that resembled Hodgkin's disease. Arch Pathol Lab Med 1992;116:862–5.

Splenic Hemangioma, Lymphangioma and Hemangioendothelioma

486. Arigad S, Jaffe R, Frand M, Izhak Y, Rotem Y. Lymphangiomatosis with splenic involvement. JAMA 1976;236:2315–7.

487. Bostick WL. Primary splenic neoplasms. Am J Pathol 1945;21:1143–65.

488. Chan KW, Saw D. Distinctive multiple lymphangiomas of spleen. J Pathol 1980;131:75–81.

489. Diebold J, Audouin J. Peliosis of the spleen. Report of a case associated with chronic myelomonocytic leukemia, presenting with spontaneous splenic rupture. Am J Surg Pathol 1983;7:197–204.

490. Falk S, Stutte HJ, Frizzera G. Littoral cell angioma, a novel splenic lesion demonstrating histiocytic differentiation. Am J Surg Pathol 1991;15:1023–33.

491. Feigenberg Z, Wysenbeek A, Aridor E, Dinstsman M. Malignant lymphangioma of the spleen. Isr J Med Sci 1983;19:202–4.
492. Garcia RL, Khan MK, Berlin RB. Peliosis of the spleen with rupture. Hum Pathol 1982;13:177–9.
493. Garvin DF, King FM. Cysts and nonlymphomatous tumors of the spleen. Pathol Annu 1981;16(Pt 1):61–80.
494. Hamoudi AB, Vassy LE, Morse TS. Multiple lymphangioendothelioma of the spleen in a 13-year-old girl. Arch Pathol 1975;99:605–6.
495. Harshman JA, Smith EB, Evans PV. Cystic lymphangiectasis of the spleen. Arch Pathol 1961;71:344–8.
496. Husni EA. The clinical course of splenic hemangioma, with emphasis on spontaneous rupture. Arch Surg 1961;83:681–8.
497. Kaw YT, Duwaji MS, Knisley RE, Esparza AR. Hemangioendothelioma of the spleen. Arch Pathol Lab Med 1992;916:1079–82.
498. Lacson A, Berman LD, Neiman RS. Peliosis of spleen. Am J Clin Pathol 1979;71:586–90.
499. Morgenstern L, Rosenberg J, Geller SA. Tumors of the spleen. World J Surg 1985;9:468–76.
500. O'Brien DM, Ghent WR, Dexter DF. Systemic cystic angiomatosis in a woman with hematuria and splenomegaly. Can J Surg 1987;30:277–9.
501. Pines B, Rabinovitch J. Hemangioma of the spleen. Arch Pathol 1942;33:487–503.
502. Pinkhas J, Djaldetti M, Vries Ade A, Safra D, Dollberg L. Diffuse angiomatosis with hypersplenism. Splenectomy followed by polycythemia. Am J Med 1968;45:795–801.
503. Ruck P, Horny HP, Xiao JC, Bajinski R, Kaiserling E. Diffuse sinusoidal hemangiomatosis of the spleen, a case report with enzyme-histochemical, immunohisto-chemical, and electron-microscopic findings. Pathol Res Pract 1994;190:708–14.
504. Schmid C, Beham A, Uranus S, et al. Non-systemic diffuse lymphangiomatosis of spleen and liver. Histopathology 1991;18:478–80.
505. Sencer S, Coulter-Knoff A, Day D, Foker J, Thompson T, Burke B. Splenic hemangioma with thrombocytopenia in a newborn. Pediatrics 1987;79:960-6.
506. Suster S. Epithelioid and spindle cell hemangioendothelioma of the spleen, report of a distinctive splenic vascular neoplasm of childhood. Am J Surg Pathol 1992;16:785–92.
507. Symmers WS. The lymphoreticular system. In: Symmers WS, ed. Systemic Pathology. 2nd ed. Edinburgh: Churchill Livingstone, 1978:740.
508. Tada T, Wakabayashi T, Kishimoto H. Peliosis of the spleen. Am J Clin Pathol 1983;79:708–13.
509. Taxy JB. Peliosis: a morphologic curiosity becomes an iatrogenic problem. Hum Pathol 1978;9:331–40.

Splenic Hemangiopericytoma

510. Jurado JG, Fuentes FT, Menendez CG, Jimenez AL, de la Riva ML. Hemangiopericytoma of the spleen. Surgery 1989;106:575–7.
511. Neill JS, Park HK. Hemangiopericytoma of the spleen. Am J Clin Pathol 1991;95:680–3.

Splenic Angiosarcoma

512. Autry JR, Weitzner S. Hemangiosarcoma of spleen with spontaneous rupture. Cancer 1975;35:534–9.
513. Bostick WL. Primary splenic neoplasms. Am J Pathol 1945;21:1143–65.
514. Chen KT, Bolles JC, Gilbert EF. Angiosarcoma of the spleen: a report of two cases and review of the literature. Arch Pathol Lab Med 1979;103:122–4.
515. Enzinger FM, Weiss SW. Soft tissue tumors. 3rd ed. St. Louis: CV Mosby, 1995:641–77.
516. Falk S, Krishnan J, Meis JM. Primary angiosarcoma of the spleen. A clinicopathologic study of 40 cases. Am J Surg Pathol 1993;17:959–70.
517. Garvin DF, King FM. Cysts and nonlymphomatous tumors of the spleen. Pathol Annu 1981;16(Pt 1):61–80.
518. Nanba K, Soban EJ, Bowling MC, Berard CW. Splenic pseudosinuses and hepatic angiomatous lesions. Distinctive features of hairy cell leukemia. Am J Clin Pathol 1977;67:415–26.
519. Silverman ML, Federman M, O'Hara CJ. Malignant hemangioendothelioma of the spleen. A case report with ultrasound observations. Arch Pathol Lab Med 1981;105:300–4.
520. Smith VC, Eisenberg BL, McDonald EC. Primary splenic angiosarcoma. Case report and literature review. Cancer 1985;55:1625–7.
521. Takato H, Iwamoto H, Ikezu M, Kato N, Ikarashi T, Kaneko H. Splenic hemangiosarcoma with sinus endothelial differentiation. Acta Pathol Jpn 1993;43:702–8.
522. Wick MR, Scheithauer BW, Smith SL, Beart RW Jr. Primary nonlymphoreticular malignant neoplasms of the spleen. Am J Surg Pathol 1982;6:229–42.
523. Wilkinson HA III, Lucas JC, Foote FW Jr. Primary splenic angiosarcoma. A case report. Arch Pathol 1968;85:213–8.
524. Wolf BC, Neiman RS, Bennington TL. Disorders of the Spleen. In: ed. Major problems in pathology, Vol. 20. Philadelphia: WB Saunders, 1989:196–9.
525. Zwi LJ, Evans DJ, Wechsler AL, Catovsky D. Splenic angiosarcoma following chemotherapy for follicular lymphoma. Hum Pathol 1986;17:528–30.

Nonvascular Sarcomas of the Spleen

526. Dehner LP. Malignant fibrous histiocytoma. Nonspecific morphologic pattern, specific pathologic entity, or both? [Editorial] Arch Pathol Lab Med 1988;112:236–7.
527. Garvin DF, King FM. Cysts and nonlymphomatous tumors of the spleen. Pathol Annu 1981;16(Pt 1):61–80.
528. Govoni E, Bazzochi F, Pileri S, Martinelli G. Primary malignant fibrous histiocytoma of the spleen: an ultrastructural study. Histopathology 1980;6:351–61.
529. Jepson W, Albert F. Primary sarcoma of the spleen and its treatment by splenectomy. Ann Surg 1904;40:80–97.
530. Matejicek F. Primary sarcoma of the spleen in a three year old child. Ann Pediatr (Basel) 1960;195:167–73.
531. Morgenstern L, Rosenberg J, Geller SA. Tumors of the spleen. World J Surg 1985;9:468–76.
532. Rappaport H. Tumors of the hematopoietic system. Altas of Tumor Pathology, 1st Series, Section 3, Fascicle 8. Washington DC: Armed Forces Institute of Pathology, 1966:386–8.

533. Roholl PJ, Kleijne J, van Basten CD, van der Putte SC, van Unnik JA. A study to analyze the origin of tumor cells in malignant fibrous histiocytomas. A multiparametric characterization. Cancer 1985;56:2809–15.

534. Rousselot LM, Stein C. Malignant neoplasms of the spleen, primary and secondary. Surg Clin N Am 1953;133:493–9.

535. Sieber SC, Lopez V, Rosai J, Buckley PJ. Primary tumor of spleen with morphologic features of malignant fibrous histiocytoma. Immunohistochemical evi-

536. dence for a macrophage origin. Am J Surg Pathol 1990;14:1061–70.

536. Wick MR, Scheithauer BW, Smith SL, Beart RW Jr. Primary nonlymphoreticular malignant neoplasms of the spleen. Am J Surg Pathol 1982;6:229–42.

537. Wood GS, Beckstead JH, Turner RR, Hendrickson MR, Kempson RL, Warnke RA. Malignant fibrous histiocytoma tumor cells resemble fibroblasts. Am J Surg Pathol 1986;10:323–35.

Inflammatory Pseudotumor of Spleen

538. Alpern HD, Olson JE, Kozak AJ. Inflammatory pseudotumor of the spleen. J Surg Oncol 1986;33:46–9.

539. Cotelingam JD, Jaffe ES. Inflammatory pseudotumor of the spleen. Am J Surg Pathol 1984;8:375–80.

540. Dalal BI, Greenberg H, Quinonez GE, Gough JC. Inflammatory pseudotumor of the spleen. Morphological, radiological, immunophenotypic, and ultrastructural features. Arch Pathol Lab Med 1991;115:1062–4.

541. Fu KH, Liu HW, Leung CY. Inflammatory pseudotumors of the spleen. Histopathology 1990;16:302–4.

542. McMahon RF. Inflammatory pseudotumor of spleen. J Clin Pathol 1988;41:734–6.

543. Monforte-Munoz H, Ro JY, Manning JT, et al. Inflammatory pseudotumor of the spleen. Report of two cases with a review of the literature. Am J Clin Pathol 1991;96:491–5.

544. Sheahan K, Wolf BC, Neiman RS. Inflammatory pseudotumor of the spleen: a clinicopathologic study of three cases. Hum Pathol 1988;19:1024–9.

545. Thomas RM, Jaffe ES, Zarate-Osorno A, Medeiros LJ. Inflammatory pseudotumor of the spleen, a clinicopathologic and immunophenotypic study of 8 cases. Arch Pathol Lab Med 1993;117:921–6.

546. Wiernik PH, Rader M, Becker NH, Morris SF. Inflammatory pseudotumor of the spleen. Cancer 1990;66:597–600.

Splenic Hamartoma

547. Beham A, Hermann W, Vennigerholz F, Schmid C. Hamartoma of the spleen with haematological symptoms. Virchows Arch [A] 1989;414:535–9.

548. Berge TH. Splenoma. Acta Pathol Microbiol Scand 1965;63:333–9.

549. Coe JI, von Drashek SC. Hamartoma of the spleen. A report of four cases. Am J Pathol 1952;28:663–71.

550. Darden JW, Teeslink R, Parrish A. Hamartoma of the spleen: a manifestation of tuberous sclerosis. Am Surg 1975;41:564–6.

551. Falk S, Stutte HJ. Hamartomas of the spleen: a study of 20 biopsy cases. Histopathology 1989;14:603–12.

552. Garvin DF, King FM. Cysts and nonlymphomatous tumors of the spleen. Pathol Annu 1981;16(Pt 1):61–80.

553. Iozzo RV, Haas JE, Chard RL. Symptomatic splenic hamartoma: a report of two cases and review of the literature. Pediatrics 1980;66:261–5.

554. Kirkland WG, McDonald JR. Hamartoma of the spleen. Report of three surgical cases. Arch Pathol 1948;45:371–9.

555. Krishnan J, Danon AD, Frizzera G. Use of anti-factor VIII-related antigen (F8) and QBEND10 (CD34) antibodies helps classify the benign vascular lesions of the spleen [Abstract]. Mod Pathol 1993;6:94A.

556. Morgenstern L, McCafferty L, Rosenberg J, Michel SL. Hamartomas of the spleen. Arch Surg 1984;119:1291–3.

557. _____, Rosenberg J, Geller SA. Tumors of the spleen. World J Surg 1985;9:468–76.

558. Pardo-Mindan FJ, Vazquez JJ, Joly M, Rocha E. Splenic hamartoma, vascular type, with endothelial proliferation. Pathol Res Pract 1983;177:32–40.

559. Rappaport H. Tumors of hematopoietic system. Atlas of Tumor Pathology, 1st Series, Fascicle 8. Washington DC: Armed Forces Institute of Pathology. 1966:380–388.

560. Ross CF, Schiller KF. Hamartoma of spleen associated with thrombocytopenia. J Pathol 1972;105:62–4.

561. Schrijver H, Verdonk GJ. Hamartoma of the spleen with inhibition of bone marrow. Acta Med Scand 1957;158:235–7.

562. Shalev O, Ariel I. Hamartoma of the spleen. A case report. Isr J Med Sci 1978;14:862–4.

563. Silverman ML, LiVolsi VA. Splenic hamartoma. Am J Clin Pathol 1978;70:224–9.

564. Teates CD, Seale DL, Allens MS. Hamartoma of the spleen. Am J Roentgenol Radium Ther Nucl Med 1972;116:419–22.

565. van Heerden JA, Longo MF, Cardoza F, Farrow GM. The abdominal mass in patient with tuberous sclerosis. Surgical implications and report of a case. Arch Surg 1967;95:317–20.

566. Videbaek A. Hypersplenism associated with hamartomas of the spleen. Acta Med Scand 1953;141:275–88.

567. Wallach JB, Nakao N. Hamartoma of the spleen. J Med Soc NJ 1962;59:75–9.

568. Zukerberg LR, Kaynor BL, Silverman ML, Harris NL. Splenic hamartoma and capillary hemangioma are distinct entities: immunohistochemical analysis of CD8 expression by endothelial cells. Hum Pathol 1991;22:1258–61.

Splenic Cysts

569. Blank E, Campbell JR. Epidermoid cysts of the spleen. Pediatrics 1973;51:75–84.

570. Bostick WL, Lucia SP. Nonparasitic, noncancerous cystic tumors of the spleen. Arch Pathol 1949;47:215–22.

571. Burrig KF. Epithelial (true) splenic cysts. Pathogenesis of the mesothelial and so-called epidermoid cyst of the spleen. Am J Surg Pathol 1988;12:275–81.

572. Cave RH, Garvin DF, Doohen DJ. Metaplastic mesodermal cyst of the spleen. Am Surg 1971;37:97–102.

573. Elit L, Aylward B. Splenic cyst carcinoma presenting in pregnancy. Am J Hematol 1989;32:57–60.

574. Fonkalsrud EW, Walford RL. Transitional cell splenic cyst excised without splenectomy. Report of a case. Arch Surg 1960;81:636–40.

575. Fowler RH. Nonparasitic benign cystic tumors of the spleen. Int Abst Surg 1953;96:209–27.

576. Garvin DF, King FM. Cysts and nonlymphomatous tumors of the spleen. Pathol Annu 1981;16(Pt 1):61–80.

577. Lifschitz-Mercer B, Open M, Kushnir I, Czernobilsky B. Epidermoid cyst of the spleen: a cytokeratin profile with comparison to other squamous epithelia. Virchows Arch 1994;424:213–6.

578. Lippitt WH, Akhavan T, Caplan GE. Epidermoid cyst of the spleen with rupture and inflammation. Arch Surg 1967;95:74–8.

579. Miracco C, De Martino A, Lio R, Botta G, Volterrani L, Luzi P. Splenic cyst lined with mucus-secreting epithelium. Evidence of an intestinal origin. Arch Anat Cytol Pathol 1986;34:304–6.

580. Morgenstern L, Rosenberg J, Geller SA. Tumors of the spleen. World J Surg 1985;9:468–76.

581. Morinaga S, Ohyama R, Koizumi J. Low-grade mucinous cystadenocarcinoma in the spleen. Am J Surg Pathol 1992;16:903–8.

582. Ough YD, Nash HR, Wood DA. Mesothelial cysts of the spleen with squamous metaplasia. Am J Clin Pathol 1981;76:666–9.

583. Rappaport H. Tumors of the hematopoietic system. Atlas of Tumor Pathology. 1st Series, Fascicle 8. Washington DC: Armed Forces Institute of Pathology, 1966:388–97.

584. Robbins FG, Yellin AE, Lingua RW, Craig JR, Turrill FL, Mikkelsen WP. Splenic epidermoid cysts. Ann Surg 1978;187:231–5.

585. Shousha S. Splenic cysts: a report of six cases and a brief review. Postgrad Med J 1978;54:265–9.

586. Sparks AK, Connor DH, Naefie RC. Echinococcosis. In: Binford CH, Connor DH, eds. Pathology of tropical and extraordinary diseases. Washington DC: Armed Forces Institute of Pathology. 1976:530–3.

587. Symmers WS. The lymphoreticular system. In: Symmers WS, ed. Systemic pathology, 2nd ed. Edinburgh: Churchill Livingstone, 1978;738–9.

588. Talerman A, Hart S. Epithelial cysts of the spleen. Br J Surg 1970;57:201–4.

589. Tang X, Tanaka Y, Tsutsumi Y. Epithelial inclusion cysts in an intrapancreatic accessory spleen. Pathol Int 1994;44:652–4.

590. Tsakraklides V, Hadley TW. Epidermoid cysts of the spleen. A report of five cases. Arch Pathol 1973;96:251–4.

Rare Lesions of Spleen

591. Bostick WL. Primary splenic neoplasms. Am J Pathol 1945;21:1143–65.

592. Daftary M, Barnett RN. Malignant teratoma of the spleen. Yale J Biol Med 1971;43:283–7.

593. Easler RE, Dowlin WM. Primary lipoma of the spleen. Report of a case. Arch Pathol 1969;88:557–9.

594. Katz JA, Mahoney DH, Shukla LW, Smith CW, Gresik MV, Hawkins HK. Endovascular papillary angioendothelioma in the spleen. Pediatr Pathol 1988;8:185–93.

595. Rappaport H. Tumors of the hematopoietic system. Atlas of Tumor Pathology. 1st Series, Fascicle 8. Washington D.C., Armed Forces Institute of Pathology, 1966:388.

596. Westra WH, Anderson BO, Klimstra DS. Carcinosarcoma of the spleen, an extragenital malignant mixed Mullerian tumor? Am J Surg Pathol 1994;18:309–15.

Metastatic Tumor in Spleen

597. Abrams HL, Spiro R, Goldstein N. Metastases in carcinoma. Analysis of 1000 autopsied cases. Cancer 1950;3:74–85.

598. Berge T. Splenic metastases. Frequencies and patterns. Acta Pathol Microbiol Scand [A] 1974;82:499–506.

599. Butler JJ. Pathology of the spleen in benign and malignant conditions. Histopathology 1983;7:453–74.

600. Cummings OW, Mazur MT. Breast carcinoma diffusely metastatic to the spleen. A report of two cases presenting as idiopathic thrombocytopenic purpura. Am J Clin Pathol 1992;97:484–9.

601. Dunn RI. Cancer metastases in the spleen. Glasgow Med J 1955;36:43–9.

602. Edelman AS, Rotterdam H. Solitary splenic metastasis of an adenocarcinoma of the lung. Am J Clin Pathol 1990;94:326–8.

603. Fakan F, Michal M. Nodular transformation of splenic red pulp due to carcinomatous infiltration. A diagnostic pitfall. Histopathology 1994;25:175–8.

604. Falk S, Stutte HJ. Splenic metastasis in an ileal carcinoid tumor. Pathol Res Pract 1989;185:238–42.

605. Gilks GB, Acker BD, Clement PB. Recurrent endometrial adenocarcinoma: presentation as a splenic mass mimicking malignant lymphoma. Gynecol Oncol 1989;33:209–11.

606. Goldberg GM. Metastatic carcinoma of the spleen resulting from lymphogenic spread: report of two cases. Lab Invest 1957;6:383–8.

607. Harman JW, Dacorso P. Spread of carcinoma to the spleen. Its relation to generalized carcinomatous spread. Arch Pathol 1948;45:179–86.

608. Henriksen E. The lymphatic spread of carcinoma of the cervix and of the body of the uterus. A study of 420 necropsies. Am J Obstet Gynecol 1949;58:924–42.

609. Hirst AE Jr, Bullock WK. Metastatic carcinoma of the spleen. Am J Med Sci 1952;223:414–7.

610. Jorgensen LN, Chrintz H. Solitary metastatic endometrial carcinoma of the spleen. Acta Obstet Gynecol Scand 1988;67:91–2.

611. Klein B, Stein M, Kuten A, et al. Splenomegaly and solitary spleen metastasis in solid tumors. Cancer 1987;60:100–2.

612. Marymount JH Jr, Gross S. Patterns of metastatic cancer in the spleen. Am J Clin Pathol 1963;40:58–60.

613. Nathanson L. Hall TC, Farber S. Biological aspects of human malignant melanoma. Cancer 1967;20:650–5.

614. Nosanchuk JS, Tyler WS, Terepka RH. Fine-needle aspiration of spleen: diagnosis of a solitary ovarian metastasis. Diagn Cytopathol 1988;4:159–61.

615. Rappaport H. Tumors of the hematopoietic system. Atlas of Tumor Pathology. 1st Series, Fascicle 8. Washington D.C.: Armed Forces Institute of Pathology. 1966:397–425.

616. Wolf BC, Neiman RS. Disorders of the spleen. In: Bennington TL ed. Major problems in pathology. Vol. 20. Philadelphia: WB Saunders, 1989;199–202.

22

IMMUNODEFICIENCY-ASSOCIATED
LYMPHOPROLIFERATIVE DISORDERS

Lymphoproliferative disorders develop with increased incidence in patients with immunodeficiencies of both acquired and congenital origin. Acquired immunodeficiency syndrome (AIDS) and immunosuppressive therapies for prevention of allograft rejection are common causes of acquired immunodeficiency. This chapter briefly reviews some of the distinctive pathologic features of lymphoproliferative disorders arising in the setting of various immunodeficiency states.

LYMPHOPROLIFERATIONS
ASSOCIATED WITH CONGENITAL
IMMUNODEFICIENCIES

Many congenital immunodeficiencies are associated with an increased risk of neoplasms; over half of associated neoplasms are malignant lymphomas (20,63). The primary immunodeficiencies most often associated with lymphoid neoplasia include X-linked lymphoproliferative syndrome, ataxia-telangiectasia, common variable immunodeficiency, Wiskott-Aldrich syndrome, and severe combined immunodeficiency syndrome (20). The incidence and type of lymphoproliferative disorder varies with the immunodeficiency condition; lymphomas, however, tend to involve extranodal sites and are usually diffuse intermediate to high-grade neoplasms, most often of plasmacytoid immunoblastic type (23). Hodgkin's disease occurring in patients with primary immunodeficiencies tends to be of mixed cellularity or lymphocyte depletion subtype (53).

In X-linked lymphoproliferative syndrome, a disease marked by profound susceptibility to diseases induced by the Epstein-Barr virus (EBV), approximately 65 percent of patients develop severe or fatal EBV-associated infectious mononucleosis, 30 percent have acquired hypoglobulinemia or agammaglobulinemia, and 25 percent develop malignant lymphoma (27). In this syndrome, lymph nodes and spleen involved by infectious mononucleosis show a marked immunoblastic proliferation associated with necrosis early in the clinical course, a marked plas-

macytoid proliferation in intermediate stages, and ultimately, lymphocyte depletion in patients who survive more than 4 weeks. In the thymus, lymphoid hyperplasia occurs early and lymphocyte depletion later; the liver shows periportal lymphoid infiltration associated with hepatitis. A hemophagocytic syndrome is seen in approximately 65 percent of the patients who die of infectious mononucleosis. The malignant lymphomas are all diffuse B-cell neoplasms, often limited to stage I and II, and have a predilection for the ileocecal region. In one series of 17 cases, 41 percent were small noncleaved cell lymphomas, 18 percent were immunoblastic lymphomas, 12 percent were small cleaved cell or mixed lymphomas, and 6 percent were unclassifiable (30a). The survival rate is approximately 50 percent, with infection being the major cause of death.

Ataxia-telangiectasia syndrome is an autosomal recessive syndrome associated with chromosomal breakdown that is characterized by both B- and T-cell immunodeficiencies. Patients often have poor thymic maturation, along with diminution of the paracortical regions of lymph nodes, due to a decrease in T cells. The risk of lymphoma has been estimated at 10 percent, accounting for approximately 50 percent of the neoplasms that develop in these patients (43). These lymphomas often occur in childhood and are heterogeneous; they include both B- and T-cell lymphomas (20), as well as Hodgkin's disease. Hodgkin's disease accounts for approximately 10 percent of the neoplasms occurring in this syndrome, and is often of the lymphocyte depletion subtype (23).

Common variable immunodeficiency syndrome (late-onset hypogammaglobulinemia) encompasses a clinically heterogeneous group of disorders characterized by markedly reduced serum levels of immunoglobulin, particularly immunoglobulin G, due to a block in the differentiation of B lymphocytes into plasma cells (31). Patients are at increased risk for non-Hodgkin's lymphomas: these occur in 1 to 7 percent of patients (16). Several histologic appearances are seen in the lymph nodes, including chronic granulomatous inflammation, reactive follicular hyperplasia, atypical lymphoid hyperplasia, and malignant lymphoma (55). The atypical hyperplasia may appear to show architectural effacement, thus mimicking lymphoma, but immunohistochemistry reveals preserved immunoarchitecture with florid expansion of the B- and T-cell compartments. The malignant lymphomas are usually diffuse intermediate to high-grade non-Hodgkin's lymphomas.

Wiskott-Aldrich syndrome is an X-linked disorder characterized by immune deficits of both B and T lymphocytes as well as macrophages. The lymph nodes and spleen often show a diminution of the T-cell areas, prominence of the stroma, presence of atypical plasma cells with and without plasmacytosis, and extramedullary hematopoiesis (62). Approximately 10 to 20 percent of patients develop lymphomas, mostly of non-Hodgkin's type (15,20). The lymphomas usually present in childhood, and are diffuse intermediate to high grade; most are large cell immunoblastic lymphomas. There is a predilection for involvement of extranodal sites, particularly the central nervous system.

Severe combined immunodeficiency may be autosomal recessive (lacking adenosine deaminase) or X-linked, and is characterized by profound defects in both T- and B-cell function. Lymph nodes, spleen, and other lymphoid tissues show a virtual absence of lymphocytes. The incidence of neoplasia is about 1 to 5 percent, of which 75 percent are non-Hodgkin's lymphomas and approximately 10 percent are Hodgkin's disease (20). The median age at diagnosis of non-Hodgkin's lymphomas is 1.6 years, with a male to female ratio of 3 to 1. Multiple sites are involved in approximately 50 percent of cases, and are usually extranodal.

LYMPHOPROLIFERATIONS ASSOCIATED WITH SECONDARY IMMUNODEFICIENCIES

Acquired Immunodeficiency Syndrome

A wide variety of lymphoid neoplasias occur in AIDS patients, including non-Hodgkin's lymphoma and Hodgkin's disease. Patients infected with human immunodeficiency virus (HIV) often have lymphadenopathy that is sometimes biopsied to rule out infection or neoplasm. Although no single histologic finding is pathognomonic of HIV

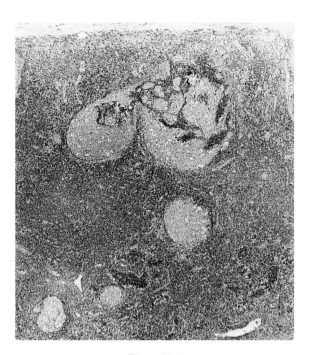

Figure 22-1
FOLLICULAR HYPERPLASIA WITH
FOLLICLE LYSIS IN HIV INFECTION
Note the multiple collections of small lymphocytes within the large, irregular germinal center at top ("follicle lysis"). Other areas of this lymph node showed more pronounced ("explosive") follicular hyperplasia.

infection, characteristic histologic findings have been identified and classified (10,18). Chadburn and colleagues (10) proposed classifying HIV-related benign lymphadenopathy into four categories: explosive follicular hyperplasia, mixed follicular hyperplasia/follicular involution, follicular involution, and lymphocyte depletion. Explosive follicular hyperplasia consists of markedly hyperplastic follicles, often with highly irregular shapes. The surrounding mantle zones are often effaced and the distinction between the germinal centers and the interfollicular areas is not clear. Follicle lysis (follicular fragmentation), in which the germinal centers are overrun by small lymphocytes along with hemorrhage, is present in approximately half of biopsies (fig. 22-1). Warthin-Finkeldy–type multinucleated cells are often present in the interfollicular areas, and collections of monocytoid B cells are often found in the sinuses. In follicular involution, the germinal centers show regressive changes and are small, hypocellular, and often hyalinized (fig. 22-2). The

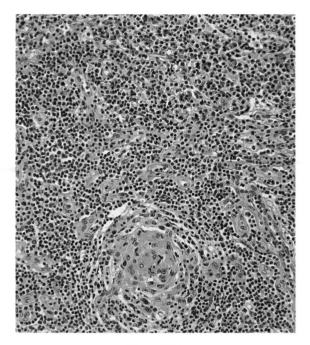

Figure 22-2
HIV-ASSOCIATED LYMPHADENOPATHY
Follicular involution is present.

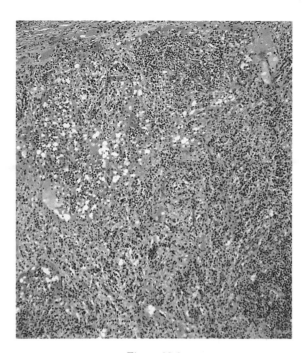

Figure 22-3
HIV-ASSOCIATED LYMPHADENOPATHY
Marked lymphocyte depletion is seen. Follicles are not seen, and sinuses appear patent.

interfollicular areas often show a mixture of small lymphocytes, histiocytes, and plasma cells. In mixed follicular hyperplasia/follicular involution, discrete areas of both explosive follicular hyperplasia and follicular involution are seen. In lymphocyte depletion, there is a loss of germinal centers and a paucity of small lymphocytes; the medullary cords and sinuses comprise a relatively large area of the lymph node (fig. 22-3). Sequential biopsies from HIV-infected patients show progression from florid follicular hyperplasia through lymphocyte depletion (10,67). Although these histologic changes do not predict progression to non-Hodgkin's lymphoma, there is a correlation between increasing lymphocyte depletion and progression to AIDS.

Non-Hodgkin's Lymphoma

Non-Hodgkin's lymphoma is by far the most frequent AIDS-associated lymphoid neoplasm (38). AIDS-associated non-Hodgkin's lymphomas represent a major complication of AIDS, and are now included within its definition (9). Approximately 3 percent of AIDS patients develop non-Hodgkin's lymphoma; the risk of developing malignant lymphoma in these patients is estimated

to be 60-fold greater than the normal population (4). The lymphomas occur in all epidemiologic groups at risk for AIDS, including homosexual or bisexual men, intravenous drug users, hemophiliacs, and transfusion recipients, but the incidence appears to be highest in hemophiliacs and lowest in those born in the Caribbean or Africa who acquired HIV by heterosexual contact. Non-Hodgkin's lymphoma is a late manifestation of HIV infection, and the risk of developing the neoplasm increases with longer survival, decreasing CD4 counts, lower mean neutrophil counts, and a prior diagnosis of Kaposi's sarcoma, cytomegaloviral disease, or oral hairy leukoplakia (4,42). In one study of over 1,000 symptomatic patients receiving antiviral therapy, there was a 3.2 percent probability of developing lymphoma at 2 years, with an additional 0.8 percent risk for each subsequent 6-month period (42). Due to the increasing number of HIV-infected patients and their longer survival, the incidence of HIV-related lymphoma is high: between 8 and 27 percent of the non-Hodgkin's lymphomas diagnosed in the United States in 1992 were HIV related (24).

Two thirds to 98 percent of patients with AIDS-associated non-Hodgkin's lymphoma present with multiple sites of extranodal involvement (34,36,70): the central nervous system, gastrointestinal tract (including anus and rectum), bone marrow, and liver are the most common, but any site, including heart, may be affected. Because of the widespread organ involvement at the time of presentation, patients are almost always clinical stage III or IV. Stage I disease is usually extranodal (stage IE), and usually involves the central nervous system or, less commonly, the gastrointestinal tract or skin (36). A higher percentage of patients present with B symptoms than do those with non-HIV–infected lymphomas (39).

Most AIDS-associated non-Hodgkin's lymphomas are either high-grade, small noncleaved cell type (particularly the non-Burkitt's subtype); plasmacytoid immunoblastic subtype; or intermediate grade, large cell type (fig. 22-3) (34,36,70). These lymphomas are almost all B lineage, expressing pan-B-cell markers such as CD19, CD20, or CD22 (36). The small noncleaved cell lymphomas almost invariably express monotypic surface immunoglobulin; only half of the large cell lymphomas express immunoglobulin.

Rare cases of low-grade lymphoma (70), solitary plasmacytoma, or multiple myeloma (8) have also been reported, but there are no data yet to suggest that these neoplasms are preferentially more common in this patient population. Several types of T-cell lymphoma have been reported, including "cutaneous T-cell lymphoma," lymphoblastic lymphoma, and post-thymic T-cell lymphoma, including the HTLV-1–associated and anaplastic large cell variants (11,25,26,34,59). However, it does not appear that T-cell lymphomas occur with increased frequency in this setting.

There are limited data to suggest that small noncleaved cell lymphoma is seen at a younger age and occurs with higher mean CD4 counts than immunoblastic lymphoma (4,54). The histologic subtype may correlate with the site affected. One study found that large cell lymphomas, including immunoblastic type, are more likely to affect extranodal sites such as gastrointestinal tract, brain, and oral cavity (fig. 22-4), while small noncleaved cell lymphomas have a predilection for lymph node, bone marrow, and muscle (51).

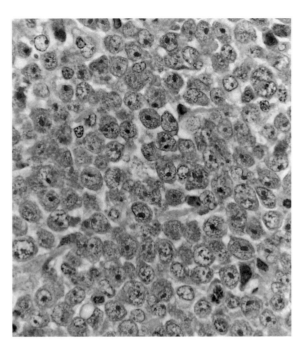

Figure 22-4
HIV-ASSOCIATED DIFFUSE LARGE CELL LYMPHOMA
This tumor arose in the gastrointestinal tract.

Almost all non-Hodgkin's lymphomas arising in the setting of AIDS contain clonal immunoglobulin gene rearrangements consistent with their B-cell origin, including most cases that lack lineage-restricted antigen expression. Some cases have differences in gene rearrangement profiles in biopsies from different sites in the same patient (47), consistent with a potential multiclonal origin similar to lymphomas arising in iatrogenic immunodeficiencies of organ allograft recipients (see below). Some hyperplastic lymph nodes from AIDS patients contain minor B-cell clones, noted by gene rearrangement analysis, in the absence of other features of malignant transformation (47). These features suggest that the hyperplastic lymphadenopathy in AIDS is a premalignant condition that predisposes to the development of non-Hodgkin's lymphoma at increased frequency, perhaps secondary to unregulated B-cell proliferation leading to secondary genetic changes.

Non-Hodgkin's lymphomas arising in the setting of AIDS have molecular and cytogenetic features similar to sporadic Burkitt's lymphoma. Up to 75 percent of cases, including small noncleaved cell, large cell, and immunoblastic lymphomas, have been reported to contain *myc* gene rearrangements with breakpoint locations typical of those seen in sporadic Burkitt's lymphoma (chapter 10) (64). The *bcl*-2 and T-cell receptor genes are invariably in germline configurations.

Patients with AIDS have defective T-cell surveillance which, combined with the ubiquitous nature of EBV infection, results in abnormally high numbers of circulating EBV-infected B cells in the peripheral blood and greater than normal numbers of EBV-infected B and T lymphocytes in lymph nodes (1,6). The identification of these EBV-infected cells has been correlated with the synchronous or metachronous development of EBV-associated non-Hodgkin's lymphoma (61). The incidence of EBV positivity among the AIDS-associated non-Hodgkin's lymphomas ranges from 40 to 67 percent, possibly varying on a geographic basis (46,61). Both EBV type 1 and 2 are found (60). EBV positivity is most likely in systemic immunoblastic lymphoma (about 80 percent), and is less frequent in small noncleaved cell (about 30 percent) or diffuse large cell (about 20 percent) lymphoma (28). Virtually all reported primary central nervous system lymphomas are EBV associated (41). EBV-positive lymphomas express EBNA-1, with the pattern of transcription of the EBNA-1 gene closer to that seen in Burkitt's lymphoma than post-transplantation lymphoproliferative disorders; they also express LMP-1, as do the post-transplantation lymphoproliferative disorders in contrast to Burkitt's lymphoma (60).

Treatment of AIDS-associated non-Hodgkin's lymphomas with intense multiagent chemotherapy has been disappointing. Currently, low-dose chemotherapy or standard-dose chemotherapy with hematopoietic growth factors is used (38). Intrathecal chemotherapy is often used for central nervous system prophylaxis. In one study, patients with high-grade, immunoblastic or small noncleaved lymphoma fared worse than those with intermediate-grade, diffuse large cell type lymphoma (36), although this finding has not been confirmed in other studies (34,39). Other prognostic factors for poor survival include a history of AIDS, Karnofsky performance status less than 70 percent, bone marrow involvement, CD4 counts less than $100/mm^3$, and extranodal disease (34,39). Patients with primary central nervous system disease have a poor prognosis, but they commonly have many of the adverse prognostic factors (39).

Hodgkin's Disease

There is no statistically significant association between HIV infection and Hodgkin's disease (37). Yet, Hodgkin's disease occurring in these patients has distinctive clinicopathologic features (35,52, 56,57). HIV-associated Hodgkin's disease affects both homosexual men and intravenous drug abusers. Almost all patients are clinical stage III or IV at presentation, with a high incidence of involvement of multiple lymph node groups and extranodal sites, including unusual sites such as liver and skin. Staging studies have revealed spread in a noncontiguous fashion, in contrast to the orderly progression found in typical Hodgkin's disease.

In contrast to the usual preponderance of nodular sclerosis Hodgkin's disease, 55 percent of cases of HIV-associated Hodgkin's disease are mixed cellularity; 30 percent are nodular sclerosis; 10 percent, lymphocyte depletion; 5 percent, unclassified; and only rare cases are lymphocyte predominance (35). The histologic appearance of HIV-associated Hodgkin's disease is similar to that seen in the general population, although there is a tendency for the tissues to contain an increased number of Hodgkin cells with a greater degree of cytologic atypia and an increased number of nonlymphoid fibrohistiocytoid stromal cells (35,52). The proportion of cases of Hodgkin's disease that contain EBV genomes in the Reed-Sternberg cells and variants is much higher in the setting of AIDS and approaches 100 percent (3,32).

Patients are usually treated with standard Hodgkin's disease regimens. Nonetheless, the clinical outcome is poor, with death usually occurring from infectious complications or progressive Hodgkin's disease.

POST-TRANSPLANTATION LYMPHOPROLIFERATIVE DISORDERS

There is an increased incidence of neoplasia in general, and lymphoproliferative disorders in particular, in patients maintained on immunosuppressive therapy after organ transplantation, including renal, cardiac, heart-lung, lung, hepatic, and bone marrow allografts. The incidence of lymphoid neoplasia varies from about 1 to 12 percent, depending mostly upon the immunosuppressive agents used and their doses and, possibly, on the type of organ transplant and characteristics of the recipient. For example, the incidence of lymphoma developing in heart transplant recipients was initially reported as 8 percent using cyclosporine as the primary immunosuppressive agent (7), but more recent experience utilizing lower doses of this agent has resulted in a significantly lower incidence of about 1 percent. In contrast, the incidence of lymphoma is 11.4 percent in heart transplant recipients treated with OKT3-containing regimens, with increased risk correlated with higher dose (65). However, the increased incidence of lymphomas associated with use of OKT3 is not seen in children (5). Additional risk factors for lymphoma may include a greater number of rejection episodes in the first 6 months following transplantation, younger age at transplantation, and pretransplant history (2,5,7).

The clinical presentation of transplant recipients who develop lymphoproliferative disorders also varies depending upon the immunosuppressive regimen, the organ transplanted, and characteristics of the recipient. The disease usually first manifests within a year of transplantation, either presenting as an infectious mononucleosis–like syndrome, often involving the head and neck, or as localized extranodal tumor masses (30,44). Virtually any site may be affected, including the allograft organ, central nervous system, liver, lung, gastrointestinal tract, soft tissue (particularly at the site of antithymocyte globulin injection), and lymph nodes. Involvement of the allograft is particularly common in heart-lung transplant recipients (50).

Post-transplant lymphoproliferative disorders may appear grossly as a solid tumor or multiple tumors, a diffuse infiltrate of the parenchymal organ, enlargement of native lymphoid tissue, or may be grossly inapparent (22,44). Histologically, the lesions consist of a diffuse proliferation of lymphoid and plasma cells with variable degrees of atypia and monomorphism (22,44). Necrosis is common, and may be extensive and geographic (fig. 22-5) or may manifest as single cell necrosis, associated with neutrophils and histiocytes. The cytologic composition is variable and ranges from highly polymorphic to monomorphic. In plasmacytic hyperplasia, which most commonly arises in the oropharynx and lymph nodes, there is retention of underlying architecture, but a diffuse infiltrate by plas-

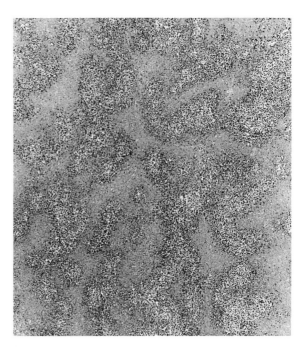

Figure 22-5
GEOGRAPHIC NECROSIS IN POST-TRANSPLANT
LARGE CELL LYMPHOMA
Note the large, pale areas of necrosis interspersed with irregular nests and cords of lymphoma cells.

macytoid lymphocytes, associated with plasma cells and sparse immunoblasts (34b). In polymorphic lesions (fig. 22-6), the entire range of B-lymphocyte forms is seen, including small lymphocytes, plasma cells, small lymphoplasmacytoid forms, plasmacytoid immunoblasts, and small and large cleaved and noncleaved lymphoid cells. The immunoblasts show varying degrees of atypia and multinucleation, particularly adjacent to areas of necrosis. Monomorphic lesions have the appearance of typical non-Hodgkin's lymphoma, of either intermediate-grade, diffuse large cell type, or high-grade plasmacytoid immunoblastic type (fig. 22-7); small noncleaved cell lymphomas are less common in this setting (44,69). Rarely, post-thymic T-cell lymphoma, low-grade non-Hodgkin's lymphoma, multiple myeloma, plasmacytoma, and Hodgkin's disease have also been reported in transplant recipients (21,34b).

Most post-transplantation lymphoproliferative lesions are B-lineage processes, expressing multiple B-cell antigens (19,44,66,69). Lesions that exhibit polymorphic histology are often polyclonal, while lesions that exhibit monomorphic

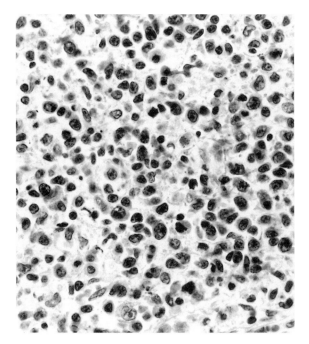

Figure 22-6
POLYMORPHIC POST-TRANSPLANT
LYMPHOPROLIFERATIVE DISORDER

Note the admixture of small lymphocytes, plasmacytoid lymphocytes, plasma cells, and occasional large lymphoid cells. This lymph node is from a child who developed widespread adenopathy following bone marrow transplantation for severe combined immunodeficiency. This particular lesion showed a mixture of kappa- and lambda-stained cells and oligoclonal bands on Southern blots hybridized with immunoglobulin light and heavy chain probes.

histology usually express monoclonal immunoglobulin or are immunoglobulin negative (fig. 22-8). In addition, the proliferating B cells express adhesion and activation markers such as CD11a (lymphocyte function antigen [LFA]-1), CD23, CD54 (ICAM-1), and CD58 (LFA-3).

The B-cell origin of post-transplant lymphoproliferations is supported by the presence of clonally rearranged immunoglobulin genes in most cases, including many lymphoproliferations that have polymorphic features and express polyclonal immunoglobulins (14,29,34b, 40). Occasional cases, including most cases of plasmacytic hyperplasia, contain no demonstrable gene rearrangements or show multiple, faint, rearranged bands consistent with polyclonal or oligoclonal proliferations, respectively (29,34b, 58). Occasional monoclonal bands are seen in conjunction with polyclonal bands, suggesting that these disorders may initially evolve from

polyclonal proliferations to monoclonal B-cell disorders (58). Analyses of tissues from different sites of the same patient frequently show different patterns of rearranged bands consistent with the multiclonal origins of these disorders (13). Rare cases of post-transplantation lymphoma express T-cell–associated markers and possess clonal beta-T-cell receptor gene rearrangements (68).

With rare exceptions, virtually all post-transplantation lymphoproliferations harbor EBV genomic DNA and RNA; this is consistent with the important etiologic role of the virus in these disorders (fig. 22-9) (48). Most cases of plasmacytic hyperplasia contain multiple EBV infection events or only a minor cell population infected by a single form of EBV (34b). In most other cases, the EBV genomes are clonal, indicating the presence of EBV in the progenitor B cell that gave rise to the neoplastic population (12,34b,45). The clonal composition of EBV DNA generally parallels that of the immunoglobulin genes (12). Evidence of abnormally high numbers of EBV-infected cells may be found in biopsies from transplantation patients who later develop lymphoma (49).

The few cytogenetic studies of post-transplant lymphoproliferative disorders show variable clonal abnormalities, generally in cases with monomorphic features. Unlike AIDS-associated lymphomas, *myc* gene rearrangements are not common but when present are exclusively associated with monomorphic lymphomas (34b,40). N-ras gene codon 61 point mutation and p53 gene mutation have also been reported in immunoblastic lymphoma and multiple myeloma, but not in polymorphic lesions (34b). The molecular and cytogenetic features are consistent with a spectrum of EBV-harboring disorders of varying clonal composition, from polyclonal mononucleosis-like proliferations to frank monoclonal lymphomas (Table 22-1). These disorders may reflect different stages of the progressive, relentless proliferation of EBV-infected B cells that escape normal T-cell surveillance in the setting of immunosuppression.

Treatment options for post-transplantation lymphoproliferative disorders range from reduction in immunosuppression to antiviral therapy (such as acyclovir) to standard chemotherapy or radiation therapy. Many lesions regress with reduced immunosuppression, particularly those

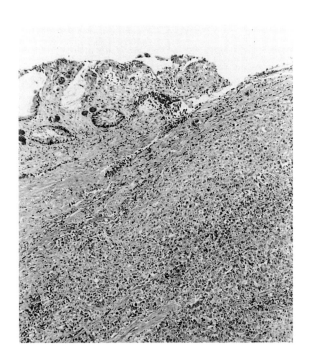
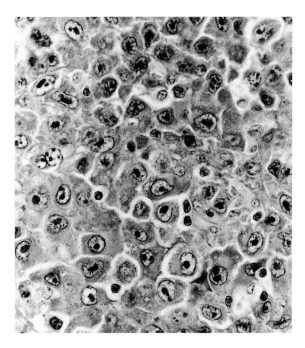

Figure 22-7
POST-TRANSPLANT IMMUNOBLASTIC LYMPHOMA PRESENTING AS A PROLAPSED HEMORRHOID
Left: The lymphoma replaces the mucosa at top, and extensively infiltrates the submucosa.
Right: The cells comprising this lymphoma include many with large, central nucleoli as well as those differentiating to plasma cells. This lymphoma was monoclonal on the basis of phenotypic and genotypic findings.

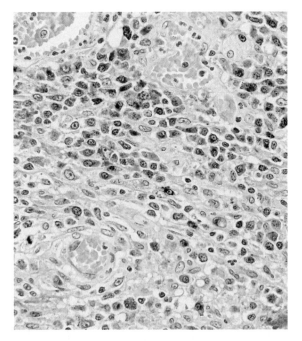
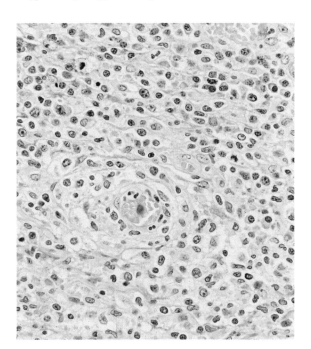

Figure 22-8
POST-TRANSPLANT LYMPHOPROLIFERATIVE DISORDER PRESENTING WITH INTESTINAL PERFORATION
Although this lesion shows a polymorphous cellular composition, many of the cells stain for kappa light chain (left) while only rare cells stain for lambda light chain (right). This patient had prior abdominal surgery for unexplained hepatosplenomegaly which was found to be secondary to bacillary angiomatosis. This intestinal resection specimen also contained cytomegalovirus which eventually led to the patient's death, i.e., there was no evidence of a lymphoproliferative disorder at postmortem examination. (Immunoperoxidase with hematoxylin counterstain)

Table 22-1

FEATURES OF POST-TRANSPLANTATION LYMPHOPROLIFERATIVE DISORDERS*

Histology	Immunoglobulin Gene Configurations	EBV DNA Status	*Myc* Gene Status	Response to Reduced Immunosuppression
Polymorphic	Germline	Nonclonal	Germline	Regression
Polymorphic	Germline/polyclonal	Clonal/nonclonal	Germline	Regression
Polymorphic	Monoclonal	Monoclonal	Germline	Most progress
Monomorphic	Monoclonal	Monoclonal	Germline	Most progress
Monomorphic	Monoclonal	Monoclonal	Rearranged	Progression

*Based on data from reference 40. Most cases are polymorphic or monomorphic.

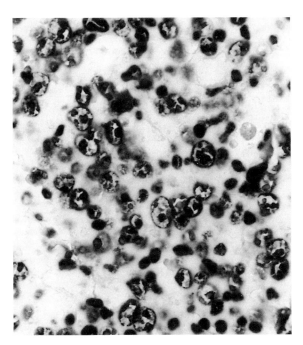

Figure 22-9

POST-TRANSPLANT IMMUNOBLASTIC LYMPHOMA

Almost all the tumor cells are positive for EBV. (In situ hybridization using biotinylated EBV EBER 1 oligonucleotide probe without counterstain)

with polymorphic histology, large numbers of T cells, and absent or weak evidence of clonality by molecular studies (Table 22-1) (40,66). Cases that tend to progress are those with monomorphic histology, sparse numbers of T cells, evidence of c-*myc* rearrangement, and significant monoclonal populations.

IMMUNOSUPPRESSIVE AGENTS OUTSIDE OF THE SETTING OF TRANSPLANTATION

Immunosuppressive agents, including steroids, azathioprine, cyclophosphamide, and methotrexate, are used for the treatment of many diseases, including malignant neoplasms and connective tissue disorders. Theoretically, use of these agents could lead to an increased incidence of malignant lymphoma by mechanisms similar to those discussed, although the level of immunosuppression is much lower than seen in AIDS or transplant recipients. One study found an increased risk for lymphoma in rheumatoid arthritis patients related to immunosuppressive therapy with azathioprine and cyclophosphamide (34a), while other reports have documented the occurrence of lymphoma in patients with connective tissue disease taking methotrexate or cyclosporine (17,33,71). In two of these reports, the neoplasms were found to be EBV positive (33,71); in some cases, the neoplasms, diffuse large cell lymphoma and Hodgkin's disease, spontaneously regressed after discontinuation of methotrexate (33).

REFERENCES

1. Arber DA, Shibata D, Chen YY, Weiss LM. Characterization of the topography of Epstein-Barr virus infection in human immunodeficiency virus-associated lymphoid tissues. Mod Pathol 1992;5:559–66.

2. Armitage J, Kormos R, Stuart R, et al. Posttransplant lymphoproliferative disease in thoracic organ transplant patients: ten years of cyclosporine-based immunosuppression. J Heart Lung Transplant 1991;10:877–87.

3. Audouin J, Diebold J, Pallesen G. Frequent expression of Epstein-Barr virus latent membrane protein-1 in tumour cells of Hodgkin's disease in HIV-positive patients. J Pathol 1992;167:381–4.

4. Beral V, Peterman T, Berkelman R, Jaffe H. AIDS-associated non-Hodgkin lymphoma. Lancet 1991;337:805–9.

5. Bernstein DL, Baum D, Berry GJ, et al. Neoplastic disorders after pediatric heart transplantation. Circulation 1993;88(5 Pt 2):II230–7.

6. Birx D, Redfield RR, Tosato G. Defective regulation of Epstein-Barr virus infection in patients with acquired immunodeficiency syndrome (AIDS) or AIDS related disorders. N Engl J Med 1986;314:874–9.

7. Brumbaugh J, Baldwin JC, Stinson EB, et al. Quantitative analysis of immunosuppression in cyclosporine-treated heart transplant patients with lymphoma. J Heart Transplant 1985;4:307–11.

8. Carbone A, Tirelli U, Vaccher E, et al. A clinicopathologic study of lymphoid neoplasias associated with human immunodeficiency virus infection in Italy. Cancer 1991;68:842–52.

9. Centers for Disease Control, Department of Health and Human Survices. Revision of the case definition of acquired immunodeficiency syndrome for national reporting—United States. Ann Intern Med 1985;103:402–3.

10. Chadburn A, Metroka C, Mouradian J. Progressive lymph node histology and its prognostic value in patients with acquired immunodeficiency syndrome and AIDS-related complex. Hum Pathol 1989;20:579–87.

11. Ciobanu N, Andreeff M, Safai B, Koziner B, Mertelsmann R. Lymphoblastic neoplasia in a homosexual patient with Kaposi's sarcoma. Ann Intern Med 1983;98:151–5.

12. Cleary ML, Nalesnik MA, Shearer WT, Sklar J. Clonal analysis of transplant-associated lymphoproliferations based on the structure of the genomic termini of the Epstein-Barr virus. Blood 1988;72:349–52.

13. _____, Sklar J. Lymphoproliferative disorders in cardiac transplant recipients are multiclonal lymphomas. Lancet 1984;2:489–93.

14. _____, Warnke R, Sklar J. Monoclonality of lymphoproliferative lesions in cardiac-transplant recipients. Clonal analysis based on immunoglobulin gene rearrangements. N Engl J Med 1984;310:477–82.

15. Cotelingam JD, Witebsky FG, Hsu SM, Blaese RM, Jaffe ES. Malignant lymphoma in patients with the Wiskott-Aldrich syndrome. Cancer Invest 1985;3:515–22.

16. Cunningham-Rundles C, Siegal FP, Cunningham-Rundles S, Lieberman P. Incidence of cancer in 98 patients with common varied immunodeficiency. J Clin Immunol 1987;7:294–9.

17. Ellman MH, Hurwitz H, Thomas C, Kozloff M. Lymphoma developing in a patient with rheumatoid arthritis taking low dose weekly methotrexate. J Rheumatol 1991;18:1741–3.

18. Ewing EP Jr, Chandler FW, Spira TJ, Brynes RK, Chan WC. Primary lymph node pathology in AIDS and AIDS-related lymphadenopathy. Arch Pathol Lab Med 1985;109:977–81.

19. Ferry JA, Jacobson JO, Conti D, Delmonico F, Harris NL. Lymphoproliferative disorders and hematologic malignancies following organ transplantation. Mod Pathol 1989;2;583–92.

20. Filipovich AH, Mathur A, Kamat D, Shapiro RS. Primary immunodeficiencies: genetic risk factors for lymphoma. Cancer Res 1992;52(Suppl):5465–67s.

21. Frizzera G. Atypical lymphoproliferative disorders. In: Knowles DM, ed. Neoplastic hematopathology. Baltimore: Williams & Wilkins, 1992:459–95.

22. _____, Hanto DW, Gajl-Peczalska KJ, et al. Polymorphic diffuse B-cell hyperplasias and lymphomas in renal transplant recipients. Cancer Res 1981;41(11 Pt 1):4262–79.

23. _____, Rosai J, Dehner LP, Spector BD, Kersey JH. Lymphoreticular disorders in primary immunodeficiencies. New findings based on an up-to-date histologic classification of 35 cases. Cancer 1980;46:692–9.

24. Gail MH, Pluda JM, Rabkin CS, et al. Projections of the incidence of non-Hodgkin's lymphoma related to acquired immunodeficiency syndrome. JNCI 1991;83:695–701.

25. Goldstein J, Becker N, DelRowe J, Davis L. Cutaneous T-cell lymphoma in a patient infected with human immunodeficiency virus, type 1. Use of radiation therapy. Cancer 1990;66:1130–2.

26. Gonzalez-Clemente JM, Ribera JM, Campo E, Bosch X, Monserrat E, Grau JM. Ki-1+ anaplastic large-cell lymphoma of T cell origin in an HIV-infected patient. AIDS 1991;5:751–5.

27. Grierson H, Purtilo DT. Epstein-Barr virus infections in males with the X-linked lymphoproliferative syndrome. Ann Intern Med 1987;106:548–45.

28. Hamilton-Dutoit SJ, Raphael M, Audouin J, et al. In situ demonstration of Epstein-Barr virus small RNAs (EBER 1) in acquired immunodeficiency syndrome-related lymphomas: correlation with tumor morphology and primary site. Blood 1993;92:610–24.

29. Hanto DW, Birkenbach M, Frizzera G, Gajl-Peczalska KJ, Simmons RL, Schubach WH. Confirmation of the heterogeneity of posttransplant Epstein-Barr virus-associated B cell proliferations by immunoglobulin gene rearrangement analyses. Transplantation 1989;47:458–64.

30. _____, Frizzera G, Purtilo DT, et al. Clinical spectrum of lymphoproliferative disorders in renal transplant recipients and evidence for the role of Epstein-Barr virus. Cancer Res 1981;41(11 Pt 1):4253–61.

30a. Harrington DS, Weisenburger DD, Purtilo DT. Malignant lymphoma in the X-linked lymphoproliferative syndrome. Cancer 1987;59:1419–29.

31. Hermans PE, Diaz-Buxo JA, Stobo JD. Idiopathic late-onset immunoglobulin deficiency: clinical observations in 50 patients. Am J Med 1976;61:221–37.

32. Herndier B, Sanchez H, Chang KC, Chen YY, Weiss LM. High prevalence of detection of EBV RNA in the Reed-Sternberg cells of HIV-associated Hodgkin's disease. Am J Pathol 1993;142:1073–9.

33. Kamel OW, van de Rijn M, Weiss LM, et al. Brief report: reversible lymphomas associated with Epstein-Barr virus during methotrexate therapy for rheumatoid arthritis and dermatomyositis. N Engl J Med 1993;328:1317–21.

34. Kaplan LD, Abrams DI, Feigal E, et al. AIDS-associated non-Hodgkin's lymphoma in San Francisco. JAMA 1989;261:719–24.

34a. Kinlen LJ. Incidence of cancer in rheumatoid arthritis and other disorders after immunosupressive treatment. Am J Med 1985;(Suppl)1A:44–9.

34b. Knowles DM, Cesarman E, Chadburn A, et al. Correlative morphologic and molecular genetic analysis demonstrates three distinct categories of posttransplantation lymphoproliferative disorders. Blood 1995;85:552–65.

35. _____, Chadburn A. Lymphadenopathy and the lymphoid neoplasms associated with the acquired immune deficiency syndrome (AIDS). In: Knowles DM, ed. Neoplastic hematopathology. Baltimore: Williams & Wilkins, 1992:773–835.

36. _____, Chamulak GA, Subar M, et al. Lymphoid neoplasia associated with the acquired immunodeficiency syndrome (AIDS): The New York University Medical Center experience with 105 patients (1981-1986). Ann Intern Med 1988;108:744–53.

37. Levine AM. Non-Hodgkin's lymphomas and other malignancies in the acquired immunodeficiency syndrome. Semin Oncol 1987;14(2 Suppl 3):34–9.

38. _____. Acquired immunodeficiency syndrome-related lymphoma. Blood 1992;80:8–20.

39. _____, Sullivan-Halley J, Pike MC, et al. Human immunodeficiency virus-related lymphoma. Prognostic factors predictive of survival. Cancer 1991;68:2466–72.

40. Locker J, Nalesnik M. Molecular genetic analysis of lymphoid tumors arising after organ transplantation. Am J Pathol 1989;135:977–87.

41. MacMahon EM, Glass JD, Hayward SD, et al. Epstein-Barr virus in AIDS-related primary central nervous system lymphoma. Lancet 1991;338:969–73.

42. Moore RD, Kessler H, Richman DD, Flexner C, Chaisson RE. Non-Hodgkin's lymphoma in patients with advanced HIV infection treated with zidovudine. JAMA 1991;265:2208–11.

43. Morrell D, Cromartie E, Swift M. Mortality and cancer incidence of 263 patients with ataxia-telangiectasia. JNCI 1986;77:89–92.

44. Nalesnik MA, Jaffe R, Starzl TE, et al. The pathology of posttransplant lymphoproliferative disorders occurring in the setting of cyclosporine A-prednisone immunosuppression. Am J Pathol 1988;133:173–92.

45. Patton DF, Wilkowski CW, Hanson CA, et al. Epstein-Barr virus-determined clonality in posttransplant lymphoproliferative disease. Transplantation 1990; 49:1080–4.

46. Pedersen C, Gerstoft J, Lundgren JD, et al. HIV-associated lymphoma: histopathology and association wtih Epstein-Barr virus genome related to clinical, immunological and prognostic features. Eur J Cancer 1991;27:1416–23.

47. Pelicci PG, Knowles DM, Arlin Z, et al. Multiple monoclonal B-cell expansions and c-myc oncogene rearrangements in AIDS-related lymphoproliferative disorders: implications for lymphomagenesis. J Exp Med 1986;164:2049–60.

48. Randhawa PS, Jaffe R, Demetris AJ, et al. The systemic distribution of Epstein-Barr virus genomes in fatal post-transplantation lymphoproliferative disorders: an in situ hybridization study. Am J Pathol 1991;138:1027–33.

49. _____, Jaffe R, Demetris AJ, et al. Epstein-Barr virus-encoded small RNA (by the EBER-1 gene) in liver specimens with post-transplant recipients with post-transplantation lymphoproliferative disease. N Engl J Med 1992;327:1710–4.

50. _____, Yousem SA, Paradis IL, Dauber JA, Griffith BP, Locker J. The clinical spectrum, pathology, and clonal analysis of Epstein-Barr virus-associated lymphoproliferative disorders in heart-lung transplant recipients. Am J Clin Pathol 1989;92:177–85.

51. Raphael M, Gentilhomme O, Tulliez M, Byron PA, Diebold J. Histopathologic features of high grade non-Hodgkin's lymphomas in acquired immunodeficiency syndrome. Arch Pathol Lab Med 1991;115:15–20.

52. Ree HJ, Strauchen J, Khan A, et al. HIV-associated Hodgkin's disease: clinicopathologic studies of 24 cases. Preponderance of mixed cellularity characterized by occurrence of fibro-histiocytoid stromal cells. Cancer 1991;67:1614–21.

53. Robison LL, Stoker V, Frizzera G, Heinitz K, Meadows AT, Filipovich AH. Hodgkin's disease in pediatric patients with naturally occurring immunodeficiency. Am J Pediatr Hematol Oncol 1987;9:189–92.

54. Roithman S, Tourani JM, Andrieu JM. AIDS associated non-Hodgkin's lymphoma (Letter). Lancet 1991;338:884–5.

55. Sander CA, Medeiros LJ, Weiss LM, Yano T, Sneller MC, Jaffe ES. Lymphoproliferative lesions in patients with common variable immunodeficiency syndrome. Am J Surg Pathol 1992;16:1170–82.

56. Schoeppel JL, Hoppe RT, Dorfman RF, et al. Hodgkin's disease in homosexual men with generalized lymphadenopathy. Ann Intern Med 1985;102:68–70.

57. Serrano M, Bellas C, Campoe, et al. Hodgkin's disease in patients with antibodies to human immunodeficiency virus. A study of 22 patients. Cancer 1990;65:2248–54.

58. Shearer WT, Ritz J, Finegold MJ, et al. Epstein-Barr virus-associated B-cell proliferations of diverse clonal origins after bone marrow transplantation in a 12-year-old patient with severe combined immunodeficiency. N Engl J Med 1985;312:1151–9.

59. Shibata D, Brynes RK, Rabinowitz A, et al. Human T-cell lymphotropic virus type I (HTLV-I)-associated adult T-cell leukemia-lymphoma in a patient infected with human immunodeficiency virus type l (HIV-1). Ann Intern Med 1989;111:871–5.

60. _____, Weiss LM, Hernandez AM, Nathwani BN, Bernstein L, Levine AM. Epstein-Barr virus-associated non-Hodgkin's lymphoma in patients infected with the human immunodeficiency virus. Blood 1993;81:2102–9.

61. _____, Weiss LM, Nathwani BN, Brynes RK, Levine AM. Epstein-Barr virus in benign lymph node biopsies from individuals infected with the human immunodeficiency virus is associated with the concurrent or subsequent development of non-Hodgkin's lymphoma. Blood 1991;77:1527–33.

62. Snover DC, Frizzera G, Spector BD, Perry GS III, Kersey JH. Wiskott-Aldrich syndrome: histopathologic findings in the lymph nodes and spleens of 15 patients. Hum Pathol 1981;12:821–31.

63. Spector BD, Perry GS III, Kersey JH. Genetically determined immunodeficiency diseases (GDID) and malignancy: report from the immunodeficiency-cancer registry. Clin Immunol Immunopathol 1978;11:12–29.

64. Subar M, Neri A, Inghirami G, Knowles DM, Dalla-Favera R. Frequent c-myc oncogene activation and infrequent presence of Epstein-Barr virus genome in AIDS-associated lymphoma. Blood 1988;72:667–71.

65. Swinnen L, Costanzo-Nordin M, Fisher S, et al. Increased incidence of lymphoproliferative disorders after immunosuppression with the monoclonal antibody OKT3 in cardiac-transplant recipients. N Engl J Med 1990;323:1723–8.

66. Thomas JA, Hotchin NA, Allday MJ, et al. Imunohistology of Epstein-Barr virus-associated antigens in B cell disorders from immunocompromised individuals. Transplantation 1990;49:944–53.

67. Turner RR, Levine AM, Gill PS, Parker JW, Meyer PR. Progressive histopathologic abnormalities in the persistent generalized lymphadenopathy syndrome. Am J Surg Pathol 1987;11:625–32.

68. Waller EK, Ziemianska M, Bangs CD, Cleary M, Weissman I, Kamel OW. Characterization of posttransplant lymphomas that express T-cell-associated markers: immunophenotypes, molecular genetics, cytogenetics, and heterotransplantation in severe combined immunodeficient mice. Blood 1993;82:247–61.

69. Weintraub J, Warnke RA. Lymphoma in cardiac allotransplant recipients. Clinical and histological features and immunological phenotype. Transplantation 1982;33:347–51.

70. Ziegler JL, Beckstead JA, Volberding PA, et al. Non-Hodgkin's lymphoma in 90 homosexual men. Relation to generalized lymphadenopathy and the acquired immunodeficiency syndrome. N Engl J Med 1984;311:565–70.

71. Zijlmans J, van Rijthoven A, Kluin P, Jiwa NM, Dijkmans B, Kluin-Nelemans JC. Epstein-Barr virus-associated lymphoma in a patient with rheumatoid arthritis treated with cyclosporine (Letter). N Engl J Med 1992;326:1363.

❖❖❖

Index*

*Numbers in boldface indicate table and figure pages.

✧✧✧